Orville Gilbert Brim is the former director of the MacArthur Foundation Research Network on Successful Midlife Development. **Carol D. Ryff** is professor of psychology and director of the Institute on Aging at the University of Wisconsin–Madison. **Ronald C. Kessler** is professor in the Department of Health Care Policy at the Harvard Medical School.

How Healthy Are We?

*The John D. and Catherine T. MacArthur Foundation Series on
Mental Health and Human Development*

STUDIES ON SUCCESSFUL MIDLIFE DEVELOPMENT

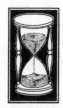

Also in the series:

Sexuality across the Life Course
Edited by Alice S. Rossi

The Parental Experience in Midlife
Edited by Carol D. Ryff and Marsha Mailick Seltzer

Multiple Paths of Midlife Development
Edited by Margie E. Lachman and Jacquelyn Boone James

Welcome to Middle Age! (And Other Cultural Fictions)
Edited by Richard A. Shweder

*Caring and Doing for Others: Social Responsibility in the Domains
of Family, Work, and Community*
Edited by Alice S. Rossi

How Healthy Are We?

A National Study of Well-Being at Midlife

Edited by

Orville Gilbert Brim, Carol D. Ryff, and Ronald C. Kessler

The University of Chicago Press
Chicago and London

Orville Gilbert Brim is the former director of the
MacArthur Foundation Research Network on Successful Midlife Development.
Carol D. Ryff is professor of psychology and director of the Institute on Aging
at the University of Wisconsin–Madison.
Ronald C. Kessler is professor in the Department of Health Care Policy
at the Harvard Medical School.

THE UNIVERSITY OF CHICAGO PRESS, CHICAGO 60637
THE UNIVERSITY OF CHICAGO PRESS, LTD., LONDON
© 2004 by The University of Chicago
All rights reserved. Published 2004
Printed in the United States of America
13 12 11 10 09 08 07 06 05 04   5 4 3 2 1

ISBN (cloth): 0-226-07475-7

The University of Chicago Press gratefully acknowledges a subvention from
the John D. and Catherine T. MacArthur Foundation in partial support of the
costs of production of this volume.

Library of Congress Cataloging-in-Publication Data

How healthy are we? : a national study of well-being at midlife / edited
by Orville Gilbert Brim, Carol D. Ryff, and Ronald C. Kessler.
    p.   cm.—(The John D. and Catherine T. MacArthur Foundation
series on mental health and development. Studies on successful midlife
development)
Includes bibliographical references and indexes.
ISBN 0-226-07475-7 (cloth : alk. paper)
1. Middle age—Psychological aspects.   2. Middle age—Social aspects.
3. Middle age—Health and hygiene.   I. Brim, Orville Gilbert, 1923–
II. Ryff, Carol D.   III. Kessler, Ronald C.   IV. Series.
BF724.6 .H69   2004
305.244'0973—dc21

2003012636

⊗ *The paper used in this publication meets the minimum requirements of the*
American National Standard for Information Sciences—Permanence of
Paper for Printed Library Materials, ANSI Z39.48-1992.

CONTENTS

Contents

ACKNOWLEDGMENTS

The editors thank the many individuals across the United States who gave their time and energy to participate in the MIDUS survey. What we know is that midlife, for many, is the busiest period of life. Thus, we are deeply grateful that so many were willing to speak to us at length about themselves, their families, their lives, and their health so that we might create a more informed story about who is, and is not, thriving in midlife and why. The many researchers who have contributed to this study, most of whom are authors of chapters in this volume, also thank the John D. and Catherine T. MacArthur Foundation for its support of the Midlife Network and the MIDUS survey. From the beginning, the MacArthur Foundation nurtured a commitment to approach midlife in all of its complexity, a task that required blending expertise from numerous scientific disciplines. Without the sustained Midlife Network support, this one-of-a-kind integrative study, which required years of planning, would never have been possible. The chapters in this book illustrate the unprecedented advances that follow from a visionary new kind of science about midlife. Finally, as editors, we thank Marty Quimby from the staff of the Institute on Aging at the University of Wisconsin–Madison for her many organizational skills and outstanding attention to detail in helping us bring this collection to completion.

CHAPTER ONE

The MIDUS National Survey: An Overview

Orville Gilbert Brim, Carol D. Ryff, and Ronald C. Kessler

Midlife has been described as the "last uncharted territory" of the life course. Extensive prior literatures have been devoted to early life and childhood, adolescence, and more recently, old age, but surprisingly little attention has been given to the middle years, which, for most individuals, constitute the longest segment of their life. The John D. and Catherine T. MacArthur Foundation established the Research Network on Successful Midlife Development (MIDMAC), directed by Orville Gilbert Brim, to advance knowledge of this neglected period of the life course. A multidisciplinary team of investigators was brought together to organize existing work on midlife development and, importantly, to generate new understanding of the challenges faced by individuals in the middle decades of life, including the contexts that create or minimize difficulties, as well as the strengths and weaknesses that midlife adults bring to their life tasks.

A major activity of the MIDMAC network was to conceive of and implement a national survey of midlife Americans. This study, known as MIDUS, which stands for Midlife in the United States, is the raison d'etre for the present volume. The central objective of this collection is to summarize the rich array of new findings generated by the MIDUS national survey. To put this endeavor in context, we first describe the background and history of the MIDMAC network, including the ideas and intentions that led to its members' creation of a national survey focused on midlife Americans.

We clarify the numerous dimensions along which this study was innovative and groundbreaking. We then briefly describe the sample, design, and measures of the MIDUS study, providing along the way links to websites and technical reports that review this material in greater detail. After the description of MIDUS, we provide an overview of the chapters that follow, highlighting their major questions and findings. This introductory chapter then concludes with a brief glimpse at the extent to which MIDUS has captured the interest of investigators across diverse scientific fields, in the United States and beyond, and what the future may hold for this one-of-a-kind study of midlife development.

At the outset, it is important to clarify our use of the terms *health* and *well-being,* as evident in our title, *How Healthy Are We? A National Study of Well-Being at Midlife.* By *health,* we endorse a multidisciplinary definition of the term that includes not only physical health but also psychological and social health. A major objective of MIDMAC was, in fact, to broaden the purview of what has traditionally been included under the rubric of health. Understanding how these multiple levels interact is part of a growing concern for integrative approaches to health (Singer and Ryff 2001a). By *well-being,* we give explicit emphasis to the positive side of these multiple levels of health. That is, we challenge the preoccupation with health conceived exclusively as illness and disease (physical or mental) and instead call for greater attention to the upside of human functioning (Ryff and Singer 1998). MIDUS provided the opportunity to measure health not just as the absence of illness but also as the presence of wellness.

HISTORY OF THE MIDLIFE NETWORK

The Research Network on Successful Midlife Development was established in 1990. Its mission was to identify the major biomedical, psychological, and social factors that permit some to flourish in the middle years, achieving good health and psychological well-being, and exercising social responsibility. Although there was explicit interest in understanding such positive midlife trajectories, the network was also interested in identifying the factors that undermine and limit good health, well-being, and social responsibility in midlife. A team of thirteen scholars from the fields of anthropology, demography, epidemiology, health care policy, medicine, psychology, and sociology was assembled to carry out this task. Over its ten-year history, MIDMAC also brought in fifteen junior scholars as network associates. Their backgrounds reflected the same diversity of fields. The chapters that follow are authored by the members and associates of MIDMAC, along with their collaborators.

The collective goals of the MIDMAC team were to (1) develop indicators (physical, psychological, social) for assessing successful midlife development; (2) establish an empirical basis of what happens in midlife—the who, what, when, where, and why of midlife events and the beliefs people hold about them; (3) identify factors that influence the course of midlife development, including illness, life stresses, work and family interactions,

and culture; and (4) illuminate the psychological and behavioral strategies that people use to understand and deal with the challenges of midlife,
thereby elaborating the variety of individual differences in how midlife
is negotiated.

These broad interests were pursued via numerous initiatives (e.g., conferences, new data collection, and analyses), many of which culminated
in topically organized edited volumes, such as *Sexuality across the Life
Course* (Rossi 1994); *The Parental Experience in Midlife* (Ryff and Seltzer
1996); *Multiple Paths of Midlife Development* (Lachman and James 1997);
Welcome to Middle Age! (And Other Cultural Fictions) (Shweder 1998);
and *Caring and Doing for Others* (Rossi 2001). With the exception of the
latter volume, scientific findings across these endeavors were based on
earlier studies, not on the MIDUS national survey. In fact, it was in working with earlier studies that the disciplinary limitations became apparent.
Rather than approach midlife one discipline at a time, where the focus is
exclusively on psychological, or social, or biomedical aspects, what was
needed was an investigation of all of these levels combined. This realization was the genesis of the plan to carry out a national survey of midlife
Americans in which information would be collected across a wide array
of topics so that the intersections of psychological, social, and biomedical
processes could be brought into focus.

Strengths of the MIDUS Survey

Creating a national survey via a multidisciplinary team approach was
innovative on multiple levels. Among the unique strengths of this integrative study, we highlight the following. First, MIDUS provided a
groundbreaking assessment of numerous psychological constructs (e.g.,
personality traits, sense of control, positive and negative affect, goal commitments, well-being) in a national sample of Americans. Such variables
define mainstream research in life-course studies of personality, affect,
and well-being (McCrae and Costa 1990; Helson 1993; Ryff, Kwan, and
Singer 2001), and the psychology of adulthood and aging (Birren and
Schaie 1996, 2001), but extant knowledge has been generated with select
samples having limited generalizability to the larger population. Thus,
MIDUS provided an unprecedented opportunity to bring core psychological constructs to a large and diverse sample of midlife Americans. The
diversity in educational level, income, and occupational status, as well as
race/ethnicity and region of the country, proved to be extremely fruitful
in the scientific findings generated.

3

Second, MIDUS afforded new directions for fields of demography, epidemiology, and sociology, where national surveys are standard fare, but where typical sociodemographic and health variables (e.g., marital status, employment status, socioeconomic standing, family structure, health status, health care utilization) are rarely linked to mainstream psychological and social constructs. MIDUS provided the opportunity to build bridges between these largely disciplinary-specific realms of knowledge.

Third, before conducting the study, the multidisciplinary team of investigators carried out painstaking pilot research, involving six separate studies (some involving national samples), to develop short-form assessments of many key psychosocial constructs. Thus, another first of MIDUS was the creation of condensed psychological assessment inventories that could be used with large population samples, where the trade-offs between sampling scope and depth of measurement must be negotiated. MIDUS demonstrated how these trade-offs can be accomplished via pilot research designed to maintain the conceptual and theoretical integrity of the constructs that personality, social, and cognitive psychologists bring to the table, but at the same time, sharply reduce the number of questions/items asked to probe such constructs.

Fourth, MIDUS made creative use of satellite studies, essentially studies within a study, so that greater depth could be obtained in certain areas. For example, a subset of MIDUS respondents not only completed the telephone interview and self-administered questionnaire given to all members of the national sample but they also participated in a diary study of daily stress, involving additional data collection over a period of eight days. The nature and scope of the satellite studies are described in greater detail later in this chapter. For now, the generic point is that the use of the satellites built around the main study provided a compelling solution to the competing forces of sampling scope, variability, and generalizability, on the one hand, and in-depth assessments of core constructs on the other. The MIDUS design encompassed both.

Finally, because of these innovations in assessment and design, MIDUS had an exceptionally expansive scientific scope. A synopsis of the substantive areas included in the study is provided in tables 1 and 2. The main categories of assessment are elaborated later in this chapter in discussion of the MIDUS measures. Here we highlight the unprecedented breadth of content in the MIDUS survey. Thus, one of the main advances of this investigation was to demonstrate that a population-level inquiry covering such wide territory could actually be done. That is, MIDUS

TABLE 1 MIDUS Content: Demographics and Psychosocial Factors

Demographics

Age, gender, race, ethnicity, marital status, education

Living Arrangements

History of institutionalization homelessness without telephone, housing tenure, neighborhood safety, marital history, current status, number of marriages, first marriage, current or recent marriage, widowhood, divorce

Childhood/Background

Country of birth, parents' country of birth, head of household (male and female), parents' education, occupational status, job classification, ever on welfare, language(s) spoken, religion, urbanicity, number of times moved, financial status of parents, regular chores and rules, number of siblings, birth order, relationship with mother and father during childhood, emotional and physical abuse

Occupational History

Age at first job, job status over past ten years, current status, job classification (industry, occupation, socioeconomic index), characteristics of current or most recent job, comparison of job status and characteristics over time, unemployment history, retirement, work-to-family spillover

Finances

Personal earnings, spouse's earnings, Social Security benefits, governmental assistance, household income assets, comparison of financial situation over time, control over financial situation, adequacy of current income, finances for retirement (pension plan, IRA, Keogh)

Spouse/Partner

Age, education, employment status, job classification, job characteristics, job security, physical health, mental health, relationship with spouse/partner, stability of relationship, communication with spouse/partner, level of support, understanding, and criticism from spouse/partner, sharing of household chores

Sexuality

Rated sexual aspects of life, comparison of sexual aspects over time, number of sexual partners over past year, number of sexual encounters over past six months, sexual orientation

Parents

Age, health during respondent's adolescence, current health status, age at death

Children and Parenting

Number of biological and nonbiological children, age, gender, relationship with children over time, assessment of contribution to family, family-to-work spillover, difficulties with child care

Psychological Assessments

Personality traits, locus of control, goal tenacity, goal strategy, planning, making sense of the past, satisfaction with life domains, disappointment with achievements, self-description (outgoing, moody, curious, optimistic, etc.), level of interdependence, rated life overall, gender roles and parenting, perceived inequalities (work, home, community), perceived discrimination

Social Networks and Support

Family, friends, neighbours, community members and organizations, emotional support, instrumental support, perceived support, support given, support received, level of interaction with network members, sense of community, problems among members of social network

Social Participation

Level of community involvement, control over community involvement, contributions to welfare of others, social obligations, volunteerism, involvement with social organizations

Religion and Spirituality

Religious affiliation, degree of religiosity/spirituality, frequency of attendance at religious/spiritual services, use of religion/spirituality for guidance

TABLE 2 MIDUS Content: Mental and Physical Health, and Beliefs about Health

Mental/Emotional Health	Physical Health	Health-Related Beliefs
Self-rated mental health, rated change over time, mental health–related disability, depression, anxiety, affect, panic attacks, psychological well-being, sense of hopelessness, stress at home, stress at work, health-related behavior, smoking history, alcohol consumption history, problems with alcohol, moderate and vigorous physical activity, prescription medications, vitamins, treatments and therapies used, substance use/abuse	Self-rated physical health, rated change over time, health-related disability and limitations, cardiovascular history, cancer history, chronic conditions, physical symptoms, somatic symptoms, height, weight, waist–hip ratio, weight change over time, self-assessed weight appropriateness, history of operations, history of hospitalizations, menstruation, menopause, control over health risk perceptions	Health risks, treatment decision-making processes, control over health, effort put into health, health care utilization, regular doctor, regular clinic, health insurance coverage, routine preventative care within past twelve months, emergency care, mental health care, psychiatrist, minister (self-help groups, etc.), alternative therapies (acupuncture, chiropractic, herbal therapy, etc.)

changed the social scientific understanding of the boundary conditions under which research is conducted. We found that through a well-crafted, engaging interview, combined with a lengthy self-administered questionnaire, it was possible to collect an unprecedented amount of information about a very large number of Americans. In that sense, MIDUS broke through long-standing barriers, implicit and explicit, of what is possible in a national survey.

The collective innovations of the study were accomplished by bringing together the scientific disciplines, represented by the MIDMAC members and associates, and through years of regular meetings and working out differences in research priorities. In the fields of sociology, demography, and epidemiology, primary resources are frequently channeled into recruiting large, representative samples. Alternately, in psychology and anthropology, greater emphasis is given to developing in-depth assessment procedures—interviews, observations, questionnaires. The net effect of these differing conceptions of quality research is that much comprehensive, detailed data collection has been carried out on small, biased samples. Studies of large, representative samples, in turn, have frequently been limited in depth of assessment, particularly in psychosocial realms. MIDUS effectively bridged these competing priorities, thereby allowing the psychologists and anthropologists in the group to investigate their questions in a diverse sample of Americans, while at the same time, sociologists, demographers, and epidemiologists had the benefit of adding new psychosocial content to their inquiries. It cannot be overemphasized that this novel synthesis required compromise and trade-offs on all sides. All players had to retreat somewhat on their own priorities for this new, integrative inquiry to work.

MIDUS SAMPLES, DESIGN, AND MEASURES

Detailed information about the MIDUS national survey is available in previous publications (Brim 2000) and at the MIDMAC website (http://midmac.med.harvard.edu/research.html). In the present chapter we provide a condensed description of this information as entrée to the researching findings that follow.

Sample: Who Was in the Study?

Overall, the MIDUS survey was administered to a national sample of 7189 non-institutionalized, English-speaking adults. All respondents, aged 25–74, were recruited by telephone to participate in the study. The rationale for the wide age range was that those in the middle years (40–60) could be compared with those younger and older. Respondents completed a telephone interview (approximately forty-five minutes in length) and a self-administered questionnaire (approximately two hours in length). Of the general population sample, which did not include twins, siblings, or city over samples, 3032 respondents completed both the telephone survey and the questionnaire. Another 453 respondents completed only the telephone survey. These data were collected primarily in 1995.

The response rate for the telephone interview was 70 percent, which is generally considered quite good for a population survey. Among the telephone respondents, 86.8 percent completed the lengthy self-administered questionnaire, yielding an overall response rate of 60.8 percent. Comparison of the MIDUS main sample with the Current Population Survey (U.S. Census Bureau 1995) revealed that the sample underrepresented those with a high school education or less and African Americans. Presumably, the lengthy content of the survey (phone and questionnaire) would not have been possible without some underrepresentation of the least educated. Alternately, by design the sample overrepresented older males so as to facilitate gender comparisons by age.

In addition, MIDUS included oversamples ($N = 757$) in select metropolitan areas. The purpose of these was to facilitate in-depth data collection for satellite studies. To investigate familial and genetic influences on questions of interest to MIDUS investigators, the study also included siblings ($N = 951$; allowing for 1614 pairs of siblings) of the main sample respondents, plus a separate sample of twins ($N = 1996$; 998

pairs). The phone interview and questionnaire mentioned earlier were also used with the sibling and twin samples. These data were collected primarily in 1995–96.

The main MIDUS sample included 339 African Americans (approximately 6.1 percent of the general population sample). To expand possibilities for investigating questions pertaining to ethnic/racial minorities, additional data were collected from minority samples in Chicago (235 Mexican Americans, 196 Puerto Ricans) and New York City (384 Dominicans, 284 Puerto Ricans, 338 African Americans). These subsamples were selected from predesignated geographic areas to allow for contrasts between high versus low socioeconomic neighborhoods, and high versus low density of members of particular ethnic/racial groups (e.g., segregated neighborhoods). Respondents completed approximately 65 percent of the material used in the national survey along with detailed descriptions of community, family, and kinship membership. These data were collected primarily in 1995–96.

Satellite Design: "Studies within a Study"

The wide sampling scope (main sample, twins, siblings, metropolitan oversamples, city-specific minority subsamples) was accompanied by a design strategy that not only collected the core MIDUS data from all respondents but also allowed for more in-depth assessment with subgroups of respondents in targeted areas. For example, a large number of the main-sample respondents ($n = 1031$) and twins ($n = 452$) also participated in the National Study of Daily Experiences (NSDE). These respondents completed a short telephone interview about their daily experiences on each of eight consecutive evenings. Such assessments provided a more textured understanding of the challenges of daily life and how they are responded to (see chap. 15 by Almeida and Horn for further details). In addition, the Boston oversample allowed for more in-depth evaluation, including laboratory-based assessments, of cognitive capacities and life management strategies among 302 MIDUS respondents (see chap. 11 by Lachman and Firth).

A further satellite involved a subsample of 724 respondents randomly selected from the larger sample who participated in an in-depth interview about "turning points" in their lives (see chap. 20 by Wethington, Kessler, and Pixley for further details). An additional, in-depth qualitative interview was conducted with 83 MIDUS respondents from around the country. These individuals provided perspectives on their own well-being—what it is and how they maintain it. They were preselected to allow a focus on individuals with low socioeconomic status (indexed by educational level) who have nonetheless been able to achieve high well-being as defined by the structured scales included in MIDUS (see chap. 10 by Markus, Ryff, Curhan, and Palmersheim).

In combination, these additional studies, built around the main MIDUS sample, allowed investigators in particular areas to cover topics in much greater detail. Such data collection in itself is not novel, but what was unique was that these individuals were embedded within a large national survey. This meant they could be compared with the full sample on a host of other variables (sociodemographic characteristics, health, well-being), which, in turn, provided further interpretive insight regarding their comparability (or uniqueness) with the main sample.

Survey Content: MIDUS Measures

Table 1 provides an overview of the many areas of assessment in MIDUS. This wide content was assembled by the multidisciplinary team of investigators. The overall survey instrument, known as the Midlife Development Inventory (MIDI), contains more than eleven hundred items. The entire instrument is available for downloading at two locations—the MIDMAC website (http://midmac.med.harvard.edu/) and the University of Michigan website (http://www.isr.umich.edu/src/midus/), where the data are archived. The main categories of assessment have been described in earlier summaries of MIDUS (Brim 2000) and are also the topic headings in tables 1 and 2. The chapters that follow provide further measurement and psychometric detail on the variables of interest in targeted analyses.

The overall profile of what we learned about those who participated in the study included their demographic characteristics (e.g., gender, age, race/ethnicity, marital status, education, income, living arrangements); current living arrangements (e.g., housing tenure, neighborhood safety); childhood and family background (e.g., parental education and occupation, birth order, number of siblings, quality of early ties to mother and father); occupational history (e.g., job status over the past ten years, current job classification, unemployment history); finances (e.g., personal earnings, household income, finances for retirement); spouse/partner relationship (e.g., sociodemographic characteristics of partner, level of support, understanding, criticism from partner); sexuality (e.g., sexual orientation, frequency of sexual experience, quality of sexual experience); parents (e.g., age, health, age at death); parental experience (e.g., number of children, their age/gender, quality of ties to them); psychological assessments (e.g., personality traits, locus of control, goal orientations, life satisfaction, perceived discrimination, perceived inequalities); social networks and support (e.g., ties to family, friends, neighbors; instrumental and emotional support, support given and received); social participation (e.g., community involvement, social obligations, volunteerism); religion and spirituality (e.g., attendance, use of religion/spirituality for guidance); mental/emotional health (e.g., depression, anxiety, psychological well-being); physical health (e.g., subjective health, chronic conditions, health symptoms, waist–hip ratio, history of hospitalization); and health behaviors and beliefs (e.g., smoking, alcohol consumption, exercise, medications, perceived risks, doctor visits, preventive care, alternative therapies). Additional examples of variables within the main categories are provided in tables 1 and 2.

Most of this information, minus the depth and detail in psychological assessments, was not new to national surveys, whether oriented to epidemiological studies of health, or to sociological assessments of family life or occupational experience. What MIDUS contributed, however, was the integration of all of these domains of assessment in a single study. That is, this was the first time a national sample had been interviewed in which the members were asked questions covering topics that were of interest to epidemiologists and occupational or family sociologists as well as questions covering topics that mental health researchers typically probe; a wide array of new territory was also brought to the study by psychologists, who rarely assess their constructs in large, national samples. MIDUS investigators were also innovative in developing entirely novel areas of assessment, for example, pertaining to work–family spillover (how work and family life influence each other in both positive and negative ways), social responsibility (perceived obligation to others, behaviors of assistance to others), and perceived inequalities (the sense that one's opportunities in life have been limited).

As noted earlier, the assessments in new areas as well as the development of short-form assessments of many psychological and social constructs were accomplished through six separate pilot studies, some with samples of more than a thousand respondents. This high level of research investment before embarking on the MIDUS study spoke powerfully to the collective commitment of the research team to find a way to bring their respective disciplines together in implementing a new kind of integrative investigation.

OVERVIEW OF THE CHAPTERS

We have organized the chapters in this volume into three main parts. Part 1 pertains to midlife perspectives on physical health. Different assessments of health are covered in these chapters, and some incorporate other levels of psychological and social health as well. Part 2 summarizes findings on emotion, quality of life, and psychological well-being in the middle years. Part 3 is organized around the contexts of midlife, such as work and family experience, or neighborhood, regional, and racial/ethnic influences. Although these overarching headings provide a clustering of the findings, the chapters themselves make evident that many authors approached their main questions in ways that allowed them to benefit from the unusually rich survey within which their interests were embedded. That is to say, the MIDUS investigators drew on the sampling strengths of the study as well as on its diverse content to add important new directions to their own particular areas of expertise.

Midlife Perspectives on Physical Health

Chapter 2 by Cleary, Zaborski, and Ayanian describes the rich array of health status indicators, health behaviors, and health attitudes in MIDUS, along with its wealth of psychological and social information. The authors use the data to examine life-course variations and gender differences in health status—questions of interest to both medical and social scientists. Their analyses included numerous health measures (e.g., subjective health, number of days in a previous month unable to work or do normal activities, whether had diagnosis of heart disease, other chronic conditions, symptom profiles, waist–hip ratio, and body mass index) as well as the amount of effort respondents devoted to their health. They were also interested in somatosensory amplification, which describes sensitivity to somatic and visceral sensations not generally regarded as symptoms of serious illness. In turn, other personality and behavioral characteristics (e.g., neuroticism, depression, tendency to seek advice, perceived control) were examined as possible predictors of amplification.

With regard to age patterns of health, Cleary, Zaborski, and Ayanian document that physical health ratings become more negative over the midlife period. Both men and women gave higher ratings to mental than to physical health, although women's scores on mental health are lower, especially in the 35–44 age group. There is also a steady increase in functional health problems with age, although women report more problems on average than do men at all ages. Women also have significantly higher odds of having numerous chronic conditions than do men. However, some of these differences drop out when adjustments are made for somatosensory amplification, which suggests that the gender differences may be due in part to sensitivity to symptoms or reporting tendencies. For both men and women, a constellation of characteristics (neuroticism, advice-seeking, low perceived control) was linked to amplification. This chapter also reviews notable variations in health status between those who are working versus not working in midlife. The authors also examine the extent to which individuals devote effort to their health, and they find both age and gender differences therein.

Chapter 3 by Marmot and Fuhrer illustrates how MIDUS investigators worked together to advance understanding of social inequalities in health, a topic whose explanation must, as they note, be approached from both biomedical and social behavioral perspectives. In fact, it is increasingly evident that the causes of the socioeconomic gradient in health lie outside the medical sector. MIDUS offered a rich array of possible intervening mechanisms, such as family background, health behaviors, social relationships, authority in the workplace, and perceived control. A previous analysis of MIDUS data (Marmot et al. 1998) had documented social gradients (using education as the key variable) in three health measures (self-reported health, waist–hip ratio, psychological well-being) and further demonstrated that these mechanisms, taken not individually but as a whole, helped to account for such differences.

This chapter probed whether there are age differences in the social gradient in health—are they, for example, of lesser magnitude in early rather than later adulthood? Using the above health measures plus measures of physical health functioning (SF-36) and depression, the MIDUS data provided no strong support for a difference in the steepness of the social gradient by age. Marmot and Fuhrer expanded the analyses to incorporate other measures of socioeconomic status (occupational prestige, household income, poverty index of one's neighborhood). These measures are correlated; thus, including all of them in the analyses clarifies the influence of each. Among women, education is strongly related to subjective health and functional health, even after adjusting for the other measures of socioeconomic status. Among men, both education and income are predictive of health outcomes. Again, no single factor explained these social gradients in health; rather it was the combination of the behavioral and psychosocial factors. However, their analyses also documented the influence of an "area effect," thereby drawing attention to contextual influences (e.g., transport amenities, quality of housing). Thus, in two separate analyses, the MIDUS data have clarified that how social inequalities in health come about involves a complex interplay between psychological, social, behavioral, and environmental factors.

Chapter 4 by Ryff, Singer, and Palmersheim also addresses social inequalities in health, but with an emphasis on the high degree of variability within each socioeconomic grade. Such variation makes clear that not all individuals at the lower end of the socioeconomic status hierarchy are in poor physical or mental health. This raises the question of what protective factors enable some individuals who lack socioeconomic advantage to maintain good health and well-being. The authors focus on good-quality social relationships and religion and spirituality, both of which have been shown in earlier research to be predictive of reduced morbidity and later mortality. MIDUS allowed for an assessment of cumulative profiles on social relationships and religion/spirituality via its questions about quality of ties to one's mother and father in childhood as well as to one's spouse/partner in adulthood, along with its measurement of the importance of religion in one's childhood environment and in one's adult life.

The authors' findings highlight gender differences in the study of protective factors vis-à-vis social inequalities, but they also reveal differences that depend on whether the focus was on physical or mental health. Positive social relationship histories emerged as a strong feature of men who have high psychological well-being, despite lacking educational advantage. Similar patterns were found with regard to health symptoms: high school–educated men who reported low symptom profiles also had positive relationship histories compared with those of less educated men who had high symptom reports. For women, social relationship histories were particularly informative in understanding those in poor health (mental and physical) who also lacked educational advantage. Among these women, negative relationship histories clearly predominated. Alternately, women of all educational and health levels were likely to have high rather than low levels of persistent religious engagement—meaning that religiosity did not emerge as an apparent protective factor for those at the low end of the educational hierarchy who were nonetheless in good health. Patterns of religious engagement for men supported the hypothesized protective influence, but only for select outcomes.

In chapter 5, Kessler, Gilman, Thornton, and Kendler use the MIDUS sample of twins and nontwin sibling pairs to conduct a behavior genetic analysis of three primary criteria of midlife success, namely, that one is in good physical health, has high psychological well-being, and lives in a socially responsible way. Their chapter first reviews earlier research on the heritability of health, which shows a wide range (e.g., they cite coefficients between .25 and .58), depending on the specific health measure under consideration. There have been no earlier studies of the heritability of psychological well-being or social responsibility, although related constructs have been examined (e.g., self-esteem, social support, altruism), with coefficients ranging from .20 to .72.

Their analyses tested and adjusted for a variety of assumptions pertaining to environmental similarity and behavioral differentiation between MZ (monozygotic-identical) and DZ (dizygotic-fraternal) twins. Using multiple measures of each of the above three constructs, the authors found the strongest evidence of heritability for multiple dimensions of psychological well-being (correlations for MZ twins were significantly higher than were those for DZ twins), with the effects being especially strong for women's reports of purpose in life. The weakest evidence for genetic effects pertained to self-reported health for males and social responsibility for females, where only one of four correlations was higher for MZ than for DZ pairs. The nontwin sibling pairs were used to evaluate the environmental effects of being a twin, which showed a modest influence on perception of self-rated health. On the basis of their findings, the authors suggest that future surveys, rather than ask single global questions about health, should keep measures of mental and physical health separate because they appear to have quite different heritability profiles.

Chapter 6 by Rossi focuses on a biological transition of notable significance to midlife women–menopause. She reviews the earlier literature and controversies on this topic and shows the need to place menopause in a larger framework of aging processes and their relationship to role performance. MIDUS provides a unique advantage over numerous studies undertaken in the past decade in that the study is not limited to women, but also includes men; nor is it limited to a narrow age range of midlife adults, but includes the full span from 25 to 74. These design features make it possible to evaluate how midlife is experienced differently by women and men as well as how unique the middle years of adulthood are relative to early adulthood and old age. More importantly, MIDUS covers all the major aspects of life: physical and mental health, personality, psychological well-being, and social roles in family, work, and community. That is, MIDUS affords a comprehensive biopsychosocial framework for investigating the menopausal experience.

For both the timing of menopause and women's reactions to it, Rossi's analysis shows wide age diversity in the three stages of the menopausal transition (premenopausal, perimenopausal, postmenopausal), thereby underscoring the misleading message that the "average" age of becoming menopausal is 50 or 51. The overwhelming majority of postmenopausal women report feeling "only relief." Very few women expressed concern about being too old to have children, but concerns were expressed about the prospect of future illness and about loss of attractiveness. Only a minority of women report elevated symptoms associated with meno-pause.

Gender differences in menopause-related symptoms (particularly sweating) were evident, but the data underscore that many younger and older women, and a minority of men, also report such symptoms. Draw-ing on strengths of the MIDUS data, Rossi then demonstrates that nu-merous factors, including a woman's history of menstrual pain, role stress at home or on the job, and somatosensory amplifications (see chap. 2), all contribute independently to elevated symptoms, as does poor mental or physical health.

Summary

Taken as a whole, the chapters in part 1 illustrate the wide scope of MIDUS interest in and assessments of health. Age and gender dif-ferences emerge as key themes across these analyses, along with vari-ations in health as a function of socioeconomic status. Areas of new findings are that social inequalities in health do not vary by age and that single psychosocial factors do not emerge as prominent interven-ing processes to account for these differences. Rather, the full scope of psychosocial variables is implicated in how differences in socioeconomic status translate to health disparities. The findings also underscore the wide variability within social strata—for example, that some individu-als with only a high school education are in good physical and mental health. The quality of their social relationships and their religious beliefs may contribute to such resilient profiles, especially among men. With regard to the MIDUS twin samples, new findings reveal high heritability coefficients for psychological well-being but low coefficients for social responsibility. Finally, MIDUS brought a comprehensive biopsychoso-cial framework to the menopausal transition, which in turn clarified that numerous factors such as role stress at home or at work, history of men-strual pain, and mental and physical health contribute to menopausal symptoms.

Emotion, Quality of Life, and Psychological Well-Being in Midlife

Chapter 7 by Mroczek begins with the observation that although positive and negative affect have been extensively studied, rarely has midlife been the focus of such research. Given age-related differences in life contexts (e.g., experience of role overload in midlife) as well as biological aging and theories of affect regulation in adulthood, he elaborates reasons for expecting that affective experience might vary from young adulthood through midlife into old age. MIDUS made it possible to investigate these questions in a sample with wide age ranges and with greater sociodemographic variability than is evident in previous psychological studies of affect in adulthood and aging. Importantly, Mroczek also brings a rich array of contextual variables to the analysis in an attempt to account for influences on affective profiles. These include background sociodemographic factors such as gender, educational level, marital status, and physical health status as well as more proximal influences such as work and relationship stress.

Mroczek finds that the general pattern for negative affect is one of decline across the three age groups and also that older men are less variable on negative affect than are midlife or young adult males. Regarding positive affect, both midlife and young adults report lower levels than do old-aged individuals, and the older respondents (both men and women) were also less variable on positive affect than were the two younger age groups. The analyses further revealed that affective profiles of midlife adults were more influenced by context than was evident for young or older adults. Most midlife adults are heavily engaged in work and relationships, and this involvement may contribute to their levels of good cheer and fulfillment as well as to their levels of distress. Finally, physical health was found to have a significant effect on both positive and negative affect across the adult years.

Chapter 8 by Kessler, Mickelson, Walters, Zhao, and Hamilton examines the links between age and major depression. Many community surveys of psychiatric disorder have consistently found a negative relationship between age and lifetime clinical depression: highest rates are usually found among young adults and lowest rates among the oldest old. The explanation for this pattern is, however, unclear. Older persons are less likely to report feeling depressed because of the stigma associated with it, or perhaps they are better able to prevent depressed mood from evolving into major depression because they are less reactive to stress. The authors use the MIDUS data to investigate the latter possibility by incorporating respondents' evaluations of stress in major life areas (physical health, work, finances, relationship with children, marriage/close relationship, sexuality). Their analyses also address links between major depression and role changes (e.g., in marital status, employment status, parenting status) over the life course.

MIDUS findings converge with the prior pattern of a negative relationship between age and depression among both men and women, although women have a significantly higher twelve-month prevalence than men. The authors also found higher prevalence among homemakers and the unemployed, although no significant differences were evident as a function of parental status. Regarding life stresses, increased age was not invariably associated with increased stress. There are increases in role loss due to widowhood, retirement, and sexuality, but there are other areas of life where stress decreases with age (job, finances, personal relationships). Supporting the view that lower prevalence of depression among the aged may be due to reduced reactivity to stress, they point to the significant drop in the percentage of older men who rate their physical health in the stressful range. Although additional data would be needed to confirm their interpretation, the authors suggest that it is unlikely such older men are actually in better health compared with younger men. What may be changing rather is that they are lowering their expectations about what constitutes health stress in later life.

Chapter 9 by Fleeson probes age variation in quality of life, thereby linking MIDUS to an extensive history of earlier U.S. surveys on the same topic. Fleeson uses this earlier literature to ask whether age trajectories in quality of life are specific to particular cohorts. That is, are they age patterns that are relatively stable across cohorts, or do they vary across historical periods? He focuses specifically on the study conducted by Campbell, Converse, and Rodgers (1976), which provides a twenty-five-year window of time during which considerable social change occurred (in values, prosperity, politics). In 1976, Americans reported the highest levels of life satisfaction with their marriage and family, and most domains showed a steady linear increase in satisfaction with age. Fleeson's question thus was whether these findings could be replicated twenty-five years later. Expanding previous queries, MIDUS added two new domains of assessment to quality of life: sexuality and contributions to others.

The MIDUS data, like the earlier study, reveal that Americans lead high-quality lives. The five domains of children, marriage, work, financial situation, and overall life show a general increase with age, but the domains of quality of marriage, relationship with children, and overall life do not begin to improve until a person's late thirties or early forties. On the other hand, contributions to others peak in midlife, sexuality substantially decreases with age, and ratings of health satisfaction showed no relationship to age. This overall pattern is consistent with the 1976 study. The two strongest predictors of overall quality of life are the quality of one's marriage/close relationship and one's financial situation. The emphasis on marriage parallels the earlier study, and in both, health did not emerge as of great importance for overall quality of life, even among older participants. Thus, despite different samples, slightly different wording of questions, and intervening social change over a twenty-five-year period, the American story of quality of life remains quite consistent.

Chapter 10 by Markus, Ryff, Curhan, and Palmersheim reports results from the in-depth qualitative study of well-being that was conducted with eighty-three MIDUS respondents from around the country. The purpose was to explore the meaning and sources of well-being with a preselected sample of high school- and college-educated men and women aged 40–59 who reported high psychological well-being in the national survey. How is well-being characterized by those who differ in educational attainment, and what are its attendant links to financial resources and health problems? The authors hypothesized that there would be some common understanding between these educational groups as to what a good life entails but that they would also differ in important ways. The college–educated, for example, were expected to describe their well-being more in terms of personal accomplishment and self-fulfillment, whereas the high school-educated were expected to give greater emphasis to their relationships with others and religious faith in describing their own well-being.

Detailed coding and analysis of open-ended responses revealed that there is clear consensus across educational levels and gender that relations with others is the most important aspect of well-being. Thus, respondents referred to their social relationships in answering multiple questions: What is a good life? Why has your life gone well? What are your hopes for the future? The respondents also agreed that well-being is strongly influenced by having physical health, being able to enjoy oneself, and developing the self. However, when the content and form of responses were examined in detail, more educational differences were apparent. Those with a college education emphasized having a purpose, seeking new opportunities, and experiencing self-enjoyment. Their narratives reflect lives structured by purpose and goals, and they see themselves acting directly on the world. Relations with others are central, but they characterize such ties in terms of influencing, advising, and respecting one another. The high school–educated, in contrast, did not focus on personal accomplishments, skills, or abilities but instead spoke more about their families, financial security, and jobs. The needs and requirements of others are what structure their everyday lives. Their sense of well-being thus involves doing what one should be doing according to the communities one is engaged in.

Chapter 11 by Lachman and Firth brings the construct of perceived control to the MIDUS agenda, asking who by age, gender, and educational level has it, and further, what are the consequences of this perception for psychological well-being and physical health? They note that previous studies have concentrated on comparisons between younger and older adults, with little attention given to the middle years, and they have generally used small, nonrepresentative samples. MIDUS examined general perceptions of sense of mastery and beliefs about external constraints, as well as perceived control within specific life domains. This chapter integrates a rich array of findings not only from MIDUS but also from the Boston oversample, and with additional links to the Whitehall II longitudinal study of British civil servants.

No age differences were evident in the general sense of mastery from young adulthood to old age, although older adults reported higher levels of perceived external constraints than did the two younger groups. Three life domains showed an upward trajectory of perceived control (work, finances, marriage), and two showed downward age trajectories (children, sex life), where respondents perceived less control with aging. Men reported higher mastery and lower constraint than did women, although with regard to specific life domains, both genders perceived the least control over their finances and sex life, and the most control over their marriage and life overall. Those with higher levels of education perceived fewer constraints and greater control over health, work, finances, and contributing to the welfare of others. Those with higher sense of control also reported higher life satisfaction and lower depression. A final set of analyses examined mediators of the sense of control and health outcomes, where the results showed that those who perceive greater control are more likely to engage in health-promoting behaviors, which are linked to better health outcomes (e.g., lower waist–hip ratio). Regarding social inequalities, their findings document that individuals with lower incomes have lower mastery and higher constraint profiles but that there is notable variability. Lower-income respondents who had higher profiles of control also had better health, suggesting that perceptions of control may serve as a possible buffer against health-compromising life stressors.

Chapter 12 by Keyes and Shapiro focuses on social well-being, an area in which MIDUS carved new scientific territory. Previous theoretical work on social well-being is in the sociodemographic literature on alienation and anomie. What is the positive alternative to these maladaptive states? In response to this query, Keyes developed and validated a multidimensional measure of social well-being, which measured the degree to which individuals perceive they are integrated into society, their acceptance of other people, their contribution to society, and their perception that society is understandable, coherent, and has the potential to improve over time (i.e., the world can become a better place). Using such instruments, their chapter focuses on how social well-being is distributed in the U.S. population by age, gender, marital status, and socioeconomic status. The key question was whether social well-being is disproportionately evident among particular sociodemographic groups.

Their findings suggest generally good social well-being in the MIDUS national sample—only about 16 percent of respondents did not report being in the top third on any dimension of social well-being, and more than 20 percent were in the top third on four or five dimensions. With regard to life-course variation, they found positive increments with age for social acceptance and social integration, but a negative profile on age decrements for social coherence and social contribution. Women reported higher social acceptance than men, but men reported higher social coherence than women. Married persons, not surprisingly, reported higher levels of social integration than did nonmarried individuals, but the never married also reported significantly higher levels of social contribution. Those with lower occupational status had lower profiles of social well-being on several dimensions compared to those with higher occupational status. The multivariate models revealed that being male, having high occupational status, and being married or never married were the strongest predictors of high social well-being, whereas low social well-being was evident primarily among females, those who were previously married, and those of low occupational status.

Chapter 13 by Horton and Shweder brings a focus on ethnic minority samples to the analysis of psychological well-being. Their specific question is whether ethnic conservatism, defined as the tendency to resist rapid and full assimilation into the mainstream Anglo-American culture, contributes to the well-being of ethnic minorities. They summarize findings from a report of the National Research Council, which showed there are protective factors such as strong family bonds that act to sustain cultural orientation and thereby protect the health and well-being of first-generation immigrants. Thus, the length of time immigrants reside in the United States has been associated with declining physical and mental health. These authors address such issues via MIDUS subsamples that include first-generation Mexican Americans in Chicago and first- and second-generation Puerto Ricans in Chicago and New York City. They measure ethnic conservatism in terms of the disposition to communicate ethnic pride to one's children, the use of Spanish language in thinking, and weak acculturation ideals. These assessments were then linked to the measures of psychological well-being, measured both in MIDUS and the ethnic/minority subsamples.

They found that first-generation Mexican Americans and Puerto Ricans who are ethnically conservative have higher well-being, particularly autonomy, purpose in life, and positive relations with others. These positive effects are strongly moderated by generational status— that is, attitudes and practices of ethnic conservatism were associated with higher psychological well-being for the first-generation but not the second-generation sample of Puerto Ricans. Thus, the authors' findings converge with the earlier National Research Council report suggesting that the longer immigrant families reside in the United States, the less are the protective benefits derived from ethnic conservatism. The authors note that the sampling strategies, which were designed to recruit individuals from highly segregated neighborhoods, may have resulted in underrepresentation of the most highly assimilated portion of these populations.

Chapter 14 by Ryff, Keyes, and Hughes continues the emphasis on psychological well-being in the ethnic/minority context. Their analyses contrast the well-being of blacks and whites in the MIDUS national survey as well as subsamples of African Americans in New York City and Mexican Americans in Chicago. Extensive prior literature on primarily white, local-community samples had documented replicable age differences on psychological well-being. Some aspects of well-being show incremental profiles with age, such as environmental mastery, whereas others show notable age decrements, such as purpose in life and personal growth, and still others, such as self-acceptance, show little age variation. For two dimensions (autonomy, positive relations with others), prior patterns vary between showing stable or age-incremental profiles. For the most part, men and women have not differed on reported well-being, with the exception of positive relations with others, on which women always score notably higher than men. This chapter also reviews earlier findings on mental health in ethnic/racial samples, which underscore compromised quality of life in the minority context but also notable areas of strength (e.g., self-esteem). MIDUS provided a first opportunity to extend that literature via the above measures of well-being.

Many of the preceding age differences were replicated in the minority samples, suggesting considerable uniformity in how well-being varies across the life course. However, these more expansive samples not only in terms of race/ethnicity but also in terms of socioeconomic variability revealed generally lower profiles of well-being among women compared to men, with the effects most pronounced in the Chicago and New York minority subsamples. One of the most provocative findings emerged from the multivariate analyses, which showed that in addition to age and gender predicting these outcomes, minority group status emerged as a strong positive predictor of well-being. That is, minority respondents are more likely to have high well-being than are majority respondents. Education was also a strong positive predictor of well-being, while perceived discrimination was a strong negative predictor. Overall, these findings underscore the presence of psychological strengths in the lives of those confronted with the stresses of minority group status.

Summary

MIDUS investigators contributed numerous advances to our knowledge of emotion, quality of life, and well-being across the decades of midlife. For the most part, findings revealed a positive portrayal of aging: older adults reported higher levels of positive affect, combined with lower levels of negative affect relative to young and midlife adults. However, the affect of those in midlife was found to be more heavily influenced by context, work, and family than was that of those who are younger or older. Similarly, age was negatively linked with major depression, with older adults showing less likelihood of this disorder. Little evidence was found to support the view that increased age translates to increased stress, although these effects may, in part, be attributable to older respondents being less reactive to stress. Ratings of specific domains of life—children, marriage, work, finances—also showed age-related improvements, beginning in a person's late thirties or early forties. Two domains, however, sexuality and contributing to others, showed a decline in quality with age. Interestingly, self-rated health did not emerge as a strong contributor to overall quality of life. Underscoring themes of social stability, the MIDUS quality-of-life findings were shown to be comparable to those obtained in a national survey twenty-five years ago.

Paralleling quality-of-life results, ratings of perceived control over work, finances, and marriage showed increments with age, although older respondents perceived less control over their sex lives and children. The general sense of mastery did not differ across age groups, but older adults perceived higher external constraint than did the two younger age groups. Men and those with more education reported higher mastery and lower constraint than did women or those with less education. Importantly, those who perceived greater control were more likely to engage in health-promoting behaviors and have better health. Returning to the theme of socioeconomic status–related variability, low-income respondents who had high-control profiles also reported better health.

When asked to characterize well-being in their own terms, MIDUS respondents gave primary importance to having good social relationships. However, educational differences were also evident, with the college-educated referring more to their life purposes, opportunities, and self-enjoyment, while the high school–educated spoke more about families, financial security, and jobs. In addition to these open-ended assessments, MIDUS provided new quantitative measures of social well-being. Older respondents reported higher levels of social integration and acceptance of others than did those in younger age groups, although the aged also reported lower profiles on contributing to society. Those most likely to have high social well-being were males, the married and never married, and individuals with high occupational status.

Finally, the ethnic/minority analyses revealed that first-generation Mexican Americans and Puerto Ricans have higher well-being than do second-generation immigrants. These findings were attributed, in part, to practices of ethnic conservatism among first-generation respondents. Age differences in psychological well-being previously found among white, majority samples were largely comparable for African and Mexican Americans. For example, there were age increments in environmental mastery but decrements in purpose in life, and no age differences for self-acceptance. A particularly novel finding was that ethnic/minority status was a positive predictor of psychological well-being, perhaps underscoring the gains in life purpose and self-regard linked to the challenges of living with racism and discrimination.

Contexts of Midlife: Work and Family Experience, Neighborhood, and Geographic Region

Chapter 15 by Almeida and Horn reports on findings from the National Study of Daily Experiences that was embedded within the larger

MIDUS survey. The authors observe that midlife has been portrayed both as a time of crisis and as the prime of life; they then ask what might day-to-day stressors contribute to these differing views. Although there has been extensive research on age differences in major life events, surprisingly little is known about daily stress. Almeida and Horn examine the nature of daily stressors in two ways: first, they code stressors into types, such as arguments or overloads; second, they evaluate the meaning of the stressor to the individual by probing the affective response to it (e.g., crying, feeling sad). On the basis of previous research, they predicted that women would report more home- and network-related stressors whereas men would report more stressors related to work tasks and overloads. Their data were based on daily reports of stress over eight consecutive days.

On average, respondents reported experiencing at least one stressor on about 40 percent of the days and multiple stressors on about 10 percent of the days. Women reported more frequent days with stressors than did men, but the genders had similar numbers of days involving multiple stressors. Age was negatively related to the frequency of experiencing daily stress in that young and midlife adults reported more frequent days of any stressors and multiple stressors than did older adults. The two younger groups also rated their stressors as more disruptive and unpleasant than did the older adults. Age was also negatively related to the majority of types of stressors (e.g., interpersonal tension, overloads), although older adults reported the highest proportion of network stressors. Overall, the most frequent daily stressor was interpersonal tension. As predicted, women reported more frequent overload, network, and child-related stressors than did men, while men had more frequent stressors involving a coworker.

Chapter 16 by Carr brings a cohort perspective to the MIDUS national survey and asks whether different cohorts of adults show different levels of well-being (environmental mastery) and self-acceptance, and if so, to what extent such differences reflect shifting access to structural opportunities (higher education, gainful employment) as well as individual strategies for accommodating work and family demands. The three cohorts considered include the silent generation (born between 1931 and 1943; ages 52–64), the baby boom cohort (1944–59; ages 37–52), and the baby bust cohort (1960–70; ages 36 and younger). Carr describes how the three cohorts have had very different occupational opportunities as labor market prospects for women have changed dramatically over these periods. Fertility rates have also dropped steadily in the United States since the mid-1960s. What are the implications of these macro-level changes in family structure, educational attainment, and industrial shifts for positive self-regard and the sense that one can manage the surrounding environment?

Carr finds that no single cohort had clear advantage in terms of psychological well-being: the oldest adults were higher in environmental mastery, but the baby bust cohort was highest in levels of self-acceptance. Each successive cohort had a higher proportion of college graduates than the last, although women's occupational status scores still lag significantly behind men's. Multivariate analyses revealed that the higher levels of self-acceptance among baby bust women could be explained by their greater access to self-esteem-enhancing resources, such as higher education, higher occupational status, and fewer family-related obstacles to their work lives. However, baby bust and baby boom women had significantly lower levels of environmental mastery, likely reflecting the intense pressures of balancing work and family life among the former. The three cohorts of men did not differ in environmental mastery, once occupational status and education were controlled for. Finally, the men of the silent generation had significantly lower levels of self-acceptance than did the men of the two younger cohorts. Moreover, cutting back on work to tend to childrearing responsibilities reduced levels of self-acceptance among the oldest men, likely reflecting a choice that went against the then prevailing norms in which men should be primary breadwinners.

Chapter 17 by Earle and Heymann provides a public policy context for an analysis of the MIDUS data, focusing on the interface of work, family, and socioeconomic status. The authors' starting point is the sweeping change in poverty policy that occurred in 1996, when the U.S. Congress ended the guarantee of income support for single parents and their children living in poverty by enacting the Personal Responsibility and Work Opportunity Reconciliation Act (PRWORA). Under the new law, the majority of welfare recipients are required to find work within two years, and individuals may not receive support for more than a total of five years in their lifetime. Earle and Heymann focus on how poor working parents manage the challenges of balancing work and family life under these conditions, emphasizing the implications for the health and well-being of their children. To explore these questions, the authors use not only data from MIDUS, which is valuable for its assessments of autonomy and decision-making in the workplace, and the number of days in which respondents changed their work schedules to meet family responsibilities; they also use the National Longitudinal Survey of Youth (NLSY), which offers information on medical conditions and illnesses among children in low-income families, and the National Medical Expenditure Survey (NMES), which provides data on whether illness caused individual family members to miss school or work and how many such cutbacks occurred over a one-year period.

Earle and Heymann's findings document that low-income families face greater caregiving responsibilities and yet fewer social supports. Low-income parents in MIDUS reported needing 3.4 work cutbacks in a three-month period for their children, compared with 1.84 cutbacks for parents not living in poverty. Single parents without a high-school diploma living in poverty had a work cutback rate three times greater than that of single parents with a high-school diploma or who were not low income. The NLSY data showed that mothers who have received Aid to Families with Dependent Children (AFDC) are significantly more likely than non-AFDC mothers to have at least one child with asthma or a chronic condition requiring time for care. Mothers who have been on AFDC for more than two years were twice as likely as mothers who had never been on AFDC to have at least one child with a chronic condition. Both MIDUS and NLSY underscored the critical differences across social class in the availability of social supports. AFDC mothers were significantly less likely to have paid sick or vacation leave than were other mothers. MIDUS data revealed that employed parents with incomes at or below 150 percent of the poverty line were significantly less likely to get help and support from co-workers, and twice as many low-income working parents stated that they could not rely on family or neighbors for help as compared to higher-income working parents. Their chapter concludes with a discussion of needed policy changes following from these findings.

Chapter 18 by Marks, Bumpass, and Jun takes a broad perspective on family roles during the middle life course and the ways those roles influence physical, mental, and social well-being. The authors note a current controversy regarding the family as a social institution—are we witnessing its demise, or its changing patterns and resilience over time? Their chapter enters this debate by first considering the distribution of those occupying marital/partner, parental, and adult child roles among those persons aged 25–74. They then link these role statuses to assessments of physical health, psychological well-being, negative affect, and generativity concern for guiding the next generation. Although such family roles have been previously linked to health outcomes in national surveys, MIDUS offered an unusual opportunity to link occupancy in various family roles to a rich and diverse array of outcomes.

Only about 1 in 10 women and 1 in 8 men in MIDUS report never having been married. Thus, despite the rhetoric about the retreat from marriage, Americans remain a largely "marrying" people. Historically, being married has been associated with better mental health than being unmarried, but research has seldom included all the relevant categories (e.g., cohabiting, remarried). Among the extensive MIDUS findings was that those in a first marriage reported less negative affect than those formerly married at all ages. Being married also appears particularly relevant to the psychological well-being and generativity of midlife men. Regarding parental status, by age 40–59, only 7.4 percent of women and 9.6 percent of men do not have children. In general, women reported less psychological well-being compared to men in comparable parenting categories, likely reflecting women's greater emotional and instrumental responsibility for children. Men's generativity is higher among those who are parents, and the psychological well-being of midlife men and women is higher among those with adult children compared to those with no children. Regarding midlife adults and their aging parents, the findings show that the mental and physical health of adult children is undermined by having unhealthy parents, particularly an unhealthy sole-surviving mother. Taken together, the findings presented by Marks, Bumpass, and Jun underscore the prominence of family life among MIDUS respondents and its clear ties to diverse indicators of health and well-being.

Chapter 19 by Rossi reviews the MIDUS findings on social responsibility in family and community life. The chapter begins with a review of current claims that Americans are turning away from civic participation in voluntary associations, are alienated from the political process, are neglectful of their family responsibilities, and have become excessively individualistic. Rossi notes the numerous times in our history when contemporary critics portrayed such fraying of the social fabric. Such critiques frequently neglect the strong and positive performance of Americans in their work roles. Amid this backdrop, the MIDUS study gave singular emphasis to the diverse ways in which Americans currently enact their social responsibility to others in family and community life. An edited volume (Rossi 2001) provides a detailed look at how Americans care and do for others. The specific focus of this chapter is on age trends in normative obligations to family and community, with characteristics of respondents' jobs used as control variables that constrain the time available to help family members or to participate in the larger community.

The key predictors of adult responsibility are found to differ both by social structural factors and by phase of the life course. Adults of low social status (indexed by education and income) are heavy providers of emotional support to family members, as they are of hands-on caregiving. If they are also married women with a number of children, they contribute time to both family and community. By contrast, it is high-income, well-educated adults who are more apt to limit their contribution in the family domain to financial assistance but provide both time and money in the community domain. Their social world extends away from the family domain to more involvement with friends, parish, and community organizations. Phase of the life course is the second axis of social differentiation: the family preoccupies the responsibilities of young people, whereas older adults show greater involvement in community affairs. Such patterns are framed from the perspective of a pluralist society best served by a diversity of arenas in which adults show social responsibility tailored to their preferences and abilities.

Chapter 20 by Wethington, Kessler, and Pixley brings the experience of "turning points" to the MIDUS study. Work and family life are likely implicated in why and how Americans see significant change in their lives, but other realms, such as health, may also contribute to turning points. In the popular literature, midlife is frequently depicted as a time of crisis and personal turmoil brought about by the realization that one is aging. In MIDUS, turning points were investigated as experiences involving fundamental shifts in meaning, purpose, or direction that included a self-reflective awareness of the significance of the change. These authors examined how such turning points are distributed across the life span, and via in-depth interviews conducted with a subset of MIDUS respondents ($n = 724$), they explored the meaning of such experiences in qualitative detail. Their chapter also summarized findings from Clausen's earlier work on turning points, which for men were primarily about career followed by marriage, and for women, were most frequently about marriage followed by career.

In the MIDUS national survey, 26 percent of Americans reported that they had had a midlife crisis, but most did not attribute such crises to aging. Rather, major life events were what posed severe threats and challenge. Turning points were somewhat more prevalent in early adulthood than in midlife. Work was the most frequently endorsed realm for experiencing such change (23 percent of men, 27 percent of women), followed by fulfilling a dream (18 percent of men, 22 percent of women). Most individuals reported positive impact from their turning points. For example, challenge and stress at work produced adaptation that, in retrospect, was construed positively, as involving a sense of personal growth.

Moreover, people reported experiencing psychological growth because they believed they had coped well with the process of change.

Chapter 21 by Markus, Plaut, and Lachman brings an entirely new contextual question to the fore: namely, to what extent are there regional differences in well-being? The underlying assumption is that culturally prevalent ideas and practices shape individual well-being, and although there are core elements in this assumption that are true for the country as a whole (e.g., beliefs in independence, self-reliance, and the work ethnic), there may also be important variation by geographic region. To explore this idea, the authors examine historical, sociological, and cultural accounts, including discourse in the media and daily interpersonal conversations (e.g., New Hampshire's license plate motto: Live Free or Die), to characterize the ethos of five of nine regions as delineated by the U.S. Census Bureau: New England, Mountain, West North Central, West South Central, and East South Central. The authors also summarize the sociodemographic features of each region (employment rates, education and income levels, racial diversity, religious affiliation) and then examine region-specific profiles on a variety of measures of well-being (focused on health, autonomy, the self, emotion, others, and social responsibility).

Their findings first underscore themes of consensus: namely, that most Americans overall believe that they are healthy and in control of their lives, that they lead lives of purpose, are satisfied with their lives, feel obligated to work and family, and perceive that their families and partners support them. Nonetheless, there are differences in well-being by geographic region. Those from New England reveal the highest levels of social well-being and positive relations with others, along with high autonomy-focused well-being. Those from the Mountain region are distinctive for their emphasis on self-satisfaction and all aspects of autonomy-focused well-being. Those from the West South Central region are distinguished by their self-focused well-being, particularly a sense of personal growth, and high emotion-focused well-being. Those from the West North Central region score high on self-focused well-being and feeling cheerful, happy, calm, peaceful, and satisfied but lowest on personal growth. Finally, those from the East South Central region score relatively low on all aspects of well-being, except social responsibility; inhabitants of this region show the highest profile of contributing to the welfare and well-being of others. Such analyses thus reveal another layer, beyond the proximal influences of work and family emphasized in preceding chapters, to geographically specific influences that also contribute to diversity in reported well-being.

Orville Gilbert Brim, Carol D. Ryff, and Ronald C. Kessler

Summary

A key innovation of MIDUS was the assessment of daily stressors among a large subsample of respondents. Consistent with largely positive life-course trajectories previously described, age was negatively related to the frequency of experiencing daily stress. Young and midlife adults also rated their stressors as more disruptive than did older adults. Providing a counterpoint to the prominence of social relations in assessments of well-being is the finding that the most frequent daily stressor was interpersonal tension. Nonetheless, only about a quarter of MIDUS respondents reported experiencing a midlife crisis, which they attributed not to aging but to major life events that posed severe threat or challenge. Work was the most frequent realm for reporting turning points for both men and women, and most of these resulted in personal growth because the persons involved were able to cope well with change.

How poor working parents manage challenges of balancing work and family life was examined using MIDUS and other national studies. For example, socioeconomic status–related adversity was illustrated by the fact that low-income parents were more likely to have a child with a chronic condition, less likely to have paid sick leave, and less likely to get help from co-workers or family and neighbors. Nonetheless, MIDUS data provided scant evidence for decline of the family as a social institution. Most American adults are, or had been, married, and most have, or had, children. Importantly, psychological benefits are associated with these roles: those who are married report less negative affect, more psychological well-being, and higher levels of generativity. Mothers, however, report less well-being than fathers, and having unhealthy parents was found to undermine the mental and physical health of midlife parents.

MIDUS offered the first national look at social responsibility in family and community life. Those with less education and income were found to be heavy providers of emotional support as well as hands-on caregiving to family members. High-income, well-educated adults, in contrast, were found to contribute to family through financial assistance but also to provide both time and money to community organizations. Family life was found to comprise most of the social responsibility of younger adults, while older individuals showed greater involvement in community affairs.

From a cohort perspective, it was found that younger cohorts of women had higher levels of self-acceptance than did older cohorts, with these differences explained, in part, by their access to greater educational and occupational attainment. However, younger cohorts also had lower levels of environmental mastery, perhaps reflecting the pressures of trying to balance work and family life. Interestingly, older cohorts of men who had cutback on their work to attend to their children were found to have lower levels of self-acceptance.

Analyses of regional differences in well-being, another novelty of the MIDUS investigation, revealed notable similarities across regions. Most Americans see themselves as healthy and purposeful, in control of and satisfied with their lives, obligated to work and family, and supported by their families and partners. Nonetheless, those from New England show the highest levels of social well-being and positive relations with others. Those in the Mountain region are particularly self-satisfied and autonomous, whereas those in the West South Central region report high emotional well-being and personal growth. Respondents from the West North Central region reported being cheerful, happy, calm, peaceful, and satisfied, and those in the East South Central region were relatively low on all aspects of well-being except social responsibility, where they showed the highest profiles of contributing to the welfare of others.

Collectively, these MIDUS findings underscore the diverse ways in which midlife individuals are influenced, both positively and negatively, by their experiences in the domains of work, family, and community. As with the preceding analyses, age, gender, and socioeconomic status provide meaningful frames for interpreting such variation, along with cohort differences and regional influences. A recurrent theme across the contexts of midlife is that individuals both are significant contributors to their family, community, and workplace and are influenced by what is occurring in these life domains.

The Presence of MIDUS across Scientific Fields

The chapters in this volume illustrate the wide array of topics investigated by those who helped conceive of and implement the MIDUS national survey. It is important to recognize, however, that these products constitute only a small part of the scientific advances following from the study. In addition to the findings described here, MIDMAC investigators have also contributed new findings to a host of other topics, including perceived discrimination and mental health (Kessler, Mickelson, and Williams 1999), social support/strain and health and well-being (Walen and Lachman 2000), early parental loss and midlife health and well-being (Maier and Lachman 2000), emotion in social relationships and health (Ryff et al. 2001), age, education, and well-being (Keyes, Shmotkin, and

Ryff 2002), contributions of work and family life to racial/ethnic and socioeconomic differences in health behaviors (Grzywacz and Marks 2001), contributions of work and family spillover to midlife drinking (Grzywacz and Marks 2000), and links between health behaviors and health beliefs (Ayanian and Cleary 1999).

There has also been extensive use of the MIDUS data set beyond those affiliated with the original MIDMAC research network, and again, topical interests traverse numerous scientific disciplines. One mark of the presence of MIDUS across fields is that publications from the study have now appeared in wide-ranging journals covering such diverse topics as public health, epidemiology, marriage and family life, aging and adult development, personality, and social psychology. Included among these journals are the following: *American Journal of Health Promotion, American Journal of Psychiatry, American Journal of Public Health, Annals of Allergy, Asthma and Immunology, Annals of Internal Medicine, Contemporary Psychology, Family Relations, International Journal of Behavioral Development, International Journal of Epidemiology, Journal of Adult Development, Journal of the American Medical Association, Journal of Evaluation in Clinical Practice, Journal of Gerontology, Journal of Health and Social Behavior, Journal of Marriage and the Family, Journal of Occupational and Environmental Medicine, Journal of Personality and Social Psychology, Journal of Research in Personality, Marriage and Family Review, Medical Care, Milbank Quarterly, Motivation and Emotion, Personality and Social Psychology Bulletin, Psychology and Aging, Social Forces, Social Psychology Quarterly,* and *Social Science and Medicine.*

Such expansive use of MIDUS in little more than five years since the data have been available speaks powerfully to current scientific priorities—particularly the growing commitment among investigators trained in specific fields to conduct more expansive inquiries that link their own areas of expertise to realms beyond. MIDUS has played an important role in carrying such "integrative science" forward. In this sense, the survey has not only helped chart the territory of midlife, in all of its biopsychosocial complexity; MIDUS has also provided a model for how to bring diverse fields together in pursuit of a synergistic whole.

It is because of the energy and excitement surrounding the MIDUS endeavor that many investigators, including, but not restricted to members of the original MIDMAC Network, implemented plans to carry this national survey forward and, importantly, extend its disciplinary boundaries even further. Their efforts have been successful in obtaining funds from the National Institute on Aging to collect another wave of data, which will occur approximately ten years after the original study, on the full MIDUS samples, including twins and siblings. The novelty of satellite studies, built around the main investigation, will also be carried forward not only to assess daily stressors and cognitive functioning now longitudinally but also to add a comprehensive array of biomarker assessments to the study. In short, the life span of this unique study continues, with hopes that its future trajectory will be long, healthy, and persistently innovative.

References

Ayanian, J. Z., and P. D. Cleary. 1999. Perceived risks of heart disease and cancer among cigarette smokers. *Journal of the American Medical Association* 28111:1019–21.

Birren, J. E., and K. W. Schaie, eds. 1996. *Handbook of the psychology of aging.* 4th ed. San Diego: Academic Press.

———. 2001. *Handbook of the psychology of aging.* 5th ed. San Diego: Academic Press.

Brim, O. G. 2000. MacArthur Foundation study of successful midlife development. *ICPSR Bulletin* 20 (4): 1–5.

Campbell, A., P. E. Converse, and W. L. Rodgers. 1976. *The quality of American life: Perceptions, evaluations, and satisfactions.* New York: Sage.

Grzywacz, J. G., and N. F. Marks. 2000. Family, work, work–family spillover and problem drinking in midlife. *Journal of Marriage and the Family* 60:336–48.

———. 2001. Social inequalities and exercise during adulthood: Toward an ecological perspective. *Journal of Health and Social Behavior* 42:202–20.

Helson, R. 1993. Comparing longitudinal studies of adult development: Toward a paradigm of tension between stability and change. In *Studying lives through time: Personality and development,* ed. D. C. Funder, R. D. Parke, C. Tomlinson-Keasey, and K. Widaman, 93–119. Washington, D.C.: American Psychological Association.

Kessler, R. C., K. D. Mickelson, and D. R. Williams. 1999. The prevalence, distribution, and mental health correlates of perceived discrimination in the United States. *Journal of Health and Social Behavior* 403:208–30.

Keyes, C. L. M., C. Shmotkin, and C. D. Ryff. 2002. Optimizing well-being: The empirical encounter of two traditions. *Journal of Personality and Social Psychology* 826:1007–22.

Lachman, M. E., and J. B. James. 1997. Charting the course of midlife development: An overview. In *Multiple paths of midlife development,* ed. M. E. Lachman and J. B. James, 1–17. Chicago: University of Chicago Press.

MacArthur Foundation Research Network on Successful Midlife Development website. http://midmac.med.harvard.edu/

Maier, H., and M. E. Lachman. 2000. Consequences of early parental loss and separation for health and well-being in midlife. *International Journal of Behavioral Development* 24:183–89.

Marmot, M. G., R. Fuhrer, S. L. Ettner, N. F. Marks, L. L. Bumpass, and C. D. Ryff. 1998. Contribution of psychosocial factors to socioeconomic differences in health. *Milbank Quarterly* 76:403–48.

McCrae, R. R., and P. T. Costa, Jr. 1990. *Personality in adulthood.* New York: Guildford Press.

Rossi, A. S., ed. 1994. *Sexuality across the life course.* Chicago: University of Chicago Press.

———. 2001. *Caring and doing for others.* Chicago: University of Chicago Press.

Ryff, C. D., C. M. L. Kwan, and B. H. Singer. 2001. Personality and aging: Flourishing agendas and future challenges. In *Handbook of the psychology of aging,* 5th ed., ed. J. E. Birren and K. W. Schaie, 477–99. San Diego: Academic Press.

Ryff, C. D., and M. M. Seltzer, eds. 1996. *The parental experience in midlife.* Chicago: University of Chicago Press.

Ryff, C. D., and B. Singer. 1998. The contours of positive human health. *Psychological Inquiry* 9:69–85.

Ryff, C. D., B. Singer, E. Wing, and G. Love. 2001. Elective affinities and uninvited agonies: Mapping emotion with significant others onto health. In *Emotion, social relationships, and health,* ed. C. D. Ryff and B. Singer, 133–75. New York: Oxford University Press.

Shweder, R. A., ed. 1998. *Welcome to middle age! And other cultural fictions.* Chicago: University of Chicago Press.

Singer, B., and C. D. Ryff. 2001a. *New horizons in health: An integrative approach.* Washington, D.C.: National Academy Press.

———. 2001b. Person centered methods for understanding aging: The integration of numbers and narratives. In *Handbook of aging and the social sciences,* 5th, ed. R. H. Binstock and L. K. George, 44–65. San Diego: Academic Press.

University of Michigan website. http://www.isr.umich.edu/src/midus/

U.S. Census Bureau. 1995. *Current population survey: October 1995.* Washington, D.C.: U.S. Department of Commerce.

Walen, H. R., and M. E. Lachman. 2000. Social support and strain from partner, family, and friends: Costs and benefits for men and women. *Journal of Social and Personal Relationships* 171:5–30.

I Midlife Perspectives on Physical Health

CHAPTER TWO

Sex Differences in Health over the Course of Midlife

Paul D. Cleary, Lawrence B. Zaborski, and John Z. Ayanian

Of the many issues studied in MIDUS, health is perhaps the area in which the most is already known. There are local and regional studies, cross-sectional and longitudinal epidemiological investigations, and many specialized studies that have attempted to characterize the determinants, correlates, and consequences of different health states. One of the many ways in which the MIDUS study is unique, however, is that it collected a rich array of health status indicators, measures of health behavior, and health attitudes in the same survey in which a wealth of psychological and social information also was collected. MIDUS is a cross-sectional study, so its data do not allow us to study change in individuals. Nevertheless, the rich array of information from different age groups allows us to characterize age differences in ways previously not possible.

Although there are many questions one might ask about the determinants and consequences of health status, medical and social scientists often have been particularly interested in how health varies over the life course and in gender and socioeconomic differences in health (Fremont and Bird 2000). In chapter 3, Marmot and Fuhrer explore socioeconomic gradients in some of the MIDUS measures and the ways those differences vary over the life course. In this chapter, we focus on the relationship between age and the different indicators of self-reported health measured in MIDUS, and assess whether and how those age differences differ by sex.

There are well-established biological differences between the genders that have different implications at different points in the life course, as well as theories about psychosocial factors that help explain either the prevalence or reported prevalence of different conditions (Cleary 1987; Doyal 2001; McDonough and Walters 2001; Verbrugge 1985; Waldron 1983, 1997; Walters, McDonough, and Strohschein 2002; Wenger, Speroff, and Packard 1993). For example, there has been extensive research on the development of cardiovascular disease in men and women (Nikiforov and Mamaev 1998; Waldron 1993) and the possible biological differences that explain the development of disease at different ages (Wenger,

Speroff, and Packard 1993). There also has been work on how psychosocial factors such as social roles and stress are related to differences in the way men and women perceive and react to different situations (Cleary 1987; Verbrugge 1985). There are no physiological measures linked to MIDUS. Thus, these data cannot explicate biological explanations of these differences. It is possible, however, to use psychosocial measures to illustrate some of the factors underlying the differences presented.

One factor that is important to consider when examining self-reported health, and specifically age and gender differences in health reports, is that different groups of respondents may have systematically different propensities to report certain states or conditions. One characteristic that has been shown in numerous studies to be related to experience and reports of health problems is somatosensory amplification. Somatosensory amplification is a term we use to describe sensitivity to, and/or increased reporting of, minor somatic and visceral sensations that are not generally regarded as symptomatic of serious disease. In this chapter, we assess how somatosensory amplification is related to age and gender differences in reports about health status. Because MIDUS also included measures of other psychological variables that might be related to reports about health, we also examined the extent to which the associations between amplification and health reports were similar to and/or explained by the relationship between such variables and reports about health status. In addition, we examined age and sex differences in effort devoted to health over the life course.

Conceptual Framework

Researchers and policy makers now recognize that traditional outcome measures such as physiologic function and mortality do not adequately reflect the variations in health that are important to individuals (Brook, McGlynn, and Cleary 1996; McDowell and Newell 1996; Patrick and Erickson 1993; Tsevat et al. 1994; Wilson and Cleary 1995). Thus, there is increasing emphasis on assessing a broader range of health indicators that reflect what often is referred to as health-related quality of life (HRQL).

HRQL refers to the various aspects of a person's life that are affected strongly by changes in health status (health-related) and that are important to the person. It is affected by symptoms as well as physical, social, role, and sexual functioning and mental health.

It is important to make a distinction between HRQL and the broader concept of quality of life. The latter encompasses much more than health

(Andrews and Withey 1976; Berg, Hallauer, and Berk 1976; Flanagan 1978; Patrick and Erickson 1993). Economic, political, cultural, and spiritual factors, as well as health, can affect overall quality of life. In this chapter, we address the narrower concept of HRQL. The terms *health status* and *health-related quality of life* can refer to slightly different concepts (Guyatt, Feeny, and Patrick 1991; Guyatt, Patrick, and Feeny 1991), but in this chapter we use the terms interchangeably.

To help select and decide how to use the HRQL measures in MIDUS to examine sex differences across the life course, we use a theoretical framework developed by Wilson and Cleary (1995). In this model, measures of health can be thought of as existing on a continuum of increasing biologic, social, and psychological complexity. At one end of the continuum are biologic measures such as serum albumin levels and hematocrit, and at the other end are more complex and integrated measures such as physical functioning and overall health perceptions. These relationships are displayed schematically in figure 1. We describe the variables we used in our analyses below in terms of this model.

Symptoms

In MIDUS, there are no direct measures of physiological factors, but we do have some self-report measures, such as body mass index and waist-hip ratio. After biologic and physiologic factors, symptom status is the next level in our model. Physical symptoms have been defined as "a perception, feeling, or even belief about the state of our body" (Pennebaker

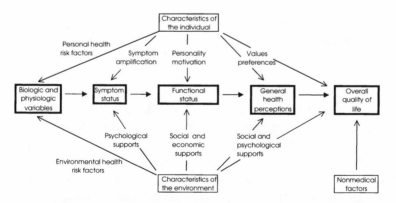

FIGURE 1. Relationships among measures of patient outcome in a health-related quality-of-life conceptual model. *Source:* Adapted from Cleary and Wilson 1995.

1982). We define a symptom as a person's perception of an abnormal physical, emotional, or cognitive state. Symptoms are assessed at the level of the organism as opposed to the level of specific cells or organs. Examples of physical symptoms are fever, nausea, pain, and fatigue; examples of emotional symptoms are feeling anxious and depressed. These are the feelings and experiences that a person typically describes to a physician. Symptom reports are influenced by complicated interactions of biologic, physiologic, and emotional factors. Also influencing the report of symptoms is the way in which the individual reacts to and processes bodily sensations—a factor difficult to measure, which probably varies greatly from person to person and is unlikely to be changed by an intervention by a physician or health care system (Barsky, Cleary, and Klerman 1992). For example, a concept called somatosensory amplification has been shown to be important in how people detect, interpret, and respond to physiological sensations (Barsky, Brener, et al. 1995; Barsky, Cleary, Brener, et al. 1993; Barsky, Cleary, et al. 1995; Barsky, Cleary, Sarnie, et al. 1993; Barsky et al. 1994). The way physicians label symptoms also can affect how individuals interpret and react to them. For example, the same symptoms may have very different consequences if they are labeled "flu" than if they are labeled "pneumonia." Thus, reported symptoms represent an integration of a large quantity of complex information, the source of which is typically the patient.

Less clearly conceptualized are emotional or psychological symptoms such as fear, worry, and frustration. Emotions and physical symptoms often vary together, and causal relationships clearly can go in both directions between these two types of symptoms (Mechanic, Cleary, and Greenley 1982; Pennebaker 1982). To include all of these different phenomena, we define a symptom as a person's perception of an abnormal physical, emotional, or cognitive state.

Functioning

The next level in our model is functional status, and like symptom status, it is an important point of integration. Among the determinants of functional status are symptom state, social factors, and psychological characteristics. Many aspects of an individual's social environment may have an important effect on his or her HRQL. In addition, individual factors such as personality and motivation are likely to be important determinants of functioning (Greenfield and Nelson 1992; Patrick 1987). A number of studies have included both clinical and functional status measures among the outcomes examined (Ayanian, Guadagnoli, and

Cleary 1995; Bombardier and Raboud 1991; Cleary et al. 1991, 1993; Laupacis, Wong, and Churchill 1991). These studies, many of which are clinical trials, demonstrate convincingly that measures of HRQL can be as sensitive to clinically important changes as are traditional clinical variables.

Health Perception

An individual's overall health perception or HRQL is a function of the importance or weight that the individual gives to various functional impairments. A construction worker or a dancer might value physical function highly and social function significantly less so. A teacher might value cognitive function much more heavily than physical function. Until these preferences are measured for individuals or particular groups, our ability to interpret changes in overall health perceptions will be limited.

In the analyses presented herein, we present measures that are representative of general health perceptions, functional status (intermediate activities of daily living and disability), symptoms (e.g., dyspnea and angina), and some measures of physiological status (e.g., high blood pressure and body mass index).

METHODS

The data reported here come from the National Survey of Midlife in the United States (MIDUS). A more complete description of the survey sample and procedures is provided in chapter 1 of this volume.

Measures

Many health status variables were assessed in the MIDUS study. One of the most commonly used measures of perceived health status is a simple question asking respondents to rate their health as excellent, very good, good, fair, or poor. This variable has been shown to have excellent construct validity, to be related to several health behaviors, and to be a strong predictor of subsequent mortality (Cleary 1997; Idler and Kasl 1991; Kaplan and Camacho 1983; Mossey and Shapiro 1982). One of the strengths of this measure is that it is a synthesis of many aspects of people's health (fig. 1). To provide a slightly more differentiated assessment in MIDUS, we created two questions—one referring specifically to physical health and the other to mental health.

Measures of functioning included number of days in the previous month the respondent was unable to work or perform normal activities, the number of days in the past month the respondent had to cutback on work or regular activities, and the respondent's difficulties with intermediate activities of daily living. Major symptoms assessed included shortness of breath related to exertion (dyspnea) and chest pain reported on exertion (angina). Dyspnea and angina were measured using adaptations of the Rose questionnaire (Rose et al. 1982), which has been validated against electrocardiogram abnormalities and mortality (Rose 1965; Rose, McCartney, and Reid 1977). We also asked whether the respondent had heart disease confirmed by a physician or had had a heart attack, reported headache symptoms, regularly took blood pressure medication, and whether they currently or ever had cancer, or any one of twenty-nine other health conditions (table 1).

We also assessed waist–hip ratio (WHR) and body mass index (BMI). WHR is often used as a crude estimate of body fat distribution. A WHR below 0.8 for women and 0.9 for men has been defined as "normal" irrespective of what the BMI is (Ledoux et al. 1997). To assess WHR, we mailed subjects a measuring tape with their survey and provided instructions on how to measure their waist and hip to the nearest quarter inch. Using those reported values, we calculated WHR as the ratio of waist to hip measures.

BMI was calculated as mass measured in kilograms divided by the squared height measured in meters. Because some values of the constituent variables were implausible, we recoded heights above 84 inches, waist measurement below 20 inches, and hip measurement below 22 or above 75 to the respective cutoff value. In addition, any WHR that was greater than four standard deviations from the sex-specific mean was recoded to be a missing value. We used those BMI data to create a variable indicating whether the person was overweight, using National Center for Health Statistics definitions (U.S. Department of Health and Human Services 1998). For men, overweight was defined as BMI greater than 27.8 kilograms/meter^2. For women the threshold was 27.3 kilograms/meter^2. Health behaviors measured included use of vitamins and exercise.

In addition, we assessed several personal beliefs or attitudes related to health. These included the amount of effort devoted to maintaining health (health effort) and reported levels of somatosensory amplification (amplification). Somatosensory amplification was measured with a five-item scale that assesses sensitivity to somatic and visceral sensations that are uncomfortable but usually minor and not generally regarded as symptomatic of serious disease (e.g., "hunger contractions," "being too hot or cold"). The scale has a four-point ordinal response format and has

TABLE 1 Prevalence of Self-Reported Conditions for Men and Women

Condition	Prevalence Female	Male	Odds Ratio (Female vs. Male) Unadjusted	Adjusted for Amplification
Anxiety, depression and other emotional problems	0.251	0.146	1.955***	1.662***
Arthritis, rheumatism, bone joint	0.230	0.173	1.425***	1.313*
Stomach problems	0.223	0.167	1.430***	1.207*
Sciatica, lumbago, backache	0.215	0.192	1.151	1.083
Hypertension	0.181	0.190	0.948	0.865
Hay fever	0.173	0.154	1.149	1.089
Urinary/bladder problems	0.163	0.103	1.704***	1.515***
Asthma, bronchitis, emphysema	0.159	0.100	1.705***	1.584***
Chronic sleep problems	0.148	0.110	1.411***	1.188
Migraine headaches	0.145	0.063	2.529***	2.244***
Foot problems	0.137	0.098	1.472***	1.364***
Skin problems	0.110	0.115	0.954	0.867
Hemorrhoids	0.106	0.114	0.931	0.816
Teeth problems	0.103	0.092	1.129	1.017
Constipation	0.091	0.029	3.314***	2.858***
Gum/mouth problems	0.086	0.068	1.280*	1.206*
Thyroid disease	0.072	0.016	4.839***	4.656***
Diabetes	0.050	0.057	0.869	0.776
Ulcer	0.045	0.035	1.293	1.087
Other lung problems	0.039	0.037	1.054	0.906
Gall bladder	0.034	0.012	2.888***	2.583***
Hernia	0.028	0.031	0.912	0.759
Multiple sclerosis, epilepsy, other neurological conditions	0.023	0.016	1.409	1.273
Lupus, other autoimmune disorders	0.019	0.005	3.451***	3.114**
Alcohol/drug problems	0.017	0.042	0.406***	0.351***
Varicose veins	0.016	0.009	1.722	1.440
Stroke	0.007	0.011	0.650	0.547
Tuberculosis	0.002	0.003	0.803	0.665
AIDS, HIV	0.002	0.003	0.667	0.555

*$p < 0.05$. **$p < 0.01$. ***$p < 0.001$.

been shown to have a test-retest reliability of 0.79 over a median interval of 74 days and an internal consistency (Cronbach's alpha) of .82 (Barsky, Brener, et al. 1995; Barsky, Cleary, Brener, et al. 1993; Barsky, Cleary, et al. 1995; Barsky, Cleary, Sarnie, et al. 1993; Barsky et al. 1994, 1988; Barsky and Wyshak 1990; Barsky, Wyshak, and Klerman 1990). Although we know a fair amount about the correlates of somatosensory amplification, there is debate about exactly what it represents. For example, it could be that persons who score high on this scale are more sensitive to common physiological sensations. That is, it could be that they simply are better at detecting physiological symptoms. Alternately, it could be that they process physiological symptoms the same as others do (as the variable name implies) but that they interpret and respond to symptoms (amplify). One way we have tried to investigate this issue is to examine whether people who have high values on this scale are more or less aware of certain physiological events. Specifically, we have investigated the extent to which this variable is related to the accuracy of the detection of cardiac arrhythmias, which can be measured objectively. Our studies in that area (Barsky, Cleary, Brener, et al. 1993) suggest that persons high on the somatosensory amplification scale are not more accurate in reporting when they have cardiac arrhythmias. Our interpretation of these results is that the scale described a tendency to interpret and respond differently to physiological sensations rather than an inherent difference in physiological sensitivity. In this study we also used the MIDUS measures of neuroticism, depression, tendency to seek advice, and low perceived control to assess whether the tendency to report symptoms is related to these other personality characteristics and behavioral dispositions.

Results

The means of responses to the self-reported global physical health question for men and women of different ages are shown in figure 2.

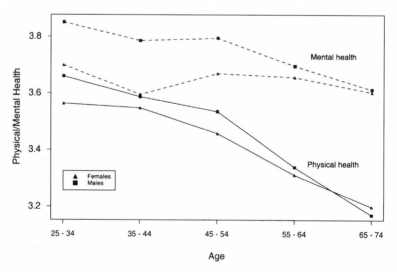

FIGURE 2. Self-assessed physical and mental health, on a scale of 1–5.

These data show that ratings of physical health become more negative over the midlife period in a relatively steady way, and that the age differences are similar for women and men, except that women tend to give a slightly lower rating for their physical health until they are older. The differences in general ratings of physical health between men and women and the differences in the change of these ratings over the life course are not statistically significant. Responses to the question about mental health show that although both men and women give higher ratings of mental health than physical health, women had significantly lower scores than men, with the lowest means being among women in the 35–44 age group. However, the differences in mental health ratings between men and women narrowed substantially after the age of 44. These findings are consistent with other studies showing that there are only small sex differences in overall ratings of physical health (Arber and Cooper 1999). They also are consistent with research showing that women tend to have much higher rates of affective disorders than do men and that these differences are most pronounced in their younger years (Kessler et al. 1993, 1994). Women also were more likely than men to report in the survey that they had anxiety, depression, or an emotional problem (table 1), and the differences were largest in the 35–44 age group (data not shown). However, the rates did not converge, as they did for self-assessed mental health.

Although simple questions about perceived health status provide a general sense of how individuals think they are doing, it is hard to interpret these measures because they reflect many different aspects of health. Another type of measure that provides a general indication of the general health status of individuals but that has a clearer interpretation is functional status. Figure 3 shows the age differences for a measure of problems with intermediate activities of daily living. These data are consistent with the data presented in figure 2 in that they show a steady increase of health problems over the ages studied, with women reporting more problems, on average, than men for all age groups.

Another way of assessing the short-term impact of health on functioning is to ask respondents how many days in the past month they were either unable to work or perform their regular activities, or had to cut back on their work or normal activities. Although these are usually asked as single questions in national surveys such as the National Health Interview Survey, we were interested in learning whether the respondent thought any reported disability was the result of physical problems, mental health problems, or a combination of the two. Furthermore, although these questions are intended to capture both work-related and

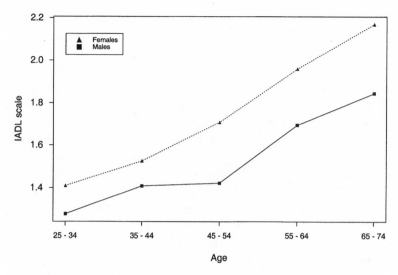

FIGURE 3. Problems with intermediate activities of daily living (IADL), on a scale of 0–4.

non-work-related disability, the interpretation of these questions depends on whether the person is working or not. Thus, we present data for each of these questions separately for those who report that they work at least part time outside the home and those who report that they do not work (figs. 4 and 5). These data reveal several striking patterns. First, for those not working, the group reporting the most days on which they were unable to perform, or had to cut back on normal activities, is women in the 45–54 age group. Most reported disability days are attributed to physical health problems by respondents, but women aged 45–54 tend to report that a higher proportion of disability days are the result of mental health problems. This is consistent with the data in figure 2 showing that women report worse mental health than do men and that these differences are more prominent in younger women. For those who report working, the pattern is quite different. Among these respondents we found less variation by age, except that fewer persons over the age of 65 report that they are unable to work because of health than do younger respondents, possibly reflecting better health states among people who choose to work after age 65. However, the gender differences are pronounced, especially for women between the ages of 25 and 54.

As indicated in figure 1, we consider symptoms and specific conditions the precursors or determinants of these more global outcomes.

Thus, to try to understand better the reasons underlying these age and gender differences in functioning, we examine a select set of more specific indicators. Two cardinal symptoms of cardiac disease that are related to functional status and general health status are dyspnea and angina. Dyspnea (fig. 6) shows a trend similar to that found for intermediate activities of daily living. Angina, however, shows a different pattern (fig. 7). For men there is a sharp increase in the prevalence of angina until about the age of 50, at which point the prevalence stops increasing. For women, on

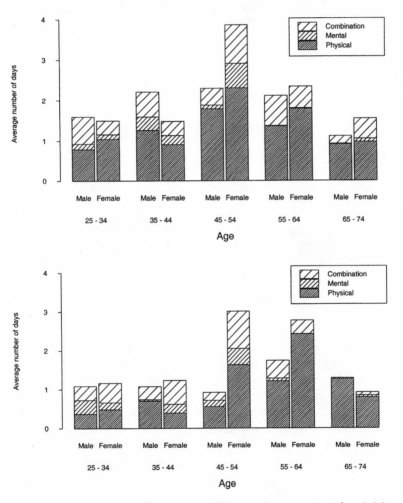

FIGURE 4. Days nonworkers were unable to carry out normal activities (top), and days nonworkers cut back on normal activities (bottom).

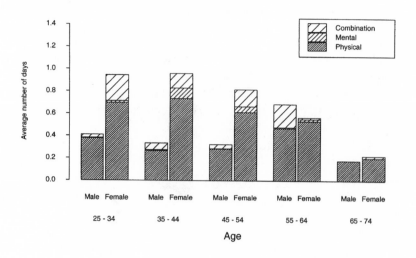

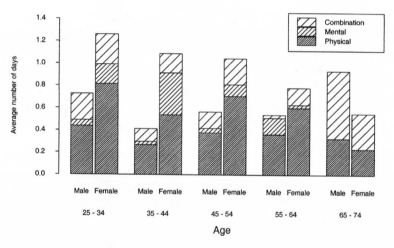

FIGURE 5. Days workers were unable to carry out normal activities (top), and days workers cut back on normal activities (bottom).

the other hand, the prevalence is very high for all age groups. In general, women, especially younger women, report more angina than do men, and the association between angina and objectively determined cardiac abnormalities is weaker in women than in men (Harris and Weissfeld 1991; Nicholson et al. 1999).

One of the most commonly detected physiological conditions that is an important marker for cardiac and general physical condition is

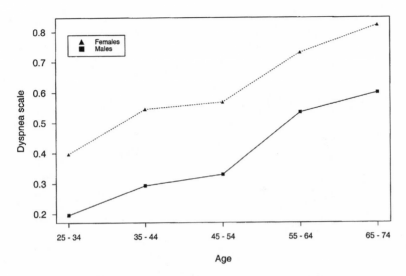

FIGURE 6. Dyspnea scale, 1–4.

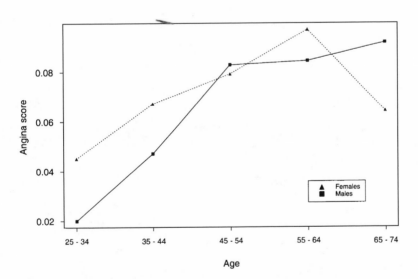

FIGURE 7. Angina combined score, 0–3.

hypertension. Although we did not obtain an independent objective measure of hypertension, such as an actual blood pressure reading, we did ask subjects whether they were taking medication for high blood pressure. Positive responses to this question increased steadily with age (fig. 8), and

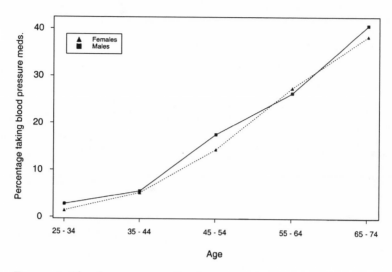

FIGURE 8. Blood pressure medication.

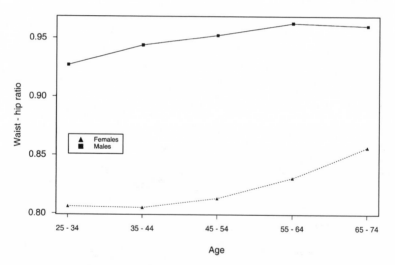

FIGURE 9. Waist–hip ratio.

the proportion of men and women responding positively is similar. There was a similar pattern for responses to a simple question about whether the person had hypertension (data not shown).

Two other measures of physical status in MIDUS that are relatively objective are waist–hip ratio (WHR) and weight, based on body mass index (BMI). WHR (fig. 9) increases steadily with age, and men generally have a higher WHR than women of the same age. Percentage overweight also tends to increase with age until about the age of 65 (fig. 10). Comparable patterns are observed in national studies using direct measurement (U.S. Department of Health and Human Services 1998).

The MIDUS survey also had a series of questions that asked respondents if they had specific medical conditions. These conditions and the prevalence for men and women are presented in table 1. Because the prevalence of many of these conditions is relatively low, we do not present age differences, but women report significantly more of many of these conditions.

Possible Determinants of Age and Gender Differences

There are substantial gender differences in amplification at all ages (fig. 11), although the differences are smaller in older age groups. To explicate the potential reporting effects in the data presented in this chapter, we recalculated the data presented in figures 4–7 and the prevalence of the chronic conditions presented in table 1, after statistically adjusting for gender differences in amplification.

Adjusting for amplification did not have a consistent impact on the size of the gender differences displayed in figure 4, but the differences in the 45–54 age group were reduced, and the difference in this age

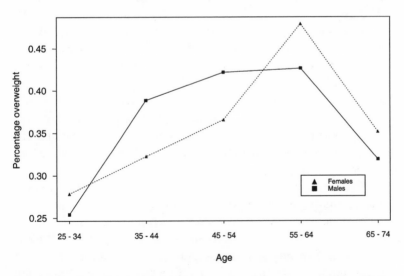

FIGURE 10. Percentage overweight (measured for men as BMI > 27.8 k/m^2; for women as BMI > 27.2 k/m^2).

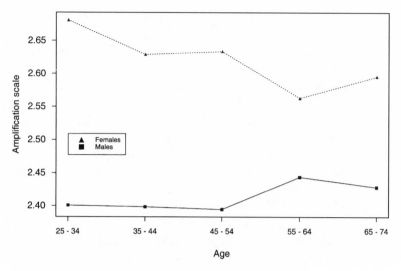

FIGURE 11. Somatosensory amplification, scale of 1–4.

group for days cutback was not significant after adjustment. Adjusting for amplification tended to reduce the sex differences shown in figure 5, but women workers were still significantly more likely to report both more days unable to work and more days cutback at work before and after adjustment.

Adjustment of dyspnea scores for amplification tended to increase the sex differences for respondents under the age of 55 and decrease the differences for those over 55. The sex differences in angina also increased for those under 55, with less consistent effects for those over 55. These effects are probably the result of the larger sex differences in amplification in younger persons (fig. 11). On average, women were significantly more likely to report dyspnea both before and after adjustment for amplification. The average sex difference for angina was not significant either before or after adjustment.

The data in table 1 (column 3, "Unadjusted") suggest that women have significantly higher odds of having asthma, bronchitis, emphysema; arthritis, rheumatism, and bone/joint problems; thyroid disease; stomach problems; urinary and bladder problems; constipation; gall bladder problems; foot problems; lupus and other autoimmune disorders; gum and mouth problems; emotional problems; migraine headaches; and chronic sleep problems. Men have significantly higher odds of having problems with drugs or alcohol. Once we controlled for the effect of amplification (column 4, "Adjusted for Amplification"), all of the odds ratios are reduced. Only the difference for sleep problems becomes statistically nonsignificant, but there are a number of conditions for which the effect is no longer statistically significant at the same critical value. These include bone and joint problems, foot problems, stomach problems, and the autoimmune disorders. The other differences persisted.

To see how much the tendency to recognize and report conditions is related to overall assessments of health, we conducted similar analyses in which self-assessed physical and mental health were the dependent variables, and we estimated gender differences after statistically controlling for amplification. For both of these variables, gender differences were not statistically significant after controlling for amplification. When we conducted similar analyses with intermediate activities of daily living as the dependent variable, adjusting for amplification, the gender difference remained significant ($p < .0001$).

There are several possible explanations for variations in amplification. One is that for a variety of biological, social, psychological, and cultural reasons, certain people learn to monitor and/or report bodily symptoms more closely than do others. An alternate explanation is that sensitivity to, and/or likelihood of reporting, symptoms is developed as a result of health experiences. To test these explanations, we first selected several health events that we thought were not likely to be influenced by symptom sensitivity or reporting tendencies. These were number of hospitalizations in the previous year, whether respondents reported being told by their physician that they had a heart problem and whether they had ever had a major heart procedure, heart attack, or cancer. We calculated correlations between each of these variables, with amplification separately for men and women. We then developed separate regression models for men and women in which the amplification score was the dependent variable and these health events were independent variables. Among women, none of the predictor variables was significantly correlated with amplification. The regression model for women with all these predictors explained less than 0.2 percent of the variance in amplification scores. In men, however, each of the events, except for having cancer, was significantly correlated with amplification. In a regression model, having had heart problems and the number of times the respondent had been hospitalized remained significant, although the model explained only about 1 percent of the variance in amplification scores among men.

Others have found that individual characteristics, such as neuroticism, are related to the reporting of physical symptoms (Ebert, Tucker, and Roth

2002). To better understand the constellation of individual characteristics that are related to amplification, we examined whether amplification also was related to neuroticism, tendency to seek advice, low perceived control, and/or depression. When we entered these variables into models predicting amplification, neuroticism, advice seeking, and perceived control were significant predictors of amplification for both men and women. Depression also was a significant predictor of amplification for women. For men, having had heart problems remained a significant predictor of amplification, but being hospitalized no longer was. In each of these models, neuroticism was the strongest predictor of amplification.

To assess the extent to which neuroticism explained variability in reporting, we re-estimated the models in which we had assessed the impact of amplification on gender differences, but now we included neuroticism. The results of these analyses suggest that the effects of amplification are related to neuroticism. For example, when we entered neuroticism into the models explaining sex differences in disability, in the three models for which amplification was a significant predictor of disability reports, neuroticism became significant and amplification was nonsignificant. A similar pattern was observed for days on which people cut back on normal activities or work because of dyspnea or angina. There were similar results for many of the conditions in table 1, but neuroticism was a significant predictor of only 17 of the 29 conditions.

Although these associations are modest, they suggest an interesting and potentially important finding regarding the determinants and consequences of different monitoring and reporting styles. That is, some of the observed differences in reported health in this and other similar surveys may be the result of gender differences in sensitivity to symptoms and/or tendency to report symptoms. These differences in reporting tendencies, in turn, may in part be responses to health or health care, although these associations appear to be relatively weak and significant only for men. A more striking pattern is that the general tendency to report symptoms appears to be related to several other personality characteristics. Specifically, those with higher neuroticism scores, greater tendency to seek advice, and low perceived control tend to have higher reports of certain types of health conditions. It also is possible, of course, that the relationship between amplification and the reporting of chronic health conditions is entirely the result of the fact that people amplify and/or have the other characteristics described (e.g., neuroticism, low perceived control, advice seeking) as a result or those conditions and that this is especially true for women.

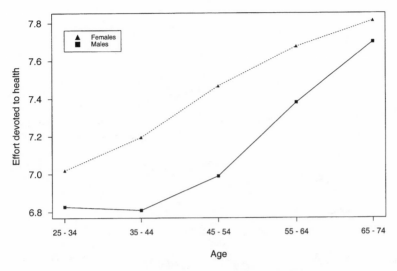

FIGURE 12. Personal effort devoted to health, scale of 0–10.

Interestingly, the adjusted measure of perceived health is not significantly different between men and women, even though there are still significant differences in several conditions and functioning, which is consistent with the findings from the British General Household Survey (Arber and Cooper 1999). It could be that such judgments are based more on conditions that have smaller differences and/or conditions that are influenced least by amplification. Because many of the conditions assessed in this study had a low prevalence and were often correlated, it was not possible to test those hypotheses.

Health Effort

There are many health behaviors and orientations that were assessed in MIDUS, but one of particular interest to us was the effort that people say they devote to different life domains. Figure 12 presents the reported effort devoted to health (on a 0–10 point scale). This variable, like many we have already presented, shows a steady increase with age and indicates that women report they devote more effort to health than do men, with the most pronounced differences in midlife.

To examine whether these trends represented actual behavioral differences or reporting tendencies, we examined the responses to questions that we thought were behavioral markers for effort devoted to health: use of vitamins as well as moderate and vigorous exercise. Data on use of

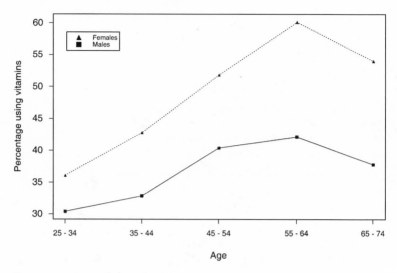

FIGURE 13. Use of vitamins.

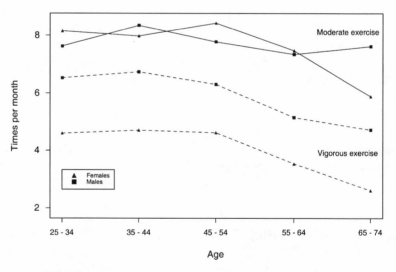

FIGURE 14. Moderate and vigorous physical exercise.

vitamins (fig. 13) are consistent with the data on effort devoted to health, except that both men and women show slight declines in the oldest age group, and the increase with age is less pronounced for men than for women. For exercise (fig. 14), reported activity generally declines with age, with vigorous exercise declining more than moderate exercise. The age differences for moderate exercise are comparable for men and women, but women tend to report engaging in vigorous exercise much less frequently than men. One possible explanation for such a large difference is that men are more likely to be engaged in work activities associated with vigorous activities. When these data are stratified by working and nonworking respondents (fig. 15), the level of vigorous exercise is comparable in nonworking men and women. However, the level of exercise is much higher in men than women among persons working outside the home.

When we estimated a regression model with effort devoted to health as the dependent variable, vitamin use and exercise were significantly related to effort devoted to health; controlling for these variables and an age–exercise interaction, there were still significant age and gender differences. Thus, individual differences in perceived effort are related to actual behaviors, such as vitamin use and exercise, and part of the increase in perceived effort over the life span may be the result of specific activities, such as taking vitamins. It may also be that although more effort is devoted to exercise among older respondents, actual rates of exercise decline. Gender differences in behaviors such as taking vitamins are consistent with the higher reported effort to maintaining health among women, but interestingly, at all ages women report less vigorous exercise. Thus, although women report more health conditions and say they devote more effort to maintaining health than men do, they may be doing less of

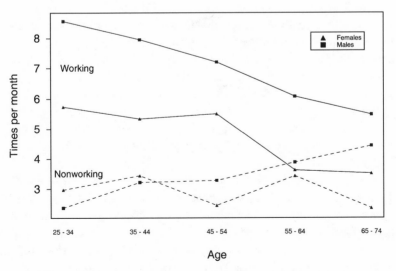

FIGURE 15. Vigorous exercise by gender and work status.

the activities (exercise) that have the most beneficial impact on their subsequent health. One possibility is that they report devoting greater effort to maintaining their health because they spend more time dealing with the conditions that are more prevalent among women. That is, all of the conditions with a higher reported prevalence in table 1 require attention and effort. When people are asked about effort devoted to health, they probably include time spent dealing with chronic conditions as well as time spent on preventive activities and exercise.

Summary and Conclusions

Much has been written about the prevalence and incidence of different conditions at different points in the life course. The MIDUS survey is unique, however, because in addition to collecting a rich array of health status indicators such as measures of health behavior and health attitudes, it also collected a wealth of psychological and social information. Thus, MIDUS data allow us to characterize age and sex differences in ways previously not possible.

Sex differences in ratings of global mental health were not significant when we controlled for amplification, suggesting that they may be due in part to sensitivity to symptoms or reporting tendencies. However, it also may simply be that the tendency to amplify is a result of mental health problems, an interpretation supported by the association between neuroticism and amplification. On a variety of more specific symptoms and the measures of functional status, women also tended to report more problems. These analyses showed that for a variety of conditions, controlling for amplification reduced the gender differences. After controlling for amplification, however, women were still significantly more likely to report having twelve of the chronic conditions asked about, and men were significantly more likely to report alcohol or drug problems. This result is consistent with other large population studies showing that women are more likely to report chronic conditions and distress than men but that men are more likely to engage in heavy drinking (McDonough and Walters 2001).

Although women report worse health on a variety of dimensions, they also report that they devote more effort to maintaining their health. These reports were consistent with analyses of more specific behaviors, such as use of vitamins. However, even when we controlled for vitamin use and exercise, there were still significant differences in reported effort. This residual effort could be because women devote more time to specific activities that were not asked about in the MIDUS survey. In addition, there are multiple interpretations of devoting effort to health. Although our intent was to assess active efforts, people might interpret their overall lifestyle when responding to such questions. Other studies have consistently found that men engage in more risky behavior and women engage in more preventive behavior as well as treatment seeking and self-care for illness (Courtenay, McCreary, and Merighi 2002; Doyal 2001; Waldron 1997).

Although these data provide important insights into possible mechanisms affecting sex differences in reports about health, they leave unanswered the question of how much of the difference is the result of biological differences and how much is the result of differences in the recognition and response to such conditions. For example, studies of the relationships among ischemic heart disease, reported chest pain, and subsequent mortality (Cohn et al. 1990; Harris and Weissfeld 1991; Nicholson et al. 1999) have been very helpful for elucidating the biological mechanisms related to reports of pain as well as the epidemiological importance of self-reports of angina. Similarly, other studies in which researchers were able to relate biological markers of disease severity to self-reports (Angel and Cleary 1984; Katz et al. 1994) have provided important information about the factors affecting the perception of, and response to, health conditions. If future studies were to include more psychological variables known to be related to the recognition and response to health conditions, such as stress and amplification, they would help illuminate some of the types of complex patterns in reported health states presented in this chapter.

One of the intriguing findings in studies of sex differences in health is that despite the higher prevalence of functional impairment (Arber and Cooper 1999) and chronic conditions, women have a substantial longevity advantage over men (Nikiforov and Mamaev 1998; Verbrugge 1985; Waldron 1983, 1993; Wylie 1984), but the reasons for this survival advantage are not fully understood. One of the most important biological differences is the greater tendency of men to develop cardiovascular disease earlier in life (Doyal 2001), but the higher cardiovascular disease mortality rates among men have not been fully explained (Nikiforov and Mamaev 1998). The relative cardiovascular risk of men and women has changed substantially over time as risk behaviors such as smoking have changed (Waldron 1993), and some have argued that the excess mortality is due in large part to factors associated with the development of industrialized societies (Nikiforov and Mamaev 1998).

One set of risks men may face more than women do are those associated with paid work (Doyal 2001), but efforts to identify environmental stressors that fully explain sex differences in mortality have not been successful (Nikiforov and Mamaev 1998; Wylie 1984). There also are potentially important social theories as to why there should be sex differences in both morbidity and mortality. For example, it has been observed that there are no societies in which women are treated as equals with men and that many women have heavy burdens of work and receive relatively little social support (Doyal 2001). However, investigations of the impact of work and multiple social roles have concluded that women's employment does not have a net negative impact on their health (Walters, McDonough, and Strohschein 2002). In fact, they may benefit from such roles through mechanisms such as increased social support (Repetti, Matthews, and Waldron 1989; Waldron and Jacobs 1989).

The data presented here illustrate the importance of taking reporting tendencies into account when analyzing self-reported data. But more importantly, they illustrate that possibly through a variety of biological, socialization, or psychological differences, women learn to monitor and respond to physical changes differently than men. They also are more likely to engage in a variety of activities that may be beneficial to health. Thus, rather than just being a reporting tendency, the tendencies revealed by the amplification scale used in this study may be indicative of learned dispositions and behavior that are beneficial for survival. More studies that combine biological and psychosocial measures would help understand these important and complex patterns.

References

Andrews, F., and S. Withey. 1976. *Social Indicators of well-being: Americans' perceptions of life quality.* New York: Plenum Press.

Angel, R., and P. Cleary. 1984. *The effects of social structure and culture on self-reports of health among Mexican Americans.* Social Science Quarterly 65: 814–28.

Arber, S., and H. Cooper. 1999. *Gender differences in health in later life: The new paradox?* Social Science and Medicine 48 (1): 61–76.

Ayanian, J. Z., E. Guadagnoli, and P. D. Cleary. 1995. Physical and psychosocial functioning of women and men after coronary artery bypass surgery. *Journal of the American Medical Association* 274 (22): 1767–70.

Barsky, A. J., J. Brener, R. R. Coeytaux, and P. D. Cleary. 1995. Accurate awareness of heartbeat in hypochondriacal and non-hypochondriacal patients. *Journal of Psychosomatic Research* 39 (4): 489–97.

Barsky, A. J., P. D. Cleary, J. Brener, and J. N. Ruskin. 1993. The perception of cardiac activity in medical outpatients. *Cardiology* 83: 304–15.

Barsky, A. J., P. D. Cleary, R. R. Coeytaux, and J. N. Ruskin. 1995. The clinical course of palpitations in medical outpatients. *Archives of Internal Medicine* 155 (16): 1782–88.

Barsky, A. J., P. D. Cleary, and G. L. Klerman. 1992. Determinants of perceived health status of medical outpatients. *Social Science and Medicine* 34 (10): 1147–54.

Barsky, A. J., P. D. Cleary, M. K. Sarnie, and G. L. Klerman. 1993. The course of transient hypochondriasis. *American Journal of Psychiatry* 150 (3): 484–88.

Barsky, A. J., P. D. Cleary, M. K. Sarnie, and J. N. Ruskin. 1994. Panic disorder, palpitations, and the awareness of cardiac activity. *Journal of Nervous and Mental Disorders* 182: 63–71.

Barsky, A. J., J. D. Goodson, R. S. Lane, and P. D. Cleary. 1988. The amplification of somatic symptoms. *Psychosomatic Medicine* 50: 510–19.

Barsky, A. J., and G. Wyshak. 1990. Hypochondriasis and somatosensory amplification. *British Journal of Psychiatry* 157: 404–9.

Barsky, A. J., G. Wyshak, and G. L. Klerman. 1990. The Somatosensory Amplification Scale and its relationship to hypochondriasis. *Journal of Psychiatric Research* 24: 323–34.

Berg, R. L., D. S. Hallauer, and S. N. Berk. 1976. Neglected aspects of the quality of life. *Health Services Research* 11 (4): 391–95.

Bombardier, C., and J. Raboud. 1991. A comparison of health-related quality-of-life measures for rheumatoid arthritis research. The Auranofin *Cooperating Group. Controlled Clinical Trials* 12 (4 suppl.): 243S–56S.

Brook, R. H., E. A. McGlynn, and P. D. Cleary. 1996. Quality of health care. Part 2: Measuring quality of care. *New England Journal of Medicine* 335 (13): 966–70.

Cleary, P. D. 1987. Gender differences in stress-related disorders. In *Gender and stress,* ed. R. C. Barnett and B. L. and G. K. Baruch, 39–72. New York: Free Press.

———. 1997. Subjective and objective measures of health: Which is better? *Journal of Health Services Research and Policy* 2 (1): 3–4.

Cleary, P. D., A. M. Epstein, G. Oster, G. S. Morrissey, W. B. Stason, S. Debussey, J. Plachetka, and M. Zimmerman. 1991. Health-related quality of life among patients undergoing percutaneous transluminal coronary angioplasty. *Medical Care* 29 (10): 939–50. Erratum published in 1992 *Medical Care* 30 (1): 76.

Cleary, P. D., F. J. Fowler, Jr., J. Weissman, M. P. Weissman, I. Wilson, G. R. Seage, C. Gatsonis, and A. Epstein. 1993. Health-related quality of life in persons with AIDS. *Medical Care* 31: 569–80.

Cohn, B. A., D. L. Wingard, R. D. Cohen, P. M. Cirillo, and G. A. Kaplan. 1990. Sex differences in time from self-reported heart trouble to heart disease death in the Alameda County Study. *American Journal of Epidemiology* 131 (3): 434–42.

Courtenay, W. H., D. R. McCreary, and J. R. Merighi. 2002. Gender and ethnic differences in health beliefs and behaviors. *Journal of Health Psychology* 7 (3): 219–31.

Doyal, L. 2001. Sex, gender, and health: The need for a new approach. *British Medical Journal* 323 (732): 1061–63.

Ebert, S. A., D. C. Tucker, and D. L. Roth. 2002. Psychological resistance factors as predictors of general health status and physical symptom reporting. *Psychology Health and Medicine* 7 (3): 363–75.

Flanagan, J. 1978. A research approach to improving our quality of life. *American Psychologist* 33: 138–47.

Fremont, A., and C. Bird. 2000. Social and psychological factors, physiological processes, and physical health. In *Handbook of Medical Sociology,* 5th ed., ed. A. Fremont, P. Conrad, and C. Bird. New York: Prentice Hall.

Greenfield, S., and E. C. Nelson. 1992. Recent developments and future issues in the use of health status assessment measures in clinical settings. *Medical Care* 30 (5 suppl.): MS23–41.

Guyatt, G., D. Feeny, and D. Patrick. 1991. Issues in quality-of-life measurement in clinical trials. *Controlled Clinical Trials* 12 (4 suppl.): 81S–90S.

Guyatt, G., D. Patrick, and D. Feeny. 1991. Postscript. *Control Clinical Trials* 12: 266S–69S.

Harris, R., and L. Weissfeld. 1991. Gender differences in the reliability of reporting symptoms of angina pectoris. *Journal of Clinical Epidemiology* 44 (10): 1071–78.

Idler, E., and S. Kasl. 1991. Health perceptions and survival: Do global evaluations of health status really predict mortality? *Journal of Gerontology* 46: S55–S65.

Kaplan, G., and T. Camacho. 1983. Perceived health and mortality: A nine-year follow-up of the human population laboratory cohort. *American Journal of Epidemiology* 117: 292–304.

Katz, J. N., E. A. Wright, E. Guadagnoli, M. H. Liang, E. W. Karlson, and P. D. Cleary. 1994. Differences between men and women undergoing major orthopedic surgery for degenerative arthritis. *Arthritis and Rheumatism* 37(5): 687–94.

Kessler, R. C., K. A. McGonagle, M. Swartz, D. G. Blazer, and C. B. Nelson. 1993. Sex and depression in the National Comorbidity Survey. Part 1: Lifetime prevalence, chronicity and recurrence. *Journal of Affective Disorders* 29 (2–3): 85–96.

Kessler, R. C., K. A. McGonagle, S. Zhao, C. B. Nelson, M. Hughes, S. Eshleman, H. U. Wittchen, and K. S. Kendler. 1994. Lifetime and 12-month prevalence of DSM-III-R psychiatric disorders in the United States. Results from the National Comorbidity Survey. *Archives of General Psychiatry* 51 (1): 8–19.

Laupacis, A., C. Wong, and D. Churchill. 1991. The use of generic and specific quality-of-life measures in hemodialysis patients treated with erythropoietin. The Canadian Erythropoietin Study Group. *Controlled Clinical Trials* 12 (4 suppl.): 168S–79S.

Ledoux, M. P., J. P. Lambert, B. A. M. D. M. Reeder, and J.-P. P. Despres. 1997. A comparative analysis of weight to height and waist to hip circumference indices as indicators of the presence of cardiovascular disease risk factors. *Canadian Medical Association Journal* 157 (1 suppl.): 32S–38S.

McDonough, P., and V. Walters. 2001. Gender and health: Reassessing patterns and explanations. *Social Science and Medicine* 52 (4): 547–59.

McDowell, I., and C. Newell. 1996. *Measuring health: A guide to rating scales and questionnaires.* New York: Oxford University Press.

Mechanic, D., P. D. Cleary, and J. R. Greenley. 1982. Distress syndromes, illness behavior, access to care and medical utilization in a defined population. *Medical Care* 20: 361–72.

Mossey, J., and E. Shapiro. 1982. Self-rated health: A predictor of mortality among the elderly. *American Journal of Public Health* 72: 800–808.

Nicholson, A., I. White, P. McFarlane, E. Brunner, and M. Marmot. 1999. Rose questionnaire angina in younger men and women: Gender differences in the relationship to cardiovascular risk factors and other reported symptoms. *Journal of Clinical Epidemiology* 52 (4): 337–46.

Nikiforov, S. V., and V. B. Mamaev. 1998. The development of sex differences in cardiovascular disease mortality: A historical perspective. *American Journal of Public Health* 88 (9): 1348–53.

Patrick, D. 1987. Patients' reports of health status as predictors of physiologic health in chronic disease. *Journal of Chronic Disease* 40: 37S–40S.

Patrick, D., and P. Erickson. 1993. *Health status and health policy. Quality of life in health care evaluation and resource allocation.* New York: Oxford University Press.

Pennebaker, J. 1982. *The psychology of physical symptoms.* New York: Springer-Verlag.

Repetti, R. L., K. A. Matthews, and I. Waldron. 1989. Employment and women's health: Effects of paid employment on women's mental and physical health. *American Psychologist* 44 (11): 1394–1401.

Rose, G. 1965. Chest pain questionnaire. *Milbank Quarterly* 43: 32–39.

Rose, G., H. Blackburn, R. Gillum, and R. Prineas. 1982. *Cardiovascular survey methods.* 2d ed. Geneva: World Health Organization.

Rose, G., P. McCartney, and D. Reid. 1977. Self-administration of a questionnaire on chest pain and intermittent claudication. *British Journal of Preventive and Social Medicine* 31: 42–48.

Tsevat, J., J. C. Weeks, E. Guadagnoli, A. N. Tosteson, C. M. Mangione, J. S. Pliskin, M. C. Weinstein, and P. D. Cleary. 1994. Using health-related quality-of-life information: Clinical encounters, clinical trials, and health policy. *Journal of General Internal Medicine* 9 (10): 576–82.

U.S. Department of Health and Human Services. 1998. *Health, United States.* PHS 98-1232. Hyattsville, Md.: Centers for Disease Control and Prevention.

Verbrugge, L. 1985. Gender and health: An update on hypotheses and evidence. *Journal of Health and Social Behavior* 26: 156–82.

Waldron, I. 1983. Sex differences in illness incidence, prognosis, and mortality: Issues and evidence. *Social Science and Medicine* 17: 1107–29.

———. 1993. Recent trends in sex mortality ratios for adults in developed countries. *Social Science and Medicine* 36 (4): 451–62.

———. 1997. Changing gender roles and gender differences in health behavior. In *Handbook of health behavior research,* ed. David S. Gochman, 303–28. New York: Plenum Press.

Waldron, I., and J. A. Jacobs. 1989. Effects of multiple roles on women's health: Evidence from a national longitudinal study. *Women and Health* 15 (1): 3–19.

Walters, V., P. McDonough, and L. Strohschein. 2002. The influence of work, household structure, and social, personal and material resources on gender differences in health: An analysis of the 1994 Canadian National Population Health Survey. *Social Science and Medicine* 54 (5): 677–92.

Wenger, N., L. Speroff, and B. Packard. 1993. Cardiovascular health and disease in women. *New England Journal of Medicine* 329 (4): 247–56.

Wilson, I. B., and P. D. Cleary. 1995. Linking clinical variables with health-related quality of life. A conceptual model of patient outcomes. *Journal of the American Medical Association* 273 (1): 59–65.

Wylie, C. M. 1984. Contrasts in the health of elderly men and women: An analysis of recent data for whites in the United States. *Journal of the American Geriatrics Society* 32 (9): 670–75.

CHAPTER THREE

Socioeconomic Position and Health across Midlife

Michael G. Marmot and Rebecca Fuhrer

Socioeconomic position is a powerful determinant of risk of death. There is ample evidence internationally for the relation between socioeconomic position and mortality (Adler and Ostrove 1999). There is much less evidence on its relation to measures of morbidity and of ability to function physically, psychologically, and socially. The MIDUS study of Americans at midlife provides the opportunity to examine the relation between socioeconomic position and measures of health and functioning. That MIDUS contains information from a range of domains pertinent to people's well-being allowed us to explore influences that may be responsible for the differences observed.

In this chapter we first summarize our initial analyses of the data from MIDUS that demonstrate the differences in health according to socioeconomic position. We then consider three additional questions that relate to health and to measures of functioning. First we ask whether the magnitude of the socioeconomic differences varies through the age range studied, 25–74. Second, we examine the predictive power of four different measures of socioeconomic position: education, household income, degree of poverty of the area of residence, and the Duncan socioeconomic index, which is based on educational attainment and income. If these measures are differently related to measures of health and functioning, the differences may convey information about potential causal pathways. Third, and related, we ask whether the different measures of socioeconomic position may relate differently to the potential mediating factors that we have identified.

BACKGROUND: THE IMPORTANCE OF THE SOCIAL GRADIENT IN HEALTH

Research results have led to three important insights that lay the basis for the findings reported in this chapter. First, inequalities in health are important but they are not limited to worse health among the socially excluded. Second, they do not arise solely as the result of differential provision and access to high-quality medical care. Third, the determinants of health, to a large extent, lie outside the medical sector. Research to understand these determinants and policies to influence them must therefore reach beyond the medical sector.

To take the first issue: social inequalities in health are now recognized to confront societies in important ways. They are on the agenda in the United States, the United Kingdom, the Netherlands, Sweden, Australia, and other countries, and the World Health Organization. In the United Kingdom, for example, the government set up an independent inquiry into inequalities in health, which reported in 1998 (Acheson 1998), eighteen years after the Black report (Townsend, Davidson, and Whitehead 1990). The statistical evidence reviewed by the independent inquiry and summarized in its report made clear that mortality and morbidity do indeed follow a social gradient. This was shown in the Whitehall studies. Among civil servants, position in the hierarchy was intimately related to risk of morbidity and mortality: higher status, lower risk (Marmot et al. 1984, 1991). The evidence does not show that there are simply health differentials between "them," the poor, and "us," the nonpoor. The poor are worse off, but among the nonpoor there is a social gradient in health and disease. Yet policy discussions commonly relate to how to improve the health status of "them" to make it more like the health status of "us." Many of the policy options put before the Independent Inquiry on Inequalities in Health dealt with poverty and strategies either to relieve poverty or to interrupt its link with ill health.

Discussions of policy options to reduce the social gradient in ill health are limited by the relative lack of understanding of the reasons why position in the hierarchy is intimately related to health risk. The MIDUS study offers further opportunity to contribute to understanding of determinants of the gradient in ill health.

The second issue relates to medical care. This is perhaps a more central discussion in the United States than it is in Europe because the differentials in access to medical care appear to be much more marked in the United States. The view summarized by the Independent Inquiry on Inequalities in Health (Acheson 1998) was that improvement of quality and access to medical care had an important part to play but that the causes of inequalities in health were primarily socioeconomic.

Both the first and second issues lead to the third: the causes of the social gradient in health lie outside the medical sector. If relative position in the hierarchy is important in addition to the effects of absolute deprivation, one must look to the social sciences for understanding of what that means and what the social and psychological processes might be that link relative social position to health.

The MIDUS study was conducted by the MacArthur Foundation Research Network on Successful Midlife Development. A subgroup of that network came together around the issue of psychosocial factors and the social gradient in health (Marmot et al. 1997). This interdisciplinary group was responsible for collecting data in MIDUS across a greater range of aspects of social and psychological characteristics than is common in more medically oriented studies. The disciplinary breadth of the network, applied to the scientific problem of inequalities in health, contributed a rich array of intervening mechanisms. The scope of the sociodemographic and psychosocial variables across multiple domains in the MIDUS study means that MIDUS provides a good vehicle for examining potential contributors to the social gradient in health. Given that MIDUS was a cross-sectional study, it cannot provide the kind of answers to etiological questions that a cohort study could provide, but it can help point in the right direction.

A particular advantage of MIDUS is that it is based on a representative sample of the U.S. population. Much of the study of mechanisms underlying inequalities in health has, of necessity, been based on more restricted populations. These restricted populations will continue to be crucial because they are amenable to intensive data collection. A study of a wider national sample provides important complementary information.

Multiple Causes of the Social Gradient in Health: The MIDUS Study

In a previous report from MIDUS, we analyzed the relation of socioeconomic status to health, using education as a measure of socioeconomic status (Marmot et al. 1998). We analyzed three different measures of health, broadly defined. In the report, we used self-reported health because it has been employed in a number of different populations and is a predictor of mortality, in addition to being an overall summary measure of health. Respondents rated their present state of physical health on a five-point scale (1, poor; 5, excellent). The scale was dichotomized to poor/fair versus moderate/good/excellent health. Second, we examined waist–hip ratio. This measurement was chosen as a more objective marker of risk of physical disease. Respondents were provided with a tape measure, a diagram, and instructions on where and how to measure the waist and hip circumference. The waist–hip ratio is calculated by dividing the waist circumference by the hip circumference; higher values indicate greater central adiposity. Central adiposity is related to development of diabetes and cardiovascular disease. Respondents in the top quintile were considered to be in the least favorable category, and this was taken as the health outcome. Third, we examined psychological well-being. This is not a measure of health in the usual sense but was included because it approaches the question of health as a positive attribute. Psychological well-being was measured with a composite score for six dimensions of positive psychological functioning (autonomy, environmental mastery, personal growth, positive relations with others, purpose in life, and self-acceptance). All three measures showed clear social gradients in health. Men and women who did not complete high school had worse health than did other groups. High school graduates were, in general, in worse health than were those with some college education, and persons who had completed college had the best health status.

We considered a number of factors that could potentially account for the link between educational status and health status: parents' education; neighborhood characteristics; smoking behavior; social relations, including marital status, support from family and friends, and a measure of strain among family and friends; decision authority and skill use in the workplace; perception of inequality; and control/efficacy, including measures of mastery and constraints. We asked if these could be mediators of the relation between socioeconomic status and health, in the sense of providing an account of why people of lower socioeconomic status have worse health. In most cases this is easily thought of as being in the causal chain; for example, people with lower education are more likely to smoke and thereby have worse health. Parental education does not lie on the causal chain in the same sense. Had it been the case that the relation between education and health could be accounted for by parents' education, the causal explanation might then have suggested that parental education might have been a "cause" of both low education and poor health.

Most of the variables listed were related to the three health outcome measures, but none taken alone provided the major explanation for the social gradient in health. Taken together, however, these variables had a substantial impact (table 1). Their importance in mediating the relation between socioeconomic status and health was assessed by computing the odds ratios of, for example, poor health in each educational group compared with the best-off group and then assessing the impact on the odds ratio of including these variables in a model. For self-reported health, for

TABLE 1 Relation of Educational Attainment and Three Health Outcome

	Women (*n* = 1544)			
	Model Adjusted for Age		Model Fully Adjusted[a]	
Variable	OR[b]	95% CI	OR[b]	95% CI
Poor/fair physical health				
Bachelor's or more	1.0		1.0	
Some college	2.63	(1.6–4.2)	1.84	(1.1–3.1)
High school	3.06	(1.9–4.9)	1.73	(1.0–3.0)
<High school	8.00	(4.7–13.5)	3.21	(1.7–6.0)
Waist–hip ratio (upper quintile)				
Bachelor's or more	1.0		1.0	
Some college	1.92	(1.3–2.9)	1.82	(1.2–2.8)
High school	1.63	(1.1–2.5)	1.40	(0.9–2.3)
<High school	3.03	(1.8–5.0)	2.33	(1.3–4.2)
Psychological well-being				
Bachelor's or more	1.0		1.0	
Some college	2.00	(1.3–3.1)	1.58	(0.9–2.7)
High school	3.41	(2.5–5.1)	2.79	(1.6–4.8)
<High school	5.91	(3.6–9.7)	3.07	(1.6–6.1)

Note: OR, odds ratio; CI, confidence intervals.

[a]Mediators: early childhood environment as measured by mother's and father's education; psychosocial work environment, measured by job characteristics of decision authority and use of skills; health behavior, measured by smoking; and degree of mastery and constraints in various aspects of life.

[b]N = 3032. Results are unweighted and expressed as odds ratio, comparing each group with the most highly educated group.

example, men with less than a high school education had an odds ratio of 6.0 of reporting themselves to be in poor health. When the variables mentioned earlier were added to the model, the odds ratio was reduced to 3.3. For women the odds ratio was reduced from 8.0 to 3.2.

We were cautious in drawing too firm conclusions from a cross-sectional study, but our interpretation of these results was that a set of early and current life circumstances appears cumulatively to make a major contribution to explaining why people of lower socioeconomic status have worse health and lower psychological well-being.

SOCIOECONOMIC DIFFERENCES IN HEALTH IN MIDLIFE: EFFECTS OF AGE AND MEASURES OF SOCIOECONOMIC STATUS
Effects of Age

It has been suggested (West 1988) that during young adulthood, social inequalities in health are of lesser magnitude than they are in older

Measures in the MIDUS National Sample

Men ($n = 1461$)			
Model Adjusted for Age		Model Fully Adjusted[a]	
OR[b]	95% CI	OR[b]	95% CI
1.0		1.0	
2.07	(1.2–3.2)	1.67	(1.0–2.7)
2.47	(1.6–3.8)	1.71	(1.0–2.8)
5.96	(3.6–9.8)	3.25	(1.8–5.9)
1.0		1.0	
1.28	(0.9–1.9)	1.15	(0.8–1.7)
1.96	(1.4–2.8)	1.70	(1.1–2.6)
2.16	(1.3–3.6)	1.47	(0.8–2.6)
1.0		1.0	
1.83	(1.3–2.7)	1.56	(1.0–2.5)
2.44	(1.7–3.5)	2.22	(1.3–3.7)
4.83	(3.0–7.6)	3.81	(2.0–7.3)

age groups. At old age, social inequalities may again be narrower in relative terms. In the first Whitehall study of British civil servants, relative differences among employment grades in mortality were less after than before retirement (Marmot and Shipley 1996). The absolute differences in mortality were greater, however, because mortality rates are higher at older ages.

There are at least three ways to view these findings. First, the lack of health inequalities at a young age may be, in part, that in such healthy groups there is little serious ill health, and therefore, little health inequalities. Second, if accumulation of disadvantage continued throughout life, one might expect health inequalities to grow wider with age. Third, if age were a leveler and the ravages of time caught up with all regardless of socioeconomic position, health inequalities might be expected to narrow in later life.

It is therefore of interest to compare the magnitude of socioeconomic differences in a number of measures of morbidity at different ages during the age period 25–74 years covered by the MIDUS sample. As an alternative, in what amounts to the same analyses in these cross-sectional data, we can examine the age trajectory of measures of morbidity during the midlife period among different socioeconomic groups.

TABLE 2 Mean Scores or Proportions of Health

Age (years)	Women			
	25–39	40–59	60–74	Interaction
Waist–hip ratio				
≥Bachelor's	0.78	0.79	0.82	
Some college	0.82	0.82	0.86	
High school	0.83	0.82	0.86	
<High school	0.84	0.86	0.88	
Linear trend in education	0.006	0.0001	0.06	>0.25
SF-36				
≥Bachelor's	91.1	86.1	74.0	
Some college	87.0	80.2	69.9	
High school	83.2	76.0	67.7	
<High school	68.0	67.3	56.2	
Linear trend in education	0.0001	0.0001	0.0002	>0.25
Poor/fair physical health				
≥Bachelor's	5.0	7.2	10.0	
Some college	16.9	15.1	15.5	
High school	13.5	17.7	24.8	
<High school	20.0	42.6	47.3	
Linear trend in education	0.02	0.001	0.001	0.22
Depression				
≥Bachelor's	15.7	17.0	10.0	
Some college	22.9	18.1	5.2	
High school	25.0	13.2	10.5	
<High school	46.7	18.5	16.2	
Linear trend in education	0.001	n.s.	0.06	0.02

Note: Interaction = *p*-value for test of differences in slope between age groups.

These are shown, using education as the measure of socioeconomic status, in table 2. We have included two further dependent variables to those outlined earlier—the physical health functioning component of the SF-36 (a health status measure) and depression. The physical functioning component of the SF-36 consisted of nine items asking respondents about vigorous and moderate activities as well as items on ability to walk, bathe, and dress oneself. The scores ranged from 0, indicating severe limitation in performing all physical activities, to 100, indicating no limitation. Depression was defined as a diagnosis during the preceding twelve months of a major depressive episode, based on the American Psychiatric Association's *Diagnostic and Statistical Manual of Mental Disorders,* revised third edition (DSM-111-R). The respondents were assessed for depression during the telephone interview by use of the World Health

Outcomes by Education and Age Group

	Men		
25–39	40–59	60–74	Interaction
0.93	0.95	0.95	
0.94	0.94	0.99	
0.94	0.99	0.97	
0.95	0.98	0.97	
0.38	0.004	0.007	0.04
93.8	89.5	82.3	
89.6	85.2	75.3	
90.5	80.5	76.6	
86.2	73.7	67.7	
0.02	0.0001	0.003	0.08
6.2	5.3	13.8	
8.2	14.5	25.0	
7.9	18.8	23.5	
31.3	36.8	37.0	
0.003	0.001	0.004	0.15
12.4	9.7	3.2	
13.5	14.5	7.8	
11.9	8.5	5.9	
18.8	15.8	6.5	
n.s.	n.s.	n.s.	>0.25

Organization's composite international diagnostic interview–short form (WHO CIDI-SF), and they were classified as yes/no.

Table 2 shows no strong support for a difference in the steepness of the social gradient by age among men or women. There is, at most, some suggestion that the social gradient in the physical health dimension of the SF-36 is wider for those in the 40–59 age span than it is for those in the 23–39 span. Looked at the other way, there is, perhaps, greater deterioration with age in the SF-36 physical health score among men with least education compared to those with most. Among women, depression decreases with age, and the social gradient diminishes. The interaction between education and age is significant.

Measures of Socioeconomic Status

The next question concerns the degree to which different socioeconomic indicators relate differently to the health outcomes. In particular, are there gender differences in the size of association? In the past the question of whether one socioeconomic measure might predict ill health better than another was seen largely as a pragmatic empirical question. To epidemiologists, more remarkable than differences among different measures of social position was that they all predicted mortality. Epidemiologists recognized that different socioeconomic measures had particular properties that made them useful. For example, work-based measures of social class are not useful for looking at persons not in the formal work force, such as housewives and older people (Goldblatt 1990). A household measure, or education, might be expected to be more related to social position for such people than occupation.

This is the perspective we take in this chapter. We have used four measure of socioeconomic position. They are, of course, correlated, but they are derived differently and serve different purposes. Two of the measures relate to the individual: educational attainment categorized into four categories from highest to lowest, and the Duncan socioeconomic index, which is based on educational attainment and income to predict occupational prestige. This index is divided into quartiles from lowest to highest (Duncan 1961; Hauser and Watten 1997). The third measure relates to the individual's household circumstances, household income, again divided into quartiles; the fourth relates not to an individual's own characteristics but to where that person lives. This measure classifies households on a poverty index according to their location by use of census information and is a combination of the proportion of households in the zip code that are below the poverty line and the proportion of unemployed persons residing in the area. This area-based measure relates to the debate in the literature about whether there are characteristics of places that predict health of residents over and above the characteristics of individuals who reside there (McIntyre and Ellaway 2000).

Lately, Bartley has pointed out that different measures of socioeconomic position have different theoretical bases and may therefore convey different information (Bartley and Marmot 2000). A measure based on work, if developed appropriately, might reflect power relations in the work place. One based on general social standing might relate more closely to lifestyle. In our analyses (see tables 7–10), we seek evidence of different pathways linking a measure of socioeconomic position to ill health.

Tables 3 and 4 show odds ratios of the four adverse health outcomes for the four socioeconomic indices. Because there were no large differences by age in the size of the association with socioeconomic status for any of the socioeconomic indices, subsequent analyses are shown for all ages adjusted for age.

In general, all four measures were associated with the four health outcomes (tables 3 and 4). For women, education appears to have a stronger relation with self-reported health and the physical component of the SF-36; the poverty index of the area and the Duncan socioeconomic index were not related to depression. In men there were no clear differences in odds ratios of having an adverse health outcome among the four socioeconomic measures.

It is useful when comparing different levels of an exposure to express the magnitude of effects relative to a baseline level. The odds ratio is one such measure, and usually the most favorable level of the exposure is taken as the baseline group. This group therefore has an odds ratio equal to 1.0, and more adverse levels of the exposure with respect to the outcome have odds ratios greater than 1.0. Thus, women who did not complete high school have 8.5 times the odds of being in poor health compared with women who completed a college education. These categories relate to readily comprehensible features of social reality. When it comes to comparing the predictive power of different measures, however, the problem arises that the distribution of the population among categories differs for the different socioeconomic measures. For example, 10.4 percent of women are in the lowest educational category, whereas approximately 30 percent of women are in the lowest household-income category and 29 percent in the highest area-of-poverty category. Therefore, in comparing predictive power of different socioeconomic measures, we are not comparing similar proportions of the population, and we might expect more extreme groups to show larger effects.

This problem was addressed in relation to time trends in social inequalities (Pamuk 1985) and in relation to international comparisons (Kunst 1997), where the same issue arises of wishing to compare similar proportions of populations. The approach taken is to use the relative index of inequality (RII) (Pamuk 1985; Mackenbach and Kunst 1997). To make fair comparisons, we score each socioeconomic measure from 0 to 1. Individual scores are assigned according to the proportion of persons who fall into a particular category. To illustrate, we place all individuals in one of four educational groups, depending on each person's educational level, ranging from less than high school to a bachelor's degree or more. For purposes of illustration, we assume

TABLE 3 Odds Ratio of Women's Adverse Health Outcomes

Variable	Waist–Hip Ratio (worst quintile)		SF-36 (worst quintile)	
	OR	95% CI	OR	95% CI
Education				
Bachelor's or more	1.0		1.0	
Some college	1.90	(1.3–2.8)	1.78	(1.2–2.6)
High school	1.61	(1.1–2.4)	2.30	(1.6–3.3)
<High school	3.21	(2.0–5.2)	5.85	(3.7–9.2)
Education RII	2.62	(1.6–4.4)	5.98	(3.7–9.7)
Household income				
Highest quartile	1.0		1.0	
Second quartile	1.86	(1.1–3.0)	1.11	(0.7–1.7)
Third quartile	1.73	(1.1–2.8)	1.37	(0.9–2.0)
Lowest quartile	3.05	(1.9–4.8)	2.74	(1.9–4.0)
Income RII	3.57	(2.1–6.1)	4.27	(2.7–6.8)
Poverty index				
Low poverty	1.0		1.0	
Intermediate	1.61	(1.1–2.3)	1.51	(1.1–21)
High poverty	1.94	(1.3–2.9)	2.14	(1.5–3.0)
Poverty RII	2.45	(1.5–4.2)	2.89	(1.8–4.6)
Duncan socioeconomic index				
Highest quartile	1.0		1.0	
Second quartile	1.18	(0.8–1.8)	1.80	(1.2–2.7)
Third quartile	0.80	(0.5–1.2)	1.21	(0.8–1.8)
Lowest quartile	1.85	(1.3–2.7)	2.41	(1.7–3.5)
Duncan RII	2.31	(1.4–3.8)	2.76	(1.8–4.3)
All four indices[a]				
Education RII	1.45	(0.8–2.8)	4.19	(2.3–7.5)
Income RII	2.55	(1.5–4.5)	2.75	(1.7–4.5)
Poverty RII	1.75	(1.0–3.0)	1.74	(1.1–2.8)
Duncan RII	1.39	(0.8–2.5)	0.97	(0.6–1.6)

Note: OR, odds ratio; CI, confidence interval.
[a]Adjusted for each other.

that 25 percent are in each group. The cut points along the 0–1 scale would then be 0.25, 0.5, and 0.75. Everyone in the lowest group would be assigned the midpoint of that group, that is, 0.125. Everyone with a high school education would be assigned the score corresponding to the midpoint of the next group, that is, 0.375; those with some college would be given the score 0.625; and those with a bachelor's degree, 0.875. Hence, the cut points are assigned according to the proportions in each category, and the scores are given by the midpoints of each category. These assignments are repeated within age strata to remove age by Category of Socioeconomic Measure (adjusted for age only)

Poor/Fair Health		Depression Diagnosis	
OR	95% CI	OR	95% CI
1.0		1.0	
2.60	(1.6–4.2)	1.16	(0.8–1.7)
3.01	(1.9–4.8)	1.13	(0.8–1.6)
8.48	(5.0–14.3)	2.12	(1.3–3.4)
8.17	(4.7–14.2)	1.75	(1.15–2.9)
1.0		1.0	
1.31	(0.8–2.1)	0.91	(0.6–1.4)
1.48	(0.9–2.3)	1.08	(0.7–1.7)
2.42	(1.6–3.7)	1.61	(1.1–2.4)
3.25	(1.9–5.5)	2.16	(1.3–3.6)
1.0		1.0	
1.60	(1.1–2.3)	1.24	(0.9–1.7)
2.29	(1.6–3.4)	1.03	(0.7–1.5)
3.16	(1.9–5.3)	1.04	(0.6–1.7)
1.0		1.0	
2.06	(1.3–3.4)	0.97	(0.6–1.5)
1.81	(1.1–2.9)	1.26	(0.9–1.8)
3.35	(2.7–5.2)	1.07	(0.7–1.6)
4.38	(2.7–7.3)	1.18	(0.7–1.9)
4.71	(2.4–9.1)	1.92	(1.0–3.6)
1.75	(1.00–3.1)	2.18	(1.2–3.8)
1.87	(1.1–3.2)	0.82	(0.5–1.4)
1.64	(0.9–3.0)	0.70	(0.4–1.2)

effects. The logistic regression model provides odds ratios for the notional top (1) and bottom (0) of the socioeconomic hierarchy. The effect is to measure the degree of inequality after taking account of the distribution of the socioeconomic variable. The odds ratio computed by using the RII is bigger than the odds ratios observed for the actual categories, provided that these odds ratios are increasing smoothly. This is because the RII represents notional individuals at the extremes, rather than those in real groups such as those with a bachelor's degree or those with less than a high school education. This "inflated" estimate of

TABLE 4 Odds Ratio of Men's Adverse Health Outcomes by

Variable	Waist–Hip Ratio (worst quintile)		SF-36 (worst quintile)	
	OR	95% CI	OR	95% CI
Education				
Bachelor's or more	1.0		1.0	
Some college	1.27	(0.9–1.9)	1.81	(1.2–2.8)
High school	1.98	(1.4–2.8)	2.11	(1.4–3.2)
<High school	2.10	(1.3–3.4)	3.86	(2.4–6.3)
Education RII	2.86	(1.7–4.7)	4.17	(2.4–7.1)
Household income				
Highest quartile	1.0		1.0	
Second quartile	1.38	(0.9–2.0)	1.63	(1.0–2.5)
Third quartile	1.63	(1.1–2.4)	2.04	(1.3–3.2)
Lowest quartile	1.51	(1.0–2.2)	3.87	(2.5–5.9)
Income RII	1.79	(1.1–2.9)	5.62	(3.3–9.6)
Poverty index				
Low poverty	1.0		1.0	
Intermediate	1.07	(0.8–1.5)	1.28	(0.9–1.9)
High poverty	1.29	(0.9–1.9)	2.32	(1.5–3.5)
Poverty RII	1.43	(0.8–2.4)	3.47	(1.9–6.2)
Duncan socioeconomic index				
Highest quartile	1.0		1.0	
Second quartile	0.89	(0.6–1.3)	1.10	(0.7–1.7)
Third quartile	1.58	(1.1–2.3)	1.55	(1.0–2.4)
Lowest quartile	1.31	(0.9–2.0)	2.03	(1.3–3.1)
Duncan RII	1.84	(1.1–3.0)	3.05	(1.8–5.3)
All four indices[a]				
Education RII	2.69	(1.5–5.0)	2.55	(1.3–4.9)
Income RII	1.31	(0.8–2.3)	3.73	(2.1–6.7)
Poverty RII	1.12	(0.6–2.0)	2.24	(1.2–4.1)
Duncan RII	0.92	(0.5–1.7)	0.94	(0.5–1.9)

Note: OR, odds ratio; CI, confidence level.
[a]Adjusted for each other.

inequalities in health should not bias the comparison among socioeconomic indicators.

Using the RII to compare predictive power of the different socioeconomic measures confirms the findings with the odds ratios: among women, education appears to have greater predictive power for self-reported health and SF-36; poverty of the area and the Duncan socioeconomic index are less predictive of depression. Among men, the RII confirms the lack of predictive power of education on depression and the ability of the other indices to predict in "bivariate" analyses, that is, adjusting only for age.

Category of Socioeconomic Measure (adjusted for age only)

Poor/Fair Health		Depression Diagnosis	
OR	95% CI	OR	95% CI
1.0		1.0	
2.07	(1.3–3.2)	1.40	(0.9–2.1)
2.49	(1.6–3.8)	0.97	(0.6–1.5)
6.11	(3.7–10.0)	1.69	(0.9–3.0)
6.54	(3.8–11.3)	1.29	(0.7–2.4)
1.0		1.0	
1.64	(1.0–2.6)	0.72	(0.4–1.2)
2.65	(1.7–2.1)	1.43	(0.9–2.3)
4.31	(2.8–6.6)	2.29	(1.5–3.6)
6.97	(4.0–12.0)	3.58	(1.9–6.5)
1.0		1.0	
1.23	(0.8–1.8)	1.13	(0.7–1.7)
2.06	(1.4–3.1)	1.38	(0.9–2.2)
2.90	(1.6–5.1)	1.58	(0.8–3.0)
1.0		1.0	
0.95	(0.6–1.5)	0.81	(0.5–1.3)
2.18	(1.4–3.4)	0.98	(0.6–1.6)
3.63	(2.3–5.6)	1.39	(0.9–2.2)
6.66	(3.79–11.8)	1.79	(1.0–3.3)
2.74	(1.4–5.3)	0.74	(0.3–1.5)
3.77	(2.1–6.8)	3.43	(1.8–6.6)
1.52	(0.8–2.8)	1.16	(0.6–2.3)
2.16	(1.1–4.3)	1.35	(0.6–2.8)

Poverty or Inequality

One of the important debates in the field of inequalities in health is the degree to which these inequalities can be explained by material differences between socioeconomic groups. Thus, if those with the lowest incomes have the worst health, this could be attributed to their disadvantaged material circumstances, which could relate to inadequate nutrition and worse housing, with damp, inadequate heating and crowding. These data show that those with lowest household incomes have highest risk of ill health, but they also show a gradient. In general, those in the second highest income quartile have worse health outcomes than do those in the highest.

TABLE 5 Relative Index of Inequality for Measures of

	Women			
	Age Only		Adjusted for Age, Race, and Mediators[a]	
	RII	95% CI	RII	95% CI
Education	2.62	(1.56–4.4)	1.85	(1.0–3.5)
Household income	3.57	(2.1–6.0)	2.24	(1.4–4.3)
Poverty index	2.45	(1.4–4.2)	1.63	(0.9–2.9)
Duncan socioeconomic index	2.31	(1.4–3.8)	1.51	(0.9–2.6)

Note: CI, confidence intervals.

[a]Mediators: early childhood environment as measured by mother's and father's education; psychosocial work environment, measured by job characteristics of decision authority and use of skills; health behavior, measured by smoking; and degree of mastery and constraints in various aspects of life.

Interpreting Analyses of Multiple Socioeconomic Indicators

At the bottom of tables 3 and 4, the RIIs have been entered in a model together. One should be wary of overinterpretation of these multivariate analyses. These four socioeconomic measures are all correlated. Hence, when all four are put into a model together, what happens to the size of the measure of effect may have as much to do with precision of the socioeconomic measurement as with the substantive importance of the concept that the measure is addressing. That, however, is a general problem, and one might have expected that it would apply more or less equally to the four health outcomes.

In women, the impression that education is most strongly related to self-reported health and SF-36 is confirmed when all four socioeconomic measures are in the model. In men, education is related strongly to these two outcomes, although not more strongly than is household income. With the other indices in the model, the Duncan socioeconomic index has no extra predictive power in women and retains it in men only for those with poor self-reported health.

Exploring the Links between Socioeconomic Status and Ill Health

In our previous analyses of the relation between education and health outcomes, we showed that no one factor accounted for the observed associations but that a combination of measures appeared to make a contribution (Marmot et al. 1998). In the present analyses, we wished to investigate the possibility that different measures of social position might be related to health outcomes through different pathways.

Socioeconomic Status, for Waist–Hip Ratio in Men and Women

	Men			
		Adjusted for		
Age Only			Age, Race, and Mediators[a]	
RII	95% CI		RII	95% CI
2.86	(1.7–4.7)		2.12	(1.2–3.8)
1.79	(1.1–2.9)		1.27	(0.7–2.2)
1.43	(0.8–2.4)		1.30	(0.7–2.2)
1.84	(1.1–3.1)		1.14	(0.6–2.0)

Statistical models of the relation between social position and health were therefore constructed that, in addition to age and race, included the following variables: mother's education, father's education, job characteristics of decision authority and use of skills, smoking, and degree of mastery and constraints in various aspects of life. Variables were included in a model if they changed the association between socioeconomic indicator and ill health by 5 percent or more. The results of these analyses are shown for the four health outcomes in tables 5–8. It is worth emphasizing that the same set of potential explanatory variables was included for each measure of social position. The aim was to assess whether different variables from among the whole group would be linked to different socioeconomic measures and hence suggest a different pathway of action.

Parents' education was included as a marker of social circumstances in which the individual was raised. Father's or mother's education enters into most of the models, suggesting that social background may, to some extent, be a determinant of health in adulthood and that it may account for some of the relation between markers of adult socioeconomic position and ill health. The fact that the relation of adult position to ill health remains, for the most part, significant after adjustment for parents' education suggests that factors from early life may not be the main determinants of the social gradient in health seen in adulthood. We had shown previously that in relation to self-reported health in MIDUS participants, mother's education was more strongly related to ill health in women, father's education to ill health in men (Marmot et al. 1998). No clear distinction is seen in these analyses, although for men, father's education enters into models as a mediator of the gradient in health more often than does mother's education.

Psychosocial factors appear also to be involved in the mediation of the relation between social position and ill health. Two classes of factors

TABLE 6 Relative Index of Inequality for Measures of

	Women			
	Age Only		Adjusted for Age, Race, and Mediators[a]	
	RII	95% CI	RII	95% CI
Education	5.98	(3.7–9.7)	3.42	(1.9–6.1)
Household income	4.27	(2.7–6.8)	2.65	(1.6–4.4)
Poverty index	2.89	(1.8–4.6)	1.75	(1.0–2.9)
Duncan socioeconomic index	2.76	(1.8–4.3)	1.38	(0.8–2.3)

Note : CI, confidence intervals.
[a]Mediators: early childhood environment as measured by mother's and father's education; psychosocial work environment, measured by job characteristics of decision authority and use of skills; health behavior, measured by smoking; and degree of mastery and constraints in various aspects of life.

TABLE 7 Relative Index of Inequality for Measures of

	Women			
	Age Only		Adjusted for Age, Race, and Mediators[a]	
	RII	95% CI	RII	95% CI
Education	8.17	(4.7–14.2)	3.18	(1.6–6.2)
Household income	3.25	(1.9–5.5)	1.62	(0.9–2.9)
Poverty index	3.16	(1.8–5.3)	1.84	(1.0–3.3)
Duncan socioeconomic index	4.38	(2.6–7.3)	1.79	(1.0–3.2)

Note: CI, confidence intervals.
[a]Mediators: early childhood environment as measured by mother's and father's education; psychosocial work environment, measured by job characteristics of decision authority and use of skills; health behavior, measured by smoking; and degree of mastery and constraints in various aspects of life.

were considered here—related to work and to other aspects of life. Both of these relate to the degree to which individuals have the opportunity to control their environment and the degree to which they feel they have mastery over it. The issue of feeling in control is explored in greater detail in chapter 11 of this volume, by Lachman and Firth. It is a matter of concern that the relation between psychosocial factors and self-reported measures of ill health could represent biased reporting: there could be a plaintive set toward negative reporting. The fact that these psychosocial factors were related also to waist–hip ratio is less easy to explain as biased reporting and makes it more likely that the observed relationships are not artifactual.

Socioeconomic Status, for SF-36 in Men and Women

	Men			
			Adjusted for	
	Age Only		Age, Race, and Mediators[a]	
RII	95% CI		RII	95% CI
4.17	(2.4–7.1)		2.27	(1.2–4.3)
5.62	(3.3–9.6)		2.77	(1.5–5.0)
3.47	(1.9–6.2)		2.26	(1.2–4.2)
3.05	(1.7–5.3)		1.44	(0.7–2.7)

Socioeconomic Status, for Fair/Poor Health in Men and Women

	Men			
			Adjusted for	
	Age Only		Age, Race, and Mediators[a]	
RII	95% CI		RII	95% CI
6.54	(3.8–11.3)		3.76	(2.0–7.2)
6.97	(4.0–12.0)		3.69	(2.0–6.7)
2.90	(1.6–5.1)		2.27	(1.2–4.2)
6.66	(3.8–11.7)		3.54	(1.9–6.7)

Not surprisingly, smoking appears to play a role in explaining the social gradient. Smoking may be present in these models both because of its own important role and because it is correlated with other health behaviors.

These analyses, shown in tables 5–8, indicate that the factors considered do appear to play some role in linking measures of social circumstances or social position to ill health. For each of these analyses we explored whether different mediators played a role in accounting for the relation between socioeconomic measure and health. No clearly different picture emerged. The mediators were more or less the same for each socioeconomic measure. The analyses shown use the same set of mediators for each table.

Interaction with Psychological Well-Being

We had previously treated psychological well-being as an "outcome," albeit one representing positive health rather than ill health. It too showed

TABLE 8 Relative Index of Inequality for Measures of

	Women			
	Age Only		Adjusted for Age, Race, and Mediators[a]	
	RII	95% CI	RII	95% CI
Education	1.75	(1.0–2.9)	1.03	(0.5–1.9)
Household income	2.16	(1.3–3.6)	1.59	(0.9–2.8)
Poverty index	1.04	(0.6–1.7)	0.93	(0.5–1.6)
Duncan socioeconomic index	1.18	(0.7–1.9)	0.72	(0.4–1.2)

Note: CI, confidence intervals.

[a]Mediators: early childhood environment as measured by mother's and father's education; psychosocial work environment, measured by job characteristics of decision authority and use of skills; health behavior, measured by smoking; and degree of mastery and constraints in various aspects of life.

TABLE 9 Relationship between Waist–Hip Ratio and SF-36, and

	Women			
	Age Only		Adjusted for Age, Race, and Mediators[a]	
	RII	95% CI	RII	95% CI
WHR–low PWB	2.02	(1.0–4.1)	1.52	(0.6–3.6)
WHR–high PWB	2.51	(1.1–5.6)	2.41	(0.9–6.5)
SF-36–low PWB	4.86	(2.5–9.2)	4.92	(2.2–10.8)
SF-36–high PWB	4.51	(2.1–9.8)	2.56	(1.0–6.7)

Notes: CI, confidence interval; WHR, waist–hip ratio; PWB, psychological well-being.

[a]Mediators: early childhood environment as measured by mother's and father's education: psychosocial work environment, measured by job characteristics of decision authority and use of skills; health behavior, measured by smoking; and degree of mastery and constraints in various aspects of life.

a social gradient: people of higher education scored better on the measure of psychological well-being. Ryff has proposed (Ryff and Keyes 1995) that well-being may act to protect individuals from breakdown in the face of adverse circumstances. Given the strong relation of socioeconomic position to ill health, we examined the relation of two of the measures of social position, education and household income, to two of the health outcomes, waist–hip ratio and SF-36 physical health, with the population further stratified as either above or below the median on psychological well-being. It seems reasonable to assume that low household income will be associated with adverse circumstances. Low education may be a measure not only of adverse circumstances but also of ability to cope.

Socioeconomic Status, for Depression in Men and Women

	Men			
			Adjusted for	
Age Only			Age, Race, and Mediators[a]	
RII	95% CI		RII	95% CI
1.29	(0.7–2.4)		0.59	(0.3–1.2)
3.58	(1.9–6.5)		2.07	(1.0–4.1)
1.58	(0.8–3.0)		1.27	(0.6–1.9)
1.79	(1.0–3.3)		0.94	(0.5–1.9)

Education Stratified by Psychological Well-Being and Gender

	Men			
			Adjusted for	
Age Only			Age, Race, and Mediators[a]	
RII	95% CI		RII	95% CI
3.50	(1.7–7.0)		2.17	(0.9–5.1)
2.17	(1.1–4.4)		2.08	(0.9–4.8)
4.99	(2.5–10.0)		2.16	(0.9–5.1)
2.04	(0.8–4.9)		1.96	(0.7–5.7)

When education is the marker of social position (table 9), there is little evidence of interaction. There is some evidence of interaction between income and psychological well-being in relation to waist–hip ratio and physical functioning (table 10). With high psychological well-being, the relation of household income to the two endpoints is weaker than when psychological well-being is low, and in most cases loses statistical significance.

DISCUSSION

These analyses from a national sample of Americans confirm the general finding that health follows a social gradient. This is seen particularly clearly in table 4: among men, for each of the four indicators of ill health, the lower the position in the social hierarchy, the higher the risk. The RII represents the slope of the relationship between socioeconomic status and ill health. Hence, the confidence intervals around the RII are roughly

TABLE 10 Relationship between Waist–Hip Ratio and SF-36, and

	Women			
	Adjusted for			
	Age Only		Age, Race, and Mediators[a]	
	RII	95% CI	RII	95% CI
WHR–low PWB	5.36	(2.6–11.2)	3.53	(1.6–7.2)
WHR–high PWB	1.98	(0.9–4.4)	1.75	(0.7–4.1)
SF-36–low PWB	6.54	(3.5–12.3)	4.73	(2.4–9.3)
SF-36–high PWB	1.55	(0.7–3.3)	0.87	(0.4–2.0)

Notes: CI, confidence interval; WHR, waist–hip ratio; PWB, psychological well-being.
[a]Mediators: early childhood environment as measured by mother's and father's education: psychosocial work environment, measured by job characteristics of decision authority and use of skills; health behavior, measured by smoking; and degree of mastery and constraints in various aspects of life.

equivalent to a test of trend. Among women, the RIIs are, in general, significantly different from 1.0, although inspection of the odds ratios shows the social gradient somewhat less clearly.

One of the questions addressed by the present analyses was possible differences in health inequalities by age. In the first Whitehall study, relative inequalities in mortality were smaller at older rather than younger ages (Marmot and Shipley 1996), and epidemiological studies of coronary heart disease show some decline in the predictive power of risk factors in this age range (Shipley, Pocock, and Marmot 1991). Putting this information together with the suggestion that inequalities in health are relatively narrow during the adolescent years led to the speculation that health inequalities might be largest in midlife. In this study, there was little evidence for difference by age in the slope in inequalities for people aged 25–74. Perhaps this age range does not provide an adequate test of the hypothesis because it excludes both adolescents and persons older than 75. Nevertheless, given the coronary heart disease experience, had there been a change in the slope of health inequalities, one might have expected to see it in this age range.

One tentative conclusion from these analyses, therefore, is that social inequalities in health do not vary greatly over the 25-to-74-year age span. This would be consistent with social circumstances affecting the health outcomes considered here, with little lag time between cause and effect.

The second issue that we addressed is the relative power of different socioeconomic indices to predict markers of ill health in men and women. We have raised three types of doubts about comparisons of size of effect,

Income Stratified by Psychological Well-Being and Gender

Men				
			Adjusted for	
Age Only			Age, Race, and Mediators[a]	
RII	95% CI		RII	95% CI
2.10	(1.1–4.1)		1.59	(0.8–3.3)
1.26	(0.6–2.7)		0.84	(0.4–2.0)
5.05	(2.5–10.0)		2.41	(1.1–5.1)
3.40	(1.3–8.6)		2.75	(1.0–7.8)

and all three relate to problems of measurement. First, when comparing different socioeconomic indices, we are in general comparing groups of different sizes. Thus, for example, 10.4 percent of women are in the lowest educational category (less than high school), whereas, 29 percent are in the highest poverty area. To correct for this problem we used the RII that can be interpreted as the odds ratio of lowest versus highest group, standardizing for the size of the groups. Measurement imprecision leads to the other two sources of doubt. One variable may appear to be more closely related to the outcome by virtue of its greater precision (and validity). Further, when several socioeconomic variables are entered into one multivariate model, one must be cautious with the interpretation of the resultant odds ratios.

With these caveats in mind, we note that education was a consistent predictor of all four health outcomes in women, and in men for all but depression. In nearly all the models that included all four socioeconomic indices, education remained a significant predictor of ill health. This relates first to the important question of health selection or reverse causation. The thrust of our analyses is based on the assumption that socioeconomic position is a determinant of ill health, rather than ill health being a prime determinant of socioeconomic position. In cross-sectional data, both directions are plausible, where socioeconomic position is measured by, for example, income. Ill health could lead to deterioration of income. It is less plausible where socioeconomic position is measured by education. It is of course possible that ill health in childhood could affect educational achievement. Where it has been studied, however, this is a minor effect (Wadsworth 1986). A more likely interpretation is that education is a measure of socioeconomic position that precedes the development of ill health. The observed relation cannot, therefore, be explained primarily by health selection.

The results further show that after taking education into account, other indices are still predictive of ill health. Household income, as an obvious marker of financial circumstances, is related to all measures of ill health in women and to all but waist–hip ratio in men. Despite the correlation between education and income, the fact that income has an independent relation with health is evidence for the effect of current social circumstances on health. For men, particularly, income shows the social gradient effect on health. Men in the worst quartile of household income have worse health than those in the top quartile, but those in the third quartile also have worse health than those in the top quartile. The significance of the RII is therefore not driven only by worse health for those at the bottom but also by a social gradient that runs across society. It is this that has given rise to the hypothesis that it is inequality rather than lack of material well-being that contributes to the gradient in health (Wilkinson 1996; Wadsworth 1986).

These analyses also show an area effect. There has been debate over the extent to which characteristics of areas may contribute to health over and above the characteristics of individuals who live in those areas—the so-called contextual as against compositional effects (Diez-Roux 1998). This has policy relevance. If apparently unhealthy areas are unhealthy because of the degree of deprivation of their residents, that conclusion has different policy implications than if an area is unhealthy because of characteristics of the area itself, such as transport, amenities, the quality of housing, or because of characteristics of the social environment such as social capital. These data are consistent with an area effect on health, more consistently seen in women, after the effect of education, household income, and the Duncan socioeconomic index have all been taken into account.

One of the stimuli for this further analysis of MIDUS data was the question of whether different socioeconomic indices would have different predictive power in men and women. The gender differences were not striking. Comparison of the bivariate and multivariate models in tables 3 and 4 suggests that much, but not all, of the strong predictive effect of education in both men and women is taken up by measures of current socioeconomic status. This is consistent with a hypothesis that part of the reason for the link between education and health is that education is a route into social circumstances in adult life. A plausible interpretation of these data, therefore, is that part of the reason people with less education have worse health is not because of their education level per se, but because they have less attractive jobs, have lower household incomes, and live in poorer areas.

Women's education shows a lower correlation with household income than does men's. Under these circumstances, the fact that, in multivariate models, education looks marginally stronger than household income as a predictor in women, and marginally less strong in men, is consistent with not all of the education effect being the result of current social circumstances.

We reported previously (Marmot et al. 1998) from these MIDUS data that no single factor explained the majority of the social gradient in health. Here we explored the hypothesis that different socioeconomic measures may have different pathways of action in their effect on health. We examined four domains as potential mediators: early childhood environment as measured by mother's and father's education; psychosocial work environment, as measured by job characteristics of decision authority and use of skills; health behavior, as measured by smoking; and degree of mastery and constraints in various aspects of life. A combination of these factors appeared to account for some of the social gradient in health. We did not, however, detect a difference among our four socioeconomic indices in the degree to which different variables appeared to mediate the relationship with health.

There is abundant evidence on the social gradient in mortality but much less on differences in morbidity. These analyses show that for a number of health outcomes, there is a clear social gradient in women, as in men. In the age range studied here, 25–74, there is no difference by age in the slope of the gradient. Although it is hazardous to draw firm conclusions from a cross-sectional study such as this, the analyses are consistent with some persisting effect of childhood circumstances on adult health, as shown by the independent relation to these health outcomes. The analyses also show, however, that social circumstances of adults are related to ill health, independent of education and mother's and father's education. These results are consistent with the view that in order to reduce inequalities in health, it is necessary to improve the quality of localities as well as to pay attention to the individuals who live and work in those areas (Acheson 1998).

ACKNOWLEDGMENTS

This research was supported by the John D. and Catherine T. MacArthur Foundation Research Networks on Successful Midlife

Development and Socioeconomic Status and Health. M.G.M. is supported by a Medical Research Council research professorship.

REFERENCES

Acheson, Sir Donald. 1998. *Independent inquiry into inequalities in health report.* London: Her Majesty's Stationery Office.

Adler, N., and J. Ostrove. 1999. Socioeconomic status and health: What we know and what we don't. In *Socioeconomic status and health in industrial nations,* ed. N. Adler, M. Marmot, B. McEwen, and J. Stewart, 3–15. New York: New York Academy of Sciences.

Bartley, M., and M. G. Marmot. 2000. Social class and power relation. In *The workplace and cardiovascular disease,* ed. P. Schnall, K. Belkic, P. Landsbergis, and D. Baker. *Occupational Medicine: State of the Art Reviews* 15(1).

Diez-Roux, A. V. 1998. Bringing context back into epidemiology: Variables and fallacies in multi-level analysis. *American Journal of Public Health* 88(2): 216–22.

Duncan, O. D. 1961. A socioeconomic index for all occupations. In *Occupations and social status,* ed. A. J. Reiss, Jr., 109–38. New York: Free Press.

Goldblatt, P. 1990. Mortality and alternative social classifications. In *Longitudinal study: Mortality and social organization,* ed. P. Goldblatt. London: Her Majesty's Stationery Office.

Hauser, R. M., and J. R. Watten. 1997. Socioeconomic indexes for occupations: A review, update, and critique. *Sociological Methodology* 27:177–298.

Kunst, A. 1997. *Cross-national comparisons of socioeconomic differences in mortality.* Rotterdam: Erasmus University.

MacIntyre, S., and A. Ellaway. 2000. Ecological approaches: Rediscovering the role of physical and social environment. In *Social epidemiology,* ed. L. F. Berkman and I. Kawachi, 332–48. New York: Oxford University Press.

Mackenbach, J. P., and A. E. Kunst. 1997. Measuring the magnitude of socio-economic inequalities in health: An overview of available measures illustrated with two examples from Europe. *Social Science and Medicine* 44:757–71.

Marmot, M. G., G. Davey Smith, S. A. Stansfeld, C. Patel, F. North, J. Head, I. White, E. J. Brunner, and A. Feeney. 1991. Health inequalities among British Civil Servants: The Whitehall II study. *Lancet* 337:1387–93.

Marmot, M. G., R. Fuhrer, S. L. Ettner, N. Marks, L. L. Bumpass, and C. D. Ryff. 1998. Contribution of psychosocial factors to socio-economic differences in health. *Milbank Memorial Fund Quarterly* 76:403–48.

Marmot, M. G., C. D. Ryff, L. L. Bumpass, M. Shipley, and N. F. Marks. 1997. Social inequalities in health: Next questions and converging evidence. *Social Science and Medicine* 44: 901–10.

Marmot, M. G., and M. J. Shipley. 1996. Do socioeconomic differences in mortality persist after retirement? Twenty-five-year followup of civil servants from the first Whitehall study. *British Medical Journal* 313:1177–80.

Marmot, M. G., M. J. Shipley, and G. Rose. 1984. Inequalities in death: Specific explanations of a general pattern. *Lancet* 1:3–6.

Pamuk, E. R. 1985. Social class inequality in mortality from 1921 to 1972 in England and Wales. *Population Studies* 39:17–31.

Ryff, C. D., and C. L. M. Keyes. 1995. The structure of psychological well-being revisited. *Journal of Personal and Social Psychology* 69:719–27.

Shipley, M. J., S. J. Pocock, and M. G. Marmot. 1991. Does plasma cholesterol concentration predict mortality from coronary heart disease in elderly people? Eighteen year followup of the Whitehall study. *British Medical Journal* 303:89–92.

Townsend, P., N. Davidson, and M. Whitehead. 1990. *Inequalities in health: The Black Report; the health divide.* London: Penguin.

Wadsworth, M. E. J. 1986. Serious illness in childhood and its association with later-life achievement. In *Class and Health,* ed. R. G. Wilkinson, 50–74. London: Tavistock Publications Ltd.

West, P. 1988. Inequalities? Social class differentials in health in British youth. *Social Science and Medicine* 27:291–96.

Wilkinson, R. G. 1996. *Unhealthy societies: The afflictions of inequality.* London: Routledge.

CHAPTER FOUR

Social Inequalities in Health and Well-Being: The Role of Relational and Religious Protective Factors

Carol D. Ryff, Burton H. Singer, and Karen A. Palmersheim

Scientific studies of social inequalities in health have proliferated in recent years (Feinstein 1993; Marmot, Shipley, and Rose 1984; Williams and Collins 1995). This literature, which links various indicators of socioeconomic status (SES) to health outcomes, documents the increased likelihood for diverse forms of disease, illness, and maladjustment among those at lower ends of the socioeconomic hierarchy. Initial epidemiological studies focused on describing SES gradients in health (e.g., Marmot, Shipley, and Rose 1984). Increasingly, however, the scientific focus has shifted toward identifying the intervening mechanisms (e.g., health behaviors, environmental conditions, psychosocial variables, biological processes) thought to account for SES-related health disparities (Adler et al. 1999). MIDUS has, in fact, been part of this inquiry—showing that midlife is a time when there are substantial socioeconomic differences in health, and further documenting the role of psychosocial factors (e.g., family background, social support, social strain, work characteristics, sense of control, perceived inequalities) in understanding health gradients (Marmot et al. 1998).

Despite evidence of SES gradients in health, it is the case that within levels of education, income, or occupational status, there are high levels of variability. That is, variability *within* socioeconomic grades is sometimes as pronounced as variability *between* SES levels, particularly as one moves down the SES hierarchy (Backlund, Sorlie, and Johnson 1999; Diez-Roux et al. 1995; Mustard et al. 1997). This within-grade variability, particularly at the low end, is the starting point for the present chapter, in which we use the MIDUS data to focus on individuals who show positive profiles of mental or physical health, despite having low educational standing. These individuals have somehow evaded the adverse health consequences associated with having limited education (i.e., a high school education or less). Thus, health-wise, they look more like those who are well educated (i.e., those who have a college degree or more). Our question is, What accounts for such positive health profiles, despite the lack of educational advantage?

To this query we bring two prior literatures, each of which suggest different categories of "protective factors" that might help explain a person's good health and well-being, despite limited educational attainment. First, we consider the benefits that ensue from the social relational world. As highlighted later in the chapter, a growing body of research, across numerous scientific fields, underscores the salubrious role of positive social relationships in the maintenance of good health, both mental and physical. Second, we consider the role of religion and spirituality as a further concomitant of positive health profiles. This realm is also accompanied by a growing literature suggesting that those with high engagement in religious/spiritual beliefs and practices have lowered profiles of morbidity and mortality.

To both the relationship and religiosity realms, we bring an emphasis on *cumulative* effects—that is, we target the possible health benefits ensuing from having long-term profiles of the above protective factors. Thus, we use concurrent and retrospective data from MIDUS to measure *persistent* (from childhood to adulthood) social relational strengths and *persistent* (from childhood to adulthood) religious/spiritual practices. The objective is to evaluate whether these characteristics are part of the life-course profiles of those who lack educational advancement but yet have good physical and mental health. We construe such lives as embodying a form of resilience (Ryff et al. 1998) vis-à-vis a world of social inequalities. That is, our inquiry probes the hypothesis that good social relationships as well as religion/spirituality are protective factors that enable some individuals to remain healthy and well despite lack of educational attainment and its associated benefits.

PROTECTIVE FACTORS: SIGNIFICANT OTHERS AND SIGNIFICANT BELIEFS
Social Relationships and Health

Across diverse disciplines, the social relational world has increasingly been linked to health outcomes. From initial work in the Alameda County study (Berkman and Syme 1979), epidemiologists have repeatedly shown that social isolation, or lack of social support, is linked to increased risk of various diseases as well as to length of life (Berkman and Breslow 1983; House, Landis, and Umberson 1988; Seeman 1996; Seeman et al. 1993). A review of eight major epidemiological studies (Berkman 1995) indicated that, in each case, mortality was significantly lower among those who were more socially integrated.

The social support literature has extended such epidemiological findings (Cohen 1988; Cohen, Underwood, and Gottlieb 2000; Cohen and
Wills 1985) by distinguishing main effects (social support is good for
health under all circumstances) versus buffering models (support from
others is particularly beneficial for health when one is confronted with
stress or adversity). This literature has also linked social support to stress
and coping (Thoits 1995), family relationships (Pierce, Sarason, and
Sarason 1996), personality (Pierce et al. 1997), and differential survival from various health challenges, including myocardial infarction
(Ruberman et al. 1984) and cancer (Spiegel and Kimerling 2001). How
significant others promote positive health behaviors and practices has
also been of increased interest (Berkman 1995; Spiegel and Kimerling
2001; Taylor, Repetti, and Seeman 1997) in efforts to account for the
routes through which the relational world influences health.

Among the most rapidly proliferating areas of research is the focus
on the physiological mechanisms through which social relationships affect health (Cohen and Herbert 1996; Kiecolt-Glaser and Newton 2001;
Ryff et al. 2001; Seeman 1996; Seeman et al. 1994, 2002; Seeman and
McEwen 1996; Uchino, Cacioppo, and Kiecolt-Glaser 1996). To advance
mechanistic understanding at the biological level, however, we must first
understand the emotional features of significant social relations (Ryff and
Singer 2001), because these likely activate intervening physiological processes. Also important is the need to monitor long-term profiles of these
socioemotional strengths or adversities through time (Ryff and Singer
2000; Singer and Ryff 1999).

Psychological research has probed the significant emotional features of
social relationships, whether in contexts of studies of attachment (Hazan
and Shaver 1994), close personal relationships (Berscheid and Reis 1998;
Reis and Patrick 1996), or marital quality (Bradbury 1998; Carstensen,
Levenson, and Gottman 1995). Measures from such emotional features
of the quality of social relationships have rarely made their way into
population-level studies, although MIDUS was fortunate to have detailed assessments in these areas (Ryff et al. 2001). Questions included
detailed items on the emotional features of key relationships (e.g., with
spouse/partner, with mother and father during childhood). Although
MIDUS data cannot address intervening physiological processes, the
study can inform understanding, at the population level, of the links
between socioemotional experience and various aspects of physical and
mental health.

Regarding the interface between social relationships and social in-equalities, such relationships can be construed as risk or protective factors for various health outcomes. On the one hand, the relational stress and conflict that may accompany economic strain or blocked life opportunities over the long term may contribute to adverse health. For other individuals, however, the relational realm may be an important source of strength and support vis-à-vis life difficulties, including those that follow from low standing in the socioeconomic hierarchy.

For example, our earlier work with a subsample of respondents from the Wisconsin Longitudinal Study revealed that those on positive relationship pathways (i.e., having good-quality relationships with parents in childhood and with spouse in adulthood) were less likely to have high allostatic load, an index of wear and tear on multiple physiological systems, compared with those on negative pathways (Singer and Ryff 1999). Importantly, these findings also demonstrated the protective benefits of positive relations in the context of persistent economic adversity. That is, individuals who had long-term economic disadvantage *but persistently good social relationships* had reduced likelihood of having high allostatic load compared with those with persistent adversity in both economic and social relational realms.

Using the MIDUS data, the objective of the present analysis is to investigate in a population-level study the extent to which persistent social relational strengths are part of the life histories of those who, despite low educational attainment, have good physical and mental health. In addition, as discussed later in this chapter, we examine the possible protective influence of religion and spirituality.

Religion/Spirituality and Health

A growing literature traversing diverse scientific disciplines (gerontology, medicine, psychology, sociology) is exploring the role of religion and spirituality in mental and physical health (Koenig 1998; Koenig, McCullough, and Larson 2001; Seybold and Hill 2001; Thoresen 1999). This work has identified multiple dimensions of religion and spirituality and explored their linkages to diverse mental and physical health outcomes. The intervening processes or mechanisms that link realms of religiosity and health have also been probed in various studies. Examples of these topics are selectively noted here as a prelude to how we used data from MIDUS to examine religion and spirituality as possible protective influences in the face of social inequalities.

The multidimensional nature of religion and spirituality has been elaborated in numerous publications, including a panel of experts commissioned by the Fetzer Institute and the National Institute on Aging. Their report (Fetzer Institute/National Institute on Aging 1999) identified ten dimensions of religion and spirituality (religious-spiritual history, preference affiliation, social participation, private practices, coping styles, beliefs and values, commitment, experiences, sense of support, and motivation for regulating and reconciling relationships) that have appeared in recent research. Further dimensions are elaborated in Hill and Hood's (1999) review of 125 measures of religion and spirituality. The similarities and differences between religion and spirituality have also received considerable attention (Hill et al. 2000). The task of linking religion and spirituality to health outcomes is thus both enriched and complicated by the diverse operational definitions of these domains.

Considerable work has focused on behavioral measures, such as church attendance, linked to health outcomes. Koenig and Larson (1998) found that people who attended church weekly (or more often) were significantly less likely to be admitted to a hospital in the previous year and had fewer hospital admissions and fewer days in the hospital than did those who attended less often. These associations remained after controlling for effects of age, sex, race, education, social support, depressive symptoms, physical function, and severity of illness. Religious attendance has also been found to predict mortality, with the relationship reduced only slightly after controlling for demographics, social support, health practices, and health conditions (Strawbridge et al. 1997; Koenig et al. 1999; Oman and Reed 1998). Three large national probability surveys from the 1970s and 1980s found that religious involvement (primarily religious attendance) was significantly associated with positive self-rated health, health satisfaction, and psychological well-being (Levin and Chatters 1998).

Numerous other studies have linked religion and spirituality to specific disease outcomes. For example, cancer mortality rates have been found to be lower among more religious groups (Dwyer, Clarke, and Miller 1990; Enstrom 1975), and a twenty-three-year longitudinal study found that those with higher degrees of religiosity experienced lower rates of death as a result of coronary heart disease, even after controlling for important risk factors (e.g., smoking; Goldbourt, Yaari, and Medalie 1993). The incidence of hypertension, a key risk factor for stroke and other cardiovascular disease, has been shown to correlate inversely with religious attendance and private religious practices (praying, reading the Bible) (Koenig et al. 1998). Seybold and Hill (2001) summarize findings across multiple studies showing salutary effects of religion and spirituality on a wide array of health measures, including those just noted and others (e.g., chronic pain, cholesterol levels, surgery-related stress, cirrhosis, emphysema, kidney failure, and so forth).

The links between religion/spirituality and mental health have also received considerable attention, generally pointing to positive associations (Larson et al. 1992; Levin and Chatters 1998). For example, Ellison (1991) reported that individuals with strong religious faith reported higher levels of life satisfaction, greater personal happiness, and fewer negative psychosocial consequences or traumatic life events. Other samples of Mexican Americans (Levin, Markides, and Ray 1996) and African Americans (Levin and Taylor 1998) revealed positive links between various indicators of religiosity (e.g., attendance, prayer) and measures of life satisfaction, happiness, or psychological distress. Kendler, Gardner, and Prescott (1997) also found that high levels of personal devotion were related to lower levels of depressive symptoms, and Koenig, George and Peterson (1997) found that depressed cancer patients with higher intrinsic religiosity scores had more rapid remissions than did patients with lower scores.

The potentially harmful effects of religion have not been neglected. Seybold and Hill (2001) describe blindly obedient versions that have been associated with child abuse or neglect, intergroup conflict, and false perceptions of control. Religion has also been associated with authoritarianism, rigidity, dogmatism, and dependence (Gartner 1996), and harmful forms of religious coping have been associated with impaired mental health and poorer resolution of negative life events (Pargament 1997). Overall, however, the larger story is one of the salutary effects of religion on mental health.

Study of the way in which religion has affected health—that is, the mechanisms through which it influences health (Seybold and Hill 2001)—has focused on lifestyle and health behaviors (e.g., abstinence from smoking, alcohol, drug use, risky sex). Psychological factors may also mediate the links between religion and health via such processes as effective coping strategies, sense of control, attribution of meaning and purpose to negative life events, and optimistic explanatory styles. The links between religion and social support and community resources have also been proposed as mechanisms. Positive emotions associated with religiosity (e.g., forgiveness, hope, contentment, love) may also affect various physiological mechanisms, possibly reducing arousal in the sympathetic nervous system and the hypothalamic-pituitary-adrenal axis or increasing immune competence.

MIDUS included various questions pertaining to religion and spirituality, including assessment of the importance of religion in one's early childhood. Thus, paralleling our social relational analyses, the focus was on the extent to which persistent religious profiles (from childhood through adulthood) might help to characterize the life trajectories of individuals who, despite limited educational attainment, have achieved high levels of health and well-being. We therefore preselected from the data set these high-functioning individuals (both high school–educated and college-educated) and then investigated whether they were similar to each other in protective factors, as well as distinguished from those at the low end of the educational hierarchy who showed poor profiles of health and well-being.

Analytic Approach and Key Predictions

Overall, our analytic approach converges with the growing interest in the study of extreme groups (Kagan, Snidman, and Arcus 1998) and the heightened emphasis on typologies in diverse areas of inquiry. Illustrations of such work include efforts to discern types of developmental trajectories (Robbins, John, and Caspi 1998), types of mental health (Singer et al. 1998), and types of well-being (Keyes, Shmotkin, and Ryff 2002; McKennell 1978; Shmotkin 1998). In the present inquiry, we begin with a focus on extreme groups—namely, those with particularly high (top 25 percent) or low (bottom 25 percent) health standing (mental and physical). Within such groups, we then create types of relationship histories (positive versus negative) and types of religion/spirituality histories (high versus low levels of involvement). The guiding hypothesis is that among those with especially good health and well-being (both high school–educated and college-educated), there will be a greater prevalence of positive relationship types and high religion/spirituality types than among those with poor health and well-being (bottom 25 percent) who have a high school education.

In addition to this prediction *within* educational groups, we also hypothesized that high school–educated individuals with good health (i.e., the resilient) would be significantly different from their same-education counterparts in poor health in the prevalence of the relationship and religious types, but would show no differences from the college-educated in good health. Because the central *between*-groups question was whether relationship and religious histories of the resilient (low education/high health and well-being) would be comparable to those of the college-educated in good health but different from those of the high school–educated in poor health, we did not include comparison of the college-educated in poor health. This latter comparison is also more difficult to pursue, given the reduced variability in health outcomes among the highly educated relative to those lower in the educational hierarchy.

METHODS
Sample

For this investigation, we selected a subsample of MIDUS respondents on the basis of multiple selection criteria. Because the aim was to explore social relationships as potential influences on the links between educational standing and health, only persons who were married, or living with a partner, were included in the analysis. In addition, the sample was stratified by educational attainment to facilitate comparison of respondents who had a high school education or less with those who had obtained a bachelor's degree or more. These selection criteria resulted in a subset of 1465 respondents from the main MIDUS sample.

Measures

Described are the items from the MIDUS survey that were used to operationalize quality of social relationships and degree of religion/spirituality. Also summarized are the procedures used to create long-term relationship and religiosity profiles. Missing data were dealt with in a consistent manner across all scales and indices. That is, a minimum of half of the items used to construct each scale or index score had to be present in order to be included in analyses.

Significant Social Relationships

Maintaining a life-course approach, we asked respondents retrospective questions that evaluated the quality of their close relationships during both childhood and adulthood. Two sets of questions were used to evaluate the valence of parental relationships experienced during childhood. Each set of questions was sequentially asked about the respondent's mother (or woman who raised him/her) and father (or man who raised him/her). The four questions used to assess level of positive relational experiences included (1) How much did s/he understand your problems and worries? (2) How much could you confide in her/him about things that were bothering you? (3) How much love and affection did s/he give you? and (4) How much time and attention did s/he give you when you needed it? Responses were obtained on a four-point scale, ranging from "a lot" to "not at all." Items were reverse-coded so that higher scores represented more positive relations. Summary scores were then calculated across sets of items for each person's mother and father, and the resulting two sums were averaged to create one score representing positive relations during childhood.

Negative parental relationships experienced during childhood were assessed via a series of three questions that explored whether, and to what extent, the respondent experienced negative and/or abusive behavior during their earlier years. The first of these three questions asked the respondent about being insulted, sworn at, or ignored. The second question inquired into whether the respondent had been pushed, slapped, or had objects thrown at him/her. And the third question explored the occurrence of more serious forms of physical abuse such being kicked, bitten, or struck with an object. Responses were obtained on a four-point scale, ranging from "often" to "never." Each set of questions was sequentially asked about the respondent's mother (or woman who raised him/her) and father (or man who raised him/her). Items were weighted to reflect greater negativity associated with more severe forms of abuse. A summary score, representing negative relations during childhood, was then calculated in a manner similar to that for positive relations, with high scores denoting a low level of negative relations (i.e., more positive relations).

To combine the positive and negative scores into an index representing "childhood relations," we divided each of the summary scores at the median. Respondents who scored at or below the median were assigned a 1, representing less positive relations, and those above the median were assigned a 2, designating more positive relations. These two variables were then added together, creating a variable that ranges from 2 to 4, representing an increasing gradient of positive relationships during childhood.

Relations during Adulthood

A respondent's relations during adulthood were assessed by use of a series of questions that inquired about the respondent's relationship with his/her spouse (or partner). Six questions explored positive features of connections with one's partner: (1) How much does your spouse or partner really care about you? (2) How much does he or she understand the way you feel about things? (3) How much does he or she appreciate

		Adulthood relations		
		Mostly negative	Mixed	Mostly positive
Childhood relations	Mostly negative	A	B	
	Mixed	C		D
	Mostly positive		E	F

Figure 1. Creation of negative and positive relationship profiles.

you? (4) How much can you rely on him or her for help if you have a serious problem? (5) How much can you open up to him or her if you need to talk about your worries? and (6) How much can you relax and be yourself around him or her? Each response set was coded on a four-point scale, ranging from "a lot" to "not at all." All of these items were reverse-coded, so higher scores reflect more positive relations during adulthood.

The following six questions explored negative relations with partners: (1) How often does your spouse or partner make too many demands on you? (2) How often does he or she make you feel tense? (3) How often does he or she argue with you? (4) How often does he or she criticize you? (5) How often does he or she let you down when you are counting on him or her? and (6) How often does he or she get on your nerves? Each question was coded on a four-point scale, with responses ranging from "often" to "never."

An index representing "adulthood relations" was created by following the same process as that used for an index of childhood relations. Again, the resulting variable ranges are from 2 to 4, representing an increasing gradient in level of positive relations during adulthood.

Cumulative Relationship Profiles

To investigate whether respondents who varied on the basis of their educational status and health outcomes differed in terms of their relationship experiences over the life course, we created cumulative relationship profiles. Cross-tabulations were employed to identify two distinct profiles—one consisting of those individuals who had experienced predominantly negative relations, and the other representing those who experienced mostly positive relations from childhood to adulthood. Figure 1 presents a schema of the distributions used to identify these two contrasting groups. The rows in the grid represent scores on the childhood relations index, which was produced from a summary of both positive and negative relations with a mother and father. The top row represents respondents who reported more negative relationships during their childhood, the bottom row designates those reporting more positive relations, and those in the middle row had mixed responses. The columns in the grid represent scores on the adulthood relations index, which summarized respondents' experience of positive and negative relations with their spouse/partner. The first column represents respondents who reported more negative relationships during adulthood, the last column designates those reporting more positive relations, and those reporting a mixed valence are represented in the middle column.

Using these cross-tabulations, we selected respondents who had experienced predominantly negative relationships during both their early and adult years (those in cells A, B, and C on the grid). The comparison group was identified as those individuals who reported more positive relations during both childhood and adulthood (cells D, E, and F on the grid).

Religion/Spirituality

Four questions were used to measure various aspects of religiosity or spirituality over the life course. One of the four questions explored religious experience during childhood: How important was religion in your home when you were growing up? Responses were obtained on a four-point scale, ranging from "very important" to "not at all important." Three questions that appraised respondents' connectedness to religion or spirituality as adults included (1) How often do you usually attend religious or spiritual services? (2) When you have problems or difficulties in your family, work, or personal life, how often do you seek comfort through religious or spiritual means, such as praying, meditating, attending a religious or spiritual service, or talking to a religious or spiritual advisor? and (3) When you have decisions to make in your daily life, how often do you ask yourself what your religious or spiritual beliefs suggest you should do? The first question was measured on a five-point scale, with responses ranging from "more than once a week" to "never." The other two questions were answered on a four-point scale, from "often" to "never." All responses were reverse-coded so that higher scores represent higher levels of religion/spirituality. A summary score was calculated to represent adult religion/spirituality across the three respective questions. This score was then divided into quartiles to obtain a variable based on a four-point scale that could be compared with the four-point scale of childhood religiosity in cross-tabulation analyses.

		Adulthood religiosity			
		Lowest quartile	2nd quartile	3rd quartile	Highest quartile
Childhood religiosity	Not at all important	A	B		
	Not very important	C			
	Somewhat important				D
	Very important			E	F

FIGURE 2. Creation of low- and high-religiosity profiles.

Cumulative Religion/Spirituality Profiles

To examine whether levels of religiosity over the life course are associated with educational background and health-related outcomes, cumulative profiles were created in a manner similar to that for social relationship histories. Again, cross-tabulations were used to identify two distinct profiles: individuals who reported low overall levels of religion/spirituality, and those reporting generally high levels of religion/spirituality. Figure 2 presents a schema of the cross-tabulations used to identify the two contrasting groups. The rows in the grid represent scores on the childhood measure of religious importance, which consisted of one question, coded on a four-point scale. The top row represents respondents who reported that religion was not at all important during their childhood, the bottom row designates those reporting it was very important, and those in the middle rows range in between. The columns in the grid represent scores on the adulthood religion/spirituality index, which resulted from summing across the three questions on religion during adult years and dividing the summed score into quartiles. The first column represents respondents who reported low levels of religion/spirituality during adulthood, the last column designates those reporting high levels, and those reporting more moderate levels of religion/spirituality are represented in the two middle columns.

From among these cross-tabulations, we selected respondents who reported lower levels of religiosity during both their early and adult years (cells A, B, and C in the grid). The comparison group was identified as those individuals who reported higher levels of religiosity during both childhood and adulthood (cells D, E, and F in the grid).

Physical Health

Three assessments of physical health were included in these analyses. A global indicator of self-reported health asked respondents to rate their health on a scale from 1 to 5, with a score of 1 indicating poor health and a 5 representing excellent health. Individuals also completed a checklist indicating which of twenty-nine chronic conditions they had experienced over the past twelve months (i.e., asthma, arthritis, diabetes, and so forth). An additional checklist measure evaluated which of nine physical symptoms respondents had experienced over the previous thirty days (i.e., headaches, back aches, difficulty sleeping). A summary score was calculated for each of the checklist measures. These scores were then reverse-coded so that higher scores reflect better physical health (fewer conditions or symptoms).

Indicators of Psychological Well-being

Three dimensions of psychological well-being—autonomy, personal growth, and purpose in life—were selected for analysis in this study. Ryff's (1989) index of psychological well-being operationalized multiple facets of positive psychological functioning. For the national survey, this was reduced to a short-form, eighteen-item instrument that encompasses the same six dimensions: self-acceptance, purpose in life, environmental mastery, positive relations with others, personal growth, and autonomy (see Ryff and Keyes 1995). We did not use the positive relations with others scale because as a mental health outcome, it is somewhat redundant with the social relational histories. Because the aim was to restrict the analysis to three aspects of physical health and three dimensions of mental health, our analyses also did not include the scales of self-acceptance and environmental mastery. These, compared with the three scales we did use, showed less variability as a function of educational standing.

Each dimension is measured using a three-item scale in which respondents indicate their level of agreement (or disagreement) on a six-point scale (strong, moderate, or slight agreement/disagreement). The scales incorporate both positive and negative items, with negative items being reverse-coded so that higher scores reflect more positive appraisals. Although the full fourteen-item and twenty-item scales for each of the six dimensions of well-being exhibit high internal (alpha) reliability (Ryff 1989, 1991), the reduced-item scales exhibit modest reliability, stemming from the decision to select items for the larger survey that maximize content validity rather than internal consistency (i.e., the separate scales revealed multifactorial structures; thus, rather than represent only single subdimensions for each scale, items were selected across subdimensions to maximize theoretical coverage). (For a more detailed discussion of psychometric properties and the item selection process, see Ryff and Keyes 1995.)

RESULTS

To reiterate, the central question guiding the analyses was whether positive social relational and high-engagement religious histories would predominate in the lives of those who rate themselves as healthy and well (both the high school–educated and college-educated) relative to those who see themselves as having poor health and low well-being (the high school–educated). The findings arrayed below first report the prevalence of positive versus negative relationship histories among our targeted health/education groups. These analyses are followed by the prevalence of the high versus low religion/spirituality histories among the same targeted groups. In each section, results for the three physical health outcomes are presented first, followed by results for the three dimensions of psychological well-being. All analyses are presented separately for men and women.

With regard to statistical comparisons, across each of the health outcomes we first compare the prevalence of positive versus negative social relationship histories (or high versus low religion/spirituality types) *within* the three health/education groups: college-educated individuals in the top quartile of each health outcome, high school–educated individuals also in the top quartile of health, and high school–educated individuals in the lowest quartile of health. The key prediction is that those in good health (both high school–educated and college-educated) would have significantly higher prevalence of positive versus negative relationship types and high versus low religion/spirituality types, whereas those in poor health would have the reverse profile (i.e., significantly higher prevalence of negative versus positive relationship histories and low versus high religion/spirituality types).

Assessment of the within-group (health/education) differences are followed by assessment of between-group (health/education) differences, where the focus is on two specific comparisons: the high school–educated in good health with the high school–educated in poor health, and the high school–educated in good health with the college-educated also in good health. The key prediction is that the two former groups should differ significantly in the prevalence of the previously described types, whereas the two latter groups should not. That is, the high school–educated in good health should have relationship and religion/spirituality profiles similar to those of the college-educated also in good health, but different from the high school–educated in poor health.

The statistical analyses performed to test these hypotheses consisted of *t*-tests for differences in proportions. Comparisons of relationship categories or religiosity categories *between* education by health, or education by well-being groups, were based on mutually exclusive and independent subgroups of the total population. Thus, for example, if we consider the population (A) of men who are only high school graduates and who score low on personal growth in contrast to the population (B) of men who are only high school graduates and score high on personal growth, we have mutually exclusive populations. Furthermore, responses on relationship or religiosity measures in population A can be assumed to be statistically independent of the analogous responses in population B. If $p^A = \{$proportion of persons in A who have negative relationship profiles$\}$ and $p^B = \{$proportion of persons in B who have negative relationship profiles$\}$, then we set a confidence interval around the difference in proportions, $p^A - p^B$, by use of standard methodology for independent populations (http://davidmlane.com/hyperstat/B9344.html). We identify the confidence level of the widest interval that does not cover 0 (corresponding to "no difference"). Then $1 -$ (confidence level of widest interval not covering 0) is the reported p value for this single comparison. This calculation is performed for all between-group comparisons.

For within-group comparisons, we employ a different procedure because of the dependence among subgroups of a given group. For example, when considering the population of men who are high school graduates and low on personal growth and then letting $p^A = \{$proportion of this population with high relationship scores$\}$ and $p^B = \{$proportion of this population with low relationship scores$\}$, it is important to observe that there is a third group within this population—a proportion p^C—those who have intermediate relationship scores. Here, $p^A + p^B + p^C = 1$. Our interest is in the difference, $p^A - p^B$. Confidence limits around $p^A - p^B$ are given by

$$[m_A/n - m_B/n] \pm c[m_A(n - m_A) + m_B(n - m_B)$$
$$+ 2m_A m_B/n]^{1/2}/n,$$

where

m_A = number of people with high relationship scores;
m_B = number of people with low relationship scores;
n = number of males who are only high school graduates
  and low on personal growth; and
c = percentage point from the standard normal distribution.

The product term $m_A m_B / n$ is a contribution as a result of the dependence between those who score high and those who score low on relationship profiles, relative to the third group, who have intermediate scores.

We identify the confidence level corresponding to the widest interval that does not cover 0, hence the largest corresponding value of c. Then, analogous to what is described in the previous paragraph, 1 − (confidence level of widest interval not covering 0) is the reported p value for this single comparison.

There are a total of 168 comparisons associated with figures 3–6. Thus, the p values of the individual comparisons can be used as indicators of degrees of separation of the proportions being compared. However, to take account of the multiplicity of comparisons, we would only declare that comparisons with associated p values of .001 or less are simultaneously significantly different at a level of .05 (Miller 1981).

Cumulative Social Relationships and Physical Health

Figure 3 consists of six graphs (A–F), each showing the percentage of respondents in various health/education subgroups (A–C for men and D–F for women) who experienced largely positive (hatched bars) or largely negative (open bars) relationship histories. Figure 3C, involving reports of physical health symptoms by men, indicates that the findings for this outcome clearly fit the guiding predictions. The figure illustrates the findings that within-group differences among men with a high school education or less who reported poor health (high levels of health symptoms), significantly more experienced predominantly negative (47.4 percent) social relationships during childhood and adulthood, compared with 25 percent who experienced more positive social relationships during childhood and adulthood. In contrast, among high school–educated men in good health (low levels of health symptoms), significantly more experienced predominantly positive (52.2 percent) than negative (22.5 percent) social relationships from childhood through adulthood. Similarly, among the college-educated men reporting low levels of health symptoms,

MEN   WOMEN

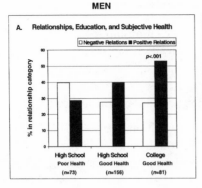
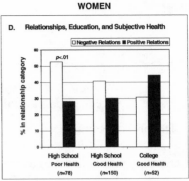
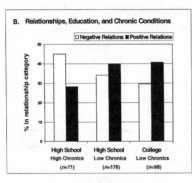
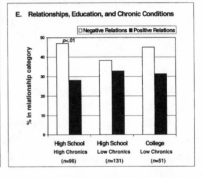
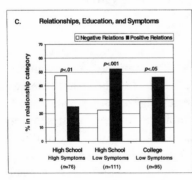
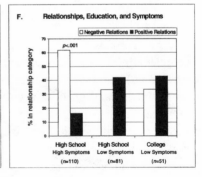

FIGURE 3. Relationships, education, and health.

significantly more experienced positive (46.9 percent) than negative (28.5 percent) social relationship histories.

Select between–group differences were also found: specifically, the high school–educated men in good health (i.e., those with low health symptoms) had a significantly higher prevalence of positive social relationship histories than did high school–educated men in poor health (52.2 percent versus 25.0 percent, p < .001). Similarly, the high school–educated men in good health also had a significantly lower prevalence of negative social histories compared with high school–educated men in poor health (22.5 percent versus 47.4 percent, $p < .001$).

Findings for subjective health for men went in the appropriate direction, with those in good health (both high school–educated and college-educated) having greater prevalence of positive versus negative relationship histories, whereas those in poor health (high school–educated) having greater prevalence of negative versus positive relationship histories. However, significant differences were evident only among the college-educated, where 53.1 percent had positive relationship histories, compared with 27.1 percent who had negative relationship histories. No between-group differences were significant for subjective health. For reports of chronic conditions among men, the results were also in the predicted direction (as described earlier), although no significant differences were obtained.

The findings for women revealed fewer significant differences overall, except for those in poor health. As predicted, those with high school education and in poor health had a significantly higher prevalence of negative than positive social relationship histories. This effect was evident for all three health outcomes: among those reporting poor subjective health, significantly more had negative (52.6 percent) rather than positive (28.2 percent) relationship histories; among those reporting high levels of chronic conditions, significantly more had negative (47.0 percent) rather than positive (28.1 percent) relationship histories; and among those reporting high levels of health symptoms, significantly more had negative (61.8 percent) rather than positive (16.3 percent) relationship histories. No other significant differences were evident in the assessment of physical health outcomes for women.

Cumulative Relationships and Psychological Well-Being

Figure 4 shows the percentage of respondents in well-being/education subgroups (A–C for men and D–F for women) who experienced largely positive versus negative social relationship histories. For men, all of the within-group comparisons were significantly different, and all were in the predicted directions. Thus, whether assessing autonomy, personal growth, or purpose in life, men in the top quartile of well-being (whether high school–educated or college-educated) had significantly higher prevalence of positive versus negative social relationship histories.

MEN **WOMEN**

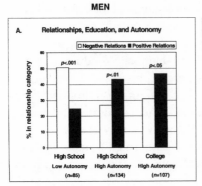

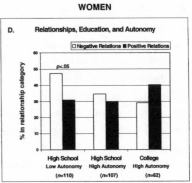

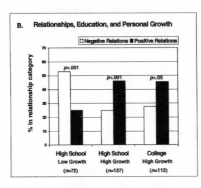

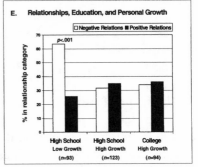

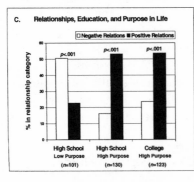

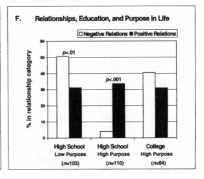

FIGURE 4. Relationships, education, and psychological well-being.

The effects were especially dramatic for purpose in life, where among the high school–educated, 53.1 percent had positive relationship histories, compared with 16.2 percent who had negative histories, and among the college-educated, 53.6 percent had positive social histories, compared with 23.6 percent who had negative relationship experiences. In contrast, among high school–educated men with low levels of purpose in life, 50.5 percent had negative relationship histories compared with 22.7 percent who had positive relationship histories.

The between-group comparisons for men further revealed that across all three aspects of psychological well-being, high school–educated men in the top quartile were significantly different from high school–educated men in the bottom quartile in the prevalence of positive versus negative relationship types. Specifically, men with high autonomy were significantly more likely to have positive relationship histories than men with low autonomy (43.3 percent versus 24.7 percent, $p < .01$), and conversely, men with low autonomy were significantly more likely to have negative relationship histories than men with high autonomy (50.6 percent versus 26.9 percent, $p < .001$). High school–educated men with high levels of personal growth were significantly more likely to have positive relationship histories than men with low personal growth (46.0 percent versus 25.0 percent, $p < .001$), and conversely, those with low personal growth were significantly more likely to have negative relationship histories than men with high personal growth (52.8 percent versus 24.8 percent, $p < .001$). High school–educated men with high levels of purpose in life were significantly more likely to have positive relationship histories than were men with low purpose in life (53.1 percent versus 22.7 percent, $p < .001$), and conversely, those with low purpose in life were significantly more likely to have negative relationship histories than were men with high purpose in life (50.5 percent versus 16.2 percent, $p < .001$).

Finally, as predicted, none of the between-group comparisons between high school–educated and college-educated men with high well-being was significantly different. Thus, these low-education men were consistently similar to those with advanced educational attainment in having higher prevalence of positive versus negative social relationship histories, at the same time that the high school–educated men were consistently different in social relationship histories from their same-education counterparts who had low levels of well-being.

For women, the analyses of psychological well-being revealed patterns similar to those found for physical health outcomes. That is, the most consistent effects were evident among the high school–educated women with low well-being, where in all instances, the prevalence of negative relationship histories was significantly higher than the prevalence of positive relationship histories: autonomy (47.3 percent versus 30.9 percent, $p < .05$), personal growth (63.5 percent versus 25.8 percent, $p < .001$), and purpose in life (50.5 percent versus 31.1 percent,

$p < .01$). Also, for purpose in life, high school–educated women in the top quartile had significantly higher prevalence of positive versus negative social relationship histories (33.7 percent versus 4.0 percent, $p < .001$). Among college-educated women, there were no significant differences in the prevalence of positive versus negative relationship histories.

Finally, with regard to between-group comparisons, there were significant differences in the prevalence of negative relationship histories among high school–educated women having low versus high levels of personal growth and purpose in life. Those reporting low levels of personal growth were much more likely to have had negative relationship histories than were those reporting high personal growth (63.5 percent versus 31.7 percent, $p < .001$). Similarly, those reporting low levels of purpose in life were much more likely to have had negative relationship histories than were those reporting high purpose in life (50.5 percent versus 4.0 percent, $p < .0001$).

Cumulative Religion/Spirituality and Physical Health

Findings for the prevalence of high versus low religion/spirituality for the various health and education subgroups are arrayed in figure 5. For these findings, we discuss the data for women first because the patterns are more consistent across health measures. As predicted, women in good health (across all three measures—subjective health, chronic conditions, health symptoms), whether high school–educated or college-educated, were significantly more likely to have high rather than low profiles of religion/spirituality from childhood to adulthood. These differences were strong (all but one were $p < .001$), involving a three- to sixfold likelihood of high versus low religious involvement.

However, the findings for high school–educated women with poor health profiles (across all three measures), although statistically significant, revealed the *opposite pattern* to what we had predicted. That is, in all instances, women in poor health were significantly ($p < .001$) more likely to have high rather than low religious involvement from childhood through adulthood. This is a pattern to which we return in discussion of the present findings. None of the between-group comparisons in the analyses for women revealed significant differences.

The data for men were somewhat similar in pattern to those for women, but they were less clear-cut. That is, only among the college-educated men in good health was there a significant difference, in the predicted direction, between the prevalence of high versus low religion/spirituality across all three measures. For high school–educated men

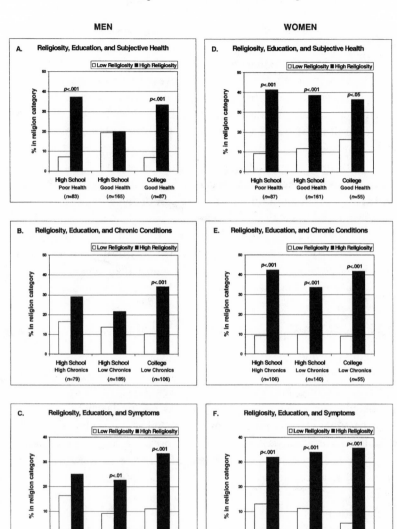

FIGURE 5. Religiosity, education, and health.

in good health, the effects were significant only for the measure of health symptoms, where significantly more men had high profiles of religiosity (22.7 percent versus 9.2 percent).

For high school–educated men with poor physical health profiles, there was a higher prevalence of high versus low religiosity across all measures, although the effects were significantly different only in the case of subjective health. Thus, like women, the low-education men in poor health revealed patterns that ran opposite to the guiding predictions: such individuals were more, not less, likely to have strong profiles of religiosity.

With regard to between-group differences, effects were evident only for subjective health. In that aspect of health, high school–educated men in poor health were significantly more likely to have high religious engagement than were high school–educated men in good health (37.3 percent versus 20.0 percent, $p < .001$), and similarly, they were significantly less likely to have low religious engagement (7.2 percent versus 19.4 percent, $p < .01$). In addition, among those reporting good health, significantly more of the high school–educated were likely to report low religious involvement than among the college-educated (19.4 percent versus 6.9 percent, $p < .001$), and concomitantly, significantly fewer among the high school–educated were likely to report high religious engagement than among the college-educated (20.0 percent versus 33.3 percent, $p < .05$).

Cumulative Religion/Spirituality and Psychological Well-Being

Figure 6 arrays the findings on the prevalence of high- versus low-religiosity types across the three dimensions of psychological well-being. Again, the findings for women revealed clear and consistent patterns. As predicted, women in the top quartile of psychological well-being (autonomy, personal growth, purpose in life), whether high school–educated or college-educated, were significantly more likely to have high rather than low profiles of religiosity. These effects were strongly significant ($p < .001$ in all cases), involving a difference in likelihood from four- to tenfold.

As with physical health outcomes, however, high school–educated women with low levels of well-being show greater, not reduced, likelihood of have high- versus low-religiosity profiles. These differences were strongly significant ($p < .001$) for all three measures of well-being.

The majority of between-group comparisons were not significant. Thus, high school–educated and college-educated women with high well-being did not differ in their likelihood of having high rather than low levels of religious engagement. With regard to differences between high school–educated respondents showing high versus low levels of well-being, only the comparisons of religiosity for personal growth were statistically significant. As predicted, high school–educated women in the top quartile of personal growth had greater likelihood of having

MEN   **WOMEN**

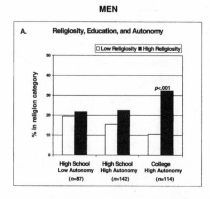

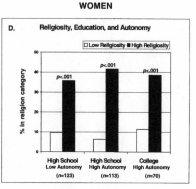

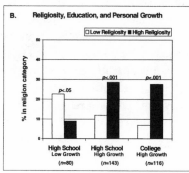

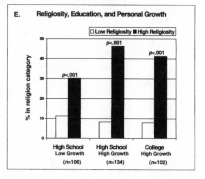

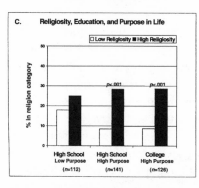

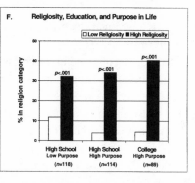

FIGURE 6. Religiosity, education, and psychological well-being.

high-religiosity profiles than did high school–educated women in the bottom quartile of personal growth (46.3 percent versus 30.2 percent, $p < .01$).

Like women, the data for men with high profiles of well-being (whether high school–educated or college-educated) were consistent and in the predicted directions. That is, there was a greater prevalence of high versus low religiosity among these men, and the effects were strongly significant ($p < .001$ in all cases but one). Among high school–educated men with low well-being, only one significant effect was obtained (for personal growth), and it was in the predicted direction. There was a significantly higher prevalence of low versus high religiosity (22.6 percent versus 8.9 percent, $p < .05$) among these men.

With regard to between-group differences, none of the comparisons between high school–educated and college-educated men was (as predicted) significantly different. In the comparison between high school–educated men with high versus low well-being, the differences for personal growth were significant. Here, those with low levels of personal growth were, as predicted, significantly more likely to have low religiosity (22.6 percent versus 11.9 percent, $p < .05$) and significantly less likely to have high religiosity (8.9 percent versus 28.7 percent, $p < .001$). In addition, for purpose in life, there was a significant difference among the high school–educated men. Those with low levels of purpose were, as predicted, significantly more likely to have low levels of religiosity than were those with high levels of purpose (17.9 percent versus 8.5 percent, $p < .05$).

Discussion

This investigation probed the life characteristics of an anomalous group in the social inequalities literature, namely, those at the low end of the socioeconomic hierarchy who are in good health and have high well-being. These individuals do not fit the generic health predictions associated with low levels of education, income, or occupational status. Our question was whether they have protective characteristics that help them avoid adverse health outcomes. We examined two such protective influences—the quality of their social relationships from childhood to adulthood, and the level of their religious engagement from childhood to adulthood.

Before reviewing and interpreting the findings, we acknowledge several issues that lie in the background of this inquiry. First, our emphasis on protective factors does not include an obvious realm of influence— namely, genetics—that may be part of the accounting for resilience (i.e., able to maintain good health and well-being) in the face of social inequalities. That we target the social environment and individuals' religious engagement is not meant to convey a view that good health at the low end of the SES hierarchy is due exclusively to external influences. Genetic factors are undoubtedly part of the story, but we note that even among those attempting to understand such influences, a growing emphasis is on "environmentally-induced genetic expression" (Singer and Ryff 2001). From this perspective, assessment of social relational and religious environments need not be seen as antithetical to interest in potential genetic influences.

Second, from public policy, if not ideological, perspectives on social inequalities and health, it is important to clarify that interest in resilience at the low end of the SES hierarchy is not an endorsement of existing differences in access to resources and opportunities. We bring into high relief those who are healthy and well, despite low educational standing, *not* to diminish problems of social inequalities but rather to probe how, in the face of them, some individuals manage to do remarkably well. Their psychosocial strengths are potentially informative not only in understanding resilience but also in conveying that health research must ultimately include both macro-level, social structural influences and micro-level, individual factors. Neither level of analysis in itself is sufficient to explain the whole story.

That said, what has our inquiry clarified? A main message is that the data both support and challenge the prediction that social relational and religious histories distinguish those in good health (both high school–educated and college-educated) from those in poor health (high school–educated). In reviewing the results, which were notably qualified by gender differences and physical versus mental health outcomes, we first focus on the social relationship histories and then the religion/spirituality histories.

For men, the findings for mental health were strongly consistent with the guiding predictions regarding relationship histories. That is, across all measures of psychological well-being, high school–educated and college-educated men in the top quartile of well-being had a strong predominance of positive versus negative relationship histories. And for high school–educated men in poor health, the opposite was evident—that is, they had a strong predominance of negative versus positive relationship histories. Analyses also revealed the predicted differences between the two high school–educated groups (those having high versus low well-being) in the prevalence of positive versus negative relationship histories, but no differences between the high school–educated men with high well-being and the college-educated (also with high well-being).

Men's physical health outcomes revealed the predicted patterns, but only for assessments of health symptoms. Here, the high school–educated men with low symptoms, like the college-educated men also with low symptoms, had a significantly greater prevalence of positive rather than negative relationship histories. Alternately, high school–educated men with high levels of health symptoms reported a greater predominance of negative rather than positive relationship histories. No effects were evident for chronic conditions, and for subjective health, it was only the college-educated in the top quartile of good health who showed the predicted predominance of positive over negative relationship histories.

For women, the predicted patterns for both physical and mental health were evident, but only for those having low levels of education and poor health. These women, who embody the essence of social inequalities in health, revealed the expected predominance of negative rather than positive social relationship histories for all health outcomes but one (subjective health). However, for women in good mental or physical health (both high school–educated and college-educated), there were no significant differences in the prevalence of positive versus negative relationship histories, with the exception of findings for purpose in life. Here, but only for high school–educated women, those in the top quartile of purpose, as predicted, showed a predominance of positive versus negative social relationship histories.

Thus, good-quality social relationships from childhood to adulthood appeared to be critical elements in understanding the salubrious health (symptoms only) and high well-being of men who had been unable to achieve educational advancement. Their relationship profiles distinguished them from other high school–educated men in poor health, while simultaneously rendering them similar to college-educated men in good health. For women, alternately, social relationship histories were informative primarily in understanding those in poor health (mental and physical) who also lacked educational advantage. Among these women, negative social relationship histories clearly predominated.

As such, these findings add to the growing literature on gender differences in how the social relational world influences health outcomes (e.g., Kiecolt-Glaser and Newton 2001; Ryff and Singer 2000; Seeman et al. 1994). They also bring such differences into the realm of socioeconomic inequalities, suggesting that the presence of social relational strengths from childhood through adulthood may be an important element in understanding the health resilience of men with low levels of education, whereas the absence of such strengths and, indeed, the persistence of relational problems may be part of understanding the compromised health and well-being of women at the low end of the educational hierarchy. This result converges with earlier studies showing that men reap greater benefits from the social relational realm than do women, who in turn may have greater health-related vulnerability vis-à-vis the hazards of social relational difficulties (Fuhrer et al. 1999; Kiecolt-Glaser and Newton 2001; Schuster, Kessler, and Aseltine 1990; Seeman et al. 1994).

Our focus on histories of religion and spirituality revealed strong and remarkably consistent patterns for women. Across all measures, both high school–educated and college-educated women in the top quartile of health and well-being revealed the hypothesized predominance of high religious involvement from childhood to adulthood. Thus, the benefit of religious engagement, especially for women with limited education, was clearly evident. However, contrary to prediction, high school–educated women in poor health or with low well-being (again, across all measures) also revealed a predominance of high religiosity from childhood to adulthood. In short, for all combinations of health and education, women were more likely to have high rather than low levels of persistent religious engagement.

For men, the findings were more qualified. Regarding physical health, the college-educated in the top quartile (good subjective health, low chronic conditions, low health symptoms) revealed the predicted predominance of high versus low religious involvement, but among the high school–educated men in good health, this effect was evident only for health symptoms. Alternatively, among high school–educated men in poor health, the outcomes for subjective health paralleled those for low-educated women discussed earlier—that is, such men were more, not less, likely to have histories of high religious involvement. Psychological outcomes among men generally supported the predicted patterns for those with high well-being (both high school–educated and college-educated): in all instances but one (autonomy for high school–educated men), there was a significant predominance of high versus low religion and spirituality. For high school–educated men with low well-being (only for personal growth), these patterns of religious engagement were significantly different. This was the one instance in which those with low well-being showed the hypothesized predominance of low rather than high religiosity.

The overall story thus is that women revealed strong profiles of religious engagement across all levels of education, health, and well-being. Such patterns make sense as a possible protective influence among those with good health and high well-being (regardless of educational level), but what do they mean for women in poor health and with compromised well-being? One possible interpretation might involve a reversal of the putative direction of influence between religion/spirituality and health outcomes. That is, among these individuals, high levels of religious engagement may be a response to, rather than an antecedent of, mental and physical health outcomes. Because of its cross-sectional nature, MIDUS cannot illuminate this possibility.

Like women, men with good health and well-being (both high school–educated and college-educated) showed a predominance of high rather than low religious involvement, but the effects were more strongly evident for psychological well-being than physical health outcomes. For men in poor health and having low well-being, the religion and spirituality histories were either not significantly different or contrary to prediction.

Overall, then, the realm of religion and spirituality fits our framework for understanding those with good health and high well-being, especially women, but it challenged our perspective regarding those at the low end of the educational hierarchy with compromised health and well-being. Many of these individuals, again, especially women, showed high levels of religious engagement. Although such beliefs and practices may offer important sources of comfort and support in their lives, their religiosity cannot be construed in these data as a factor that has helped keep them healthy and well.

There are many avenues for extending and refining the questions that guided this chapter. As noted earlier in the text, longitudinal tracking of social relationship and religious profiles through time, rather than constructing them retrospectively as done herein, is important to test the view that persistently positive or negative experience in these realms, and its associated neurobiology, is consequential for health. Cross-time analyses will also be necessary to disentangle the directional influences, including possible reciprocal relations between relationships and health, or religiosity and health.

References

Adler, N. E., M. Marmot, B. S. McEwen, and J. Stewart, eds. 1999. Socioeconomic status and health in industrialized nations: Social, psychological, and biological pathways. *Annals of the New York Academy of Sciences* 896: 1–501.

Backlund, E., P. D. Sorlie, and N. J. Johnson. 1999. A comparison of the relationships of education and income with mortality: The National Longitudinal Mortality Study. *Social Science and Medicine* 49: 1373–84.

Berkman, L. F. 1995. The role of social relations in health promotion. *Psychosomatic Medicine* 57: 245–54.

Berkman, L. F., and L. Breslow. 1983. *Health and ways of living.* New York: Oxford University Press.

Berkman, L. F., and S. L. Syme. 1979. Social networks, host resistance, and mortality: A nine-year follow-up study of Alameda County residents. *American Journal of Epidemiology* 100: 186–204.

Berscheid, E., and H. T. Reis. 1998. Attraction and close relationships. In *Handbook of social psychology,* 4th ed., ed. D. T. Gilbert, S. T. Fiske, and G. L. Lindzey, 2: 193–281. Boston: McGraw-Hill.

Bradbury, T. N., ed. 1998. *The developmental course of marital dysfunction.* Cambridge: Cambridge University Press.

Carstensen, L., R. W. Levenson, and J. M. Gottman. 1995. Emotional behavior in long-term marriage. *Psychology and Aging* 10: 140–49.

Cohen, S. 1988. Psychosocial models of the role of social support in the etiology of physical disease. *Health Psychology* 7: 269–97.

Cohen, S., and T. B. Herbert. 1996. Health psychology: Psychological factors and physical disease from the perspective of human psychoneuroimmunology. *Annual Review of Psychology* 47: 113–42.

Cohen, S., L. Underwood, and B. H. Gottlieb, eds. 2000. *Social support measurement and intervention: A guide for health and social scientists.* New York: Oxford University Press.

Cohen, S., and T. A. Wills. 1985. Stress, social support, and the buffering hypothesis. *Psychological Bulletin* 98: 310–57.

Diez-Roux, A. V., F. J. Nreto, H. A. Tyroler, L. D. Crum, and M. Szklo. 1995. Social inequalities and atherosclerosis: The atherosclerosis risk in community study. *American Journal of Epidemiology* 141 (10): 960–72.

Dwyer, J. W., L. L. Clarke, and M. K. Miller. 1990. The effect of religious concentration and affiliation on county cancer mortality rates. *Journal of Health and Social Behavior* 31: 185–202.

Ellison, C. G. 1991. Religious involvement and subjective well-being. *Journal of Health and Social Behavior* 32: 80–99.

Enstrom, J. E. 1975. Cancer mortality among Mormons. *Cancer* 36: 825–41.

Feinstein, J. S. 1993. The relationship between socioeconomic status and health: A review of the literature. *Milbank Quarterly* 71: 279–322.

Fetzer Institute/National Institute on Aging. 1999. *Multidimensional measurement of religiousness/spirituality for use in health research: A report of the Fetzer Institute/National Institute on Aging working group.* Kalamazoo, Mich.: John E. Fetzer Institute.

Fuhrer, R., S. A. Stansfeld, J. Chemali, and M. J. Shipley. 1999. Gender, social relations and mental health: Prospective findings from an occupational cohort (Whitehall II study). *Social Science and Medicine* 48: 77–87.

Gartner, J. 1996. Religious commitment, mental health, and psychosocial behavior: A review of the empirical literature. In *Religion and the clinical practice of psychology,* ed. E. P. Shafranske, 187–214. Washington, D.C.: American Psychological Association.

Goldbourt, U., S. Yaari, and J. H. Medalie. 1993. Factors predictive of long-term coronary heart disease mortality among 10,059 male Israeli civil servants and municipal employees: A 23-year mortality follow-up in the Israeli Ischemic Heart Disease Study. *Cardiology* 82: 100–121.

Hazan, C., and P. R. Shaver. 1994. Attachment as an organizational framework for research on close relationships. *Psychological Inquiry* 5: 1–22.

Hill, P. C., and R. W. Hood, Jr., eds. 1999. *Measures of religiosity*. Birmingham, Ala.: Religious Education Press.

Hill, P. C., K. I. Pargament, R. W. Hood, M. E. McCullough, J. P. Swyers, D. B. Larson, and B. J. Zinnbauer. 2000. Conceptualizing religion and spirituality: Points of commonality, points of departure. *Journal for the Theory of Social Behavior* 30: 51–77.

House, J. S., K. R. Landis, and D. Umberson. 1988. Social relationships and health. *Science* 241: 540–45. http://davidmlane.com/hyperstat/B9344.html.

Kagan, J., N. Snidman, and D. Arcus. 1998. The value of extreme groups. In *Methods and models for studying the individual*, ed. R. C. Cairns, L. R. Bergman, and J. Kagan, 65–79. Thousand Oaks, Calif.: Sage Publications.

Kendler, K. S., C. O. Gardner, and C. A. Prescott. 1997. Religion, psychopathology, and substance use and abuse: A multimeasure, genetic-epidemiologic study. *American Journal of Psychiatry* 154: 322–29.

Keyes, C. L. M., D. Shmotkin, and C. D. Ryff. 2002. Optimizing well-being: The empirical encounter of two traditions. *Journal of Personality and Social Psychology* 82: 1007–22.

Kiecolt-Glaser, J. K., and T. L. Newton. 2001. Marriage and health: His and hers. *Psychological Bulletin* 127: 472–503.

Koenig, H. G., ed. 1998. *Handbook of religion and mental health*. San Diego: Academic Press.

Koenig, H. G., L. K. George, H. J. Cohen, J. C. Hays, D. G. Blazer, and D. B. Larson. 1998. The relationship of religious activities and blood pressure in older adults. *International Journal of Psychiatry in Medicine* 28: 189–213.

Koenig, H. G., L. K. George, and B. L. Peterson. 1997. Religiosity and remission of depression in medically ill older patients. *American Journal of Psychiatry in Medicine* 155: 536–42.

Koenig, H. G., J. C. Hays, D. B. Larson, L. K. George, H. J. Cohen, M. E. McCullough, K. G. Meador, and D. G. Blazer. 1999. Does religious attendance prolong survival? A six-year follow-up study of 3,968 older adults. *Journal of Gerontology* 54A: M370–M376.

Koenig, H. G., and D. B. Larson. 1998. Use of hospital services, religious attendance, and religious affiliation. *Southern Medical Journal* 91: 925–32.

Koenig, H. G., M. E. McCullough, and D. B. Larson, eds. 2001. *Handbook of religion and health*. New York: Oxford University Press.

Larson, D. B., K. A. Sherrill, J. S. Lyons, F. C. Craigie, S. Thielman, M. A. Greenwold, and S. S. Larson. 1992. Associations between dimensions of religious commitment and mental health reports in the *American Journal of Psychiatry* and *Archives of General Psychiatry* 1978–1989. *American Journal of Psychiatry* 149: 557–59.

Levin, J. S., and L. M. Chatters. 1998. Religion, health, and psychological well-being in older adults: Findings from three national surveys. *Journal of Aging and Health* 10: 504–31.

Levin, J. S., K. S. Markides, and L. A. Ray. 1996. Religious attendance and psychological well-being in Mexican Americans: A panel analysis of three-generations data. *The Gerontologist* 36: 454–63.

Levin, J. S., and R. J. Taylor. 1998. Panel analyses of religious involvement and well-being in African Americans: Contemporaneous vs. longitudinal effects. *Journal for the Scientific Study of Religion* 37: 695–709.

Marmot, M. G., R. Fuhrer, S. L. Ettner, N. F. Marks, L. L. Bumpass, and C. D. Ryff. 1998. Contribution of psychosocial factors to socioeconomic differences in health. *Milbank Quarterly* 76: 403–48.

Marmot, M. G., M. J. Shipley, and G. Rose. 1984. Inequalities in death: Specific explanations of a general pattern? *Lancet* 1: 1003–6.

McKennell, A. C. 1978. Cognition and affect in perceptions of well-being. *Social Indicators Research* 5: 389–426.

Miller, R. G. 1981. *Simultaneous statistical inference.* 2d ed. New York: Springer-Verlag.

Mustard, C. A., S. Derksen, J. M. Berthelot, M. Wolfson, and L. L. Roos. 1997. Age-specific education and income gradients in morbidity and mortality in a Canadian province. *Social Science and Medicine* 45: 383–97.

Oman, D., and D. Reed. 1998. Religion and mortality among the community-dwelling elderly. *American Journal of Public Health* 88: 1469–75.

Pargament, K. I. 1997. *The psychology of religion and coping.* New York: Guildford Press.

Pierce, G. R., B. Lakey, I. G. Sarason, and B. R. Sarason. 1997. *Sourcebook of social support and personality.* New York: Plenum Press.

Pierce, G. R., B. R. Sarason, and I. G. Sarason. 1996. *Handbook of social support and the family.* New York: Plenum Press.

Reis, H. T., and B. C. Patrick. 1996. Attachment and intimacy: Component processes. In *Social psychology: Handbook of basic principles,* ed. E. T. Higgins and A. Kruglanski, 367–89. Chichester, U.K.: Wiley.

Robbins, R. W., O. P. John, and A. Caspi. 1998. The typological approach to studying personality. In *Methods and models for studying the individual,* ed. R. B. Cairns, L. R. Bergman, and J. Kagan, 135–60. Thousand Oaks, Calif.: Sage Publications.

Ruberman, W., E. Weinblatt, J. D. Goldberg, and B. S. Chaudhary. 1984. Psychosocial influences on mortality after myocardial infarction. *New England Journal of Medicine* 311: 552–59.

Ryff, C. D. 1989. Happiness is everything, or is it? Explorations on the meaning of psychological well-being. *Journal of Personality and Social Psychology* 57: 1069–81.

———. 1991. Possible selves in adulthood and old age: A tale of shifting horizons. *Psychology and Aging* 6: 286–95.

Ryff, C. D., and C. L. M. Keyes. 1995. The structure of psychological well-being revisited. *Journal of Personality and Social Psychology* 69 (4): 719–27.

Ryff, C. D., and B. H. Singer. 2000. Interpersonal flourishing: A positive health agenda for the new millennium. *Personality and Social Psychology Review* 4: 30–44.

———, eds. 2001. *Emotion, social relationships, and health.* New York: Oxford University Press.

Ryff, C. D., B. Singer, G. D. Love, and M. J. Essex. 1998. Resilience in adulthood and later life: Defining features and dynamic processes. In *Handbook of aging and mental health: An integrative approach,* ed. J. Lomranz, 69–96. New York: Plenum Press.

Ryff, C. D., B. H. Singer, E. Wing, and G. D. Love. 2001. Elective affinities and uninvited agonies: Mapping emotion with significant others onto health. In *Emotion, social relationships, and health,* ed. C. D. Ryff and B. H. Singer, 133–75. New York: Oxford University Press.

Schuster, T. L., R. C. Kessler, and R. H. Aseltine. 1990. Supportive interactions, negative interactions, and depressed mood. *American Journal of Community Psychology* 18: 423–38.

Seeman, T. E. 1996. Social ties and health: The benefits of social integration. *Annals of Epidemiology* 6: 442–51.

Seeman, T. E., L. F. Berkman, D. Blazer, and J. Rowe. 1994. Social ties and support and neuroendocrine function: The MacArthur Studies of Successful Aging. *Annals of Behavioral Medicine* 16: 95–106.

Seeman, T. E., L. F. Berkman, F. Kohout, A. LaCroix, R. Glynn, and D. Blazer. 1993. Intercommunity variation in the association between social ties and mortality in the elderly: A comparative analysis of three communities. *Annals of Epidemiology* 3: 325–35.

Seeman, T. E., and B. S. McEwen. 1996. Impact of social environment characteristics on neuroendocrine regulation. *Psychosomatic Medicine* 58: 459–71.

Seeman, T. E., B. H. Singer, C. D. Ryff, G. D. Love, and L. Levy-Storm. 2002. Social relationships, gender, and allostatic load across two age cohorts. *Psychosomatic Medicine* 64: 395–406.

Seybold, K. S., and P. C. Hill. 2001. The role of religion and spirituality in mental and physical health. *Current Directions in Psychological Science* 10: 21–24.

Shmotkin, D. 1998. Declarative and differential aspects of subjective well-being and implications for mental health in later life. In *Handbook of aging and mental health: An integrative approach,* ed. J. Lomranz, 15–43. New York: Plenum Press.

Singer, B. H., and C. D. Ryff. 1999. Hierarchies of life histories and health risk. *Annals of the New York Academy of Sciences* 896: 96–115.

———. 2001. *New horizons in health: An integrative approach.* Washington, D.C.: National Academy Press.

Singer, B., C. D. Ryff, D. Carr, and W. J. Magee. 1998. Life histories and mental health: A person-centered strategy. In *Sociological methodology 1998,* ed. A. Raftery, 1–51. Washington, D.C.: American Sociological Association.

Spiegel, D., and R. Kimerling. 2001. Group psychotherapy for women with breast cancer: Relationships among social support, emotional expression, and survival. In *Emotion, social relationships, and health,* ed. C. D. Ryff and B. H. Singer, 97–122. New York: Oxford University Press.

Strawbridge, W. J., R. D. Cohen, S. J. Shema, and G. A. Kaplan. 1997. Frequent attendance at religious services and mortality over 28 years. *American Journal of Public Health* 87: 957–61.

Taylor, S. E., R. L. Repetti, and T. Seeman. 1997. Health psychology: What is an unhealthy environment and how does it get under the skin? *Annual Review of Psychology* 48: 411–47.

Thoits, P. A. 1995. Stress, coping, and social support processes: Where are we? What next? *Journal of Health and Social Behavior* (extra issue): 53–79.

Thoresen, C. E. 1999. Spirituality and health: Is there a relationship? *Journal of Health Psychology* 4: 291–300.

Uchino, B. N., J. T. Cacioppo, and J. K. Kiecolt-Glaser. 1996. The relationship between social support and physiological processes: A review with emphasis on underlying mechanisms and implications for health. *Psychological Bulletin* 119: 488–531.

Williams, D., and C. Collins. 1995. U.S. socioeconomic and racial differences in health: Patterns and explanations. *Annual Reviews of Sociology* 21: 349–86.

CHAPTER FIVE

Health, Well-Being, and Social Responsibility in the MIDUS Twin and Sibling Subsamples

Ronald C. Kessler, Stephen E. Gilman, Laura M. Thornton, and Kenneth S. Kendler

One of the special design features of MIDUS was the augmentation of the general population sample to include nationally representative subsamples of twins and nontwin sib-pairs (Kendler et al. 2000). The respondents in these subsamples were administered the same interview and questionnaires as other MIDUS respondents and also received a separate short interview that asked them about the extent to which they were treated similarly or differently from their sibs during their childhood years. Twins were also asked a series of questions about biological similarity that allowed us to classify them as either identical monozygotic (MZ) or nonidentical dizygotic (DZ). Finally, cheek scrape samples were collected from twins and sibs to extract DNA for future molecular genetic analyses. Although no results are yet available from the molecular genetic analyses, behavior genetic analyses have been completed for all three of the central MIDUS outcome domains of self-reported health, psychological well-being, and social responsibility. These behavior genetic analyses are the focus of this chapter.

The analyses reported here are limited to univariate investigations of heritability. Heritability is the percentage of variance in observed variables as a result of between-respondent variation in genes. Documentation of significant heritability is a necessary first step before performing more complex multivariate behavior genetic analyses and molecular genetic analyses. As described in more detail later in the chapter, the estimation of heritability in behavior genetic analyses is usually based on comparisons of the similarities of scores on observed variables in pairs of MZ twins versus DZ twins (Loehlin 1989). Greater similarities in the former than the latter are taken as evidence of genetic influences, because MZ twins share 100 percent of their genes identically by descent, whereas DZ twins share, on average, 50 percent of their genes. A variety of tests described later in this chapter are typically made to rule out competing explanations before concluding that genes are at work. These tests deal with the possibility that MZ twins might be treated more similarly than DZ twins or that

MZ twins might want to differentiate themselves more than DZ twins. When information from nontwin sib-pairs is included in these analyses, it becomes possible to evaluate the effects of being a twin, because nontwin sibs are the same as DZ twins in sharing an average of 50 percent of their genes. Finally, special types of structural equation models can be used to estimate the relative influences of genes and environment in explaining variance in specific outcomes and to perform multivariate analyses (Neale and Cardone 1992).

The Heritability of Self-Reported Health

Previous studies comparing MZ and DZ twins have consistently shown that a variety of physical illnesses are heritable. For example, in the NAS-NRC twin study (Jablon et al. 1967), Kendler and Robinette (1983) estimated that the heritability of ischemic heart disease is .37 and that the heritabilities of diabetes and hypertension are both .58. Similar findings have been reported by a number of other investigators on the basis of analyses of other twin samples and documenting significant heritabilities of ischemic heart disease (Carroll et al. 1985; Nora et al. 1980), hypertension (Borhani et al. 1976; Carroll et al. 1985; Lichtenstein et al. 2000; Selby et al. 1991), a variety of cancers (Hemminki, Dong, and Vaittinen 1999; Holm, Hauge, and Harvald 1980; Page et al. 1997; Partin et al. 1994; Schneider, Williams, and Chaganti 1986), and obesity (Allison et al. 1994, 1996; Fabsitz, Sholinsky, and Carmelli 1994; Selby et al. 1990; Stunkard 1991; Stunkard, Foch, and Hrubec 1986; Turula et al. 1990).

The heritability of self-reported health has been a subject of much less research. Measures of self-reported health, which are the health measures included in MIDUS, are important because they significantly predict survival even after adjusting for the effects of diagnosed health problems (Mossey and Shapiro 1982). In addition, summary measures of self-reported health are useful proxies for overall objective health, because self-reported health is strongly predicted by a combination of medical morbidities, physical and psychological symptoms, and measures of functional status (Barsky, Cleary, and Klerman 1992; Fylkesnes and Forde 1992; Jylha et al. 1986; Moum 1992).

Two aspects of self-reported health are considered in this chapter: self-rated health perceptions and functional status. Self-rated health perceptions were assessed with global questions that asked about overall health and then separately about physical health and mental health. Global questions like these are widely used in health surveys, although it is rare to ask separate questions for physical and mental health. We are aware of only one study that estimated the heritability of global self-rated health. This study was performed in four age cohorts of the Swedish Adoption/Twin Study of Aging (Harris et al. 1992). Evidence for statistically significant heritability was found in the older cohorts (.25) but not in the younger cohorts. This specification is interesting in light of previous evidence that there is a statistically significant inverse relationship between self-rated health and age, controlling for objective measures of physical health and psychological distress (Levkoff, Cleary, and Wetle 1987).

Functional status, the second aspect of self-reported health considered here, is the extent to which health limits routine daily activities. Two groups of investigators have estimated the heritability of functional status. Yashin et al. (1998) assessed multiple domains of functional status in a sample of Danish twins and showed that the correlations of these measures among twins were significantly stronger for MZ than DZ twins. The estimated heritability of functional status was approximately .30 for both males and females. Miles (1997), in a separate small study of MZ and DZ twins, documented the existence of significant familial aggregation of self-reported functional status based on substantial correlations between the scores of respondents with their cotwins. However, the sample was so small that no data were reported on differences in the correlations of MZ and DZ twin-pairs or on the estimated heritability of self-reported functional status.

In comparison with the scant amount of literature on the heritability of self-reported physical health, a large number of studies have investigated the familial aggregation of self-reported psychiatric disorders. These studies consistently find that most commonly occurring psychiatric disorders are moderately heritable (Kendler, Walters, et al. 1995). For depression, the mental disorder that has been the subject of the most extensive behavior genetic studies, the majority of familial aggregation of the disorder has consistently been shown to be the result of genes (e.g., Kendler et al. 1993; Kendler, Pedersen, et al. 1995; McGuffin et al. 1996). Genes also appear to play an important role in the familial aggregation of generalized anxiety disorder and phobias (Kendler et al. 1992a, 1992b). A number of studies have also estimated the heritability of dimensional scales of nonspecific psychological distress and have found consistent evidence of significant heritability (e.g., Kessler et al. 1992; Silberg et al. 1990).

The Heritability of Psychological Well-Being

Ryff (1989) proposed a multidimensional model of psychological well-being that included six dimensions: self-acceptance, personal growth, purpose in life, positive relations with others, environmental mastery, and autonomy. Although we are unaware of any studies that have examined the familial aggregation of these six dimensions as a set, there has been some research on the heritability of constructs related to two of these dimensions: self-esteem and social support.

Self-esteem is a personality characteristic that is strongly related to the Ryff dimension of self-acceptance. Two studies have examined the heritability of self-esteem using twin data (Kendler, Gardner, and Prescott 1998; Roy, Neale, and Kendler 1995). Both found that twin concordance for self-esteem was explained by a combination of genetic and individual-specific environmental factors. In the earlier of these studies, based on a sample of same-sex female twins, additive genetic factors accounted for 53 percent of the variance; in the latter study, based on same-sex and opposite-sex pairs, the estimated heritability was approximately .30 for both males and females. There was no evidence in either study that shared environmental influences were related to twin concordance for self-esteem.

Several studies have examined the heritability of various aspects of social support, including measures of support that are conceptually identical to the Ryff and Keyes dimension of positive relations with others (Bergeman et al. 1990; Kendler 1997; Kessler et al. 1992). Heritability estimates for measures of positive social relations have consistently been significant in these studies and in the range .25–.50.

Although they are less closely mapped onto individual dimensions in the Ryff model of psychological well-being, commonly studied dimensions of personality, such as neuroticism, extraversion, conscientiousness, openness to experience, and agreeableness, have all been shown to have heritabilities in the range .20–.40 (Heath et al. 1992; Loehlin 1992; Viken et al. 1994). This is indirectly relevant to the investigation of well-being because Schmutte and Ryff (1997) showed that these dimensions of personality are strong correlates of the well-being dimensions considered here.

The Heritability of Social Responsibility

Four domains of social responsibility proposed by Rossi (2001) are considered in this chapter: normative altruistic obligation, civic-job obligation, primary obligation, and contribution to others. The only previous studies that examined the heritability of any of these dimensions focused on the personality trait of altruism (Loehlin and Nichols 1976; Matthews et al. 1981; Rushton et al. 1984) and estimated the heritability of this construct to be between .40 and .72. As noted in the previous subsection, personality characteristics that one might expect to be related to social responsibility, such as conscientiousness and extraversion, have also been shown to be heritable. One might expect, therefore, that there is at least some evidence for significant heritability of social responsibility.

SAMPLE AND METHODS
Sampling Procedures for the Twin and Sib Samples

Twin-pairs were recruited using a separate two-part sampling design from the main MIDUS sample. The first part of the design involved screening a representative national sample of approximately 50,000 households for the presence of a twin. This was done as part of ongoing national omnibus surveys conducted by ICR/AUS Consultants and Bruskin Associates. Respondents who indicated that twins resided in the household or that they themselves were part of a twin-pair were asked permission to be contacted by our research team for inclusion in MIDUS. One-seventh (14.8 percent) of respondents reported the presence of a twin in the family, of which 60.0 percent gave permission to be contacted for the twin study.

The second part of the twin sample design involved student recruiters from the University of Michigan contacting the twins to participate in MIDUS. Cooperating twins were asked to provide contact information for their cotwins, who were also recruited by the students. The final response rate for twin pairs (i.e., the probability of obtaining complete interviews from both members of the pairs detected in the 50,000 screening interviews) varied dramatically, depending on whether the initial person contacted in the screening interview was a member of a twin pair (60.4 percent response rate) or the relative of twins (20.6 percent response rate). This dramatic variation is due to the fact that the relatives of twins were often reluctant to provide contact information, whereas the twins themselves were much more willing to participate in the survey and to contact their cotwins to encourage them to participate. The final MIDUS twin sample included 794 twin-pairs from 763 distinct families, with 29 families contributing two twin pairs and one family contributing three pairs.

Nontwin sib-pairs were recruited in a different manner. We began by sending a postcard to all MIDUS respondents, telling them of our interest in including siblings in the survey. The card asked respondents to provide contact information for their siblings and to communicate with their siblings about participation before a recruiter made a contact attempt. Because the family study was a secondary aim of the project, no follow-up procedures were employed to increase the low proportion of eligible

MIDUS respondents who provided names and addresses of their siblings (19.7 percent). As with the twin sample, though, the cooperation rate of siblings was much higher once they were contacted (69.3 percent). In total, 529 original MIDUS respondents returned the postcards, providing us with contact information for their siblings. There were 1372 siblings listed on these return postcards, 951 of whom completed the MIDUS survey. The number of additional siblings recruited from any single family ranged from one to six. These included one additional sibling from 272 families, two from 146 families, three from 75 families, four from 22 families, five from 10 families, and six from 4 families.

Of the 951 sibs who completed the MIDUS telephone interview, all but 81 also completed the mail questionnaires. As described later in the chapter, in the discussion of the analysis method, the data were analyzed for pairs of respondents. As a result, sibships in which complete data were collected on four or six sibs were divided up into either two or three randomly constituted pairs. We deleted the data from one random sib in sibships with complete data on three, five, or seven sibs. The remaining data in the sibships that originally had five or seven sibs were then organized into two or three random sib-pairs. The resulting dataset contained 1220 sibs that were divided into 610 sibling pairs. Although the majority of sibling pairs came from distinct families, there were 82 families (16.1 percent) that contributed two pairs of siblings, and 9 families that contributed three pairs of siblings.

Zygosity Determination

At the time of initial recruitment into the survey, same-sex twins were administered a number of standard questions about whether they were identical (MZ) or fraternal (DZ). (Opposite-sex twins are always DZ.) None of these questions yields a perfect assessment of zygosity. The latter can only be obtained by performing molecular genetic analysis. Because the molecular genetic analysis of the MIDUS twin data did not begin until well after we performed the initial behavior genetic analyses, a classification rule was developed based on comparison with data from members of the Virginia Twin Registry (VTR) who were previously included in molecular genetic analyses. Eight self-report measures about whether the twins were identical or fraternal were included both in MIDUS and in the VTR. These variables were used to estimate a logistic regression equation in the VTR data to predict zygosity that used a classification of MZ and DZ based on molecular genetic analysis. The coefficients from this prediction equation were then used to generate predicted probabilities of being

MZ versus DZ in the MIDUS data. A strong classification (defined as a predicted probability of being MZ either less than 10 percent or greater than 90 percent) was obtained for 86 percent of the pairs, while a likely classification (defined as a predicted probability of being MZ outside of the 40 percent to 60 percent range) was obtained for an additional 10.5 percent. The remaining 3.5 percent were excluded from the study.

Measures

Four measures were used as indicators of self-reported health. Three focused on self-rated health perceptions and the fourth on functional status. The first of the three self-rated health measures asked about overall health without distinguishing mental and physical. The wording was as follows: "How would you rate your health these days on a 0–10 scale where 0 is the worst possible health and 10 is perfect health?" Separate single-item questions were then asked about rating physical health and mental health as either poor, fair, good, very good, or excellent (coded 1–5). The functional status scale was made up of responses to a question about how much health problems "limit you in doing each of the following activities." Response categories were a lot, some, a little, and not at all (coded 1–4). Seven representative intermediate activities of daily living were included in the assessment (e.g., bending, kneeling, or stooping; lifting or carrying groceries). Responses were summed into a scale with a 7–28 range. All four self-reported health measures were standardized to have a mean of 0 and variance of 1 in the nationally representative component of the MIDUS sample. Means and variances were not constrained to be equal across the twin and sib subsamples, making it possible to study between-subsample differences in means and variances.

Short forms of the six Ryff–Keyes psychological well-being scales (Ryff and Keyes 1995) were used to measure psychological well-being. As noted in the introduction, these six dimensions (with illustrative items in parentheses) include the following: (1) self-acceptance ("I like most parts of my personality"); (2) personal growth ("I think it is important to have new experiences that challenge how I think about myself and the world"); (3) purpose in life ("Some people wander aimlessly through life, but I am not one of them"); (4) positive relations with others ("People would describe me as a giving person, willing to share my time with others"); (5) environmental mastery ("In general, I feel that I am in charge of the situation in which I live"); and (6) autonomy ("I judge myself by what I think is important, not by the values of what others think is important"). The questions asked respondents to indicate how strongly they agreed or disagreed with each of the statements. Response options included agreeing or disagreeing either strongly, somewhat, or only a little. A "don't know" category was also included as the midpoint on the 1–7 scale, with 1 being "strongly agree" and 7 being "strongly disagree." Each of the six dimensions was measured with either three or four items that were selected on the basis of extensive pilot work to be optimal indicators of the more extensive scales developed by Ryff and Keyes (1995). As with the measures of self-reported health, these scales were standardized to have a mean of 0 and a variance of 1 in the nationally representative component of the MIDUS sample.

Social responsibility, finally, was assessed with scales developed by Rossi (2001) to tap four key dimensions of social responsibility. The first three of these four dimensions were assessed by asking respondents to "rate how much obligation you would feel" in each of a number of hypothetical situations on a 0–10 scale, where 0 means "no obligation at all" and 10 means "a very great obligation." The scales with representative items in parentheses include the following: (1) normative altruistic obligation ("to volunteer time or money to social causes you support"); (2) normative civic and job obligation ("to testify in court about an accident you witnessed"); and (3) normative primary obligation ("to raise the child of a close friend if the friend died"). Four items were used to measure each of the first two dimensions and eight to measure the third. The fourth measure was a singe-item question about (4) contributions to others ("How would you rate your contribution to the welfare and well-being of other people these days?"). Responses were recorded on a 0–10 self-anchoring scale, where 0 represented "the worst" and 10 represented "the best." As in the health and psychological well-being domains, each social responsibility scale was standardized to have a mean of 0 and a variance of 1 in the nationally representative component of the MIDUS sample.

Analysis Methods

The logic of behavior genetic analysis of twin data hinges on comparing similarities in measured variables of MZ twins, who share 100 percent of their genes identical by descent, and other sib-pairs, usually same-sex DZ pairs, who share, on average, 50 percent of their genes. Differences in similarity are interpreted as the result of genetic influences (Loehlin 1989). This interpretation implicitly assumes that environmental factors are not more similar for MZ twins than for other sib-pairs. This "equal-environment" assumption is plausible for narrowly defined environmental exposures, such as fluoride in water or lead in house paint.

However, the assumption can be called into question for broader environmental variables, such as preferential treatment of one twin by parents, which might be less likely to occur in MZ pairs than in other sib-pairs (Rowe 1983). As described in the first part of the results section, a special investigation of this issue was undertaken before computing correlations. In addition, a special analysis was undertaken of a second plausible possibility that could lead to differential nongenetic influences on differential similarities of MZ twins in comparison to other sib-pairs: the possibility of behavioral differentiation based on twin status (Plomin and Daniels 1987). The notion here is that MZ twins, because of their physical similarities, might be more inclined to differentiate themselves than other sibs might be.

Once the equal-environment assumption and twin differentiation assumption were investigated and either adjusted for (in the case of the equal-environment assumption, which, as described in the first part of the results section, was found to be violated) or shown not to be a problem (in the case of the twin differentiation hypothesis), twin and sibling resemblance on the outcome measures was assessed in two ways. The first consisted of a simple comparison of Pearson correlations for similarities in the outcomes among MZ twin-pairs, same-sex DZ pairs, and same-sex nontwin sib-pairs. If strong genetic influences were at work in explaining variance in these measures in the population, we would expect the correlations to be much larger for MZ pairs than for same-sex DZ and sibling pairs, but we would not expect to find any difference between same-sex DZ and nontwin sib-pairs. If being a twin itself affects similarity for reasons unrelated to genes, then we would expect to find stronger correlations in same-sex DZ pairs than nontwin pairs. If the relevant genes were not the same in males and females, we would expect higher correlations in same-sex versus opposite-sex pairs. It is also possible that the genes are the same but have different effects in same-sex male versus same-sex female pairs.

The second method used to study twin and sibling resemblance was linear structural equation analysis (Neale and Cardone 1992). The goal was to reproduce the within-pair variances and covariances of the eight subsamples with maximum parsimony. The eight subsamples included separate male and female same-sex MZ, DZ, and nontwin sib-pairs as well as opposite-sex DZ and nontwin pairs. There are three observed pieces of information in each of the eight matrices (two variances and one covariance), for a total of twenty-four pieces of information that we seek to reproduce. We began the modeling by assuming that four broad classes of influences contribute to these observed variances and covariances: (1) additive genes, which we denote as A ("additive" in the sense that we assume the effect to be twice as strong for MZ pairs than other pairs because MZ twins share 100 percent of their genes rather than the average of 50 percent for other sib-pairs); (2) common environmental influences, which we denote as C, that affect the similarity of all twin-pairs and sib-pairs equally; (3) special twin environment influences, which we denote as T, that lead twins (whether MZ or DZ) to be more similar to each other than nontwins are; and (4) an individual-specific environmental component, which we denote as E, that represents all the unique experiences an individual has that are not shared with his or her siblings. The models were subsequently expanded to allow for gender differences in parameter values as well as for special genetic (A′) and common environmental (E′) effects that are different for males than females. All models were fit using the Mx software package (Neale 1991). Comparative model fit was assessed using both the Akaike information criterion (AIC; Akaike 1987) and the Bayesian information criterion (BIC; Schwarz 1978). However, because these two criteria always yielded the same conclusions about the best-fitting models in this particular investigation, only the AIC is reported here. The model with the lowest AIC is defined as having the best balance of fit and parsimony.

RESULTS
The Equal-Environment Assumption

Given the importance of the equal-environmental assumption to the accurate interpretation of twin data, we began by testing the validity of this assumption. This was done by using a standard method that begins with questions included in the twin questionnaire that asked twins about three aspects of environmental similarity during their childhood years: how often they played together, how often they were dressed identically, and how often they were placed in the same classroom in school. We recognize that these are only superficial marker items of the complex ways in which twins are treated similarly or differently. Nonetheless, items similar to these have been shown to be sensitive in previous research comparing the environments of MZ and DZ twins.

We found that MIDUS MZ twins repeatedly reported significantly greater similarities than did same-sex DZ twins on all three measures, which is consistent with the previous research. This was expected. However, the research question of real interest was whether these greater similarities in childhood experiences are relevant to the outcomes under consideration in this chapter. Not all environmental similarities are meaningful ones. If, for example, being dressed in identical clothing as children is unrelated to adult health, well-being, and social responsibility, then the greater similarity of MZ than DZ in this experience is irrelevant for our purposes. To evaluate this issue, we estimated a series of linear regression equations in which MZ-DZ differences in similarity on outcome variables were related to differences in similarity of childhood experiences. This analysis of differences in similarity required us to begin by computing the absolute value of within-pair differences on the outcome measures and using these difference scores as dependent variables in regression analyses that treated the twin-pairs as units of analysis. Predictors included a dummy variable coded 1 for MZ pairs and 0 for DZ pairs and the average within-pair scores on the three questions regarding similarity of childhood environmental experiences. The critical test was whether these three scores significantly predicted within-pair similarities in the outcomes after controlling for zygosity.

We would expect a mostly positive sign pattern of associations of the scores with the outcomes if the equal-environment assumption were violated, because similarity in childhood experience should predict similarity in the outcomes. As shown in table 1, a pattern of this sort was found with 27 (64 percent) of the 42 coefficients positive. However, this sign pattern was confined to having similar playmates (86 percent of coefficients positive), while there was no meaningful preponderance of positive coefficients for the effects of being in the same school classroom (57 percent) or dressing identically (50 percent). Consistent with the sign patterns, 36 percent of the coefficients for similar playmates are significant at the .05 level, and all of these significant coefficients are positive in sign. Only 7 percent of the coefficients for the other predictors are significant, and the sign pattern of these coefficients is inconsistent.

On the basis of these results, we concluded that the equal-environment assumption is violated for the outcomes considered here. It is worth noting that this violation is small in magnitude, with correlations averaging only .07 for the relationships between similarity in childhood playmates and similarity in the outcomes. Nonetheless, because the childhood experience measures are nothing more than crude indicators rather than fine-grained measures of environmental similarity, the disattenuated correlation could be substantial. In an effort to adjust for this bias to the extent possible in the data, we weighted the twin data so that the distribution of the MZ twins on responses to the question about childhood playmates was set equal to the distribution found among same-sex DZ twins. All further

TABLE 1 Assessment of the Equal-Environment Assumption in
Same-Sex Twin-Pairs

	Childhood Similarities			
	Playmates	School Class	Dress	$F^a_{3,582}$
Self-reported health				
Health perception	.11*	−.03	−.05	1.85
Self-rated physical health	.12*	−.03	−.03	1.59
Self-rated mental health	.08	.05	.07	3.96*
Functional status	.13*	−.01*	−.09	4.34*
Social responsibility				
Normative altruism obligation	.09	.00	.01	1.00
Normative civic and job obligation	.04	.13*	.03	5.53*
Normative primary obligation	.15*	−.05	−.01	2.42
Contribution to others	−.08	.00	.00	0.65
Psychological well-being				
Autonomy	.09	.01	−.03	1.04
Environmental mastery	.05	.50	−.04	1.06
Personal growth	.05	−.05	.06	1.55
Positive relations with others	.08	.07	.02	3.08*
Purpose in life	.14*	.05	−.01	2.35
Self-acceptance	−.02	.06	.05	2.06

Notes: Results are based on a series of fourteen separate linear regression equations with twin-pairs as the unit of analyses, each including a dummy variable for zygosity and the three childhood similarity measures to predict the absolute value of the difference in the outcome scores between cotwins. A total of 594 twin-pairs were included in the analysis. The coefficients reported in the table are standardized linear regression coefficients.

[a]The *F*-tests evaluate the joint significance of the three childhood similarity measures in predicting the outcome.

*Significant at the .05 level, two-sided test.

results reported in this chapter are based on analyses of these weighted data. To the extent that this adjustment was inadequate, the analyses presented later in the chapter overestimate the effects of genes because excess similarities of MZ pairs in comparison to DZ pairs will be interpreted as the result of genetic influences rather than environmental influences.

Behavioral Differentiation Based on Twin Status

Another important issue to consider before turning to an analysis of genetic influences is the possibility that MZ twins might be more likely than DZ twins to make themselves distinct from their cotwins by consciously selecting environmental experiences that are different from those selected by their identical brother or sister. If one twin chooses to play baseball, in such a scenario, the other would avoid baseball at all costs. If this kind of systematic differentiation occurs, it would violate the assumptions of the models considered here by introducing a systematic

TABLE 2 Within-Pair Correlations of

	MZ	
	Male	Female
Self-reported health		
Health perception	.26*	.38*
Self-rated physical health	.20*	.38*
Self-rated mental health	.18*	.26*
Functional status	.19*	.31*
Social responsibility		
Normative altruism obligation	.35*	.26*
Normative civic and job obligation	.37*	.45*
Normative primary obligation	.14*	.26*
Contribution to others	.25*	.07
Psychological well-being		
Autonomy	.30*	.39*
Environmental mastery	.35*	.37*
Personal growth	.24*	.47*
Positive relations with others	.35*	.35*
Purpose in life	.22*	.39*
Self-acceptance	.39*	.47*
(*n*)	(149)	(186)

*Significant at the .05 level, two-sided test.

negative correlation within MZ pairs. This bias, in turn, would lead to an underestimation of genetic effects. We would not expect a direct bias of this sort with respect to the health outcomes considered here. There is no reason to believe, for example, that one cotwin will decide to choose poor mental health to differentiate himself from his mentally healthy cotwin, but such a possibility is more plausible for some aspects of well-being and social responsibility. For example, if one twin in a pair takes on the role of leader and develops a very high level of environmental mastery, this might lead his cotwin to respond by taking on the role of follower and developing a low level of environmental mastery. Similar processes could occur with respect to such aspects of social responsibility as normative primary obligations (i.e., one twin becomes the family caregiver, while the cotwin develops a low sense of familial obligation).

We know that differentiation processes of this sort occur in families (Plomin and Daniels 1987). However, as with the equal-environment assumption, the important question for our purposes is whether these processes are more pronounced for MZ twins than for DZ twins or nontwin sibs in ways that affect the outcomes of consideration here. To evaluate this question, we turned to an inspection of the variances of the outcome measures. Greater within-pair differentiation among MZ twins will lead

Outcomes Stratified by Zygosity and Sex

DZ			Nontwin Sibs		
Male	Female	Opposite	Male	Female	Opposite
.22*	.30*	.05	.11	.15*	−.01
.26*	.33*	.12	.10	.38*	.09
.22*	.18*	.10	.17	.09	.10
.24*	.34*	.17*	.15	.43*	.17*
.25*	.38*	.08	.13	.16*	.13*
.27*	.26*	.11	−.02	.18*	.24*
.20*	.33*	.11	.11	.09	.06
.10	.06	.10	.12	.07	.12*
.01	.13	−.03	.14	.03	.04
.07	.04	.12	.21*	.06	
.27*	.29*	.13	.18*	.05	.28*
.21*	.15*	.06	.03	.10	.22*
.06	.30*	.06	.10	.12	−.16*
.10	.16*	.08	.03	−.02	.16*
(103)	(156)	(200)	(128)	(192)	(290)

to variances being higher, even if means are similar for MZ twins in comparison to DZ twins and nontwin siblings. An analysis was performed that examined means and variances of the ten outcome variables within sex for MZ, same-sex DZ, and same-sex nontwin sib-pairs. No evidence was found for meaningful differences either in means or in variances across these three subsamples for any of the outcomes either for male pairs or for female pairs. On the basis of this consistent result, we put aside concerns that greater behavioral differentiation among identical twins might introduce bias into our analyses of these outcome domains.

Correlations

The within-pair correlations for measures in all three outcome domains are reported in table 2 separately by sex for MZ twins (weighted to adjust for violation of the equal-environment assumption), DZ twins, and nontwin sib-pairs. Conventional twin analyses work largely with same-sex pairs of MZ and DZ twins and generally do not distinguish male pairs from female pairs. As a result, there is only one critical comparison in such analyses: between MZ pairs and DZ pairs. As described in the section on analysis methods, evidence of higher correlations in the former than the latter are taken to mean that genetic influences are at work based on the assumption that greater similarity in genetic makeup is the only factor that differentiates MZ pairs from DZ pairs (i.e., the assumption that environmental similarity is identical for MZ and DZ pairs).

The results in the first four rows of table 2 present comparisons between MZ and same-sex DZ pairs by sex. Every correlation is positive, and 84 percent are significant at the .05 level, showing that there is meaningful familial aggregation for these outcomes. However, the correlations are modest in magnitude, with a range of .01–.47, and the majority in the range of .20–.40. There is mixed evidence for genetic effects. The weakest evidence is in the self-reported health domain for males and the social responsibility domain for females, in each of which only one of the four correlations is higher for MZ than DZ pairs. The strongest evidence is in the psychological well-being domain, where five of six correlations are higher for MZ rather than DZ male pairs and six of six for MZ rather than DZ female pairs. It is important to note that the well-being MZ–DZ correlation differences are quite substantial in most cases, with eight of the twelve MZ correlations more than twice as large as the DZ correlations. Differences as large as this are important if they are the result of more than sampling error, because they go beyond the 2:1 ratio we would expect on the basis of additive genetic effects, raising the possibility of nonadditive genetic effects. Evidence for genetic effects is intermediate in the self-reported health domain among females and the social responsibility domain for males, in each of which three of the four correlations are higher for MZ than DZ pairs, but with differences almost always less than a 2:1 ratio.

The inclusion of nontwin sib-pairs in the analysis also allows us to evaluate the environmental effects of being a twin by comparing correlations for MZ twins with those for nontwin sibs. This can be done for each of the 14 outcomes separately for male, female, and opposite-sex pairs, for a total of 42 comparisons. An inspection of the last six columns of table 2 shows a clear trend for higher correlations among same-sex twins than same-sex nontwin sibs (71 percent of comparisons), but not among opposite-sex twins compared with opposite-sex sibs (29 percent of comparisons). One potentially important biasing factor here is that cotwins are always the same age, but nontwin siblings differ in age. To control for this potential bias, we recomputed the sib-pair correlations for pairs that do not differ by more than three years in age. The same general pattern continued to hold as the one seen in table 2.

It is interesting to compare differences in correlations to get a rough sense of the relative importance of genetic influences (MZ versus same-sex DZ) compared with environmental influences of being a twin (DZ versus nontwin sibs). In the case of self-rated health among males, for example, the MZ–DZ difference is .04 (.26–.22), suggesting that there is no meaningful genetic effect on this outcome. The DZ-sib difference, in comparison, is .11 (.22–.11), suggesting that environmental experiences associated with being a twin have a modest influence on perceptions of self-rated health. A systematic comparison of this sort across all fourteen outcomes both for male and female same-sex pairs shows that the MZ–DZ difference is larger than the DZ-sib difference in roughly half the cases, while the DZ-sib difference is larger than the MZ–DZ difference in the other half. This rough comparison suggests that environmental effects of being a twin are as common as genetic effects for this set of outcomes.

Heritability

A comprehensive series of structural equation models was fit to the eight 2 × 2 covariance matrices of each outcome measure. An illustration is presented in table 3 for one of the outcomes—self-rated mental health. A total of twenty-three models were fit to the covariance matrices for this outcome. These represent all logically possible models that could be identified and were substantively plausible for these data. The most complex model, with eleven parameters, is model AA'DD'TE. This model allows for additive (A) and nonadditive (D) genetic effects that are the same for men and women as well as for sex-specific additive (A') and nonadditive (D') genetic effects, sex-specific effects of being a twin (T), environmental effects that are unique to individuals (E), and constant variance across subsamples. Other less complex models included subsets of these parameters either with or without a common environment (C) parameter.

It is noteworthy that none of these models included both nonadditive genetic effects (D) and common environmental effects (C). This is because nonadditive genetic effects only make sense to estimate when the MZ correlation is more than twice as large as the same-sex DZ correlation. In cases of this sort, a model that includes all additive environmental and genetic effects always estimates a value of 0 for C. Importantly, to identify a model including D, it is necessary to constrain C to some fixed value, which is usually set to 0. It is important to note that there can be situations in which nonadditive genetic effects and common environmental effects are both at work. However, a model including parameters for both of these influences cannot be estimated with the data available to us here. As a result, a model that includes a D effect should be interpreted as indicating the existence of nonadditive genetic effects but leaving uncertain whether or not there are also common environmental effects.

TABLE 3 Summary Evaluations of

Model	χ^2	df	AIC	Male				
				A	A'	C	C'	D
AA'CTE	16.3	15	−13.7	.02	.00	.16		
ACC'TE	16.3	15	−13.7	.02		.16	.00	
ACTE	16.3	16	−15.7	.02		.16		
ACTE[a]	18.0	20	−22.0	.17		.02		
ACE	17.1	18	−18.9	.05		.15		
ACE[a]	18.8	21	−23.2	.23		.01		
ATE	17.7	18	−18.3	.24*				
ATE[a]	18.1	21	−23.9	.20*				
CTE	17.6	18	−18.4			.19*		
CTE[a]	19.4	21	−22.6			.11*		
AE	18.7	20	−21.3	.23*				
AE[a]	18.8	22	−25.2	.25*				
CE	22.1	20	−17.9			.16*		
CE[a]	22.2	22	−21.8			.15*		
TE	26.9	20	−13.1					
TE[a]	27.1	22	−16.9					
E	53.9	22	9.9					
E[a]	53.9	23	7.9					
AA'DD'TE	17.6	14	−10.4	.19	.05			.00
ADTE	17.6	16	−14.4	.24				.00
ADTE[a]	18.1	20	−21.9	.20				.00
ADE	18.3	18	−17.7	.25*				.00
ADE[a]	18.8	21	−23.2	.25*				.00

Notes: Results are based on a series of twenty three separate structural equation models, each of which attempted to fit the covariance structure of the eight subsample matrices with the series of parameters specified in the first column of the table. The AE model is the best-fitting model based on the AIC. A, additive genetic effect; A', sex-specific additive genetic effect; D, nonadditive genetic effect; D', sex-specific nonadditive genetic effect; C, common environmental effect; C', sex-specific common environmental effect; T, environmental effect of being a twin; and E, individual-specific environmental effect.

[a]Models in which parameters were constrained to be equal for males and females.
*Significant at the .05 level, two-sided test.

The best-fitting model for self-rated mental health is the AE model that constrains the coefficients to have the same values for males and females. The AIC of −25.2 for this model is considerably lower than that for any other model, indicating that the preference for this model over others is not sensitive to minor differences in model fit. The estimate for A is .25, which means that 25 percent of the variance in self-rated mental health is estimated to be the result of additive genetic effects. The remaining 75 percent of the variance is estimated to be the result of individual-specific

Univariate Model Fit

			Explained Variance				
				Female			
D'	T	E	A	C	D	T	E
	.03	.79*	.18	.01		.07	.74*
	.03	.79*	.18	.01		.07	.74*
	.03	.79*	.18	.01		.07	.74*
	.05	.76*	.17	.02		.05	.76*
		.79*	.25*	.01			.74*
		.76*	.23	.01			.76*
	.00	.75*	.17*			.09	.74*
	.05	.75*	.20*			.05	.75*
	.00	.81*		.07		.15	.78*
	.09	.81*		.11*		.09	.81*
		.77*	.26*				.74*
		.75*	.25*				.75*
		.84*		.15*			.85*
		.85*		.15*			.85*
	.18*	.82*				.20*	.80*
	.19*	.81*				.19*	.81*
		1.00*					1.00*
		1.00*					1.00*
.00	.01	.75*	.16		.03	.08	.73*
	.01	.75*	.14		.05	.08	.73*
	.05	.75*	.20		.00	.05	.75*
		.75*	.18		.10		.72*
		.75*	.25*		.00		.75*

environmental effects. It is instructive to go back to the fourth line in table 2 to compare the correlations with the model parameters in order to see the way in which constraints are being imposed. The fact that sex-specific effects are assumed not to exist in the best-fitting AE model means that the three male versus female same-sex pair comparisons in table 2 were judged to be insignificant as a set. This, in turn, means that the .18 MZ male correlation and the .26 MZ female correlation were averaged in the model to a correlation of approximately .22. The fact that the environmental effect of being a twin is assumed not to exist in the AE model means that the DZ and nontwin sibling correlations were also averaged and treated as a single correlation. A comparison of the averaged MZ correlation (.22) and the pooled correlation for the other six subsamples (.12) yields a ratio close to 2:1, which is consistent with a genetic effect that linearly extrapolates to a common environmental effect of 0. In other words, if 100 percent of genetic similarity leads to a

TABLE 4 Model Statistics and Standardized Estimates

	Model	χ^2	df	AIC
Self-reported health				
Health perception	ATE	22.9	18	−13.2
	ADE	22.9	18	−13.1
Self-rated physical health	CTE	16.0	18	−20.0
Self-rated mental health	AE[a]	18.8	22	−25.2
Functional status	CE	60.3	20	20.3
	CTE	55.7	18	19.7
Social responsibility				
Normative altruism obligation	AE[a]	31.2	22	−12.8
	CTE[a]	29.6	21	−12.4
Normative civic and job obligation	AE[a]	55.4	22	11.4
Normative primary obligation	CTE[a]	17.5	21	−24.5
Contribution to others	CE	11.9	20	−28.1
	AE	11.2	20	−28.8
Psychological well-being				
Autonomy	ADE	17.1	18	−18.9
Environmental mastery	ADE[a]	26.7	21	−15.3
Personal growth	AE	29.5	20	−10.5
	AE[a]	33.2	22	−10.8
Positive relations with others	AE[a]	12.3	22	−31.7
Purpose in life	AE	13.7	20	−26.3
Self-acceptance	ADE[a]	27.3	21	−14.7

Notes: Best-fitting models were selected using the AIC. See footnote b in table 3 for definitions of symbols. Additive and nonadditive genetic variance components are combined in a single measure of heritability (H).

[a]Models in which parameters were constrained to be equal across sexes.

* Significant at the .05 level, two-sided test.

.22 correlation and 50 percent genetic similarity reduces the correlation by .10 (i.e., from .22 for MZ to .12 for all other sib-pairs), then a linear extrapolation would lead to the conclusion that 0 percent genetic similarity would reduce the correlation by another .10, resulting in an effect of common environment equal to .02 (i.e., the observed .12 correlation in the pooled non-MZ subsamples minus the extrapolated .10 based on a comparison between the averaged MZ correlation) and the pooled non-MZ correlation. An effect of .02 is nonsignificant with a sample of the size analyzed here, leading to the conclusion that only additive genetic effects are involved in the familial aggregation of self-reported mental health.

The same model-fitting logic was applied to the remaining outcomes, and a best-fitting model was selected for each. Summary results are

of Best-Fitting Models for Each Outcome

Explained Variance							
Male				Female			
H	C	T	E	H	C	T	E
.00		.26*	.74*	.37*		.03	.60*
.34*			.66*	.40*			.60*
	.03	.18*	.78*		.37*	.00	.63*
.25*			.75*	.25*			.75*
	.12*		.88*		.36*		.64*
	.07*	.17*	.76*		.37*	.00	.63*
.30*			.70*	.30*			.70*
	.15*	.09	.76*		.15*	.09	.76*
.37*			.63*	.37*			.63*
	.08*	.12*	.80*		.08*	.12*	.80*
	.17*		.83*		.07*		.93*
.25*			.75*	.11*			.89*
.27			.73*	.37*			.63*
.33*			.67*	.33*			.67*
.33*			.67*	.43*			.57*
.38*			.62*	.38*			.62*
.32*			.68*	.32*			.68*
.19*			.81*	.39*			.61*
.41			.59*	.41*			.59*

reported in table 4. In cases where the best-fitting model had an AIC less than one point lower than that of competing models, the results for the competing models are also reported in the summary table. Results are reported for a total of nineteen models across the fourteen outcomes. Consistent with the pattern seen in table 2, evidence for a statistically significant genetic effect is more consistent in the psychological well-being domain (100 percent of models) than in either the self-reported health domain (50 percent) or the social responsibility domain (50 percent). The magnitudes of the significant genetic effects—with additive and nonadditive effect size estimates combined in the table into a total heritability (H) estimate—are fairly consistent across the three domains: .25–.40 for self-reported health, .11–.43 for psychological well-being, and .25–.37 for social responsibility. It is important to note that in interpreting this range, measurement error is included in the total estimate of variance. If only 70–80 percent of the variance in the observed outcomes is reliable, heritabilities in the .11–.43 range represent between 14 percent and 61 percent of true score variance.

Even with adjustments for plausible levels of measurement error, the majority of variance in all but a few of the outcomes is estimated to be environmental. In only 50 percent of the models, however, is this variance estimated to be responsible for a significant part of familial aggregation (i.e., significant C or T) effects. In the others, only individual specific environmental influences appear to be at work. It is noteworthy, though, that a significant nonadditive genetic effect is found in one-third of the models that omit common environmental effects. As noted in the last subsection, it is not possible to estimate nonadditive genetic effects and common environmental effects in the same model, given the structure of the data being analyzed here. As a result, the possibility of common environmental effects cannot be ruled out in these cases.

More than half of the best-fitting models include variance estimates that are significantly different for males and females. In general, the heritability estimates are larger for females than males (five of six) in sex-specific models that include significant genetic effects. There is no consistent pattern of sex differences, in comparison, in the magnitudes of common environmental effects in sex-specific models that include sig-nificant common environmental components (three with males larger and three with females larger). Taken together, these results mean that the effects of unique environmental experiences are generally larger for males than females in models that allow sex differences in parameter estimates (seven of nine).

Discussion

The results are broadly consistent with previous studies in finding significant heritabilities of self-rated health and certain aspects of psychological well-being. However, the results also go beyond these ear-lier studies both in specifying some previously documented associations and in finding significant heritabilities for aspects of well-being and so-cial responsibility that have not previously been the subject of behavior genetic research.

Before turning to a comment on the specific results, it is important to note that three of the outcomes in table 4 have two models that have very similar AIC values, although the parameters in these models are very different in their implications. These three outcomes are health per-ception, normative altruistic obligation, and contribution to others. One model for each of these outcomes includes a term for a genetic effect but no term for a common environmental effect, while the other model includes a term for a common environmental effect but not for a genetic effect. This kind of situation often occurs in analyses of data obtained from moderately sized samples in which there are true modest effects of both genes and common environment. In cases of this sort, there is not enough statistical power to detect both effects, and stochastic factors can lead to one model being favored over the other. It is important to keep this sensitivity of results in mind when interpreting the findings.

The finding that the MIDUS global measure of self-rated health is heritable is consistent with previous research reviewed in the introduction. However, unlike previous studies, MIDUS also included separate questions about self-rated physical and mental health. Only self-rated mental health was significantly heritable. It is understandable that self-rated mental health would be heritable in light of the substantial evidence for the heritability of psychiatric disorders that was reviewed in the introduction. However, the failure to find significant heritability of self-rated physical health is surprising in light of the fact, noted in the introduction, that a number of chronic physical illnesses are known to be heritable. Apparently the perceptions that influence self-rated physical health are sufficiently independent of heritable physical illnesses not to show significant heritability.

Given this important difference in the determinants of self-rated physical health and self-rated mental health, it would seem wise for future health surveys to keep the two measures separate rather than combine them into a single global self-rated health question. The Center for Disease Control's Behavioral Risk Factor Surveillance System Survey is currently the only major ongoing health survey in the United States that asks separately about self-rated physical health and mental health. It would be useful if other major health surveys followed this lead in expanding the assessment of self-rated health to distinguish physical and mental components.

Our failure to find that self-reported functional status is heritable is inconsistent with the one study reviewed in the introduction that investigated this issue. As with self-rated physical health, this failure is surprising in light of evidence that many of the serious physical illnesses that are largely responsible for impairments in the domains assessed in MIDUS (e.g., difficulties climbing a flight of stairs or carrying a bag of groceries) are heritable. It is conceivable that the wide age range of the sample is at least partly responsible for this result, because the causes of limitations in physical functioning among younger people tend to be acute (e.g., a broken leg) and environmentally determined, thus diminishing the effects of heritable factors.

The finding that all six dimensions of psychological well-being are heritable extends the results of previous studies that documented heritabilities of some correlates of these dimensions. Importantly, common environmental effects are absent for all six measures of well-being. Although environmental factors are largely responsible for variance in all the aspects of well-being, these factors are associated with unique environmental experiences rather than with experiences that sibs share in common.

The finding of significant heritabilities for social responsibility, finally, is consistent with evidence reviewed in the introduction for the heritability of altruism. It is interesting to note that genetic effects were limited to perceptions of responsibility regarding community and civic life (normative altruistic obligation and normative civic and job obligation). There was no genetic influence, in comparison, on feelings of responsibility to close friends and relatives (normative primary obligation). Familial factors of a nongenetic kind played the key role for these more personal obligations. However, the caution noted at the beginning of this section has to be invoked in considering this specification. With a sample of the size available here and both genetic and common environmental effects of modest size, stochastic factors alone could explain this seeming specification. Independent replication is needed before concluding that social responsibility to close loved ones is less heritable or more strongly affected by common environmental factors than is community or civic social responsibility.

We are unaware of any research that has systematically investigated male-female differences in heritabilities in these outcome domains. It is noteworthy that the higher heritabilities for women than men are largely concentrated in the psychological well-being domain, with the largest difference being the much greater heritability among women than men for purpose in life. An obvious speculation is that this might be related to gender differences in role expectations involving affiliative rather than instrumental activities. There is no way to evaluate this possibility, though, with the MIDUS data. Serious investigation of this topic would require information to be obtained about differences in the nature of the purpose perceived by male and female respondents who report that they have a strong purpose in life. An expanded investigation of this sort in future research is warranted in light of the strong gender difference in the heritability of purpose in life.

Caution is needed in interpreting the heritability estimates presented here because of violation of the equal-environment assumption. Although we attempted to compensate for this violation by weighting the data, this was only a rough adjustment because of the coarseness of the measures of within-pair similarity in childhood environment. Some sense of the magnitude of the uncertainty introduced by this problem can be obtained by evaluating the implications of the equal-environment assumption for the estimation of genetic effects. This is possible because it is not necessary to assume that the environments of MZ and DZ twins are equally similar to identify the models examined here. It is merely necessary to assume that the MZ : DZ environmental similarity ratio (ESR) is known. Although this ratio is set to 1 : 1 when the equal-environment assumption is made, it can also be set to any other fixed value. If ESR is set to 2 : 1, then the A and C parameters are collinear, in which case separate effects of genes and common environment cannot be estimated. When ESR is less than 2 : 1, however, separate estimates of A and C can be obtained.

To investigate the sensitivity of the results reported here to the equal-environment assumption, best-fitting models that contained significant genetic effects were re-estimated a number of times, with ESR values varied across the range between 1.0 and 2.0. As expected, the estimated heritability of the outcomes decreased and the standard error of the heritability estimate increased as the ESR approached 2 : 1. Most heritability estimates became nonsignificant when ESR exceeded 1.5 : 1. This means that the assumption that genetic influences exist hinges on our willingness to assume that within-pair environmental similarity is less than 50 percent greater among MZ twins than among non-MZ twins and sibs. This assumption has to take into account the fact that genetic similarity of MZ twins can elicit similarities in environmental response that should be considered aspects of genetic influence rather than aspects of environmental exposure (Scarr and McCartney 1983).

It is possible to get a more direct estimate of the effects of common environments net of genes by working with research designs that vary environments and hold genes constant. The design used in this chapter, in comparison, varied genetic similarity (i.e., MZ twins who share 100 percent of their genes compared with DZ twins and sibs who share an average of 50 percent of their genes) and treated environmental similarity as a residual category. An example of a design that varies environments and controls genes is one that compares half-sibs (who share 25 percent of their genes, on average) with pairs of cousins who are the offspring of identical twins. This is an informative comparison because these cousins are genetically the same as half-sibs (i.e., they share 25 percent of their genes, on average, compared with 12.5 percent for most cousins) because they have the "same" mother in terms of genes. However, we would expect true half-sibs to be more similar if common environment plays a part in the outcomes under investigation because half-sibs are raised in the same household whereas cousins are not.

The half-sib design is rarely used in behavior genetics research because it has low power to estimate genetic effects (25 percent versus 12.5 percent shared genes, on average, for cousins who are versus those who are not the offspring of identical twins). An adoption design is much more powerful in this regard because, at least theoretically, it completely separates genetic effects from environmental effects. However, as a practical matter, the adoption design is limited in a number of ways. Some parents, especially fathers, are unknown and cannot be used in adoption studies. Adoption agencies try to match the racial-ethnic characteristics of children who are being adopted with the characteristics of their adopted parents so that their genes and environments are not strictly independent. Adoption samples are usually unrepresentative because many adoption agencies are unwilling to cooperate with genetic researchers. And the range of environments in adoptive families is quite restricted, because adoption agencies try to choose good homes for their adoptees.

In light of these considerations, many behavior geneticists have concluded that the discordant MZ-cotwin design is the preferred approach for performing studies that examine environmental influences on outcomes like those considered in this chapter in a way that accounts for genetic effects. This design uses the logic of a matched case-control design (Schlesselman 1982) in which pairs of identical twins are used to "control" for genes in studying the effects of environmental factors on within-pair differences in outcomes. It is impossible in this design to evaluate the effects of environmental experiences that are always shared by twins, such as the early death of a parent or other childhood adversities. Adoption designs are much better suited to evaluate those effects in a way that excludes the possibility of genetic effects. However, the effects of experiences that are not always shared by cotwins, such as getting good grades in school, on later outcomes, such as adult socioeconomic achievement and the health consequences of this achievement, can be evaluated in this design in a way that is uniquely able to exclude the possibility of bias as a result of uncontrolled genetic influences. Planned future analyses of the MIDUS data to investigate predictors of the outcomes considered here will use this design in a confirmatory mode. That is, they will attempt to replicate results about the effects of predictors found in the more conventional analyses of the full MIDUS sample by using the discordant MZ-cotwin design applied to the 335 MIDUS MZ twin-pairs. This approach could be especially useful in studying the predictors of psychological well-being, because the results presented in this chapter suggest that the environmental determinants of these outcomes are largely unique and, therefore, ideally suited to investigate with the discordant MZ-cotwin design.

References

Akaike, H. 1987. Factor analysis and AIC. *Psychometrika* 52:317–32.

Allison, D. B., S. Heshka, M. C. Neale, D. T. Lykken, and S. B. Heymsfield. 1994. A genetic analysis of relative weight among 4,020 twin pairs, with an emphasis on sex effects. *Health Psychology* 13:362–65.

Allison, D. B., J. Kaprio, M. Korkeila, M. Koskenvuo, M. C. Neale, and K. Hayakawa. 1996. The heritability of body mass index among an international sample of monozygotic twins reared apart. *International Journal of Obesity and Related Metabolic Disorders* 20:501–6.

Barsky, A. J., P. D. Cleary, and G. L. Klerman. 1992. Determinants of perceived health status of medical outpatients. *Social Science and Medicine* 34:1147–54.

Bergeman, C. S., R. Plomin, N. L. Pedersen, G. E. McClearn, and J. R. Nesselroade. 1990. Genetic and environmental influences on social support: The Swedish Adoption/Twin Study of Aging. *Journal of Gerontology* 45:101–6.

Borhani, N. O., M. Feinleib, R. J. Garrison, J. C. Christian, and R. H. Rosenman. 1976. Genetic variance in blood pressure. *Acta Geneticae Medicae et Gemellologiae* 25:137–44.

Carroll, D., J. K. Hewitt, K. A. Last, J. R. Turner, and J. Sims. 1985. A twin study of cardiac reactivity and its relationship to parental blood pressure. *Physiology and Behavior* 34:103–6.

Fabsitz, R. R., P. Sholinsky, and D. Carmelli. 1994. Genetic influences on adult weight gain and maximum body mass index in male twins. *American Journal of Epidemiology* 140:711–20.

Fylkesnes, K., and O. H. Forde. 1992. Determinants and dimensions involved in self-evaluation of health. *Social Science and Medicine* 35:271–79.

Harris, J. R., N. L. Pedersen, G. E. McClearn, R. Plomin, and J. R. Nesselroade. 1992. Age differences in genetic and environmental influences for health from the Swedish Adoption/Twin Study of Aging. *Journal of Gerontology* 47:213–20.

Heath, A. C., M. C. Neale, R. C. Kessler, L. J. Eaves, and K. S. Kendler. 1992. Evidence for genetic influences on personality from self-reports and informant ratings. *Journal of Personality and Social Psychology* 63:85–96.

Hemminki, K., C. Dong, and P. Vaittinen. 1999. Familial risks in cervical cancer: Is there a hereditary component? *International Journal of Cancer* 82:775–81.

Holm, N. V., M. Hauge, and B. Harvald. 1980. Etiologic factors of breast cancer elucidated by a study of unselected twins. *Journal of the National Cancer Institute* 65:285–98.

Jablon, S., J. V. Neel, H. Gershowitz, and G. F. Atkinson. 1967. The NAS-NRC twin panel: Methods of construction of the panel, zygosity diagnosis, and proposed use. *American Journal of Human Genetics* 19:133–61.

Jylha, M., E. Leskinen, E. Alanen, A. L. Leskinen, and E. Heikkinen. 1986. Self-rated health and associated factors among men of different ages. *Journal of Gerontology* 41:710–17.

Kendler, K. S. 1997. Social support: A genetic-epidemiologic analysis. *American Journal of Psychiatry* 154:1398–1404.

Kendler, K. S., C. O. Gardner, and C. A. Prescott. 1998. A population-based twin study of self-esteem and gender. *Psychological Medicine* 28:1403–9.

Kendler, K. S., M. C. Neale, R. C. Kessler, A. C. Heath, and L. J. Eaves. 1992a. Generalized anxiety disorder in women. A population-based twin study. *Archives of General Psychiatry* 49:267–72.

———. 1992b. The genetic epidemiology of phobias in women. The interrelationship of agoraphobia, social phobia, situational phobia, and simple phobia. *Archives of General Psychiatry* 49:273–81.

———. 1993. A longitudinal twin study of personality and major depression in women. *Archives of General Psychiatry* 50:853–62.

Kendler, K. S., N. L. Pedersen, M. C. Neale, and A. A. Mathe. 1995. A pilot Swedish twin study of affective illness including hospital- and population-ascertained subsamples: Results of model fitting. *Behavior Genetics* 25:217–32.

Kendler, K. S., and C. D. Robinette. 1983. Schizophrenia in the National Academy of Sciences–National Research Council Twin Registry: A 16-year update. *American Journal of Psychiatry* 140:1551–63.

Kendler, K. S., L. M. Thornton, S. E. Gilman, and R. C. Kessler. 2000. Sexual orientation in a U.S. national sample of twin and nontwin sibling pairs. *American Journal of Psychiatry* 157:1843–46.

Kendler, K. S., E. E. Walters, M. C. Neale, R. C. Kessler, A. C. Heath, and L. J. Eaves. 1995. The structure of the genetic and environmental risk factors for six major psychiatric disorders in women: Phobia, generalized anxiety disorder, panic disorder, bulimia, major depression, and alcoholism. *Archives of General Psychiatry* 52:374–83.

Kessler, R. C., K. S. Kendler, A. Heath, M. C. Neale, and L. J. Eaves. 1992. Social support, depressed mood, and adjustment to stress: A genetic epidemiologic investigation. *Journal of Personality and Social Psychology* 62:257–72.

Levkoff, S. E., P. D. Cleary, and T. Wetle. 1987. Differences in the appraisal of health between aged and middle-aged adults. *Journal of Gerontology* 42:114–20.

Lichtenstein P., N. V. Holm, P. K. Verkasalo, A. Iliadou, J. Kapiro, M. Koskenvuo, E. Pukkala, A. Skytthe, and K. Hemminki. 2000. Environmental and heritable factors in the causation of cancer: Analyses of cohorts of twins from Sweden, Denmark, and Finland. *New England Journal of Medicine* 343:78–85.

Loehlin, J. C. 1989. Partitioning environmental and genetic contributions to behavioral development. *American Psychologist* 44:1285–94.

———. 1992. *Genes and environment in personality development.* Newbury Park, Calif.: Sage Publications.

Loehlin, J. C., and R. C. Nichols. 1976. *Heredity, environment, and personality: A study of 850 sets of twins.* Austin: University of Texas Press.

Matthews, K. A., C. D. Batson, J. Horn, and R. H. Rosenman. 1981. "Principles in his nature which interest him in the fortune of others . . . ": The heritability of empathic concern for others. *Journal of Personality* 49:237–47.

McGuffin, P., R. Katz, S. Watkins, and J. Rutherford. 1996. A hospital-based twin register of the heritability of DSM-IV unipolar depression. *Archives of General Psychiatry* 53:129–36.

Miles, T. P. 1997. Population-based, genetically informative sample for studies of physical frailty and aging: Black elderly twin study. *Human Biology* 69:107–20.

Mossey, J. M., and E. Shapiro. 1982. Self-rated health: A predictor of mortality among the elderly. *American Journal of Public Health* 72:800–808.

Moum, T. 1992. Self-assessed health among Norwegian adults. *Social Science and Medicine* 35:935–47.

Neale, M. C. 1991. *Statistical modeling with Mx.* Richmond: Department of Psychiatry, Medical College of Virginia/Virginia Commonwealth University.

Neale, M. C., and L. R. Cardone. 1992. *Methodology for genetic studies of twins and families.* Dordrecht, The Netherlands: Kluwer Academic Publishers.

Nora, J. J., R. H. Lortscher, R. D. Spangler, A. H. Nora, and W. J. Kimberling. 1980. Genetic-epidemiologic study of early-onset ischemic heart disease. *Circulation* 61:503–8.

Page, W. F., M. M. Braun, A. W. Partin, N. Caporaso, and P. Walsh. 1997. Heredity and prostate cancer: A study of World War II veteran twins. *Prostate* 33:240–45.

Partin, A. W., W. F. Page, B. R. Lee, M. G. Sanda, R. N. Miller, and P. C. Walsh. 1994. Concordance rates for benign prostatic disease among twins suggest hereditary influence. *Urology* 44:646–50.

Plomin, R., and D. Daniels. 1987. Why are children in the same family so different from one another? *Behavioral and Brain Sciences* 10:1–16.

Rossi, A. S. 2001. Domains and dimensions of social responsibility: A sociodemographic profile. In *Caring and doing for others: Social responsibility in the domains of family, work, and community,* ed. A. S. Rossi, 97–134. Chicago: University of Chicago Press.

Rowe, D. C. 1983. A biometrical analysis of perceptions of family environment: A study of twin and singleton siblings. *Developmental Psychology* 17:203–8.

Roy, M. A., M. C. Neale, and K. S. Kendler. 1995. The genetic epidemiology of self-esteem. *British Journal of Psychiatry* 166:813–20.

Rushton, J. P., D. W. Fulker, M. C. Neale, R. A. Blizard, and H. J. Eysenck. 1984. Altruism and genetics. *Acta Geneticae Medicae et Gemellologiae* 33:265–71.

Ryff, C. D. 1989. Happiness is everything, or is it? Explorations on the meaning of psychological well-being. *Journal of Personality and Social Psychology* 57:1069–81.

Ryff, C. D., and C. L. Keyes. 1995. The structure of psychological well-being revisited. *Journal of Personality and Social Psychology* 69:719–27.

Scarr, S., and K. McCartney. 1983. How people make their own environments: A theory of genotype greater than environment effects. *Child Development* 54:424–35.

Schlesselman, J. J. 1982. *Case-control studies: Design, conduct, analysis.* New York: Oxford University Press.

Schmutte, P. S., and C. D. Ryff. 1997. Personality and well-being: Reexamining methods and meanings. *Journal of Personality and Social Psychology* 73:549–59.

Schneider, N. R., W. R. Williams, and R. S. Chaganti. 1986. Genetic epidemiology of familial aggregation of cancer. *Advances in Cancer Research* 47:1–36.

Schwarz, G. 1978. Estimating the dimensions of a model. *Annals of Statistics* 6:461–64.

Selby, J. V., B. Newman, C. P. Quesenberry, Jr., R. R. Fabsitz, D. Carmelli, F. J. Meaney, and C. Slemenda. 1990. Genetic and behavioral influences on body fat distribution. *International Journal of Obesity* 14:593–602.

Selby, J. V., B. Newman, J. Quiroga, J. C. Christian, M. A. Austin, and R. R. Fabsitz. 1991. Concordance for dyslipidemic hypertension in male twins. *Journal of American Medical Association* 265:2079–84.

Silberg, J. L., A. C. Heath, R. C. Kessler, K. S. Kendler, M. C. Neale, and L. J. Eaves. 1990. Genetic and environmental effects on self-reported depressive symptoms in a general population twin sample. *Journal of Psychiatric Research* 24:197–212.

Stunkard, A. J. 1991. Genetic contributions to human obesity. *Research Publications: Association for Research in Nervous and Mental Disease* 69:205–18.

Stunkard, A. J., T. T. Foch, and Z. Hrubec. 1986. A twin study of human obesity. *Journal of American Medical Association* 256:51–54.

Turula, M., J. Kaprio, A. Rissanen, and M. Koskenvuo. 1990. Body weight in the Finnish Twin Cohort. *Diabetes Research and Clinical Practice* 10:S33–S36.

Viken, R. J., R. J. Rose, J. Kaprio, and M. Koskenvuo. 1994. A developmental genetic analysis of adult personality: Extraversion and neuroticism from 18 to 59 years of age. *Journal of Personality and Social Psychology* 66:722–30.

Yashin, A. I., I. A. Iachine, K. Christensen, N. V. Holm, and J. W. Vaupel. 1998. The genetic component of discrete disability traits: An analysis using liability models with age-dependent thresholds. *Behavior Genetics* 28:207–14.

CHAPTER SIX

The Menopausal Transition and Aging Processes

Alice S. Rossi

For the past decade or so there has been increasing attention paid to menopause in both research and the media. In 1992, Jane Brody, science writer for the *New York Times,* reported that "menopause, long mired in myth and controversy and shrouded by a cloak of embarrassed silence, is fast becoming the leading women's health issue of the decade" (Brody 1992). Gail Sheehy (1992) considered menopause to be the "last taboo," surrounded by a conspiracy of silence so great that women did not discuss their fear that they might be menopausal even with their close women friends. Sheehy, like many other authors, was dedicated to ridding society of that taboo. Today, along with menopause, we find open discussion in print and social circles of many other previously taboo subjects. The same widespread public attention given to menopause has also been focused on breast cancer, vaginal infections, hysterectomy, abortion, and male sexual impotence, to name a few. Not long ago, ads for sanitary napkins or tampons were so discrete that a child would never know what they were used for, whereas today tampon ads on television stress comfort and absorbability in frank terms. Ads for Viagra display men and women of all ages engaged in caresses and wearing postcoitally satisfied smiles. A friend reports both shock and amusement to find a cluster of brightly colored, blown-up condoms hanging as a mobile in her gynecologist's waiting room.

Clearly, menopause is out of the closet. Yet there is no evidence that in the past women did not discuss such matters among their female kin and close friends, nor has there been any evidence that the majority of women undergoing the menopausal transition today typically experience enormous discomfort or functional impairment specifically linked to the physiological changes that attend this normal transition in women's lives. The image of a woman embarrassed at a dinner party (or a board meeting) by perspiration running down her face in rivulets as a result of an intense hot flash is hardly a widespread phenomenon, although to read earlier medical journal articles about menopause, one might be led to assume it was very prevalent among women in their forties and fifties. Menopausal symptoms in the gynecological literature cover a wide range, from physical symptoms such as hot flashes, insomnia, night sweats, vaginal dryness, and faulty or impaired memory, to psychological symptoms such as irritability, moodiness, and depression. How prevalent these sorts of symptoms were among middle-aged women could not be gauged by such medical reports, however, because they were based on clinical samples. Women who did not experience menopausal problems simply did not approach their physicians for help, and hence they were not among the cases described in gynecological journal articles and medical textbooks.

A very different portrait emerges from recent research based on samples of normal, healthy midlife women. An important five-year longitudinal study in the Pittsburgh area that tracked healthy middle-aged women from the time they were menstruating regularly (premenopausal stage) to the time their menstruation had ceased entirely (postmenopausal stage) concluded that "taken together, these results suggest that natural menopause is a *benign event* for the majority of middle-aged healthy women" (Matthews et al. 1990, emphasis added). Similar findings were reported from a comparable study in the Boston area (Avis and McKinlay 1991). This conclusion from small regional metropolitan samples is consistent with our findings from the national MIDUS survey.

What does concern women today, and has become an increasing focus in medicine and the pharmaceutical industry, is the use of hormone replacement therapy (HRT). Estrogen replacement has long been prescribed by gynecologists for women undergoing the menopausal transition, primarily to reduce the incidence of hot flashes and the night sweats that often impair a good night's sleep. The use of HRT more than doubled between 1982 and 1992, and continued to increase until the past few years (Wysowski, Golden, and Burke 1995). What is new is the shift from short-term reliance on hormone replacement for a few years in midlife to reliance on hormone replacement for all the decades of life remaining for postmenopausal women. The rationale for recommending this prolonged reliance was the presumed negative effect of estrogen depletion on bone and vascular health after the cessation of menses.

One prominent gynecologist and founder of the North American Menopause Society, Wulf Utrian, predicted an "impending epidemic" of heart attacks and bone fractures as a result of the growing numbers of baby boomers who are entering late middle and old age. These medical problems, he contended, could overwhelm the health care system unless something was done to reduce these "menopause-linked problems"

(Wall Street Journal, September 12, 1991). Utrian's major recommendation has been long-term replacement therapy during all of a woman's postmenopausal years. Even the lead article in the first issue of a new journal, *Journal of Women's Health,* in 1992 provided a review of estrogen therapy by a woman epidemiologist that concluded with the recommendation that hormone supplements should be used by almost all postmenopausal women from ages 50 to 85, because they "may be needed to maintain an active and full life" (Bush 1992). On the first page of this same first issue was a full-page ad from Wyeth-Ayerst Laboratories, manufacturer of Premarin, the dominant synthetic estrogen on the market and one of the most frequently prescribed medications in the United States. The ad urged women to "start early and continue long-term for maximum osteoporosis benefits" and claimed that Premarin use by postmenopausal women reduces the risk of hip and wrist fractures by 62 percent. In the past, estrogen use tended to be of short duration, taken during the few years some women were discomforted by hot flashes brought on by hormonal changes. In more recent years, the pharmaceutical industry and many physicians have been urging that hormonal replacement continue to be used among postmenopausal women for upward of thirty years, a decided boon assuring great financial benefits to the drug firms producing such pills and gels. In the absence of adequate scientific evidence, however, there seems meager justification for such a regimen.

Whether long-term hormone therapy prevents bone fractures and cardiovascular disease to an extent that overrides the risk of breast or endometrial cancer has been under investigation in several clinical trials, testing whether estrogen alone or in combination with one of the three major progestin regimens is helpful or harmful. Early on, the expectation was that estrogen would be a magical preventive of heart attacks, strokes, and bone fractures and, in some quarters, that the drug would also assure prolonged youthful looks and moist vaginas. That optimistic view has been qualified as results from these trials are reported, results that have led to great concern and confusion for many women. Women with an intact uterus who take estrogen alone (typically Premarin, a synthetic estrogen derived from horse urine) for prolonged periods of time run the risk of endometrial cancer. Estrogen taken with a progestin carries the risk of breast cancer and breakthrough bleeding. Cell biologist Dominique Toran-Allerand (2002) cautions that Provera, the most commonly prescribed synthetic progestin, tends to block the beneficial actions of estrogen and may even have harmful effects of its own by binding to receptors of other steroid hormones.

Warnings about the risks of hormone replacement were increasing by the year 2000, with the publication of results from the three-year Postmenopausal Estrogen/Progestin Intervention (PEPI) study conducted between 1989 and 1994, a randomized, double-blind, placebo-controlled clinical trial designed to compare the effects of estrogen alone or in combination with a progestin (Meyer 2000). The PEPI study did not demonstrate any significant health benefits; in fact, it suggested that postmenopausal women with any established heart disease or risk factors for the disease should *not* take estrogen for any prolonged period of time.

For the past decade, high hopes were held for resolving many questions about HRT for postmenopausal women through a very large scale study, the Women's Health Initiative (WHI) program of research. A major arm of this program was a randomized, controlled prevention trial in which 16,608 postmenopausal women aged 50–79, with an intact uterus at baseline, were recruited by forty U.S. clinical centers during the years 1993–98. A total of 8506 women in the trial received the most commonly used combined hormone preparation in the United States, Prempro, a pill composed of 0.625 mg/day of conjugated equine estrogen and 2.5 mg/day of medroxyprogesterone acetate, while 8201 women received a placebo tablet. This was the first randomized trial to directly address whether estrogen plus progestin has a favorable or unfavorable effect on coronary heart disease. Before this trial, observational studies had suggested a 40 percent to 50 percent reduction in risk of coronary heart disease among users of either estrogen or, less frequently, the combination of estrogen and progestin. Reduced hip fracture was an additional expected health benefit, because observational studies had suggested hormone therapy slowed down the loss of bone mineral density. Invasive breast cancer was the primary potentially adverse outcome of hormone usage.

The WHI trial was originally designed to last 8.5 years, but it was abruptly terminated after a mean of 5.2 years of follow-up, in late spring 2002, as a result of the finding from follow-up testing that risks exceeded the health benefits of hormone therapy. Clinical outcomes showed negative effects for coronary heart disease, breast cancer, stroke, and pulmonary embolism. Some slight positive health effects were found for colorectoral cancer, endometrial cancer, and hip fracture (Writing Group for the WHI Investigators 2002). The analysis of data from the trials prompted the data and safety monitoring board of the study to conclude that the combined estrogen-progestin therapy does not have a risk–benefit profile consistent with the requirements for a viable intervention for the prevention of chronic disease, and therefore it should not be initiated or continued for the prevention of coronary heart disease in postmenopausal women.[1]

Termination of the WHI trial caused a widespread flurry of news coverage, thousands of frantic phone calls by women to their physicians, and gleeful reactions by some women's health advocacy groups that have been critical of the overmedicalized approaches to women's health issues for the past several decades. Still other researchers and physicians have pointed out that because of the WHI trial's design limitations, its termination must be kept in perspective. Prempro was the only hormone combination administered, with no variation in dosage level, and on a constant daily basis. It cannot be concluded that the same risk–benefit ratio would be found if a natural estrogen, such as 17β-estradiol, or a natural micronized progesterone were being tested, or if dosage level was varied in keeping with individual patients' health profiles (e.g., by tests of a woman's own hormonal secretion levels or bone density or aspects of her health history). As Toran-Allerand (2002) pointed out, "giving [synthetic] hormones in a pattern different from the normal physiological situation is likely to result in abnormal responses." Nor should women with severe menopausal symptoms that impair their ability to function well or to maintain a high quality of life conclude that personally tailored hormonal therapy on a short-term basis is too risky a step to take (Duenwald 2002).

With so many mixed messages and dire warnings, it is little wonder that many women are seeking alternatives to the usual synthetic hormone therapies. Many postmenopausal women concerned about poor bone density hope to prevent or treat osteoporosis with biophosphates, selective estrogen receptor modulators, exercise, and changes in their diets. Others turn to alternative drugs available off the shelf in health food stores, despite risk of the poor quality of such medications, most of which do not have FDA approval. In consultation with their physicians, other women try various types of progestins now available: the most common, medroxyprogesterone acetate, is derived from plants; another is derived from synthetic androgen; an even more recent product is a natural progesterone—micronized progesterone—available in either tablet or vaginal gel. The hope for the gel is that such topical treatment would bypass circulation of the progesterone through the bloodstream, a drawback to taking tablets by mouth.

But all such alternatives are accompanied by many unanswered questions (Harvard Women's Health Watch 2000). And just as the pharmaceutical industry advertised widely in support of the view that

Premarin should be taken from menopause until death, so too the herbal supplement industry has heeded the call and marketed heavily to urge the purchase of all manner of women-only products, from women-only nutrition bars, to cereals fortified with vitamins for women, even to topical creams such as Femgest, which promises to deliver progesterone to the body for women of childbearing years as well as for women experiencing pre- through postmenopause. As science writer Alex Kuczynski (2002) put it, the products are for "anyone with two X chromosomes over age 15."

As this discussion implies, the understanding and treatment of menopause and its aftermath have occurred mainly within a medical model: something wrong in the body calls for medication. Feeling depressed? Take Prozac. Migraine headaches? Take Midrin. Cholesterol too high? Take Pravacol or Welchol. A variety of pills are available for almost every departure from a hoped-for healthy, strong, and active body. Increasingly larger numbers of adults have been persuaded that buying a pill, cream, or gel provides a solution more easily adopted than increasing exercise regimens, or reducing or giving up alcohol, tobacco, and carbohydrate consumption.

In the past there have been other models for understanding and interpreting menopause. We briefly consider two of them. The first is a psychoanalytic model, well represented by the work of Helene Deutsch in the 1930s and 1940s. Her perspective on menopause is hardly shared by anyone today: menopause as the end of women's fertility. Deutsch considered menopause an invariant psychosexual stressor that stirred up previous developmental issues that triggered regression and led to menopausal symptoms of depression and irritability. Her view is best exemplified by her claim that menopause is a time of disappointment and mortification because a woman's life as a bearer of future life has ended and she therefore experiences menopause as a "partial death—as servant of the species" (Deutsch 1945).

By the 1960s, with the waning of such psychoanalytic views, quite another model came to the fore: a sociocultural model of menopause that emphasized not the biological cessation of the menses but the "empty nest" stage in women's lives, which coincided with menopause—that time in midlife when the last child leaves the parental nest and a woman's central role in life, as mother, effectively ends some fifteen years before her husband faces a comparable central role loss with retirement. Pauline Bart used her research on depression among middle-aged women to argue against the cultural pressure on women to channel their energies narrowly into childrearing. Her argument was based on two major factors that had changed the scenario of women's lives: an increased longevity, which meant a long life still ahead after menopause and child-leaving; and effective contraceptive usage, which permitted a smaller number of desired births with no risk of menopausal babies. Bart (1971) urged greater continuity of employment for married women as the solution for the midlife depression induced by role loss.

From a broad historical perspective, both the psychoanalytic and the sociocultural models were theories rooted in special historical circumstances of the first half of the twentieth century, an era demographer Kingsley Davis has described as the "breadwinner era," when, for the first time in human history, cultural pressure was on women, especially in the urban middle class, to restrict their lives to home and children, and on men to be the sole breadwinner of the family (Davis and van den Oever 1982). Before 1870 and since 1950, women have played a significant role in economic and domestic production in addition to their critical role in childbearing and childrearing. Only as productive work shifted away from home and farm to factory and office in the last quarter of the nineteenth century did the cult of domesticity take hold, keeping urban middle-class women "in their place" at home. At the same time, unions pressed for wages for men sufficient to allow them to be the sole earners in working-class families. Since the 1950s, however, each decade has seen an increasing proportion of women entering and remaining in the work force. Women's "two-shift day" (Hochschild 1989) is nothing new in the long stretch of human history. Psychoanalytic theories of the variety represented by Helene Deutsch's analysis of menopause flourished during the era that was the cult of domesticity's heyday. The feminist renascence of the 1960s rejected that domesticity cult and argued that equality of the sexes could not be reached unless women attained economic power as co-breadwinners with their husbands.

It is easier to identify key features of past historical eras than to identify the key features of one's own time and place. But it is important, in setting the stage for an analysis of menopause and what it means in women's lives, to note several major new features of American life today compared with that of a half-century ago. First in importance are the implications of the greatly extended life span that we now enjoy, with good health possible for many years in old age. Menopause at age 50 is no longer associated with impending death; there are several decades of healthy active life ahead. That we now consider menopause a "midlife" passage rather than a prelude to death indicates as much.

Second, marriage and childrearing are no longer the only roles available to women in adulthood. Increasingly, more women opt to remain single, childless after marriage, or single after divorce, without the social stigma that had been associated with such choices in the past. And if women do have children, their number and spacing are increasingly under women's control. For most women today, a last child is born a decade before menopause, thereby changing the subjective meaning of menopause. The end of menstruation becomes a release from hormonal cycling and period messiness rather than a cause for grief because of the loss of fertility. If there are any lingering feelings of regret about the ending of one's fertile years, they are more apt to be felt in connection with terminating the nursing of a last desired child or opting for a tubal ligation, rather than in connection with menopause per se.

A related point concerns a misleading notion of what middle-aged women feel about menopause in high-fertility societies, such as the Middle Eastern Muslim and African societies. Western researchers were surprised to find not negative but positive reactions to menopause among their Arab informants (Datan, Antonovsky, and Maoz 1981). Why, if their society valued fertility so highly, would women have such positive feelings about its ending? Pronatalism, I suspect, is far more valued by men in such societies than by women themselves. With no effective contraceptive control over the timing and number of pregnancies, such women carry enormous burdens at high risk to their own health and stamina. Far from being surprised, I found their comments completely understandable: as two Arab women who had had six or more pregnancies explained, "Thank God, that's all behind me," and "menopause is God's reward for a life of service."

Third, there is now greater continuity to the multiple roles women occupy across the life course. Involvement in the community and the workplace is increasingly a constant across life for women today. Short-term maternity leave for one or two births amounts to a total of less than a year of temporary withdrawal from the labor force. Hence retirement for women in our time is not from mothering but from employment, much as it is for men. Retirement itself has taken on new meaning, less threatening than it was to our grandparents and great grandparents, thanks to Social Security and private pension plans, medical benefits under Medicare, and returns from personal investments. Indeed, it is a special mark of the elderly today that they are more independent and financially secure than any previous cohort of elderly adults has been in our history. In fact, increasing numbers of the elderly are currently in the happy circumstance of being able to help their children and grandchildren financially rather than being in need of such help themselves. By the same token, this means less pressure on middle-aged children: they may need to provide psychological and social help to elderly parents, but most are spared the burden of financially supporting them.

Fourth, the "empty nest" when a last child leaves the parental home carries a different meaning than in the past: for many parents, seeing their child off to college is more traumatic and involves more change in household management than does attending an adult child's marriage or move to his or her own apartment. An unexpected change in my household when my oldest child left for college was the realization that we needed to resort to baby-sitters for the younger children for the first time in several years, which we experienced as a step backward in domestic management. If there was any moment of sadness in my experience of child-leaving, it was the summer day I emerged from a luggage store carrying a new monogrammed suitcase as a gift for my son, who was leaving for college that fall: I suddenly collapsed in tears on a bench in the mall, sobbing over his impending departure.

One last important feature of our times is the vastly increased ease of communication between the generations in a family, which is now possible thanks to cell phones, e-mail, air travel, and the rescheduling of many holidays to permit three-day weekends, all of which reduces the sense of lost contact with one's grown children once they live some distance from the parental home. There is hardly a day that either I or my husband do not find an e-mail message from one or the other of our three children, now midlife adults in their forties. One of the unexpected aspects of this frequent contact with our middle-aged children is an awareness of the aging changes that now preoccupy them. Coping as my husband and I are with much more frail bodies and chronic health problems, we forget all those early signs of aging we coped with in our forties: root canal, tooth extractions, and crowns; back and joint pains from exertion in house or garden or a game of golf; bifocal or trifocal glasses; undesired weight gain or enlarged waistlines; the realization that overindulgence in food and drink was becoming more difficult to snap back from; and so forth. The insight we have gained from these e-mail exchanges with our children is this: the older one becomes, the better we *think* we were at younger ages!

It is an assumption underlying our perspective on the menopausal transition in women's lives that the social and psychological significance of this midlife passage lies more in the experience of aging than in the loss of fertility assumed by psychoanalytic theories such as Deutsch's, or the role loss attending the empty nest stage of family life assumed by earlier sociologists, or the discomfort associated with menopausal symptoms that a medical model focuses on.

A focus on aging also argues for attention to men as well as women in research on midlife. This alerts us to one of the major sources of stress and worry in the lives of middle-aged adults: the expectation that they perform at work when they are 50 just as they were able to do at 30, which they know in their bones is possible only with much greater effort and stress. This may be of particular significance in American lives today because the pace of work is much faster than in any other Western society. Americans work longer hours under greater pressure for increasing productivity and with fewer days of vacation than citizens of any European nation. As one telling example, the average annual number of paid vacation days for employed adults in the United States is 12, compared with 28 days in Britain, 35 in Germany, and 42 in Italy (Shapiro 1999). Also, the number of hours Americans work each week has climbed sharply, while working hours in most other Western countries are falling: Americans work 350 more hours a year than do adults in European countries (Greenhouse 1999).

It is precisely by placing menopause in the larger framework of aging processes and their relationship to role performance that the MIDUS national survey provides a unique advantage over numerous other studies of menopause that have been undertaken in the past decade and more. As reported later in this chapter, these new studies are premised largely on a medical model and trace changes in body function relevant to the hormonal changes during menopause as well as related psychological symptoms and beliefs about what menopause will be like for women. By contrast, the MIDUS data set is not limited to women but includes men as well, nor is it limited to any narrow age range of midlife adults but includes the full span of years from 25 to 74. Such sex and age variables permit an analysis of whether and how midlife is experienced differently by women than by men, and how unique the middle years are compared with those of early adulthood and old age. Most important of all, our data cover all the major aspects of life: physical and mental health, personality, psychological well-being, social roles in family, work, and community. Our data also include ratings of the level of satisfaction in seven major domains of life: health, finances, sex life, current job, relations to spouse or intimate partner, relations with children, and overall contribution to the welfare of others.

These diverse measures of life domains are of particular relevance to-day because the boundaries between our roles have become increasingly blurred (Wuthnow 1998): stress at home resulting from an ill child or a serious argument with a partner can spill over into job performance; aggravation at work often spills over into tension at home; a health problem brought to the attention of a doctor may have its roots not in a malfunctioning body part but in stress at work or at home. Cell phones used while commuting between home and workplace, and lab top computers used while traveling add further to this blurring of boundaries between family, work, and leisure-time activities, crowding out time for meditation and decompression from the pressures of work or family responsibilities. Social and technological changes such as these mean that it is important as never before to define social science topics in a multidisciplinary framework appropriate to the complex lives of contemporary adults. This is precisely what the biopsychosocial theoretical framework underlying the design of the MIDUS survey encourages us to do.

PREVIEW

In keeping with this biopsychosocial framework, in this chapter I place the menopausal transition onto the larger life-course trajectory from early adulthood to early old age. In doing this, I hope better to pinpoint what is unique to midlife and to chart the age range during which the menopausal transition unfolds, the level of symptoms women report, the way they feel about the cessation of menstrual cycling, and the extent to which they worry about several aspects of aging. I ask whether it is menopausal stage, chronological age, general physical or emotional health, or role stress that matters most, and where the data permit, I compare the reports of women with those of men. Multivariate analysis traces the sources of the menopausal stress indicators reported by women, in which we draw upon a rich array of predictor variables: social-demographic characteristics (e.g., education, marital and parental status, income); ratings of physical and emotional/mental health; perceived changes in body shape and functional capacity in recent years; and measures of the level of stress in work and family roles. The analysis demonstrates the importance of defining problems in a multidimensional way, because I show that at least one of the variables in each of the domains—demographic, health, social roles—independently affects the level of reported symptoms.

After this concentrated attention to menopause, I shift to the broader array of changes that men and women report have occurred in their

163

bodies over the past five years—physical fitness, energy level, figure/
physique, and weight—as well as objective measures of hip, waist, height,
and weight. Again, the data permit us to compare men and women, and
trends across a wide range of ages.

I then shift the focus of the analysis from past change to anticipated
concerns about aging, with particular attention to the worry about becoming less attractive as one gets older, an issue that Gail Sheehy's qualitative interviews with middle-aged women identified as a highly significant
concern of many women in midlife: their fear of losing their sex appeal,
of fading "into the woodwork" or "becoming invisible" to use some of
Sheehy's colorful prose (Sheehy 1992). Unfortunately, we missed an opportunity in the design of MIDUS to address this issue of anticipated loss
of attractiveness because we only asked women, and not men, about this
fear, thus revealing by this omission that we may have shared the probably
erroneous assumption in our culture that "looks" matter only to women.
With the rapid rise in the sales of men's cosmetics, more color and variety in men's fashions, and men's use of cosmetic surgery in recent years,
this assumption does not hold, if it ever did. In the analysis of attractiveness concerns, I give special attention to women's reports about their
sex lives—frequency of sex with a partner and degree of satisfaction with
their sex lives—a domain where presumably feelings of attractiveness and
perceived recent changes in their bodies may affect them.

STAGES OF THE MENOPAUSAL TRANSITION

The labels we use in referring to the beginning and ending of a woman's
menstrual history—menarche and menopause—can be easily misunder-
stood, and they are in fact used in a number of distinct ways. In social
discourse, menarche can be viewed as an *event,* referring to a young girl's
first menstrual period—an event often experienced and remembered
with a mixture of pride and dismay, but sure to be announced however
discretely to close girlfriends and mothers. Despite the shift from private
to public discussion of many previously taboo topics, as noted earlier in
the chapter, our society has no special private or public rituals to mark
the occasion of a girl's first menstrual period. It was highly unusual and
very surprising to me when a close friend reported a very special family
occasion when her daughter had her first period, celebrated by a special
ride around the house on her father's shoulders and serving her a first-
ever small glass of wine. My own first experience was special in another
way: that same spring day my aunt brought her newborn son to our house
for a week's stay, and I carried the tiny infant around the house proudly

but awkwardly due to the bulky pad between my legs for the first time, thinking to myself that I too would soon be capable of bearing a child. Both of these examples are exceptions. More typical than either of them was the point made by social historian Joan Brumberg to the effect that menarche is defined in our society with reference not to fertility but to personal hygiene or "sanitary protection," as early ads put it when sanitary napkins came on the market after the development of cellucotton during World War I (Brumberg 1997). The beginning of menstruation has become a hygienic, not a maturational, event.

But at least it is an event definable at its first occurrence, and it is preceded and followed during some six or more years by other developmental changes: breast buds and body hair develop prior to menarche, and regular ovulation may not develop for up to two years after a first menses (a phenomenon known as postmenarcheal adolescent sterility). The age at menarche has dropped significantly over time: for most of our history as a species, the age at menarche is estimated to have been around 16, a first birth at 19. Over the past century, with improved nutrition and accumulation of body fat, the age at menarche has gradually dropped to an average of 12.6 years of age in developed societies. By 14 or 15 years of age, most girls today are ovulating regularly, with the result that unprotected sex has a much higher probability of resulting in pregnancy than it did for girls this age in the past.

By contrast, menopause is not an event but a *process* that unfolds over time, its final stage known only in retrospect; in customary medical usage, a woman is defined as postmenopausal when she has not had a menstrual period for a full year. The years preceding this final stage— the perimenopausal stage—are marked by three types of changes in the menstrual cycle: changes in the time interval between periods (becoming shorter or longer than usual, with occasional skipped months), changes in the duration of the menstrual flow, and changes in the amount of blood loss. The duration of the change from premenopausal to postmenopausal stages may take an average of seven to eight years.[2]

The term *menopause* is often used in two different senses: *menopausal woman* sometimes describes a woman currently undergoing changes in the nature of her menstrual periods—what we classify as a perimenopausal woman; other times the term refers to a woman who no longer menstruates at all—a postmenopausal woman. This varied usage probably reflects the fact that the termination of menstruation cannot be known in advance, only retrospectively. When I use the term *menopause* in an unqualified way, I am referring to the whole seven or eight years of the passage from pre- to postmenopausal stages. Otherwise I rely on more stage-specific usage.

PHYSIOLOGY AND TIMING OF MENOPAUSE

The full story cannot yet be told of what specific factors trigger the timing of the onset and termination of menstruation in women's lives. The considerable variation over historic time in the age of menarche, as noted earlier, has been largely attributed to nutritional enrichment of our diets, dramatically illustrated by the extremely rapid rate at which menarcheal age dropped in Japan after World War II. Menopausal age is a function of the number of oocytes in the ovaries. There are upward of half a million follicles in the fetal ovary, the majority of which are lost through atresia before birth (Byrd 1993). Unlike a male, who produces millions of sperm throughout his life, the human female has no capacity for oogenesis that parallels male spermatogenesis. Only 400 to 500 oocytes will ripen during the female's entire reproductive span. In each menstrual cycle, a number of follicles are stimulated to mature, with only one (or occasionally two or three in the case of fraternal twins or triplets) reaching full maturation under the influence of follicle-stimulating and follicle-luteinizing hormones. But the quality of the oocytes vary by the age of the mother: in the years before women become even perimenopausal, the older the age of the mother, the greater is the probability of spontaneous abortion of usually defective embryos, premature birth of low-birth-weight babies, more difficult deliveries, higher perinatal mortality (death of an infant soon after birth), and genetic/chromosomal defects in the fetus that survives full-term gestation. Maximum fertility, with good outcomes in terms of infant and maternal health and fitness, occurs in a woman's mid to late twenties (Richardson and Nelson 1990).

Independent of the quality of the oocytes remaining, women run an increasing risk of failure to conceive when they postpone childbearing into their late thirties and forties. Research by Richardson, Senikas, and Nelson (1987) suggests that it is not age but menopausal stage that affects the number of follicles remaining in the ovaries: in an age-matched sample of women at three stages of the menopausal transition, they found dramatic changes as a function of menopausal stage, not age per se: a tenfold greater number of follicles remained among premenopausal women than perimenopausal women *of the same age,* and virtually no follicles remained in the ovaries of postmenopausal women of any age. In the few instances of postmenopausal women who still had ovarian follicles, the follicles typically showed signs of degeneration.

Menopause is a unique human female characteristic. Over the course of the life span, most physiologic functions, such as vital capacity, cardiac or breathing capacity, or bone density, show a very slow and gradual departure from maximum function among adults in their thirties to their midsixties. On these physiologic functions it is only in the late sixties that radical depletion of capacity tends to occur. Whereas few women are fertile beyond their fifties, human males remain fertile until their midsixties, although the quality of sperm goes down as men get older. Male fertility drops to about 20 percent of maximum function by age 80.

Why human females are so unique in the timing of reproductive senescence has been subject to theoretical controversy. Similar timing does not occur in species genetically close to our own such as the common chimpanzee: a chimp female is still capable of reproduction when she dies. Only a few other female mammals live beyond their fertile years, including the African elephant, the opossum, the ringed seal, and the short-finned pilot whale (Finch 1990, 166). The pilot whale, for example, has a life expectancy at complete cessation of reproduction of about fourteen years (Kasuya and Marsh 1984). It does not seem likely that menopause is any recent historical development of the human female. Kim Hill and Magdalena Hurtado, in a detailed demographic and genealogical study of the Ache foragers in South America (Hill and Hurtado 1991; Hurtado et al. 1992), found that among the Ache women, the mean age at last birth is 42 years, but the mean life expectancy at this age is for an additional 23 years. If our hunting and foraging ancestors survived to early adulthood, their chances for survival to an old age were very good, just as they are in our time. We have often been misled on this point because of the tendency to calculate expected longevity *from birth*. This is misleading because in the past, infant mortality and infectious diseases among children took so high a toll.

If menopause is not to be explained on the grounds of changes in the length of the human life course, what is the more likely explanation? Many anthropologists (e.g., Hrdy 1999; Konner 2002; Lancaster and King 1985) have based their explanations on sociobiological assumptions of inclusive fitness theory (Hamilton 1966; Trivers 1972). The key idea in this view stems from the very special characteristic of human childrearing: the very long period of total dependency on care by others. Other mammals obtain food by their own efforts once they are weaned. Humans are unique in that they require others to provide sustenance for them during infancy and childhood, a very slow and prolonged period of growth and development (Lancaster and Lancaster 1983). This was as true thousands of years ago as it is today; hence natural selection processes favored the survival of those born to women young enough to provide for them until the offspring in turn could reproduce. Over long stretches of time, children of older mothers would not survive to produce children of their own. Across hundreds of generations, the genes that would be transmitted would be those from women who terminated childbearing at younger ages. This theory is often referred to as a *grandmother thesis,* on the argument that at some point in life, "the increases in fitness that can be attained through investment in grandchildren is greater than that expected by continuous direct reproduction" (Hill and Hurtado 1991, 318). This thesis puts too much emphasis on the role of grandmothers as direct caretakers of grandchildren; other data on foraging societies suggest that older women played a more significant role in providing food to daughters and grandchildren than in direct caregiving of the grandchildren (Hurtado et al. 1992). The underlying natural selection explanation in terms of differential survival of children born to young mothers compared with those born to older mothers also helps to explain why male fertility persisted to much older ages. In almost all known societies, mothers carry the major burden of childrearing, sometimes assisted by female members of their social group or kindred. There was no comparable natural selection pressure on males for an early age of reproductive senescence, so male fertility declines in a gradual manner along with other physiological attributes.

Timing and Reaction to Menopause

We turn now to MIDUS data on women's experience of menopause. Figure 1 shows the distribution of the three stages of the menopausal transition across the life course of women from 30 to 74 years of age. To say the "average" age at becoming postmenopausal is 50 or 51 years can be misleading unless one notes the very broad span of years during which women move from being premenopausal to postmenopausal. This means that in any one five-year age group there are women who are premenopausal, others who are perimenopausal, and still others postmenopausal. Note, for example, that one in four women in their thirties is already perimenopausal, or that one in four women in their early forties is already postmenopausal. The sharpest change between five-year age groups is between women in their early versus late fifties: the percentage who are postmenopausal jumps from 69 percent to 92 percent during these few years.

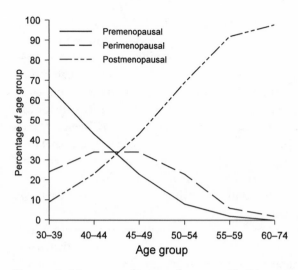

FIGURE 1. Menopausal stage of women 30–74 years of age.

TABLE 1 Surgical Menopause and Tubal Ligation, by Age

	Age					
	25–29	30–39	40–49	50–59	60–69	70–74
Percentage who have had surgical menopause[a] among postmenopausal women	—	40.6	39.1	33.3	30.3	30.4
N	(0)	(32)	(110)	(237)	(198)	(79)
Percentage who have had tubal ligation[b]	8.7	20.5	36.8	23.4	13.0	8.3
N	(173)	(336)	(367)	(333)	(238)	(97)

[a]Defined as the removal of uterus and/or both ovaries.
[b]Some 19 percent of premenopausal women report having had tubal ligation, 30 percent of perimenopausal women, and 20 percent of postmenopausal women.

Menopause as a result of surgery has been on the rise in recent years because of the increased incidence of hysterectomies, which explains most of the cases of postmenopausal women among the younger age groups. One-third of postmenopausal women in the MIDUS sample have had their uterus removed (hysterectomy) and/or both ovaries removed (oophorectomy). The distribution of the cases of surgical menopause by age group is shown in table 1. Note that surgical menopause is somewhat more typical of women under 50 than over 50 years of age. Of special interest is the addition in this table of another form of sterilization, tubal ligation, which prevents pregnancy but not menstruation (Chandra 1998). Women in their forties report the highest incidence of tubal ligation—37 percent. Many women now in their forties used estrogen/progestin contraceptive pills in their earlier years. Gynecologists typically advise women over 40 to shift from pills to other contraceptive methods. Rather than resorting to the barrier contraceptive methods of condoms or diaphragms, many women in their forties, convinced that they have no desire for further births, prefer tubal ligation, leaving their sex lives as unencumbered and spontaneous as the pill had assured. Table 1 also indicates that even 1 in 10 women under 30 and 1 in 5 in their thirties have had tubal sterilization. These figures suggest that many women have taken control of their fertility in a very direct manner, while avoiding any interference in normal endocrine functioning that hysterectomies and oophorectomies entail—further evidence of the dissociation of menopause with fertility issues. Tubal ligation is even more common in other countries than in the United States: estimates in 1994 were that some 138 million women of reproductive age throughout the world relied on tubal sterilization, more women than used any other contraceptive method. Follow-up studies of such women find fewer than 3 percent regret having had the procedure or wish they could reverse it (Chi and Jones 1994).

Subjective Feelings about Menopause

Women respondents were asked what their subjective feelings were about the time when "menstrual periods stop altogether," a question put not only to postmenopausal women but to all the women in the study, so some respondents were looking back in time, others ahead in time. Table 2 shows that the overwhelming majority of postmenopausal women

TABLE 2 Subjective Feelings about Menopause by Menopausal Stage and Type of Menopause among Postmenopausal Women (percentage)

	Menopausal Stage		Type of Menopause	
Subjective Feeling[a]	Postmenopausal[b]	Peri/Premenopausal	Natural	Surgical
Only relief	61.6	45.7	58.5	68.3
No particular feeling	23.0	25.4	25.5	16.5
Mixed feelings	13.6	25.6	14.1	13.8
Only regret	1.8	3.3	1.8	1.4
	100.0	100.0	100.0	100.0
N	(704)	(708)	(434)	(218)

[a]The question read: "Women have different feelings about the time when their menstrual periods stop altogether. Which of the following statements best describes your feelings about this? Please answer whether or not your periods have already stopped."

[b]Essentially the same distribution of responses is found if cases are restricted to women who became postmenopausal "off-time," i.e., under the age of 40.

TABLE 3 Degree of Worry Women Express about Getting Older,
on Three Issues (percentage)

Issue	Not at All	A Little	Some or a Lot	N
"Being too old to have children"	82.0	7.8	10.2	(1507)
"Being less attractive as a woman"	36.3	34.6	29.1	(1527)
"Having more illness as you get older"	21.6	38.0	40.4	(1525)

Note: Participants were asked the following question: "Women sometimes worry about the future and getting older. How much do you worry about each of the following?"

reported feeling "only relief" and a mere 2 percent "only regret." If anything it was the peri- and premenopausal women who were more inclined to report an anticipation of "mixed feelings, some regret and some relief." Table 2 also shows that women who experienced a surgical menopause were even more likely to express "only relief" than were women who experienced a natural menopause, an interesting finding in light of the fact that the former category includes more women who became infertile at quite young ages. One surmises an important factor in their "relief" is being able to put behind them whatever reproductive pathology was involved in surgical termination of fertility.

It is possible that our question format stimulated more positive responses of "relief" because it asked about cessation of menstruation ("when your periods have stopped altogether"), not menopause, and made no direct reference to being unable to have children. Although menstruation is a constant reminder of the potential for pregnancy, it is also the source for many women of physical discomfort, mood changes, and some restriction of activities. If this is what they had in mind when responding, then it is not surprising that they felt relief rather than regret. A more direct test of subjective feelings about the loss of fertility can be gauged by three questions we asked about getting older, one of which was worry about being too old to have children. (The question read, "Women sometimes worry about the future and getting older. How much do you worry about each of the following?") Table 3 shows the distribution of responses among the three areas of concern—being too old to have children, being less attractive, and having more illness as you get older.

Very few women express any concern about being too old to have children: 4 in 5 report "not at all"; only 1 in 10 expresses a moderate to high level of concern. The greatest worry for these women was the prospect of having more illness as they got older, with 4 in 10 reporting high concern, and only 1 in 5 no concern at all. Potential loss of attractiveness runs a close second to future illnesses in the level of worry women

TABLE 4 Worry about Being Too Old to Have a Child, by Age
and Parental Status (percentage)

Parental Status	25–29	30–39	40–49	50–59	60–69	70–74
No children	71.8	75.6	16.3	5.9	0.0	0.0
N	(78)	(74)	(49)	(36)	(21)	(13)
One or more children	33.7	29.1	9.3	3.5	0.0	0.0
N	(95)	(254)	(312)	(286)	(206)	(79)

Note: The respondents had expressed at least "some worry."

reported. (We reserve, to a later section, further analysis of the concern for attractiveness.)

The real significance of these concerns about aging is best seen when we consider a woman's age and her parental status. Table 4 shows that both characteristics are strong determinants of concern for being too old to conceive and bear a child. As this table shows, it is childless women under 40 years of age who report high concern about being too old to have children. With the contemporary trend toward older ages at marriage and childbearing, particularly among educated women who seek to establish themselves in careers before taking on family responsibilities, this is an understandable concern, aware as they are of the decreased odds of becoming pregnant and the increased risk of fetal defects. The increase in reliance on artificial fertilization in recent years is a telling indicator of the reality behind such concerns among childless women in their late thirties and early forties. Note too that even among women under 40 who have at least one child, approximately 30 percent feel some concern about aging effects on fertility. These are most likely women who have kept open the option of having an additional child. All told, however, passing one's fortieth birthday is clearly a threshold beyond which very few women wish to have children, a subjective report consistent with the high incidence of tubal ligation, as well as with the finding that menopause is both anticipated and experienced more with relief than regret.

Menopausal Symptoms

Despite the relief women express about menopause, it does not follow that there are no physical or psychological symptoms associated with this midlife transition. The MIDUS survey embedded a variety of acute symptoms in its modules on physical health, including five that are typically found in menopausal inventories: hot flashes (or flushes; both terms are used interchangeably), sweating a lot, insomnia, irritability, and discomfort during intercourse. The inventory of symptoms was

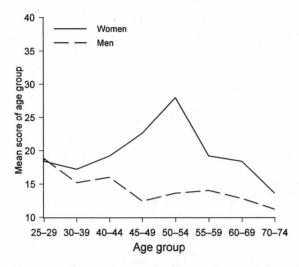

FIGURE 2. Mean score on symptoms by age and sex (means are converted to a 0–100 scale). Sex differences are significant only in the 45–54 age range.

responded to by both men and women, so we can observe sex differences across the life course. Figure 2 shows the means on the five-symptom score by sex and age, and indicates a significant increase in symptoms among women between the ages of 45 and 54, the primary years of the menopausal transition. By contrast, men show little change, only a slight nonsignificant decline in symptom score between early adulthood and old age.

Interpretation of the summary score is facilitated by examining the percentage of specific symptoms, four of which are shown in figure 3. The graphs showing the percentage of hot flashes, insomnia, and sweating a lot indicate the same profile for women as does the summary score in figure 2, with the percentage peaking in the 45–54 age range, hardly surprising because a flash episode typically involves perspiring and often causes sleep disturbance. Physiologically such symptoms indicate vascular reactions to erratic changes in endocrine secretion. The more psychological variable—irritability—shows a similar profile of decline with age for both men and women, reflecting, one surmises, both the waning of intense physical activity of more youthful years and the equanimity that comes with greater life experiences by one's elderly years.

The sharpest difference between men and women is the profile shown for sweating a lot. Frequent sweating is at its peak among men under 40,

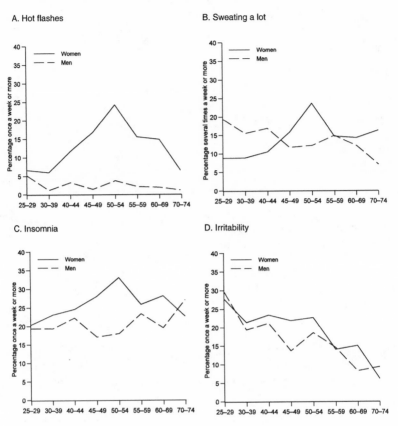

FIGURE 3. Percentage of the high frequency of four symptoms during the past thirty days, by age and sex.

declining in their middle years just at the age it increases sharply among women. The difference in this age-related profile of sweating between men and women brought a smile of recognition to me when first noted, reminiscent as it was of personal experience: in our thirties my husband was the "hotter" partner, wanting the thermostat of an electric blanket and of a room turned down, while I wanted a higher temperature. In our early fifties, I was the "hotter" partner, wanting open windows and lower room and blanket temperatures. Fortunately, American manufacturers came to the rescue, with dual controls on electric blankets that permitted us to weather the difference in temperature preferences and remain in the same bed. There would surely be a financial bonanza for any manufacturer who could produce blankets that not only warm one up but also cool one down,

TABLE 5 Frequency of Hot Flashes by Menopausal Stage among
Middle-Aged Women Aged 40–55 (percentage)

Frequency of Hot Flashes	Stage of Menopausal Transition		
	Premenopausal	Perimenopausal	Postmenopausal
Not at all	81.0	54.1	51.0
One or more times a month	13.8	32.2	23.5
One or more times a week	4.2	8.9	13.3
Almost every day	1.0	4.8	12.2
	100.0	100.0	100.0
N	(116)	(146)	(239)
Once a week or more	5.2	13.7	25.5

for those baby-boomer women in midlife who are now experiencing hot flushes and night sweats.

But what of the general population of young men and women in earlier adulthood? Perhaps men report more sweating because they engage in more vigorous physical activity either at work or, by participating in strenuous sports, at play. Further analysis, however, discounts this possibility, because in multivariate analysis regressing the sweating variable on age, education, and a scale on vigorous and moderate physical activity "enough to work up a sweat" (either job or leisure related), the physical exercise scale is not statistically significant. Rather, it is youth and low education that are significant predictors of sweating for men, and middle age and low education for women (data not shown).

On the protypical menopausal symptom of hot flashes, there is great variation among women in any age group or stage of the menopausal transition. Table 5 shows the prevalence of hot flashes by menopausal stage among women between 40 and 55 years of age. Note that fully half of the middle-aged peri- and postmenopausal women report no hot flashes. Only 12 percent of the postmenopausal women between 40 and 55 years of age report having flashes "almost every day," a far cry from the media image of the woman at a dinner party with perspiration running down her face and slipping off her chin. Our results are much closer to those found in an early Minnesota longitudinal study of women in which only 1 in 10 middle-aged women reported "severe" hot flashes (Voda 1982).

Our MIDUS survey found that only a third of postmenopausal women report any current use of hormone replacement, and such hormone usage is only weakly associated with a lower incidence of frequent hot flashes: 11 percent of hormone users and 15 percent of nonusers report hot flashes twice a week or more. So too we find that hormone use shows no effect on frequency of insomnia or sweating a lot. I suggest several possible interpretations for these results. For one, hormone use may provide only minimal help in the alleviation of hot flashes. For another, women may resort to hormone replacement for reasons other than symptom alleviation. Some may do so in response to media and medical suggestions that HRT can help in avoiding heart attacks or bone fractures. It is also possible that there are long-standing characteristics of women that predispose them to hormone use but for which HRT provides little or no relief. I return to this issue later in the chapter.

Multiple Predictors of the Five-Symptom Scale

I draw on the substantive diversity of variables in the MIDUS survey for an analysis of what predicts high scores on the five-symptoms score. Correlational and factor analyses of the five symptoms did not show any one underlying latent construct to the measure, which is hardly surprising in light of the age and sex differences we have already noted, but this also suggests that a number of individual attributes and life experiences, quite apart from age and sex, may trigger an elevation of these symptoms. In table 6, I draw on a variety of measures, including sociodemographic variables; several measures that tap health; perceived changes in the body over the past five years and somatic amplification (more on this scale below); plus two scales that measure the extent to which men and women experience stress in their daily lives at work and at home. This regression analysis is restricted to employed adults so that we can compare the effect of work versus home stress on symptom elevation.

The somatic amplification scale has its origins in medical and psychiatric research. The scale is a modified version of the private body consciousness scale developed by Miller, Murphy, and Buss (1981), with items tapping individual differences in subjective sensitivity to internal body states—for example, heartbeat and hunger—or low tolerance for stimuli from the external environment, such as loud noises or temperature extremes of hot or cold. My expectation was that women might be more alert than men to internal body processes as a consequence of their monthly experience of menstrual cycle fluctuation and greater sensory acuity (Pennebaker 1982). The somatic amplification scale does in fact show a significant sex difference: women are more attuned to internal body messages than men are. But there is no reason to think that somatic amplification does not also play a role in men's symptoms scores.

TABLE 6 Regression of Five-Symptom Score on Health, Body Decline
and Sensitivity, and Role Stress, among Employed Adults, by Sex
(standardized beta coefficients)

Predictor Variables	Women	Men
Sociodemographic variables		
Age[a]	.098***	−.102**
Education	−.106***	−.034
Married/cohabiting (1=yes, 0=no)	−.015	−.019
Number of biological children	−.024	−.064*
Health, body decline, sensitivity		
Physical health rating[b]	−.110***	−.100**
Emotional/mental health rating[b]	−.168***	−.094**
Somatic amplification scale[c]	.170***	.182***
Body decline score[d]	.121***	.145***
Social-role stress		
Work-role stress[e]	.049	.100***
Home-role stress[e]	.117***	.082**
R^2	.209***	.166***
N	(984)	(1080)

[a]Because several symptoms among women peak in midlife, a dummy variable is used for age in the equations for women (1 = 40–59 yrs, 0 =<40 or >59) and a continuous age variable for men.

[b]Single-item ratings of physical health and emotional mental health are 0=very poor to 5=excellent.

[c]The somatic amplification scale consists of five self-ratings on awareness of things happening in the body: hating to be too hot or too cold, bothered by loud noises, low tolerance for pain, and quick to sense hunger contractions. High scores indicate high sensitivity to body sensations.

[d]The body decline score has a 0–4 range, one point for each of four items rated as "worse now" than five years ago: energy level, physical fitness, physique/figure, and weight (0=none of four worse now; 4=all four judged worse now).

[e]The work stress scale consists of three items indicating the frequency that respondents report having too many demands on them, not enough time to get everything done, and a lot of interruptions on the job. The home stress scale consists of four items, comparable to the work stress items but referring to "at home," plus one item on not being able to control the amount of time spent on tasks. "At home" was used rather than "in your family" so that the items applied to adults living alone as well as to married or cohabiting adults.

$*p < .05. **p < .01. ***p < .001.$

Judging by the size of the standardized beta coefficients shown in table 6, somatic amplification is the most significant predictor of symptoms among men, on a par with mental health rating among women. Independent of the age pattern that differentiates men from women (linear decline for men, midlife peak for women, age effects that remain significant), poor physical and mental health, low education, and high somatic amplification each contribute significantly to elevated symptoms. Both men and women who rate aspects of their body as worse now than five years ago are also significantly more likely to report elevated symptoms.

One of the most interesting findings shown in table 6 is a sex-differentiated effect of role stress: for men, stress in their work role has more effect than stress at home on symptoms levels, whereas for women, home-role stress has the greater effect, and work-role stress, though positive, is not statistically significant. Even in our day, most men invest more heavily in work roles than do women, and women invest more in home and family than men do. Even in dual-earning couples, economic responsibility is heavier on husbands than on wives, because the men typically earn significantly more than their wives. Role investment involves both time and energy expenditure, which may aggravate role stress response, in this instance by elevating such symptoms as insomnia and irritability. Many women who experience menopause-related hot flashes report that anxiety or nervousness often triggers the onset of a hot flash. A former gynecologist of mine in Baltimore, a woman then in her sixties, reported that she experienced hot flashes only while driving at high speed on expressways, something she was as nervous about at the age of 64 as she had been at 34.

In both the Massachusetts and Pittsburgh longitudinal studies, the researchers report that women who at baseline indicated negative views of menopause were significantly more likely at follow-up to report that they were depressed, irritable, or troubled with hot flashes or night sweats with insomnia than were women who rejected negative views of menopause in the baseline survey (Avis and McKinlay 1991; Matthews et al. 1990). This finding was interpreted as confirming the theory that social expectations produce the discomforting symptoms, that expectations become a self-fulfilling prophecy.

An alternate explanation is that women who experience more than average discomfort in connection with their menstrual periods may be the women whose expectations about menopause are not self-fulfilling prophecies at all but realistic extrapolations from personal experience with menstruation to anticipated experience during the menopausal years. Table 7 confirms this counter-interpretation. Among postmenopausal women, the menstrual pain levels they reported experiencing in earlier stages of their lives is a significant predictor of the five-symptoms score, net of most of the predictor variables familiar from table 6.

Our findings are consistent with Ann Voda's (1982) earlier study of the menopausal hot flash, in which women kept a two-week daily record of the frequency and intensity of their hot flashes. Voda found that many women with high frequency and severity of hot flash episodes in midlife

TABLE 7 Regression of Five-Symptom Score, including Menstrual Pain Rating, among Postmenopausal Women (standardized beta coefficients)

Predictor Variables	Postmenopausal Women
Menstrual pain scale[a]	.115***
Physical health rating	−.060
Emotional/mental health rating	−.187***
Somatic amplification scale	.130***
Body decline score	.135***
Home-role stress	.180***
Education	−.062*
R^2	.234***
N	(695)

[a] A two-item scale based on assessments of the amount of discomfort experienced before and during menstrual periods, from "none at all" to "a lot." Ratings are current for menstruating women, retrospective for postmenopausal women. Scale range: 0=low to 8=high.

*$p < .05$. ***$p < .001$.

voluntarily reported a history of premenstrual headaches, and those with high heat intolerance attending hot flashes also reported cold intolerance during their younger years.[3] This finding suggests some continuity across phases of individual reproductive histories, perhaps reflecting a long-standing predisposition to either thermoregulatory problems or vascular instability or both.

In a regression analysis performed using data from postmenopausal women, I found that negative affect (e.g., feeling sad, fidgety, hopeless), neuroticism (worrying a lot, moody, nervous, not calm), and high levels of somatic amplification were independent contributors to hot flash frequency. The negative affect scale refers to "the last 30 days," but it is highly correlated with the more long-standing personality predisposition to neuroticism ($r = .60$) and somatic amplification ($r = .28$). With these more long-standing characteristics in the equation, current hormone use showed no effect on hot flash frequency (data not shown).

RECENT CHANGES IN THE BODY
Self-Ratings of Body Changes over the Past Five Years

I turn now to what respondents told us about changes in their bodies over the course of the previous five years, guided by the question of whether men and women show the same or a different profile in these perceptions of change, how these changes differ by stage of life from early adulthood to old age, and what, if any, other factors besides age and sex predict whether adults feel their bodies have gotten better or worse. At

TABLE 8 Assessment of Conditions of Body Now Compared with Five
Years Ago, by Sex (percentage)

Aspect of Body		Women	Men
Physique/figure	Better now	17.3	16.0
	No change	36.0	43.5
	Worse now	46.7	40.5
		100.0	100.0
Physical fitness	Better now	19.2	16.7
	No change	37.0	39.6
	Worse now	43.8	43.7
		100.0	100.0
Weight	Better now	18.4	18.4
	No change	35.4	46.2
	Worse now	46.2	35.3
		100.0	100.0
Energy level	Better now	17.5	13.7
	No change	40.3	45.8
	Worse now	42.3	40.4
		100.0	100.0
	Base N	(1530)	(1449)

appropriate points, I report some actual measures of changes by age and sex in terms of waist and hip measurements, and weight as indexed by body mass index, which measures weight relative to height (technically calculated by weight in kilograms divided by the square of height in meters).

Respondents rated four aspects of their bodies: physique/figure, energy level, weight, and physical fitness. Table 8 reports the full marginal distributions on these four aspects of body change by sex. Note that fewer than 1 in 5 men and women think *any* of these four aspects of their bodies are "better now" than five years ago. On all four factors, more men than women say their bodies have shown no change. The sharpest difference by sex is on weight and physique/figure: the modal response for men is no change, for women, worse now, particularly in relation to weight; 46 percent of men say "no change," to 35 percent of women. These percentages are precisely the reverse of the percentages for those responding "worse now"—which is the response of more women than men (46 percent versus 35 percent, respectively).

An obvious reason for these high reports of "worse now" is the simple fact that most of our respondents are in their middle years, with much smaller proportions of the sample in early adulthood or old age. Figure 4 shows the profiles of men and women for the same four body aspects across the life course, in terms of the percentage reporting that they

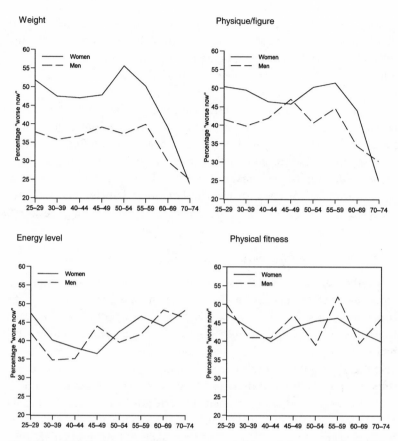

FIGURE 4. Body change for the worse over the past five years, in weight, physique/figure, energy level, and physical fitness, by age and sex.

are "worse now" than five years ago. The most dramatic age and sex differences concern weight and physique/figure. Women clearly either are more critical of their weight or have in fact shown greater weight gain than men in early adulthood and their middle years. Among women in their early fifties, a full 56 percent report that their weight is "worse now" than five years ago, a profile mirrored in women's assessments of their figure as well. Interestingly, these poor self-assessments plunge downward among older adults on both weight and figure; in the case of women, from the high of 56 percent in their early fifties to less than half that (24 percent) among older women in their early seventies.

Energy-level judgments show little sex difference, just a linear increase in "worse now" judgments from the early thirties through the early seventies for both sexes. That men and women in their late twenties give themselves poorer ratings than do those in their thirties may be the result of the realization of those in their late twenties that they don't have quite the bounce they remember from their late adolescence and early twenties.

It is at first puzzling that negative assessments of weight and figure go down so dramatically in the older years. To some degree, older adults may simply move beyond cultural pressures to retain youthful appearances. On the other hand, it is likely that there is a selection factor at work among older adults: very heavy or obese older adults run greater risks of cardiovascular diseases, stroke, and late-onset diabetes, and more of them die, leaving fewer overweight and obese survivors among the oldest respondents in a survey.

Objective Measures of Body Change

Further interpretive cues may be found in sex and age differences on more objective measures of body characteristics. Respondents' packets contained a tape measure and a sketch of a body that showed exactly where respondents were to measure their hips and waists. These self-report measures are clearly not as valid as objective measurements of height and weight by a health professional. It is known that overweight subjects in self-report studies tend to underestimate their weight and that all subjects tend to overestimate their height (Bray 1992; Palta et al. 1982). This suggests that analysis using self-report measures to estimate the prevalence of overweight or obesity is likely to be conservative. Two studies illustrate this tendency: the NHANES III (1984–94) study, in which weight and height were measured by health professionals, showed a prevalence of obesity of 22.5 percent in adults, one-third higher than the prevalence rates using self-reports in a telephone survey (Mokdad et al. 1999).

Figure 5 shows the differences between men and women across the life course in average hip and waist measurements. (These figures are shown in the familiar terms of inches to permit readers to easily gauge their own measurements against the average for their age and sex.) The most striking contrast seen in figure 5 is the very large difference between hip and waist measurements of women compared with those of men, projecting the image of the rounded hourglass contours of the female body and the more squarish contours of the male body.

It is often claimed that slim waists relative to hip measurements are an index of female fertility potential (along with clear skin and shining hair)

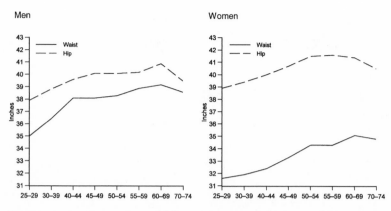

FIGURE 5. Average waist and hip measurements by age and sex (in inches).

and that childbearing has the effect of enlarging a woman's waistline compared with her hips. I found no evidence of this in the MIDUS data. We compared women who had no children with those who did in each of the eight age groups shown in figure 5 and found, if anything, a reverse pattern. For example, childless women in their late fifties had larger waistlines than did women the same age who had given birth to two children (35.1 inches versus 33.5 inches). The major characteristic of women who had large families (four or more children) was not merely larger waistlines; they were heavier at all ages than were women who had had only one child or no children (data not shown).

The second major feature of figure 5 is the steady increase in both waist and hip measurements from the late twenties through the sixties for both men and women, followed by a sharp downturn in these measurements among the oldest respondents, a finding consistent with the second interpretation offered earlier of some selection factor at work, although at later ages than shown in the perceived changes in the body reported in figure 4. One last point to note is that there is much greater variance in hip and waist measurements of women than of men, a consistent pattern across all eight age groups, as illustrated by the standard deviation on waist measurements of those in their late forties: for women, a standard deviation of 7 inches, for men, 4.8 inches.

A more direct view of objective age and sex differences in body shape and heft is provided by the body mass index (BMI). Figure 6 provides such data. Figure 6A shows the mean BMI by age and sex, with an interesting sex difference in the ages at which weight gain is increasing most sharply.

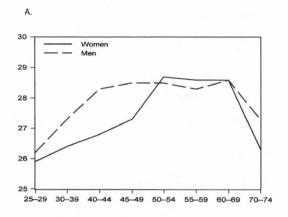

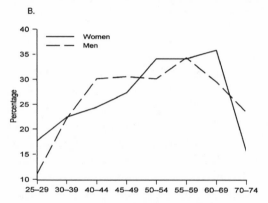

FIGURE 6. (A) Average BMI by age and sex. (B) Percentage defined as obese by the National Academy standards (BMI of 30 or more), by age and sex.

For men, the weight gain occurs between their late twenties and early forties; for women, the sharpest increase is between their late forties and midfifties, precisely the years spanning the menopausal transition. Figure 6A also shows the consistent drop in the oldest men and women, similar to the pattern shown previously.

Average BMIs hide as much as they reveal. Whether an individual's BMI is 26 or 28 represents a rather small increment tipped toward being slightly overweight. Analysts of the National Health and Nutrition Examination Studies use a BMI of 27.8 for men and 27.3 for women as the cutoff criterion for defining overweight, and a BMI of 30 or more for defining obesity (Kuczmarski et al. 1994). The average weights shown in figure 6A fall largely between a BMI of 26 and 28.5, but there is

considerable variance around such averages, with significantly large proportions of adults who are not just overweight but obese. The age and sex
profiles on obesity are shown in figure 6B: the percentage of obese persons increases with age for both men and women, but the sharpest upturn
occurs during early midlife for men, late midlife for women. Slightly more
than a third of women in their fifties and sixties are obese. The strong
relationship of obesity with age alerts us to the importance of adjusting
for age in any discussion of secular trends toward more obesity in the U.S.
population. The data in figure 6 suggest that although the baby-boomer
generation has given far more attention to physical fitness than did their
parents (with dieting, jogging, aerobic exercise, swimming, squash, and
such), they nevertheless show marked increases in weight by midlife.

Ali Mokdad and his research associates (1999) report similar results
on obesity prevalence in the United States. Using data from telephone
surveys conducted annually between 1991 and 1998, they report a rise in
obesity with age from 12 percent among 18- to 29-year-olds, to a peak
among adults in their fifties of 24 percent, then dropping to 15 percent
among adults over 70, a profile very like that shown in the MIDUS data.
These prevalence figures are from the 1998 survey. The trend from 1991
to 1998 shows increasing obesity in just these seven years in all segments
of the population, but with particularly sharp increases among young
adults, college graduates, Hispanics, and those residing in the southeast-
ern Atlantic states.

A question that is important to confront is whether the weight gain
shown by age in the last several figures is properly interpreted in a largely
maturational sense. Clearly the Mokdad series shows both maturational
and cohort trends. Internal to the MIDUS data set, we can take a step
further in an assessment of this issue, because respondents reported not
only their current weight but their weight when they were 21 years of age.
Figure 7 shows both current weight and recalled weight at 21 years of age
by both sex and current age of the respondents.

In figure 7, weight at 21 years of age shows a downward slope across
the age groups. Consistent with the trend across surveys shown in the
Mokdad study, younger adults in the MIDUS sample weigh significantly
more than younger adults did fifty years ago, as reflected by the recalled
youthful weight of our oldest respondents. An average woman in 1995
in her late twenties reports she weighed 136 when she was 21, whereas
our oldest respondents report having weighed 123 pounds when they
were 21, a difference of 13 pounds between these birth cohorts. The
contrast among men is roughly similar, 169 versus 157 pounds, for a

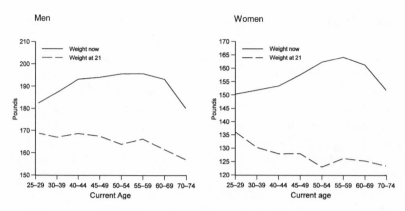

FIGURE 7. Current weight versus weight at age 21, by current age and sex (in pounds).

weight difference between these cohorts at age 21 of 12 pounds. Note, too, the enormous bulge in the graph between current weight of today's midlifers compared with what they reported for their weight at 21: a 30-pound gain for women, 32 for men. Clearly dieting, jogging, tennis, and swimming do not compensate for the sedentary occupations, rich diets, and hours of TV watching and web surfing of recent years.

In the future, adults may experience even greater weight problems, as suggested by the fact that the youngest respondents are heavier than members of preceding cohorts of young adults. Several factors contribute to this trend toward fatter youth: the dropping of physical education in so many of the nation's schools; the sedentary lifestyle implicit in the fact that children between the ages of 6 and 11 watch television an average of twenty-five hours a week; the popularity of computer and video games, which add even further to this more sedentary lifestyle; and the warnings to children by dual-earning parents that they remain indoors after school, or the children's supervision by after-school centers or babysitters, who may hesitate to take them outdoors (Brody 2000a, 2000b). Diet change in recent decades holds particular relevance for the health of future cohorts. Jane Brody reports from several studies that Americans have shown a 28 percent increase in sugar consumption in just fifteen years (Brody 2000a). This is a particular problem for children and teenagers undergoing their most significant period of healthy bone formation. With each five-year period from ages 1 through 19, children's milk consumption has dropped and carbonated soda consumption has risen. Between 15 and 19 years of age, when bone formation is at a critical stage, a teenager's soda consumption is nearly double that of milk, the best source of calcium and vitamin D. This nutritional profile of today's children and adolescents holds ominous warnings of vulnerability to osteoporosis in their later years. Trends like these imply not only that we will see a less healthy middle-aged population in the future but that today youngsters have less mental alertness and poorer health. For example, studies have shown that physically active youngsters do better in school and have fewer coronary risk factors like high blood pressure and high cholesterol.[4]

Public health journals and government reports have described this trend toward ever-increasing weight in the U.S. population as a serious "epidemic." What to do about it is far from certain. Clearly Americans have themselves tried to lose weight by dieting. At any given point in time, about 50 percent of American women and 25 percent of American men are dieting, but many if not most of such diets are unsuccessful, because weight gain typically occurs after going off the diet. Many adults resort to periodic bouts of serious dieting, resulting in a history of considerable weight fluctuation. Recent research on weight fluctuation, from the Framingham Heart Study, has shown weight fluctuation to be strongly associated with adverse health outcomes, especially among 30- to 44-year-old adults, the age group in which dieting is most common (Lissner et al. 1991).

Another cautionary tale about weight loss is found in challenges to the frequent claim that weight loss in obese persons paves the way to increased longevity. Reviews of the evidence from existing studies on this issue do not support the claim (Williamson and Pamuk 1993): obese adults who lost a great deal of weight did not live longer than obese adults who had not lost any weight. Research findings like these suggest that a wiser course to follow than frequent short-term bouts of dieting is to adopt a lifestyle, at as young an age as possible, that emphasizes physical exercise on a regular basis and a cuisine that concentrates on milk, fowl and fish, an array of fresh vegetables and fruits, and minimizes the consumption of sodas, fatty meat, high-sugar-content cereals, or frozen dinners. It is no easy task to persuade parents, teachers, and youngsters themselves to make such changes, against the massive pressures and temptations that numerous food processors and restaurants parade across the television screens by the dozens every day in most American homes.

Returning now to respondents' ratings of change in their bodies over the past five years, I raise the interesting question of to what extent adults pass such judgments on the basis of reports of their weight (using BMI

TABLE 9 Regression of Body Decline Score on Physical and
Psychological Characteristics, by Sex (standardized beta coefficients)

Predictor Variables	Women	Men
Physical characteristics		
Physical health rating	−.093*	−.143***
Body mass index (BMI)	.272***	.221***
Total exercise score[a]	−.141***	−.177***
Psychological characteristics		
Emotional/mental health	−.068*	.019
Neuroticism scale[b]	.101***	.097***
Age	−.114***	−.082**
R^2	.176***	.140***
N	(1411)	(1358)

[a] A four-item scale on the frequency of moderate and vigorous physical activity "long enough to work up a sweat" during the summer and winter, each ranging from "never" to "several times a week or more."

[b] A four-item scale on the extent to which respondents say they are moody, worrying, nervous, and (not) calm.

* $p < .05.$ ** $p < .01.$ *** $p < .001.$

rather than simply weight itself in order to correct for height), and what other factors are involved in the judgment that their bodies have changed for the worse in recent years. Table 9 brings together an array of predictor variables covering both physical and psychological characteristics of respondents, controlling for age, which we have already seen to be strongly related to both body change and BMI.

It is immediately clear from the standardized beta coefficients shown in table 9 that weight plays an equally important role in judgments about changes in their bodies for both men and women; that is, BMI is the most statistically significant predictor of the body decline scores. Independent contributions are also made by ratings of overall physical health: those with excellent health report less change for the worse than do those in very poor health. Closer analysis shows that physical fitness and energy level are the most significant, rather than weight and figure, as shown in table 9 (data not shown). By contrast, both men and women who engage in moderate or vigorous exercise are less inclined to report worsening conditions of their bodies.

The regression analysis also alerts us to the importance of psychological attributes; an elevated score on the neuroticism scale predicts greater body change for the worse. It should be noted, however, that the neuroticism scale does not measure a clinically diagnosed mental illness. Adults who score high on this scale are not "neurotic" in any technical psychiatric sense; they may simply be worrying types subject to mood changes or may have an easily excitable temperament (the items in the scale tap precisely these characteristics—nervousness, worrying, moodiness, and, reverse-coded, not calm). Some aspects of the tendency to neuroticism have genetic roots, and therefore the tendency is likely to be a long-standing characteristic of the adult. (In an analysis of the neuroticism scale, using data from the MIDMAC sample of twins, we estimate the heredity component to be 56 percent.) A high score on such a scale could have an effect on self-assessments by exaggerating even minor personal faults or body sensations or, in an ironic twist, by avoiding the enticement of an inflated sense of self-esteem that a consumer culture encourages.

One particular sex difference is suggested by the contrast between men and women in the influence of physical as opposed to emotional/mental health: men's rating of their physical health has more impact on their sense of body decline than such a rating has for women; by contrast, only women's emotional health impacts on their sense of body decline, which is not true for men. In more detailed regression analysis not shown here, a comparable analysis on the component items in the body decline score shows even stronger differences than that shown in table 9. It is on figure/physique that the difference between the sexes is sharpest: physical health is a significant predictor of worsened condition of the physique of men but not women, and whereas emotional/mental health affects women's reports of a worsening of their figures, it does not affect men's. It is tempting to interpret this difference in terms of social context: the cultural emphasis on women's looks may impact more deeply on women's emotional state in assessing change in their bodies; by contrast, more men hold jobs that require physical fitness and stamina, with the result that poor physical health is more significant to men's assessment of changes in their bodies.

Worry about Loss of Attractiveness

At this point it is appropriate to return to the measures in MIDUS of women's self-reported worries about getting older. Recall that in table 3 we found few women concerned about being unable to have children as they got older, with the exception of younger women who had not yet had a child. Loss of attractiveness, by contrast, was a source of worry to two out of three women. The first question I pose is whether age makes a difference here: at what age do women report the highest worry about loss of attractiveness, and do unmarried women express more concern

TABLE 10 Worry about Loss of Attractiveness with Age, among Women, by Age and Marital Status (percentage expressing at least some worry)

Marital Status	25–29	30–39	40–49	50–59	60–69	70–74
Married or cohabiting	66.4	78.4	71.7	60.7	50.8	30.0
N	(110)	(208)	(219)	(196)	(126)	(40)
Not married or cohabiting	77.4	70.5	69.0	66.4	42.3	25.3
N	(62)	(122)	(145)	(128)	(104)	(51)

than married women? Table 10 provides the answers to both questions: age clearly plays a larger role than marital status, with the percentage reporting some worry on this score declining among married women from 66 percent among the youngest to 30 percent among the oldest women, with an even greater contrast among the women who are neither married nor cohabiting, a drop from 77 percent to 25 percent.

There is an interesting interaction between age and marital status among the younger women: unmarried women in their late twenties show the highest worry percentage (77 percent), whereas among married women it is women in their thirties with the highest worry level (78 percent). A divorce-prone society may be particularly susceptible to heightened concern for one's looks, either to keep a spouse or to improve one's chances for a new one when returning to the singles scene at an older age. For unmarried or divorced women, the youthful images of self that are particularly revered in American society impose additional pressure to look younger than they are.

It is unfortunate that we neglected to include any question about loss of attractiveness for men in the MIDUS sample. There is only indirect evidence that men are showing an increasing concern for their looks, as witness the increased resort to male cosmetics, fashion diversity, cosmetic surgery (particularly liposuction reduction of the abdomen), and efforts to forestall or cover up baldness, or, in some social niches of society, to prefer a shaved head over thinning hair. Strenuous exercise to build upper arm biceps preoccupies thousands of men in health spas. Interestingly, even male G.I. Joe dolls for boys have shown an increasing emphasis on the size of upper arm biceps: when the doll first appeared in 1964, the proportionate width of his biceps was equivalent to 12.1 inches; then in 1974 they were bulked up to 15.2 inches. In his most recent incarnation in 1998, an appropriately renamed G.I. Joe Extreme has an incredible 26.8-inch bicep, a size even in excess of those attained by advanced bodybuilders.

Jackson Katz (1999) claims that one source of this trend toward greater attention to physical size and shape in male figures is a reaction to women's challenge to male dominance in so many spheres of life—in education, the workplace, and sports—over the past twenty-five years. Elizabeth Fox-Genevese argued a somewhat similar theme, pointing out that men are becoming frustrated by a world in which they have lost a good deal of control through an erosion of their socioeconomic advantages and the social irrelevance to their major roles of their physical superiority (Fox-Genevese 1991). Today's action figure toys for young boys, if they are taken as a male ideal, have little prospect of being translated into the boys' later adult lives except through bravado acts of high risk-taking in active sports, or in symbolic form by risk-taking in the stock market or casinos. Alas, it must be left to future contacts with MIDUS respondents or other surveys of adults to investigate the extent to which men of various ages report worry about the loss of attractiveness as they age, what predicts high or low levels of such concern, and how their profile compares with that shown here for women.

More pertinent to the analysis of women's attractiveness worries is an interesting finding from an analysis of HRT among postmenopausal women in the MIDUS sample (Keating et al. 1999). My co-authors of this medical journal article are all physicians or medical researchers in public health. When they analyzed the MIDUS data on HRT use, these authors expected that women with cardiac risk factors or diabetes mellitus would be highly likely to rely on hormone replacement therapy, but women with these conditions were less, not more, apt to report HRT. To my colleagues' surprise, the single psychological variable that predicted current hormone use was worry about attractiveness. There are echoes here of the claim made in Robert Wilson's early 1966 thesis in *Feminine Forever* that estrogen was the magical drug that assured continued sexual attractiveness well past midlife. Contemporary women seem more responsive to appeals to their femininity than to physicians' claims that medical risk factors should prompt reliance on estrogen replacement.

The next step in this analysis is to explore in greater depth what determines whether women worry about the loss of attractiveness as they get older, and to do so with attention to the likely difference between young and middle-aged married women. The results of this multivariate analysis are shown in table 11. In addition to physical measures and an expanded set of psychological variables, I introduce socioeconomic status measures here, on the expectation that higher economic status may trigger heightened concern for attractiveness among middle-aged women, knowing as they must that many middle-aged, high-earning men have many opportunities to meet and attract younger professional and business women of

TABLE 11 Regression of Worry about Attractiveness among Young and Middle-Aged Married Women (standardized beta coefficients)

Predictors	Young (25–39)	Middle-Aged (40–59)
Socioeconomic status		
Respondent's education	.043	.043
Respondent's personal earnings	−.001	−.009
Spouse's earnings	.075	.145**
Body		
Physical health rating	.070	−.015
Body decline score	.067	.110*
BMI	−.058	−.101*
Psychological		
Emotional/mental health	−.025	−.040
Neuroticism scale	.163**	.108*
Troubled marriage scale[a]	.098+	.150*
Self-acceptance scale[b]	−.195**	−.190***
R^2	.115	.166
N	(333)	(412)

[a] A five-item scale based on extent of disagreement with spouse concerning money matters, household tasks, and leisure-time activities; how often respondents thought their relationship was in trouble during the past year; and how likely they thought it was they might separate in future.

[b] A three-item psychological well-being scale, based on extent to which respondent agreed or disagreed with self-descriptive statements: "I like most parts of my personality", "When I look at the story of my life, I am pleased with how things have turned out so far", and "In many ways I feel disappointed with my achievements in life" (reverse-coded).

$+p < .10.$ $*p < .05.$ $**p < .01.$ $***p < .001.$

equal status, intelligence, and shared interests. Middle-aged women have seen the young trophy wives, usually the second wives, of their husbands' colleagues; they have seen their women friends be replaced by younger wives, and they know such women could replace them as well.

The major story told by the findings reported in table 11 is consistent with these expectations: among young married women in their late twenties and thirties, the major predictors of worry about attractiveness are all psychological variables: high scores on neuroticism, a troubled marriage, and low self-acceptance are the strongest predictors of such women's worry about loss of attractiveness as they get older. The same three psychological variables are also significant among older women in their forties and fifties, but now these variables are joined by status and physical variables in predisposing them to concern for their looks. As predicted, it is women married to high-earning spouses, whose marriages are troubled, and who report a worsening condition of their bodies in recent years, who are most worried about their looks. It is not the case, however, that being overweight is a factor here; in fact, it is low BMI women who are more worried than high BMI women, suggesting that many middle-aged women who are overweight have accepted their condition, given up the fight against the bulge, and no longer worry about loss of attractiveness. (Perhaps their husbands are as overweight as they are!)

In an effort to explore these findings in greater depth, I undertook a special analysis of the married middle-aged women who reported high worry about loss of attractiveness and tried to ascertain what character-ized those women in this special group who relied on hormone therapy compared with those who did not. The hormone-users in this special group showed a slight tendency to be married to men ten or more years older than themselves, a profile that suggests some of these hormone-using women were themselves younger trophy wives, whose husbands would be particularly concerned about their wives' retaining the youthful looks that had attracted them in the first place. This adds to the interpre-tation that hormone use is resorted to by women more for the purpose of retaining a youthful appearance than for coping with medical risk fac-tors. In light of the abrupt termination of the major WHI clinical trial on HRT, many middle-aged American women may have been wiser than physicians and medical researchers in rejecting the idea that hormone re-placement was a beneficial means of protecting heart and uterine health as they age.

SEX, ATTRACTIVENESS WORRY, AND THE MENOPAUSAL TRANSITION

To tie together some of the themes explored in this chapter, I turn now to the MIDUS measures on the sex lives of women in midlife. The key questions in this analysis are whether worry about attractiveness or perception of a body changing for the worse plays a role in either frequency of sex or satisfaction with sex lives generally, and whether the stage of menopausal transition has any bearing on women's sex lives. On this latter question, the issue is whether it is menopausal status or chronological age that relates to a lowering of sex frequency or satisfaction among older women.

Table 12 shows a decline in sex frequency among married or cohabiting women between 40 and 60 years of age by the stage of their menopausal transition: 61 percent of premenopausal women report having sex once a week or more, whereas this figure drops to 41 percent among post-menopausal women. But when we look at the regression of sex frequency, using beta coefficients, we readily see that it is not menopausal stage per

TABLE 12 Frequency of Sex and Menopausal Stage

Frequency of Sex, by Menopausal Stage, among Married/Cohabiting
Women Aged 40–59 (percentage)

	Premenopausal	Perimenopausal	Postmenopausal
Once a month or less	17.8	25.3	34.2
Two or three times a month	21.5	22.1	24.9
Once a week or more	60.7	52.6	40.9
	100.0	100.0	100.0
N	(76)	(95)	(237)

Regression of Sex Frequency on Age, Postmenopausal Stage, Body Decline,
and Physical Health (standardized beta coefficients)

Age	−.407***
Postmenopausal stage[b]	.044
Body decline score	−.064*
Physical health rating	.005
R^2	.198***
N	(845)

[a]Item read "Over the past six months, on average, how often have you had sex with someone?"
[b]Dummy variable on menopausal stage: 1=postmenopausal; 0=peri- or premenopausal.
*$p < .05.$ ***$p < .001.$

TABLE 13 Regressions of Frequency of Sex, and of Overall Satisfaction
with Sex Life, on Age, Postmenopausal Stage, and Worry about
Attractiveness (standardized beta coefficients)

Predictor Variables	Sex Frequency	Sex Life Satisfaction[a]
Age	−.399***	−.243***
Postmenopausal stage	−.037	−.036
Worry about attractiveness	−.049*	−.128***
R^2	.175***	.173***
N	(1425)	(1425)

[a]Satisfaction with sex life is an overall single rating of 0–10, where 0 means "worst possible" and 10 means "best possible."
*$p < .05.$ ***$p < .001.$

se but age and reports of body decline in recent years that are the significant predictors: it is the older women and those reporting a worsening condition of their bodies who report less frequent sex. Menopausal status contributes no independent effect, nor does the women's report of the general condition of their physical health.

Finally, table 13 shows that menopausal stage has no effect on either sex frequency or sex-life satisfaction. Both behavior and satisfaction decline significantly with age, with an added influence of worry about loss of attractiveness. That some accommodation is made to declining sex drive is suggested by the fact that frequency is more strongly affected by age than is general satisfaction with the domain of sex in one's life. By contrast, worrying about the loss of attractiveness shows greater influence on satisfaction than on sex frequency, perhaps reflecting the fact that satisfaction is an individual's judgment, whereas frequency of sex is a function of desire on the part of two partners in a relationship.

CONCLUSION

Contrary to much recent attention to the problems associated with menopause, the 1995 MIDUS survey does not demonstrate any pervasive trauma during this normal transition in women's lives. In the contemporary period, menopause is not subjectively associated with the end of fertility, because the last wanted birth takes place long before most women experience the first signs of menopause. An increasing proportion of women take control of their fertility in a more direct sense by having their fallopian tubes tied, and typically they do so years before they go through the menopausal transition.

A small minority of women report elevated symptoms typically associated with menopause. Only 12 percent of postmenopausal women in their fifties report having the prototypical menopausal symptom of hot flashes "almost every day." Nor are the symptoms of sweating, insomnia, hot flashes, irritability, or discomfort during intercourse restricted to women during the menopausal transition: many younger and older women, and a minority of men report such symptoms as well. Our findings show echoes of those Bernice Neugarten found a very long time ago in her analysis of a wide range of symptoms that gynecologists took to be linked to menopause but which she showed were often found among young women in their twenties and thirties (Neugarten and Kraines 1964).

More importantly, there are other variables that are strong predictors of such symptoms. We have identified several, including long-standing characteristics such as a history of menstrual period pain; high sensitivity to internal and environmental factors such as high or low temperatures, loud noises, or hunger contractions; and role stress at home or on the job—all of which contribute independently to elevated symptoms, as does poor mental or physical health.

Additional findings reported in this chapter help to place menopause in a larger life-course framework and to identify other characteristics of heightened significance during the middle years. The analysis of both self-reports and objective body measurements underlines the general point that past research has overinterpreted aging symptoms as being menopause induced. Our analysis of body decline showed an acute awareness of changes in physique, physical fitness, and energy level consistent with the gradual decline in functional capacity over the age of 30 for both men and women.

It is worth repeating that we regret not having asked men about whether and to what extent they worry about their looks as they get older. Not only would this tell us an important story about men's perceptions of aging, but it would stimulate interest in research that could illuminate social behavior that seems aimed at hiding one's actual age, again something that seems to obsess men as well as women in our society.

Yet another question that begs for new research is what the criteria are by which men judge female attractiveness. Do such criteria change as men get older? With the media so heavily focused on adults under 40, there is little to go on in thinking about the criteria that older men and women hold to. A related question is how women's views of themselves are affected by their perception of men's criteria in judging them. A personal experience highlights this point. It took me some ten years to persuade my mother to give up her high-heeled shoes and wear sturdy comfortable walking shoes that would make it easier for her to get around in light of her knee and hip problems. Though sympathetic to her self-perception that her legs and slim feet had long been among her most attractive features, it was hard to be sympathetic to her defense of the high heels—"What would men think of me in such dowdy shoes?" She was then 86 years of age, but she had little patience for my answer that men would think she was a sensible woman!

In this chapter I have demonstrated that menopause for most women is indeed a benign event that past medical and psychoanalytic perspectives had led us to misinterpret. This is not to belittle in any way the difficulties experienced by a minority of women who do suffer anguish and physical discomfort in midlife (I include myself among them), as they cope with severe mood fluctuation, insomnia, and hot flashes while fulfilling obligations to others in their families and on their jobs. In coping with menopause and other aspects of aging, women are dealing with their unique biology, personal menstrual history, particular life situations, ways that others perceive and treat them, especially their close women friends, co-workers, and intimate partners, and expectations flowing from the high cultural emphasis on youth and sexual attractiveness in American society.

We think there is a special need to give focused attention to the impact that the cultural emphasis on youth and sexual attractiveness has on women, and on men as well. The notion that one should perform at 50 or 60 as one did at 30 is not limited to job performance; it applies to sexual performance and athletic performance as well. Something strikes us as very unnatural and wrong-headed about a society that encourages pill-taking from childhood to old age: pills to active youngsters that keep them quiet and attentive at school; steroids to young athletes that build muscle-bound bodies but trigger aggressive behavior; tranquillizers and pep pills to get us through a fast-paced work day and sedatives to sleep at night; Viagra to perform sexually; Premarin or Prempro to look younger if not to avoid coronary disease or osteoporosis; and Prozac to ease depression in old age. There are deeply rooted economic and political pressures underlying the social institutions that reinforce the pill-popping habits in American society, and they go far beyond the ability of a social survey to identify and explore. Nonetheless, I hope that with the help of our findings from the rich MIDUS data set, we have paved the way for many new research paths toward a deeper understanding of the middle years in the lives of women—and men.

NOTES

1. The larger WHI study was designed to test more than the health effects of the estrogen-progestin combination, and these different arms continue at the forty clinical centers: they include studies of the effect of low-fat diets, and calcium and vitamin D supplementation, and a study of the effects of estrogen alone in women who have had a hysterectomy. Unless unexpected risks emerge as the latter arm proceeds, these trials are expected to continue until March 2005.

2. The operational definitions of the three stages of the menopausal transition in the MIDUS data set are as follows. Women considered to be in the *postmenopausal stage* answered yes when asked if their menopausal periods had stopped permanently, "not counting a temporary stop because of such things as pregnancy, birth control, extreme dieting, or medication." In addition to these 666 women, we added 53 cases of women who did not answer the question but were between 55 and 74 years of age, by which time 92 percent or more women are postmenopausal. This yields a total of 719 postmenopausal women. Women considered to be in the *perimenopausal stage* were identified by one of two criteria: (1) their periods are not permanently over, that is, they have menstruated at least once in the previous three months but their periods are less regular, lighter, or heavier than a year ago (287 women); and (2) they said that their periods were not permanently over, but they have not menstruated during the previous three months and they think this may be "the beginning of menopause" (10 cases), for a total of 297 perimenopausal women. Women considered to be in the *premenopausal stage*

were so classified if they met one of three criteria: (1) their periods were not permanently over, they have menstruated during the past three months, and they report no change in cycle length or menstrual flow (395 cases); (2) they report their periods are not permanently over but they have not menstruated during the past three months due to pregnancy, dieting, or side effects of medication (28 cases); and (3) they did not answer the question whether their periods were over permanently or not, but all were under 40 years of age and not classifiable as perimenopausal (25 women). This yields a total of 448 premenopausal women.

3. Voda conducted the study in the American Southwest several decades ago. Several of the women interviewed reported that the major stimulus encouraging them to air condition their cars and homes was precisely the discomfort of sweating associated with hot flashes and night sweats, which they had found intolerable when they were in their midforties (Voda 1982).

4. Ruth Clifford Engs (2000) argues that in American history, physical fitness movements go along with moral and religious movements, creating three cycles that focus on "clean living." These extremist moral crusaders, along with health zealots, overdo their proscriptions for clean living, which leads to a countermovement whose members reject such pleas and indulge instead in drinking, smoking, more sex, and a sedentary life. Engs predicts that today's baby-boomer parents, along with evangelical adherents, may produce not like-minded children but an upcoming generation of youth who reject public health messages or parental examples in favor of self-indulgence. But the weight profile we have shown in today's midlifers does not suggest they are providing very good examples of fitness to their children.

REFERENCES

Avis, N. E., and S. M. McKinlay. 1991. A longitudinal analysis of women's attitudes toward the menopause: Results from the Massachusetts Women's Health Study. *Maturitas* 13:66–79.

Bart, P. 1971. Depression in middle-aged women. In *Women in sexist society*, ed. V. Gornick and B. K. Moran, 99–117. New York: Basic Books.

Bray, G. A. 1992. An approach to the classification and evaluation of obesity. In *Obesity*, ed. P. Bjorntrop and B. N. Brodoff. Philadelphia: J. B. Lippincott.

Brody, J. E. 1992. Menopause: The new awareness. *New York Times*, May 19 and 20. Two feature articles on consecutive days.

———. 2000a. Added sugars are taking their toll on health. *New York Times*, September 12, Science News, D8.

———. 2000b. Fitness gap in America's recipe for fat-youth. *New York Times*, September 19, Science News, D8.

Brumberg, J. J. 1997. *The body project: An intimate history of American girls.* New York: Random House.

Bush, T. L. 1992. Feminine forever revisited: Menopausal hormone therapy in the 1990s. *Journal of Women's Health* 1:1–4.

Byrd, W. 1993. Fertilization, embryogenesis, and implantation. In *Textbook of reproductive medicine*, ed. B. R. Carr and R. E. Blackwell, 1–15. Norwalk, Conn.: Appleton and Lange.

Chandra, A. 1998. *Surgical sterilization in the United States: Prevalence and characteristics, 1965–95.* U.S. Department of Health and Human Services, National Center for Health Statistics, series 23, no. 20.

Chi, I-Cheng, and D. B. Jones. 1994. Incidence, risk factors, and prevention of post-sterilization regret in women: An updated international review from an epidemiological perspective. *Obstetrical and Gynecological Review* 49:722–32.

Datan, N., A. Antonovsky, and B. Maoz. 1981. *A time to reap: The middle age of women in five Israeli subcultures.* Baltimore: Johns Hopkins University Press.

Davis, K., and P. van den Oever. 1982. Demographic foundations of new sex roles. *Population and Development Review* 8:495–511.

Deutsch, H. 1945. *The psychology of women.* Vol. 2. New York: Grune and Stratton.

Duenwald, M. 2002. Hormone therapy: One size, clearly, no longer fits all. *New York Times,* July 16, Science News, 1, 6.

Engs, R. C. 2000. *Clean living movements: American cycles of health reform.* New York: Praeger.

Finch, C. E. 1990. *Longevity, senescence, and the genome.* Chicago: University of Chicago Press.

Fox-Genevese, E. 1991. *Feminism without illusions: A critique of individualism.* Chapel Hill: University of North Carolina Press.

Greenhouse, S. 1999. Running on empty: So much work, so little time. *New York Times,* September 5, News of the Week, 1, 4.

Hamilton, W. D. 1966. The moulding of senescence by natural selection. *Journal of Theoretical Biology* 12:12–45.

Harvard Women's Health Watch. 2000. HRT forum: Progestins. September, 3–5.

Hill, K., and A. M. Hurtado. 1991. The evolution of premature reproductive senescence and menopause in human females: An evaluation of the "grandmother" hypothesis. *Human Nature* 2:313–50.

Hochschild, A. 1989. *The second shift: Working parents and the revolution at home.* New York: Viking.

Hrdy, S. B. 1999. *Mother nature: A history of mothers, infants, and natural selection.* New York: Pantheon.

Hurtado, A. M., K. Hill, H. Kaplan, and I. Hurtado. 1992. Trade-offs between female food acquisition and child care among Hiwi and Ache foragers. *Human Nature* 3:185–216.

Kasuya, T., and H. Marsh. 1984. Life history and reproductive biology of the short-finned pilot whale, *Globicephala macrorhynchus,* off the Pacific Coast of Japan. *International Whaling Commission* 6:259–310.

Katz, J. 1999. Men, masculinities and the media: Some introductory notes. *Wellesley Center for Women Research Report* (Wellesley, Mass.) 2:16–17.

Keating, N. L., P. D. Cleary, A. S. Rossi, A. M. Zaslavsky, and J. Z. Ayanian. 1999. Use of hormone replacement therapy by postmenopausal women in the United States. *Annals of Internal Medicine* 130:543–53.

Konner, M. 2002. *The tangled wing.* 2d ed. New York: W. H. Freeman.

Kuczmarski, R. J., K. M. Fiegal, S. M. Campbell, and C. L. Johnson. 1994. Increasing prevalence of overweight among U.S. adults: The National Health and Nutrition Examination Surveys, 1960–1991. *Journal of the American Medical Association* 272:205–11.

Kuczynski, A. 2002. Menopause forever. *New York Times,* June 23, Sunday Styles, 1–2.

Lancaster, J. B., and B. J. King. 1985. An evolutionary perspective on menopause. In *In her prime: A new view of middle aged women,* ed. V. Kerns and contributors, 13–20. South Hadley, Mass.: Bergin and Garvey.

Lancaster, J. B., and C. S. Lancaster. 1983. Parental investment: The hominid adaptation. In *How humans adapt: A biocultural odyssey,* ed. S. Ortner, 33–65. Washington, D.C.: Smithsonian Institution, Government Printing Office.

Lissner, L., P. M. Odell, R. B. D'Agostino, J. Stokes III, B. E. Kreger, A. J. Belanger, and K. D. Brownell. 1991. Variability of body weight and health outcomes in the Framington Heart Population. *New England Journal of Medicine* 324:1839–44.

Matthews, K. A., R. R. Wing, L. H. Kuller, E. N. Meilahan, S. F. Kelsey, E. J. Costello, and A. W. Caggiula. 1990. Influences of natural menopause on psychological characteristics and symptoms of middle-aged healthy women. *Journal of Consulting and Clinical Psychology* 58:345–51.

Meyer, V. 2000. Hormones and heart disease: Medical bias disregards best evidence. *Network News,* September/October, 1, 4. Published by the National Women's Health Network, Washington, D.C.

Miller, L. C., R. Murphy, and A. Buss. 1981. Consciousness of the body: Private and public. *Journal of Personality and Social Psychology* 41:397–406.

Mokdad, A. H., M. K. Serdula, W. H. Dietz, B. A. Bowman, J. S. Marks, and J. P. Kopolan. 1999. The spread of the obesity epidemic in the United States, 1991–1998. *Journal of the American Medical Association* 282:1519–22.

Neugarten, B. L., and R. D. Kraines. 1964. Menopausal symptoms in women of various ages. *Psychosomatic Medicine* 27:266–73.

Palta, M., R. J. Prineas, R. Berman, and P. Hannan. 1982. Comparison of self-reported and measured height and weight. *American Journal of Epidemiology* 115:223–30.

Pennebaker, J. W. 1982. *The psychology of physical symptoms.* New York: Springer-Verlag.

Richardson, S. J., and J. F. Nelson. 1990. Follicular depletion during the menopausal transition. In *Multidisciplinary perspectives on menopause,* ed. M. Flint, F. Kronenberg, and W. Utian, 13–20. New York: Academy of Sciences.

Richardson, S. J., V. Senikas, and J. F. Nelson. 1987. Follicular depletion during the menopausal transition: Evidence of accelerated loss and ultimate exhaustion. *Journal of Clinical and Endocrinological Metabolism* 65:1231–37.

Shapiro, E. 1999. The life of leisure. *Wall Street Journal,* January 11, special section, The Millennium, R38.

Sheehy, G. 1992. *The silent passage: Menopause.* New York: Random House.

Toran-Allerand, C. D. 2002. Letter to the editor. *New York Times,* July 12.

Trivers, R. L. 1972. Parental investment and sexual selection. In *Sexual selection and the descent of man,* ed. B. Campbell, 80–120. Chicago: Aldine.

Voda, A. M. 1982. Menopausal hot flash. In *Changing perspectives on menopause,* ed. A. M. Voda, M. Dinnerstein, and S. R. O'Donnell, 136–59. Austin: University of Texas Press.

Williamson, D. F., and E. R. Pamuk. 1993. The association between weight loss and increased longevity: A review of the evidence. *Annals of Internal Medicine* 119: 731–36.

Wilson, R. A. 1966. *Feminine forever.* New York: M. Evans and Co.

Wuthnow, R. 1998. *Loose connections: Joining together in America's fragmented communities.* Cambridge: Harvard University Press.

Writing Group for the Women's Health Initiative Investigators. 2002. Risks and benefits of estrogen plus progestin in healthy postmenopausal women. *Journal of the American Medical Association* 288:321–33.

Wysowski, D. K., L. Golden, and L. Burke. 1995. Use of menopausal estrogens and medroxyprogesterone in the United States, 1982–1992. *Obstetrics and Gynecology* 85:6–15.

II Emotion, Quality of Life, and Psychological Well-Being in Midlife

CHAPTER SEVEN

Positive and Negative Affect at Midlife

Daniel K. Mroczek

The past decade has seen tremendous growth in research on emotional development. Children and older adults remain the staples of these studies and theories (Thompson 1999; Lawton 1996; Magai and McFadden 1996; Schaie and Lawton 1996), although many positions are life span in outlook (Carstensen and Turk-Charles 1994; Lawton et al. 1992; Lewis and Haviland 1993; Malatesta and Kalnok 1984; Mroczek, in press; Schulz and Heckhausen 1998). Other traditions, although not explicitly developmental, have nonetheless considered the ways that emotions might be influenced by age-graded events over the course of adulthood (e.g., Lazarus 1991). Rarely, however, has midlife been the focus of research on affect. How do midlife adults differ from younger or older persons with respect to positive and negative affect? Using the Midlife in the United States survey (MIDUS), we took a first step toward answering these questions.

The current study stems from two basic questions. First, were there mean or variance differences on positive and negative affect between midlife adults and younger or older persons? Emotions are sensitive to changes in people's life contexts, and because many unique contextual changes occur during midlife (childrearing, career-building), it is reasonable to hypothesize that shifts may occur either in absolute levels of key affect variables or in their variances. Second, were associations between key correlates of affect, especially contextual variables, different for people at midlife when compared with those for people who were younger or older?

Level of Affect at Midlife

Why would we expect differences in affect means or variances between midlife adults and adults of other ages? First, life-span developmental theory holds that many psychological variables should remain sensitive to contextual influences throughout the life course (Baltes 1987; Baltes and Nesselroade 1973; Baltes, Reese, and Nesselroade 1977; Bronfenbrenner

1979; Wohlwill 1973). The life-span approach suggests that variables such as affect are subject to the developmental tenet of plasticity, referring to the ability of constructs to remain supple and malleable throughout the life span (Baltes 1987). Positive and negative affect are among the types of variables that should be responsive to the contextual changes manifested at different ages. These age-graded changes in life contexts should give rise to age-graded differences in affect. Midlife is a period when such contextual changes occur in the form of increased time demands and competition between work and family (Havinghurst 1972), potentially altering levels of positive and negative affect. With respect to the direction of the effect, it is possible to imagine overload as a negative influence, minimizing positive affect while maximizing negative affect, but it is also possible to picture the overloads of midlife as a strengthening force for some, producing better mental health and with it heightened positive affect and diminished negative affect. This chapter attempts to answer this question by inspecting mean levels of affect over different age groups in the MIDUS. In a previous study we established that within the MIDUS, positive affect has a positive correlation with age, and negative affect an inverse relationship (Mroczek and Kolarz 1998). Thus, from previous work on the MIDUS, we know the general direction of the age–affect associations, although until the present study, mean levels had not been reported.

Besides life-span theory, there are other bodies of work on affect that have relevance for midlife. Using individual growth modeling and a twenty-three-year longitudinal study, Charles, Reynolds, and Gatz (2001) established that negative affect declines as people age, although persons high in neuroticism decline at a slower rate than those low on this personality trait. Charles, Reynolds, and Gatz (2001) also documented that positive affect generally remains stable as we age and that persons high in the personality trait extraversion are more stable than others. Gatz and colleagues have reported that young adults display higher levels of negative affect (in the form of anxiety and depression) than do midlife adults and, in turn, that older adults report less than those at midlife (Gatz, Kasl-Godley, and Karel 1996; Gatz and Hurwicz 1990). Gatz also proposes a diathesis-stress mechanism for understanding affect and mental health in adulthood (Gatz, Kasl-Godley, and Karel 1996; Gatz 1998). She holds that both vulnerability (which is influenced by genetic dispositions) and external challenges contribute to the affective response to stress. However, she also proposes that age has an impact on this diathesis-stress process, through changes in neurotransmitter functioning that occur with aging (e.g., Panksepp and Miller 1996) as well as through age-graded changes in the probability of certain stressors, such as the deaths of family members and friends (Gatz, Kasl-Godley, and Karel 1996). Gatz's model has relevance for the study of affect at midlife because it appears that midlife may also bring certain age-graded changes in the likelihood of particular stressors. As noted earlier, work and family demands are often maximized during the middle years. In its emphasis on age-graded stressors, Gatz's model has relevance for middle age and may help to explain differences in level of affect between midlife adults and adults of other ages.

In accentuating the interplay of biological and environmental events and the ways in which each changes over the life span to influence affect, Gatz suggests that in adulthood, emotions are the product of complex processes that stem from both internal and external sources. Many other models of emotion in adulthood emphasize complex processes as well. For example, Labouvie-Vief and Blanchard-Fields (1982) hold that the association between affect and cognition becomes more complex as we proceed through adulthood. As the two domains become better integrated, the result is increased control of one's emotions. Indeed, recent empirical work on emotion regulation has hinted that the link between cognition and emotion is more porous than previously believed (Gross 1998). Although most tests of the Labouvie-Vief and Blanchard-Fields (1982) hypothesis have focused on young–old comparisons (e.g., Labouvie-Vief, DeVoe, and Bulka 1989), it is not unreasonable to speculate that the processes giving rise to greater emotion regulation have their roots in midlife. The process by which affect and cognition become restructured, more connected, and better regulated may well begin during the middle years.

Similarly, Carstensen (1995) has suggested that changes in affect regulation occur among older adults partly as a result of shifts in the relative salience of cognition versus emotion as we grow older. These shifts are the result of a sense of limited time and of heightened awareness that ending points are drawing nearer as we age (Carstensen, Isaacowitz, and Turk-Charles 1999; Lang, Staudinger, and Carstensen 1998). Like the ideas of Labouvie-Vief and colleagues, Carstensen's theory implies greater emotional complexity among older adults. The beginnings of such complexity may be visible among midlife adults as well.

In addition, the theories of Labouvie-Vief and Carstensen suggest processes that not only foster greater emotional complexity but also contribute to a greater sense of integration and maturity. It is at midlife that such integration and maturity may first manifest themselves, altering levels of affect in the process. Indeed, other theories lend support to the notion that midlife is a time when people blossom into more mature and integrated beings, although few have linked these midlife changes to emotion. For example, Erikson (1963) portrayed midlife as a time when individuals attempt to leave a generative gift to the world in the form of deeds, creative expressions, or childrearing (cf. McAdams and de St. Aubin 1998). This generativity requires a maturity and perspective that rarely come before midlife and that may have an impact on emotion via the kinds of mechanisms proposed by Labouvie-Vief and Carstensen (Labouvie-Vief, DeVoe, and Bulka 1989; Carstensen 1995).

Affect Variability and Midlife

Midlife adults may diverge from younger and older adults in other ways as well. Affect variability may decrease or increase in midlife. Why would we expect a shift in variance? As noted earlier, as a result of neurochemical changes in the brain that result in lowered levels of acetylcholine and dopamine, the brain is less arousable in older age than in youth (Panksepp and Miller 1996). These changes have formed the basis of various hypotheses about emotional arousability and aging, each suggesting that emotions should become less extreme or less intense with age (Gatz, Kasl-Godley, and Karel 1996; Panksepp and Miller 1996). Midlife may mark the first period during which these biological changes become observable through decreased variability in positive and negative affect. If this arousability hypothesis is correct, affect variability should decrease with age, meaning that midlife adults should have smaller variances than younger adults but larger variances than their older counterparts. From this perspective, midlife adults should simply be in the middle of a lifelong decline in affect variability.

Other theoretical perspectives, however, suggest increased variability in affect with age. As people grow older, the contextual factors that influence them often diverge (Baltes 1987). In youth, people share many common contexts (e.g., most young people are in school, thus providing a common frame of experience). As they move away from youth, however, people from a common cohort go in separate directions, and the resulting divergent experiences may increase the individual differences between them, in turn increasing affect variability. Midlife, marking the period during which many people have finished school, started a career and family, and forged an identity of their own, may represent the earliest point in the life span where we may observe such increased variability.

There is another reason to expect increased variability in affect at midlife. As mentioned earlier, it is possible to conceive of the time demands and overloads of midlife as a negative influence for some people but as a strengthening force for others. This may produce divergent levels of affect among those at midlife, with some people experiencing quite low positive and high negative affect as a result of overload, and others experiencing the opposite as they draw strength from the stimulation that multiple demands may bring. If individuals at midlife are pulled in opposite directions, we would predict greater affect variability among them, and less variability among both younger and older adults. By examining and testing differences in positive and negative affect variances across younger, midlife, and older adults in the MIDUS, we may be able to determine which perspective has the most empirical support.

Differential Associations among Affect and Contextual Variables at Midlife

In addition to potential age differences in means and variances, the associations between affect and its main correlates vary over the course of adulthood. Are the associations between key explanatory variables and affect the same in midlife as they are in youth or older adulthood? Contextual variables in particular may show varying associations with affect variables over the course of adulthood. Work-related stress, for example, may give rise to higher negative and lower positive affect among young people, who generally have less control over their jobs than do midlife and older adults and who tend to be near the bottom of the seniority ladder. On the other hand, a lack of seniority may lead to a weak association between work stress and affect. Less seniority may mean less responsibility, hence less hassle and worry, even when work stress increases. By contrast, midlife adults tend to have jobs with greater seniority and responsibility as compared with younger adults, creating an increase in the association between work stress and affect. A midlife adult with heavy work responsibilities (and who perhaps is also dealing with family responsibilities—hence overload) may react to increased work stress with increased negative and decreased positive affect. The strength of the stress–affect association should therefore be greater among midlife adults if this scenario is correct. Within older adults, however, the relationship between work stress and affect may be weak or nonexistent. In the MIDUS, many of the oldest adults were retired or near retirement, or were in extremely senior positions. As Super (1990) has argued, many adults nearing retirement undergo a transformation in which work is removed from a central position in their lives. Work becomes less pivotal to one's overall identity and self-concept, and may be less likely to foster stress. If this is the case, we would expect a weaker relationship between work stress and affect among older adults than among midlife or younger adults.

Work stress is but one example of how an association may vary at different points along the life span. Other stress-based contextual variables, such as relationship discord, may also show similar age-graded differences in affect. Through years of experience, midlife and older adults may be more skilled at working through relationship issues in ways that do not heighten distress. Indeed, Carstensen, Gottman, and Levenson (1995) demonstrated that older adults were able to resolve conflicts in ways that minimized negative affect. In the MIDUS, the association between relationship stress and negative affect may be stronger in younger adults (who have not yet acquired such skills) and weaker in midlife and older adults. Such an age-graded difference in this association may reflect greater maturity of the type referred to earlier, a maturity that begins to blossom in midlife.

The MIDUS covered a wide age range (25–74), allowing researchers a unique opportunity to examine differential, age-graded associations over a wide stretch of the adult portion of the life span. By comparing the relationships between affect and key explanatory variables *within* age groups representing younger, midlife, and older adults, we will be able to assess differential associations. Few studies have considered such differential relationships, and fewer still have considered differences in variances. Nonetheless, the body of literature on age and affect comprises a valuable knowledge base regarding emotion in adulthood.

Age Differences in Affect in Adulthood

What has the extant literature revealed about affect at midlife? Few empirical studies of affect in adulthood have focused on age as an explanatory variable, and of those, only a handful used samples that included the midlife range. Most of these studies were atheoretical and simply tested whether an age–affect association existed. There was little speculation about potential maturational processes that might underlie changes in affect over the adult life span. For example, Diener, Sandvik, and Larsen (1985) provided evidence showing that midlife and older adults report less intense affect when compared with that reported by younger adults and adolescents. Similarly, Costa et al. (1987) reported that both negative and positive affect were higher among younger adults when compared with that of midlife and older adults. These early studies, while valuable, were mainly descriptive in tone.

Later empirical investigations were more theory-driven and concerned with maturational and developmental processes that produce changes in affect over the life span (Diener et al. 1999; Magai 2001). For example, Ryff (1989) based her empirical investigations on a theoretical formulation that emphasized maturity and integrated functioning. She found that persons at midlife were not different from older adults in terms of affect balance (negative affect subtracted from positive affect) but that both groups had a higher balance than young adults. Like Ryff, Gatz, and colleagues approached the issue of affect from a more theoretically informed viewpoint (the diathesis-stress perspective) and reported higher negative affect among younger adults (Gatz, Kasl-Godley, and Karel 1996; Gatz and Hurwicz 1990). Rossi and Rossi (1990), in discussing how intergenerational relationships mature, reported a steady decline in both positive and negative affect in a sample of people ranging in age from 19 to 92. Midlife adults displayed lower levels of both types of affect than did younger adults, but higher levels than older persons. Finally, Mroczek and Kolarz (1998), using the MIDUS sample and drawing on several of the aforementioned viewpoints, found that positive affect increased (at an accelerating rate) from the ages of 25 to 74, but that negative affect declined over the same age range. We must keep in mind, though, that all of the documented effects of age on emotion are small. Age usually accounts for no more than 2 percent of the variance in either positive or negative affect. Further, most of these investigations were cross-sectional (with the exception of Charles, Reynolds, and Gatz 2001), so we cannot rule out cohort explanations.

It is clear that recent studies of affect and adulthood have stood on more theory than have earlier investigations. Further, a distinct trend has emerged. In most of the previously mentioned studies, persons at midlife reported more positive and less negative affect than did younger adults, but less positive and more negative affect than older adults. This empirical evidence contradicts earlier viewpoints that portrayed midlife as a stress-filled time of crisis (Levinson 1978). Rather, the middle years may open a period when people begin moving toward more emotional balance and maturity.

Current Study

In this study, we first documented mean and variance differences in positive and negative affect between younger, midlife, and older adults.

Then we turned to the question of differential associations between affect and key explanatory variables across these three groups of adults. In posing this second question, we considered a broad collection of factors that reflected changing contexts or were sensitive to context. These were physical health, work and relationship stress, and marital status, along with two variables that are generally fixed over adulthood: gender and educational level. Inclusion of these variables was a novel aspect of the present study in that much of the theory and research reviewed in the previous sections had not considered a wide array of contextual influences. The multitude of variables available on the MIDUS allowed a broader consideration of contextual factors than had previous investigations. Additionally, few previous studies had used a sample as large or as representative as the MIDUS.

We emphasized contextual factors because more than other types of variables, they have the potential to exert different effects on affect within different parts of adulthood. For example, physical health can change quickly and unexpectedly over the course of adulthood, creating contexts that have differential effects on affect. Illnesses that are unexpected in youth, such as cancer, may have a different effect than those same illnesses would have in the middle or older years, when such illnesses are more common. Additionally, stressors can vary in their impact across adulthood (e.g., the aforementioned example on work stress). A stressor that is quite taxing during one period of adulthood may have little or no impact in another period.

We first considered mean and variances for positive and negative affect over three age groups that represented younger, midlife, and older adults. Additionally, age differences in means and variances were also examined separately for men and women because of the well-known gender difference on positive and negative affect (Mroczek and Kolarz 1998). The two affect variables were then regressed (within each of the three age groups) on gender, marital status, education, and physical health. After consideration of these results, the two stress variables (work and relationship stress) were added to the equation, again for each age group. The analysis followed this order because relatively fixed sociodemographic factors such as gender, education, and marital status, although undoubtedly sensitive to context, likely set the stage for the effects of more strongly contextualized variables such as work and relationship stress. In sum, these analyses provided a description of affect in midlife as well as insights into the variables that differentially impact positive and negative affect at different ages.

METHODS

All data were from the Midlife in the United States survey (MIDUS), conducted by the John D. and Catherine T. MacArthur Foundation Research Network on Successful Midlife Development. All measures were from the survey instrument used for the MIDUS, the Midlife Development Inventory (MIDI). The MIDI was created by the Midlife Research Network for special use on the MIDUS. It had both a telephone and mail portion.

Sample

Persons who completed both the phone and mail portions of the MIDI were used in the current analyses, for a total number of 2984. However, many questions that involved work and relationship stress were irrelevant for those not employed or not in relationships. The total sample dropped to 1937 for analyses that used these stress variables, representing those MIDUS respondents who were working and were in a relationship.

Measures

Our key variables, positive and negative affect, were assessed independently by using Watson and Tellegen's (1985) argument that the two are separate dimensions. Frequency measures of positive and negative affect, each six items in length, were included on the MIDI. These scales are described in greater detail by Mroczek and Kolarz (1998). Despite their brief length, both scales have respectable alphas: .87 for positive affect and .91 for negative affect. Summed scores were created from these items. Nearly every participant responded to all six items for each scale, but among those who did not, mean substitution was used (within scales) only if the participant responded to at least four items. Scores ranged from 6 to 30 for both positive and negative affect.

Age ranged from 25 to 74 on the MIDUS. The purpose of this particular investigation was to document various differences in affect between distinct periods of adulthood. This required the division of our age range into partitions representing young, middle, and older adulthood. After the discrete definitions of midlife suggested by Schaie and Willis (1996) and Willis and Reid (1999), age was categorized as follows: young adulthood was defined as the ages 25–34, inclusive; middle adulthood as 35–64, inclusive; and older adulthood as 65–74, inclusive. The numbers of people in these categories were 578, 1895, and 287 for young, midlife, and older persons, respectively. The boundary between young and midlife adults, age 35, reflects a point at which most people have married (and perhaps divorced) and established themselves in a career or job. Most individuals age 35 and older have negotiated the key work and relationship tasks of youth and are fairly labeled midlife adults. The boundary between midlife and older adults, age 65, represents the official retirement age in the United States but also reflects a psychological turning point as well for many people (Schaie and Willis 1996). It is the point at which people are considered senior citizens, and thus MIDUS participants age 65 and above are fairly labeled older adults.

As mentioned earlier, gender, marital status, education, and physical health were also included in the present investigation. Respondents reported education by indicating the level of schooling they had attained. The variable consisted of twelve levels, anchored on the low end by "some grade school" and at the high end by "graduate or professional degree." Marital status was assessed by use of a single item that simply asked whether one was married, never married, separated, divorced, or widowed. The item was dichotomized, with 1 representing currently married persons and 0 representing all others. Physical health was assessed by use of a single-item, global self-rating of general physical health at present, which was Likert-scaled and ranged from 1 to 5. Higher scores indicated better self-reported health.

Two types of context-based stress were assessed. One measured work and financial strain, and the other indexed relationship discord. Taken from different sections of the MIDI, these measures were built by use of several items that asked about various stressful events and situations. The four work/finance questions asked whether a person (1) had recently been laid off, (2) was experiencing serious ongoing problems with someone at work, (3) was undergoing other serious stress at work, or (4) felt no control over finances. The questions that comprised the relationship stress scale asked whether a person (1) was in the worst possible marriage or relationship, (2) felt no control over his or her relationship, and (3) described his or her relationship as poor. Each of the work and relationship items were dichotomized and then summed to create the two stress scales.

RESULTS

As noted earlier, the current study had two main goals. The first set of analyses documented basic differences in reported level of affect across adulthood. These analyses also took account of gender differences. The second set of analyses probed the effects of contextual influences on

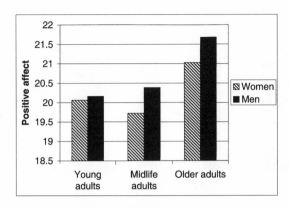

FIGURE 1. Mean positive affect by age group.

affect across three different periods of adulthood. Did variables that were associated with positive and negative affect within youth continue to be associated within midlife and, in turn, within older adulthood?

Age and Gender Differences in Means and Variances
Means

Figure 1 displays mean positive affect for younger, midlife, and older adults, by gender. Differences in these six means were tested using a two-way factorial ANOVA, which indicated a significant overall effect, $F(5, 2979) = 7.11$, $p < .0001$. The main effect associated with age group was significant, $F(2, 2979) = 11.33$, $p < .0001$, as was the main effect for gender, $F(1, 2979) = 10.94$, $p < .001$. The interaction between age and gender was not significant. Scheffé post-hoc tests revealed that midlife adults were significantly different from older adults but not from younger adults. Post-hoc tests also revealed that younger and older adults were significantly different from each other.

Note the general age pattern in figure 1. Young adults (ages 25–34) reported the least amount of positive affect, while the oldest adults (65–74) reported the most. Midlife adults, although not significantly different from younger adults, nonetheless showed an interesting pattern. Women in midlife appeared to decrease in positive affect, while men showed an uptick. Among the oldest adults, both women and men were elevated, although women were not as high. The main effect for gender was significant, although it was clear that midlife and older adults were accounting for that difference. Young women and men appeared no different in level of positive affect. Also, despite the visual appearance of

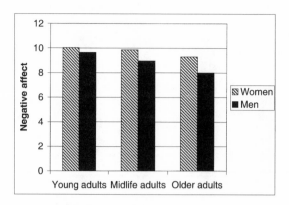

FIGURE 2. Mean negative affect by age group.

an interaction between age group and gender, there was no significant interaction. Nonetheless, the main effects of age and gender were clearly visible, and they indicated that midlife may not necessarily bring higher levels of positive affect. There was no overall mean difference between midlife adults and their younger counterparts.

With regard to negative affect, there was a much clearer picture. Figure 2 displays means for negative affect for young, midlife, and older adults. A two-way factorial ANOVA indicated a significant effect, $F(5, 2985) = 11.85$, $p < .0001$. The main effect associated with age group was significant, $F(2, 2985) = 10.18$, $p < .0001$, as was the main effect for gender, $F(1, 2985) = 34.92$, $p < .0001$. Again, the interaction between age and gender was not significant. Scheffé post-hoc tests revealed that all age groups were significantly different from one another.

The general pattern shown in figure 2 is one of decline in negative affect over the three age groups, along with a gender difference (women scored higher than men on negative affect in all age groups). This pattern was different from that observed for positive affect. Rather than being a point of transition where affect changes direction, midlife seemed to have no distinctive role with regard to absolute level of negative affect. Both men and women decreased on negative affect across the age range, although men appeared to decrease a bit more, and these declines were steady from youth through midlife and into older age.

Variances

Figure 3 displays variances for positive affect by gender and age group. Pairwise comparisons among these six variances were investigated by

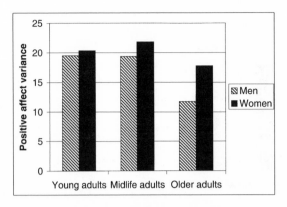

FIGURE 3. Variances in positive affect by age group.

using the significance test for variances, the F_{max} test (Kirk 1968). Note the general trend with respect to age and positive affect. Older women and men were less variable than were midlife or younger adults. The variances of these two latter groups were not significantly different from one another, but both were different from older adults. Younger men were significantly more variable than older men, $F_{max}(1, 288) = 1.67$, $p < .05$; and midlife men were significantly more variable than older men, $F_{max}(1, 946) = 1.65$, $p < .05$. Younger women were significantly more variable than older women, $F_{max}(1, 289) = 1.15$, $p < .05$; and midlife women were significantly more variable than older women, $F_{max}(1, 947) = 1.23$, $p < .05$. Note that among younger and midlife adults, there was not much difference in variance between the genders. Yet among older adults, men appeared less variable than women.

Figure 4 shows variances for negative affect, by gender and age group. Again, we found that older adults were less variable on negative affect as they were on positive affect. Younger men were significantly more variable than older men, $F_{max}(1, 289) = 1.79$, $p < .05$; midlife men were significantly more variable than older men, $F_{max}(1, 946) = 1.72$, $p < .05$. Younger women were significantly more variable than older women, $F_{max}(1, 288) = 1.21$, $p < .05$; midlife women were significantly more variable than older women, $F_{max}(1, 947) = 1.31$, $p < .05$. Note that women were more variable than men across each of our age groups, although the difference seemed less pronounced among younger adults.

These results are consistent with the models offered by Gatz, Kasl-Godley, and Karel (1996) and Panksepp and Miller (1996). Both groups argue that emotions in older adults should be less arousable than they are

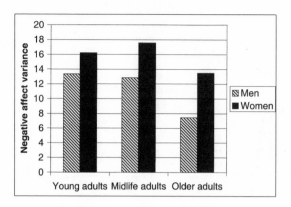

FIGURE 4. Variances in negative affect by age group.

in younger adults. Indeed, we found that older adults were significantly less variable on both positive and negative affect. Further, the significant differences were between older adults and the other two groups of adults. Midlife and younger adults did not differ from one another with respect to affect variability. If the decreased arousability model is correct, these MIDUS data suggested that older adults account for the effect. Midlife adults certainly appeared no less variable than young adults.

Differential Associations across Adulthood Groups

Having documented basic differences in affect means and variances over our adulthood groups, we turned our attention to differential associations. Were the patterns of association the same across our adulthood groups? We regressed the two affect variables on key explanatory variables within our three age categories. Such an examination allowed us to determine if particular variables were more important at midlife than at other times during adulthood. As noted earlier, we concentrated on age-graded differences in the associations between contextual factors and affect.

The top of table 1 shows regressions of positive affect on the initial set of explanatory variables (gender, education, marital status, and physical health). One element in this table stands out. All four predictors were significant among midlife adults, whereas among younger and older adults only physical health was a significant covariate. Better physical health was associated with greater positive affect across the entire (25–74) age range. However, not even one of the other three predictors was associated with positive affect in either young or older adulthood. In midlife, on the other

TABLE 1 Regressions of Positive and Negative Affect on Explanatory Variables by Adulthood Categories

	Young Adults ($N = 578$)	Midlife Adults ($N = 1895$)	Older Adults ($N = 287$)
Positive affect			
Gender	.20 (.36)	−.52 (.20)**	−.46 (.48)
Education	.01 (.08)	−.08 (.04)*	−.13 (.09)
Marital status	.35 (.36)	.56 (.22)**	.78 (.48)
Physical health	1.31 (.20)***	1.28 (.10)***	1.14 (.21)***
R^2	.075	.086	.103
Negative affect			
Gender	.17 (.32)	.70 (.17)***	1.00 (.38)*
Education	−.03 (.07)	−.06 (.03)	−.08 (.07)
Marital status	−.14 (3.2)	−.70 (.18)***	−.61 (.39)
Physical health	−.98 (.18)***	−1.15 (.09)***	−1.22 (.17)***
R^2	.058	.118	.212

Notes: Gender: 1 = women, 0 = men; married: 1 = married, 0 = not married; young adults, 25–34; midlife adults, 35–64; older adults, 65–74. The first number in each group is the b coefficient; the number in parentheses is the standard error.
*$p < .1$. **$p < .01$. ***$p < .001$.

hand, each of these factors was associated with positive affect. Women and better-educated persons reported less and married people reported more positive affect in midlife.

We observed a similar pattern with regard to negative affect. Better physical health was associated with less negative affect over all three age groups, but again this was the only variable that had a cross-adulthood effect. Women reported higher levels than men in midlife and older age, but not in younger adulthood (this effect was visible in fig. 2 as well). Education, though, had no effect across any of the age groups. Finally, at midlife, married people reported less negative affect than unmarried people, an effect that was not present among the younger or older group. This mimics the pattern detected for positive affect.

These results showed that physical health had a significant impact on both affects across the broad range of the adult years covered in the MIDUS. This effect seemed to transcend age. Gender, education, and marriage, however, had effects that were present only in midlife. The effects observed for gender must be interpreted cautiously, because we tested for a gender–age interaction in the aforementioned ANOVA, and it was not significant. Note that gender had an effect on both affect variables only among midlife adults. Among older adults, women reported higher negative affect than men, but there was no effect for positive affect. Only in midlife did gender have an impact on both affect variables. It is tempting

TABLE 2 Regressions of Positive and Negative Affect on Explanatory Variables by Adulthood Categories, Adding Relationship and Work Stress

	Young Adults (N = 403)	Midlife Adults (N = 1354)	Older Adults (N = 180)
Positive affect			
Gender	.03 (.42)	−.56 (.23)*	−1.10 (.52)*
Education	.09 (.09)	−.01 (.05)	−.12 (.09)
Marital status	−.86 (.52)	.02 (.42)	.78 (1.56)
Physical health	1.30 (.23)***	1.18 (.12)***	.84 (.24)***
Relationship stress	−.79 (.64)	−1.61 (.40)***	−4.99 (1.03)***
Work stress	−1.11 (.31)***	−1.04 (.17)***	1.97 (1.00)
R^2	.117	.115	.239
Negative affect			
Gender	.19 (.38)	.83 (.19)***	1.22 (.45)**
Education	−.09 (.08)	−.12 (.04)**	−.08 (.08)
Marital status	−.07 (.47)	−.55 (.36)	.63 (1.33)
Physical health	−.78 (.21)***	−1.03 (.10)***	−.96 (.21)***
Relationship stress	1.08 (.58)	.89 (.34)**	1.94 (.89)*
Work stress	1.04 (.31)***	.62 (.15)***	.68 (.85)
R^2	.085	.131	.210

Notes: Gender: 1 = women, 0 = men; married: 1 = married, 0 = not married; young adults, 25–34; midlife adults, 35–64; older adults, 65–74. The first number in each group is the b coefficient; the number in parantheses is the standard error.
* $p < .1.$ ** $p < .01.$ *** $p < .001.$

to think that perhaps these gender effects reflect strain emanating from trying to balance family and career. Women at midlife, perhaps as a result of reasons stemming from societal structures and expectations, may have been more susceptible to stress overload. However, table 2, in which work and relationship stress are added to the models, shows that this is not the case.

As shown in table 2, we added indicators of work and relationship stress to the equations. Note that N decreased for each age category in moving from table 1 to 2. This was because those who responded to the work stress items were those who were working. Those not working, such as retired persons, would have skipped some or all of the items that comprised the work stress variable. The same was true of those who were not in a relationship. Lack of data as a result of these reasons lowered N in the second phase of analysis, reducing the comparability of the two sets of regressions. It may therefore be preferable to interpret the two phases as distinct analyses rather than as one building on the other.

Table 2 shows regressions of affect on the initial four indicators, along with relationship and work stress. The top half of table 2 displays results for positive affect. Among both midlife and older adults, relationship stress was inversely related to positive affect, net of the other five variables in the equation. Work stress was also inversely related to positive affect among midlife and younger adults. As shown in the bottom half of table 2, we observed a similar pattern for negative affect. Greater relationship stress was associated with greater negative affect among midlife and older adults, whereas work stress was associated with negative affect among midlife and younger adults.

It was interesting that both stress variables were related to both affects among midlife adults but not among their younger and older counterparts. Among younger adults, relationship stress did not have an effect on either positive or negative affect. Keep in mind that the young adults in the MIDUS were probably less likely to be in relationships than were midlife or older adults, and thus they may have been less likely to answer the relationship questions. Nonetheless, those younger people who were in relationships and who reported relationship stress were not necessarily lower on positive affect or higher in negative affect. Relationship discord may have a lighter impact among adults aged 25–34 when compared with midlife or older adults. Perhaps this was because individuals younger than 35 are less likely to have children, or are less committed to their relationship, or have not been with their partner as long as midlife or older adults. Additionally, young adults experiencing relationship discord may have been less likely to encounter some of the issues confronting midlife and older adults who experience such problems. For example, midlife and older couples are more likely to share assets, such as a house, that add an element of complexity to relationship difficulties.

With regard to work stress, note that for both positive and negative affect, midlife and younger adults shared the same pattern. Positive affect was lowered and negative affect was heightened by work stress. The older adults in this analysis were those that were still performing some work for pay. Keep in mind that many older adults did not answer the work stress questions because they were not working and so the questions were irrelevant. Nonetheless, among those older adults who were still working, work stress appeared to have no impact at all on either affect variable.

Midlife and younger adults seem to share a common encumbrance with regard to work stress. The process of finding a job or launching a career and then maintaining it throughout midlife perhaps creates work-related burdens that foster higher negative and lower positive affect. However, by the older years, work may cease to be a source of affective grief. If older adults know that they will not remain much longer in a given job or career (e.g., Super 1990), then the ensuing decline in future orientation may free people from becoming unduly bothered by the petty trials and tribulations of the workplace.

Discussion

The present investigation centered on two questions. First, were there age differences in affect means and variances when contrasting midlife adults to other adults? Second, were the parameters that defined the relationships between affect and its predictors different across several eras of adulthood?

Data from the MIDUS provided ambiguous answers to the first set of questions. We did find mean differences. However, with regard to positive affect, midlife looked like an extension of young adulthood; with respect to negative affect, midlife appeared to simply represent the midpoint of a life-span decline. When we examined variances, midlife adults were more similar to younger than older adults. Older adults had significantly smaller affect variances than either midlife or younger adults, both of whom had variances of comparable size. It was not clear that midlife was a unique period of adulthood in terms of affect means or variances. Older adulthood, by contrast, appeared to usher in mean and variance shifts, although it was not clear whether these were aging or cohort effects. The age decline in mean negative affect was consistent with prior empirical findings (e.g., Costa et al. 1987; Rossi and Rossi 1990), although our results for positive affect were unique to the MIDUS sample (see also Mroczek and Kolarz 1998). Interestingly, the decline in both affect variances observed among older adults was consistent with biologically based theories of arousability (Gatz, Kasl-Godley, and Karel 1996; Panksepp and Miller 1996). Lower arousability in the oldest MIDUS participants may belie these significantly lower variances.

The answer to the second question was a clear yes. The relationships between affect and key explanatory variables were different over the three groups of adults. Those variables that were associated with affect in midlife were not necessarily those that were related to affect in young or older adulthood. The significant effects of education and marriage were exclusive to the middle years. More importantly, midlife was the only age group in which both stress indicators had a significant effect on affect.

These latter findings signal an interesting possibility. Midlife adults may be more influenced by context than younger or older adults. Perhaps careers, relationships, and families dominate their lives more than they dominate the lives of adults of other ages. As a result, midlife adults may find themselves more heavily engaged in the contexts that bring about stress, or at least have greater investments in those activities that bring about stress. For example, work and the money it brings take on greater importance when children need to be clothed and fed, retirement funds need building, and mortgages require financing. Relationships may take on greater importance in midlife as the shakier marriages begin to fall apart, as the demands of child-raising strain relationships, and as the prospect of losing a partner in later life begins to loom on the not too distant horizon. Midlife adults are heavily engaged in their work and relationships, and this involvement may be a source of tension as well as fulfillment. In the MIDUS, work and relationship stress had greater impact on affect during the midlife years than at other times, a finding consistent with the interpretation offered earlier in the chapter. As Havinghurst (1972) argued, midlife brings unique challenges, stressors, and demands. Midlife can often be a time of overwhelming responsibilities, especially with regard to work and family. As our findings demonstrated, these context-based stressors indeed had a unique impact on affect, but the impact took the form of differential associations, not differences in mean levels or variances.

We would like to draw attention to one additional finding. Note that among midlife adults, educational level was significantly associated with less positive affect before we added the stress variables. This was interesting, because higher educational attainment was paired with lower levels of positive affect. Better-educated people reported less positive emotion. However, after introducing the two stress variables into the model, the effect was rendered nonsignificant. In essence, people with higher educational attainment tended to have higher levels of work and relationship stress, and thus lower levels of positive affect. In other words, there was nothing about midlife itself that created the inverse association between education and positive affect. A contextual shift that was based in midlife was responsible for this effect.

With respect to negative affect, note that the reverse effect occurred. Among midlife adults, education was not initially significant, but when the contextual stress variables were added, it became significant. Midlife adults with higher levels of education had lower levels of negative affect but only when stress was controlled. This means that stress was masking the effect of education. People with higher levels of education had lower levels of negative affect, but they also had higher levels of stress. Thus, when stress was in the model (and was thus held constant), the education–affect association was able to emerge.

These context-based differential associations were all very interesting, and they shed light on the ways in which midlife was unique with respect to affect in the MIDUS. Additionally, midlife adults were clearly better off from an affective perspective than were young adults. They had higher levels of positive affect than did younger adults (at least men did) and lower levels of negative affect (a cross-gender finding). Midlife adults in the MIDUS were moving in the right direction, even in the face of stronger associations between work and relationship stress and affect. However, midlife adults were not nearly as well off as older adults, who had the lowest levels of negative and highest levels of positive affect in the MIDUS sample. Keep in mind that our oldest adults were age 74 on the high end, and it is unclear that affect remains at these levels past age 75 (Smith et al. 1999).

Differences in mean levels and variances were what made older adults unique with regard to affect. Midlife adults, on the other hand, were distinguished by a number of differential associations between affect and explanatory variables; this was the most novel element of emotion during the middle portion of adulthood. Of course these differential associations were not likely to have been caused by midlife itself but rather by contextual shifts that happen to take place in midlife. Nonetheless, we found that affect during the middle years was not distinguished by differences in level or variability but rather by the way that affect was related to key correlates. The MIDUS midlife adults were not more cheerful or distressed than other groups of adults, but the factors that provoked cheer and distress within them were different. It was this that gave affect at midlife a unique character.

REFERENCES

Baltes, P. B. 1987. Theoretical propositions of life-span developmental psychology: On the dynamics between grown and decline. *Developmental Psychology* 23:611–26.

Baltes, P. B., and J. R. Nesselroade. 1973. The developmental analysis of individual differences on multiple measures. In *Lifespan developmental psychology: Methodological issues,* ed. J. R. Nesselroade and H. W. Reese, 219–51. New York: Academic Press.

Baltes, P. B., H. W. Reese, and J. R. Nesselroade. 1977. *Lifespan developmental psychology: Introduction to research methods.* Monterey, Calif.: Brooks Cole.

Bronfenbrenner, U. 1979. *The ecology of human development.* Cambridge: Harvard University Press.

Carstensen, L. L. 1995. Evidence for a life-span theory of socioemotional selectivity. *Current Directions in Psychological Science* 4:151–55.

Carstensen, L. L., J. M. Gottman, and R. W. Levenson. 1995. Emotional behavior in long-term marriage. *Psychology and Aging* 10:140–49.

Carstensen, L. L., D. M. Isaacowitz, and S. Turk-Charles. 1999. Taking time seriously: A theory of socioemotional selectivity. *American Psychologist* 54:165–81.

Carstensen, L. L., and S. Turk-Charles. 1994. The salience of emotion across the adult life span. *Psychology and Aging* 9:259–64.

Charles, S. T., C. A. Reynolds, and M. Gatz. 2001. Age-related differences and change in positive and negative affect over 23 years. *Journal of Personality and Social Psychology* 80:136–51.

Costa, P. T., Jr., A. B. Zonderman, R. R. McCrae, J. Cornoni-Huntley, B. Z. Locke, and H. E. Barbano. 1987. Longitudinal analyses of psychological well-being in a national sample: Stability of mean levels. *Journal of Gerontology* 42:50–55.

Diener, E., E. Sandvik, and R. J. Larsen. 1985. Age and sex differences for emotional intensity. *Developmental Psychology* 21:542–46.

Diener, E., E. M. Suh, R. E. Lucas, and H. L. Smith. 1999. Subjective well-being: Three decades of progress. *Psychological Bulletin* 125:276–302.

Erikson, E. 1963. *Childhood and society.* 2d ed. New York: W. W. Norton.

Gatz, M. 1998. Toward a developmentally informed theory of mental disorder in older adults. In *Handbook of aging and mental health: An integrative approach,* ed. J. Lomranz, 101–20. New York: Plenum Press.

Gatz, M., and M.-L. Hurwicz. 1990. Are de people more depressed? Cross-sectional data on CES-D factors. *Psychology and Aging* 5:284–90.

Gatz, M., J. E. Kasl-Godley, and M. Karel. 1996. Aging and mental disorders. In *Handbook of the psychology of aging,* 4th ed., ed. J. E. Birren and K. W. Schaie, 367–82. New York: Academic Press.

Gross, J. J. 1998. The emerging field of emotion regulation: An integrative review. *Review of General Psychology* 2:271–99.

Havinghurst, R. J. 1972. *Developmental tasks and education.* 3d ed. New York: McKay.

Kirk, R. E. 1968. *Experimental design: Procedures for the behavioral sciences.* Belmont, Calif.: Brooks Cole.

Labouvie-Vief, G., and F. Blanchard-Fields. 1982. Cognitive aging and psychological growth. *Ageing and Society* 2:183–209.

Labouvie-Vief, G., M. DeVoe, and D. Bulka. 1989. Speaking about feelings: Conceptions of emotion across the life span. *Psychology and Aging* 4:425–37.

Lang, F. R., U. M. Staudinger, and L. L. Carstensen. 1998. Perspectives on socioemotional selectivity in late life. *Journal of Gerontology: Psychological Sciences* 53B:P21–P30.

Lawton, M. P. 1996. Quality of life and affect in later life. In *Handbook of emotion, adult development and aging,* ed. C. Magai and S. H. McFadden, 327–48. San Diego: Academic Press.

Lawton, M. P., M. H. Kleban, D. Rajagopal, and J. Dean. 1992. Dimensions of affective experience in three age groups. *Psychology and Aging* 7:171–84.

Lazarus, R. S. 1991. *Emotion and adaptation.* New York: Oxford University Press.

Levenson, R. W., L. L. Carstensen, and J. M. Gottman. 1994. The influence of age and gender on affect, physiology, and their interrelations: A study of long-term marriage. *Journal of Personality and Social Psychology* 67:56–68.

Levinson, D. J. 1978. *The seasons of a man's life.* New York: Knopf.

Lewis, M., and J. M. Haviland. 1993. *Handbook of emotions.* New York: Guilford.

Magai, C. M. 2001. *Emotions over the lifespan*. In *Handbook of the psychology of aging*, 5th ed., ed. J. E. Birren and K. W. Schaie, 399–426. San Diego: Academic Press.

Magai, C., and S. H. McFadden. 1996. *Handbook of emotion, adult development and aging*. San Diego: Academic Press.

Malatesta, C. Z., and M. Kalnok. 1984. Emotional experience in younger and older adults. *Journal of Gerontology* 39:301–8.

McAdams, D. P., and E. de St. Aubin. 1998. *Generativity and adult development*. Washington, D.C.: American Psychological Association.

Mroczek, D. K. In press. Age and emotion in adulthood. *Current Directions in Psychological Science*.

Mroczek, D. K., and C. M. Kolarz. 1998. The effect of age on positive and negative affect: A developmental perspective on happiness. *Journal of Personality and Social Psychology* 75:1333–49.

Panksepp, J., and A. Miller. 1996. Emotions and the aging brain: Regrets and remedies. In *Handbook of emotion, adult development and aging*, ed. C. Magai and S. H. McFadden, 3–26. San Diego: Academic Press.

Rossi, A. S., and P. H. Rossi. 1990. *Of human bonding: Parent–child relations across the life course*. New York: Aldine de Gruyter.

Ryff, C. D. 1989. Happiness is everything, or is it? Explorations on the meaning of psychological well-being. *Journal of Personality and Social Psychology* 57:1069–81.

Schaie, K. W., and M. P. Lawton. 1998. Preface. In *Annual review of gerontology and geriatrics*, ed. K. W. Schaie and M. P. Lawton, xi–xvi. New York: Springer-Verlag.

Schaie, K. W., and S. L. Willis. 1996. *Adult development and aging*. New York: Harper Collins.

Schulz, R. 1985. Emotion and affect. In *Handbook of the psychology of aging*, 2d ed., ed. J. E. Birren and K. W. Schaie, 531–43. New York: Van Nostrand Reinhold.

Schulz, R., and J. Heckhausen. 1998. Emotion and control: A lifespan perspective. In *Annual review of gerontology and geriatrics*, ed. K. W. Schaie and M. P. Lawton, 185–205. New York: Springer-Verlag.

Smith, J., W. Fleeson, B. Geiselmann, R. A. Settersten, and U. Kunzman. 1999. Sources of well-being in very old age. In *The Berlin aging study: Aging from 70 to 100*, ed. P. B. Baltes and K. U. Mayer, 450–71. Cambridge: Cambridge University Press.

Super, D. E. 1990. A life-span, life-space approach to career development. In *Career choice and development: Applying contemporary theories to practice*, 2d ed., ed. D. Brown, L. Brooks, and Associates, 197–261. San Francisco: Jossey-Bass.

Thompson, R. A. 1999. The individual child: Temperament, emotion, self, and personality. In *Developmental psychology: An advanced textbook*, 4th ed., ed. M. H. Bornstein and M. E. Lamb, 377–410. Mahwah, N.J.: Lawrence Erlbaum Associates.

Watson, D., and A. Tellegen. 1985. Toward a consensual structure of mood. *Psychological Bulletin* 98:219–35.

Willis, S. L., and J. D. Reid. 1999. *Life in the middle*. San Diego: Academic Press.

Wohlwill, J. F. 1973. *The study of behavioral development*. New York: Academic Press.

CHAPTER EIGHT

Age and Depression in the MIDUS Survey

Ronald C. Kessler, Kristin D. Mickelson, Ellen E. Walters,

Shanyang Zhao, and Lana Hamilton

Community surveys of psychiatric disorder have consistently found a negative relationship between age and lifetime clinical depression (Cross-National Collaborative Group 1992; Blazer et al. 1994; Kanowski 1994), with the highest rates usually found among young adults and the lowest rates usually found among the oldest old. However, the substantive plausibility of this finding has been called into question on the basis that cumulative lifetime risk cannot decrease with age. This means that there cannot be a negative relationship between age and lifetime disorder in the population in equilibrium (Robins et al. 1984).

Several methodological interpretations have been advanced to explain the observed negative relationship between age and depression. One is that recall error increases with age, leading to an apparent decrease in depression, even though true lifetime depression actually increases with age (Simon and Von Korff 1992). Simulation shows that a fairly modest increase in recall error with age could explain a negative relationship between age and lifetime depression of the size observed in most community surveys (Giuffra and Risch 1994). However, this hypothesis is inconsistent with the fact that the negative relationship between age and depression is found not only for lifetime depression but also for current depression.

A second methodological interpretation, this one accounting for the negative relationship between age and current depression, is that unwillingness to admit being depressed is positively associated with age. This hypothesis is consistent with evidence of a positive association between age and the perceived stigma of mental illness (Link and Cullen 1986). However, it is inconsistent with the fact that the negative relationship between age and current depression is between age and a diagnosis of major depressive episode, not age and depressed mood. That is, older people are not less likely to report feeling depressed. In fact, they report higher mean levels of depressed mood than do people in midlife (Jorm 1987; Kessler et al. 1992). Older people are, however, less likely than others to have the cluster of associated signs and symptoms required to meet criteria for a psychiatric diagnosis of major depression. There is no reason to think that unwillingness to admit these associated signs and symptoms, such as loss of energy or problems with sleep, increases with age.

A related methodological possibility is that nonresponse errors as a result of confusion increase with age. This is especially likely among the oldest old but could occur with increasing age throughout the age range. However, even though an increase of this sort has been documented empirically (Colsher and Wallace 1989), the available evidence suggests that it is much too small to explain the age gradient of reported depression.

The fact that depressed mood increases with age beginning in midlife whereas major depression decreases with age means that the probability of depressed mood evolving into major depression decreases with age over the second half of the life cycle. This pattern could be the result of either methodological or substantive factors. The most plausible methodological interpretation is related to the fact that the structured diagnostic interviews used in community surveys to assess major depression are incapable of distinguishing between the somatic symptoms caused by depression and those caused by physical illness (Robins 1985). This lack of discriminating power is addressed in structured diagnostic interviews by using the conservative strategy of excluding somatic symptoms that might have been the result of organic causes in determining whether respondents meet criteria for major depression. Underreporting bias is introduced by this rule whenever respondents mistakenly interpret somatic symptoms as the result of physical illness when they are actually part of a depressive episode, an error that is thought to increase with age because older people are more likely than others to have a co-occurring physical illness. However, a recent study by Heithoff (1995) suggests that this bias is not large enough to explain the observed association between age and depression. This investigation reanalyzed data from a large community survey (Robins and Regier 1991) to determine the magnitude of the increase in late-life DSM-III (American Psychiatric Association 1980) major depression when the organic exclusion rules were relaxed and somatic symptoms were included in making diagnostic decisions, even if respondents reported that these symptoms were the result of physical illness or injury or medications. The prevalence of depression did not increase appreciably when this change was made, which argues against the importance of confusion about somatic symptoms as an explanation for the negative relationship between age and major depression.

A case could be made for a substantive interpretation of the finding that major depression decreases with age, even though depressed mood increases with age beginning in midlife. According to this interpretation, older people are better able to prevent depressed mood from evolving into major depression. Any number of processes could bring about such an effect. Perhaps the most plausible is that the increased life experience, maturity, or wisdom that comes with age (Baltes 1993; Gove, Ortega, and Style 1989; Staudinger, Smith, and Baltes 1992) leads to a decrease in the tendency to make cognitive distortions of the sort that are thought to underlie some episodes of major depression (Abramson, Metalsky, and Alloy 1989).

An alternate possibility is that selection is more important than individual change in explaining the apparent increase with age in the ability to prevent depressed mood from evolving into major depression in community samples. Rather than people becoming more wise or more in control of their emotions with age, according to this argument, persons who are prone to depression might be selected out of the community population with age because of high relative risks of early death or institutionalization (Murphy et al. 1987), leading to an ever more mentally healthy group of survivors. This hypothesis is consistent with evidence from prospective studies that depression is a significant risk factor for both physical morbidity (Stoudemire 1995) and early mortality (Bruce and Leaf 1989).

Whether due to individual change or to selection, the last two interpretations imply that there is a change with age in the predisposition to depression among persons in the community population. Although this hypothesized diathesis could be studied at a number of different levels, the most highly developed approach in survey research involves the stress reactivity paradigm. We know from this work that the majority of episodes of major depression are provoked by stressful life experiences (Brown and Harris 1978) and that a substantial part of individual difference in risk of major depression is the result of differential reactivity to stress (Kessler 1997). Within the context of this approach, the last two interpretations lead to the prediction that the impact of stressful experiences on major depression decreases with age and that this explains much of the negative relationship between age and depression. We evaluate this prediction in this chapter.

In addition, we consider the possibility that it is differential exposure to stress rather than differential stress-reactivity that explains the negative relationship between age and major depression, a possibility also considered at the level of the daily stressor, by Almeida and Horn in chapter 15. Although it is true that stress in some domains increases with age (e.g., declining physical health, increasing exposure to death of loved ones), there are other domains in which the opposite is true. Both the roles and the role-related stresses associated with employment (Osipow, Doty, and Spokane 1985) and childrearing (Pasley and Gecas 1984) decrease for most people with age beginning at midlife. Financial adversity also decreases for many people with age, beginning in midlife, due to a combination of increased income and savings and decreased expenses. Furthermore, the accumulation of life skills with age helps many older people avoid exposure to some of the stresses that they would have been exposed to at earlier ages (Brandtstadter and Renner 1990). On the basis of these considerations, we evaluate the possibility that the negative relationship between age and major depression is the result of a decrease with age in exposure to depressogenic life experiences.

METHODS

The current report is based on data from the nationally representative subsample of 3032 MIDUS respondents who completed both the telephone and mail components of the basic survey. Weights are used to correct for discrepancies between the sample and the population on a series of U.S. Census variables.

The outcome of interest is past-year depressive episode defined according to the criteria in the third edition revised of the American Psychiatric Association's (APA) *Diagnostic and Statistical Manual of Mental Disorders* (DSM-III-R; APA 1987). The diagnosis requires that a person experience a period of at least two weeks of either depressed mood or anhedonia most of the day, nearly every day, and a series of at least four other associated symptoms typically found to accompany depression, including problems with eating, sleeping, energy, concentration, feelings of self-worth, and suicidal thoughts or actions. The diagnosis was operationalized in a screening version of the major depression section of the World Health Organization's (WHO) Composite International Diagnostic Interview (CIDI; WHO 1990, 1997). WHO field trials (Wittchen 1994) and other methodological studies (Blazer et al. 1994) have documented good test–retest reliability and clinical validity of the CIDI diagnosis of DSM-III-R major depression.

We consider the relationship of major depression both with *roles* that may change over the life course (marital status, employment status, parenting status) and with respondent evaluations of *stresses* in each of six major life areas (physical health, work situation, finances, relationship with children, marriage or close relationship, and sexuality).

The measure of marital status distinguishes the married from the never married, separated/divorced, and widowed. Respondents who reported that they were cohabiting were coded as married even if they reported being never married, separated/divorced, or widowed.

The measure of employment status distinguishes the employed from homemakers, the retired, and those in all other employment categories. MIDUS respondents were allowed to endorse more than one employment category (e.g., they could report that they were employed homemakers or disabled students or retired people who were currently working, and so forth). However, we coded employment status so that a single master status was assigned to each respondent. First, those who reported that they were currently working were coded as employed. Those who defined themselves as unemployed or other (e.g., temporarily laid off, on maternity or sick leave, permanently disabled, part-time students) were coded as unemployed, whether or not they also described themselves as homemakers or retired. Those who defined themselves as retired were coded as retired, whether or not they also described themselves as homemakers. Those who defined themselves only as homemakers were coded as homemakers. The twenty-seven full-time students in the sample who endorsed no other employment category were excluded from all analyses because they were so few in number.

The measure of parenting status is a simple dichotomy that distinguishes respondents who have one or more living children from those with no living children. A more refined classification scheme was originally explored that included information about number of children in each of three age ranges (0–12, 13–19, 20+). However, no evidence was found that variation in number or age of children, or the cross-classification of number by ages of children, increased our ability to predict major depression among either women or men or that these more refined variables interacted with age in predicting major depression among either women or men.

The stress measures are based on respondent ratings on a worst-to-best self-anchoring scale. Respondents were asked to think about each of the six areas of life assessed in these measures and to rate their situation in that area on a 0–10 scale, where 0 means "the worst possible situation" in that area and 10 means "the best possible situation." Although these rating scales do not directly assess stress in each domain, researchers have shown that satisfaction with various life domains is strongly related to stress (Baruffol, Gisle, and Corten 1995; Hall, Matthews, and Keeler 1984), suggesting that dissatisfaction with one's current situation in life may be an indicator of stress in that particular domain.

The physical health question simply asked for a rating of "your health." The work situation question asked respondents to "think of the work situation you are in now, whether part-time or full-time, paid or unpaid, at home or at a job" and to rate their "work situation" on the 0–10 worst-to-best scale. The finances question asked for a rating of "your financial situation." The sexuality question asked for a rating of "the sexual aspect of your life." The questions about marriage/close relationships and children were only asked of a subsample rather than the entire sample of respondents. The marriage/close relationship question (hereafter referred to as the marriage question) asked people who were married or living with a partner how they would rate their marriage or close relationship, whereas the children question asked parents to rate their "overall relationship with" their children.

Analysis Procedures

The analysis began by excluding the respondents who were full-time students with no other employment status, leaving 2993 (1310 men and 1683 women) for analysis. We then examined the bivariate relationship between age and major depression. This relationship was found to be significant and negative for both men and women. Age variation in the distribution and impact of roles and stresses on major depression was examined next. Finally, we used demographic rate standardization (Iams and Thornton 1975) to compare the relative contributions of differential exposure and differential reactivity to roles and stresses in explaining the observed age differences in major depression.

The models reported throughout the chapter were estimated with ordinary least squares (OLS) regression using weighted data. As noted later in the chapter, logistic regression could have been used instead of OLS. As it happened, all results were replicated with logistic regressions, and the substantive conclusions reported here remained unchanged. Presentation of results in terms of OLS was chosen because it created advantages in interpreting the results involving demographic rate standardization. Significance tests were adjusted for the use of weights by assuming a design effect of 1.2 for all univariate and multivariate analyses. This assumption is based on preliminary investigation of design effects on total sample means across a wide range of variables in the MIDUS data. Because design effects are generally smaller for multivariate than univariate statistics

TABLE 1 Relationship between Age and Twelve-Month DSM-III-R
Major Depressive Episode, by Sex

Age	Men[a]			Women[b]		
	%	SE	n	%	SE	n
25–34	12.1	(2.1)	(317)	20.7	(2.5)	(452)
35–44	11.2	(1.8)	(400)	22.6	(2.4)	(439)
45–54	11.1	(1.9)	(273)	16.0	(2.1)	(303)
55–64	7.4	(1.8)	(165)	9.8	(1.8)	(292)
65–74	3.3	(1.5)	(155)	10.4	(2.5)	(197)
Total	10.0	(0.9)	(1310)	17.3	(1.1)	(1683)

[a] $\chi^2_{(4)} = 9.7$, $p < .05$.
[b] $\chi^2_{(4)} = 25.7$, $p < .001$.

and are smaller in subsamples than total samples, the simplifying assumption of a constant design effect based on total sample univariate analyses is likely to be conservative (Kish 1965).

RESULTS

The Bivariate Relationship between Age and Major Depression

Table 1 shows prevalence estimates of twelve-month DSM-III-R major depression as estimated from the screening version of the CIDI. The sample-wide prevalence estimate of 14.1 percent is higher than the estimates in surveys that use the full CIDI rather than a screening version to assess depression (e.g., Blazer et al. 1994). This reflects the fact that the full CIDI has exclusion criteria that result in a lower prevalence estimate. Despite this difference, we find, consistent with previous research (Kessler et al. 1993, 1994), that women have a significantly higher estimated twelve-month prevalence of depression than do men ($\chi^2(1) = 26.8$, $p < .001$) and that there is a significant negative relationship between age and depression among both men ($\chi^2(4) = 9.7$, $p < .05$) and women ($\chi^2(4) = 25.7$, $p < .001$).

The Effects of Roles on Depression

Previous research has shown that social roles are strongly related to depressed mood (Lennon and Rosenfield 1992; McLanahan and Adams 1987; Mirowsky and Ross 1986). Married people in most community surveys have lower mean scores on continuous measures of depressed mood than do the unmarried, whereas employed people have lower mean scores than homemakers and the unemployed. These relationships are generally stronger among men than women. Research on the effects of having children is varied. Although most studies show that people with dependent children have higher mean levels of depressed mood than do others, other studies show that this association is stronger for women than men, and still others have found that the effect of children becomes weaker for women but stronger for men as the children grow older. It is not clear whether these associations are entirely the result of the effects of roles on depression. Selection processes could also be at work. Consistent with this possibility, we know that depression is a significant predictor of early childbearing (Kessler et al. 1997), marital timing and stability (Kessler and Forthofer 1999), and employment status (Ettner, Frank, and Kessler 1997).

Less is known about the relationships of social roles with major depression. In an effort to study this in the MIDUS data, we estimated a series of recursive regression equations in which information about social roles was used to predict twelve-month major depression. We also investigated whether the effects of social roles on depression vary with age. We recognize that the implicit assumption in these analyses, that roles influence depression but depression does not influence roles, is simplistic. However, we have no realistic way of identifying a more complex specification with the MIDUS data.

We began with bivariate analyses of the effects of marital status, employment status, and parenting status on depression. As described earlier in the section on measures, the analysis of parenting led to the decision to make only a simple dichotomous distinction between those who had one or more living children and those who had none. The analysis of marital status distinguished the married/cohabiting from noncohabiting persons who were never married, separated/divorced, or widowed. The analysis of employment status distinguished the employed from homemakers, retired persons, and other unemployed individuals. More detailed distinctions were not significant either in predicting depression or in documenting interactions with age in predicting depression.

The next step in the analysis was to examine the age gradient in these roles. Results are shown in table 2 (below, pp. 236–37). We see that there are significant age differences in all the roles. The percentage of men who are married increases with age. Among women, the percentage who are married increases with age up through the midfifties and then decreases. There is a similar increase and then decrease after age 54 for the percentage of both men and women who are separated/divorced. The percentage of those who never married, in comparison, decreases consistently with age, while the percentage of the widowed increases with age. The last of these trends is much more pronounced among women, both because men tend to die earlier than women and because widowed men are much more likely to remarry than widowed women.

The percentage of men who are employed is 95 percent in the youngest age group and declines over the age range. Among women, in comparison, the percentage employed in the youngest age group is much lower (74 percent), and it increases through the women's midforties before declining. This sex difference is consistent with what we know about delays in female labor force participation as a result of childbearing and childrearing. The percentage of women who describe themselves as a homemaker is higher in the youngest age group than in any other age group over the next three decades; the percentage then rises again in the oldest age group. Predictably, the percentage of retired persons increases steadily with age among both men and women, while the percentage in other unemployed statuses decreases in the older groups. The percentage of respondents who have ever had a child, finally, is lowest in the youngest age group and is fairly consistent across the other four age groups in the sample.

The next step was to use linear regression to estimate the additive and joint effects of age, employment status, marital status, and parental status on past-year depression. Linear regression was used instead of logistic regression in order to avoid the suppression of linear interactions that occurs in logistic models. Regression diagnostics showed that the problem of predicted values lying outside the range of the outcome, which can occur when a linear model is used to predict a skewed dichotomous outcome, did not occur with these data.

The regression analysis began with a series of global tests to evaluate the significance of interactions. Although some significant three-way and two-way interaction terms among the three role measures were found, they did not significantly increase the variance over the main effects model, and the number of significant interaction terms was not more than one would expect to find based on chance. On the basis of these results, our final model included only additive effects of roles and age.

The parameter estimates of the additive model are shown in table 3 (see p. 238). The first set of coefficients in the table is for marital status. The omitted category is married. Controlling for age and the other roles in the model, the separated/divorced have a significantly higher prevalence of twelve-month depression than do the married among both men and women. There is no significant difference between the never married

TABLE 2 Relationships between Age

		25–34		35–44	
		%	SE	%	SE
Men					
Marital status	$\chi^2_{(12)} = 167.8, \; p < .001$				
Married/cohabiting		60.3	(3.1)	77.3	(2.4)
Separated/divorced		7.9	(1.8)	15.2	(2.1)
Widowed		0.0	(—)	0.5	(0.4)
Never married		31.7	(3.0)	7.0	(1.4)
Employment status	$\chi^2_{(8)} = 593.3, \; p < .001$				
Working		94.8	(1.4)	91.3	(1.6)
Retired		0.5	(0.4)	0.4	(0.3)
Other unemployed		4.7	(1.3)	8.3	(1.5)
Parenting status	$\chi^2_{(4)} = 137.0, \; p < .001$				
Children		54.5	(3.2)	84.1	(2.1)
No children		45.5	(3.2)	15.9	(2.1)
Women					
Marital status	$\chi^2_{(12)} = 338.3, \; p < .001$				
Married/cohabiting		60.9	(3.1)	65.4	(2.7)
Separated/divorced		14.4	(2.2)	24.4	(2.5)
Widowed		0.2	(0.3)	1.0	(0.5)
Never married		24.5	(2.6)	9.2	(1.6)
Employment status	$\chi^2_{(12)} = 540.3, \; p < .001$				
Working		73.7	(2.7)	81.1	(2.3)
Homemaker		17.0	(2.3)	10.7	(1.8)
Retired		0.0	(—)	0.0	(—)
Other unemployed		9.3	(1.9)	8.3	(1.6)
Parenting status	$\chi^2_{(4)} = 92.2, \; p < .001$				
Children		71.3	(2.8)	89.9	(1.8)
No children		28.7	(2.8)	10.1	(1.8)

Notes: Employment status was classified hierarchically. For those with multiple responses, the order of category assignment was "working," "other unemployed," "retired," and "homemaker." Due to small sample size, men who reported "homemaker" were reclassified as "other unemployed."

and the married. Widowed men have a significant elevated rate of depression, but this is not true among women. These results are consistent with previous studies in finding that risk of depression is elevated by marital separation and divorce (Aseltine and Kessler 1993) and that the depressogenic effect of widowhood is significantly greater among men than women (Umberson, Wortman, and Kessler 1992).

The next set of coefficients in the table is for employment status. The omitted category is employed. Homemakers, among women, and persons in the other unemployed category, among both men and women, and Social Roles, by Sex

		Age			
45–54		55–64		65–74	
%	SE	%	SE	%	SE
76.5	(2.4)	80.4	(2.6)	82.6	(3.3)
17.5	(2.2)	11.7	(2.2)	6.1	(2.1)
0.6	(0.4)	4.6	(1.4)	5.6	(2.0)
5.4	(1.3)	3.4	(1.2)	5.7	(2.0)
92.1	(1.5)	64.3	(3.2)	22.0	(3.6)
1.9	(0.8)	31.6	(3.2)	77.1	(3.6)
6.0	(1.4)	4.1	(1.3)	1.0	(0.9)
89.9	(1.8)	89.1	(2.1)	90.0	(2.6)
10.1	(1.8)	10.9	(2.1)	10.0	(2.6)
68.6	(2.6)	66.3	(2.8)	57.6	(4.2)
24.6	(2.5)	15.5	(2.2)	9.3	(2.4)
2.8	(1.0)	12.7	(2.0)	32.0	(3.9)
3.9	(1.1)	5.5	(1.4)	1.2	(0.9)
72.4	(2.6)	54.9	(3.0)	19.5	(3.3)
14.3	(2.0)	14.6	(2.1)	21.9	(3.5)
3.1	(1.0)	24.3	(2.6)	57.7	(4.2)
10.3	(1.8)	6.2	(1.4)	0.9	(0.8)
92.7	(1.5)	90.7	(1.8)	93.0	(2.2)
7.3	(1.5)	9.3	(1.8)	7.1	(2.2)

have significantly higher prevalences of depression than do the employed. There is no significant difference in depression between the retired and the employed. These results are consistent with previous research documenting adverse effects of unemployment (Kessler, Turner, and House 1989), elevated rates of depression among homemakers (Blazer et al. 1994; Rosenfield 1989), and no significant adverse aggregate effect of retirement on depression (Midanik et al. 1995).

The final coefficient in the table compares respondents who have a child with those who do not. There is no significant difference in the prevalence of depression between these two groups, either among men or women. As noted earlier, previous research has yielded inconsistent results about this relationship, so it is not surprising that the pattern here is

TABLE 3 Linear Regressions of Twelve-Month DSM-III-R Major
Depressive Episode on Social Roles and Age, by Sex

	Men		Women	
	b	SE	b	SE
Marital status				
Married/cohabiting	0.00	(—)	0.00	(—)
Separated/divorced	0.10***	(.02)	0.11***	(.03)
Widow	0.14*	(.07)	0.05	(.04)
Never married	0.03	(.03)	0.00	(.04)
Employment status				
Working	0.00	(—)	0.00	(—)
Homemaker	—	(—)	0.08**	(.03)
Retired	0.02	(.03)	0.03	(.04)
Other unemployed	0.17***	(.03)	0.08*	(.04)
Parenting status				
Children	0.00	(—)	0.00	(—)
No children	−0.01	(.02)	0.05	(.03)
Age				
25–34	0.10**	(.04)	0.12**	(.04)
35–44	0.08*	(.04)	0.14***	(.04)
45–54	0.08*	(.04)	0.07	(.04)
55–64	0.04	(.03)	0.01	(.04)
65–74	—	(—)	—	(—)
	$R^2 = .04$		$R^2 = .04$	
	$F_{(10,1449)} = 5.5,$		$F_{(11,1522)} = 4.3,$	
	$p < .001$		$p < .001$	

*$p < .05$. **$p < .01$. ***$p < .001$.

not significant. It is consistent with previous research that the regression coefficient for women is stronger than for men. It is somewhat surprising, on the other hand, that we failed to find significant specifications depending on the number and ages of children or, among women, in comparing homemakers with the employed, because these specifications have generally been found in previous research on depressed mood (Bromberger and Matthews 1994; Brown and Bifulco 1990; Hock and DeMeis 1990).

The Effects of Stress on Depression

Previous research has shown that stressful life experiences are powerful predictors of major depression (Kessler 1997). In an effort to study this relationship in the MIDUS data, we estimated a series of recursive equations in which the 0–10 rating scales of stress in six major life domains were used to predict twelve-month depression and to investigate whether the effects of stress on depression vary with age.

We began by performing preliminary analyses of the functional form of the relationships between each of the rating scales and depression. In every case we found a significant relationship that could be adequately described by a dichotomy that distinguished respondents who reported problems in that area of life from those who did not. Thus, individuals with a score of 0 to 5 on physical health, work situation, marriage, and sexuality, or a score of 0 to 4 on children, or 0 to 3 on finances were coded as having a stress in that particular area of life.

We then examined the age gradient in exposure to these dichotomously coded stresses. As shown below in table 4, three broad patterns can be observed in this gradient. The most common is an increase in stress from early adulthood to midlife and then a decrease from midlife to older age. This pattern is found for nearly half the entries in the table, including stresses in the areas of physical health, marriage, and children among men and physical health, work situation, and children among women. The second most common pattern is a steady decrease in stress across the full age range. This is found for work situation and finances among men and for finances and marriage among women. The third pattern is a steady increase in stress throughout the age range, which is found for sexuality among both men and women.

We next estimated a series of interaction models to determine whether the effects of these dichotomously measured stresses on past-year depression vary significantly across the age range of the sample. A number of significant interactions were found. Final models were then estimated in which the slopes of the stresses were constrained to be equal across the age groups where significant differences had not been found and allowed to vary across those where significant differences had been found. Only an additive specification was considered.

Table 5 (on pp. 242–43) shows the results of a model that includes the effects of the significant stress measures controlling for roles. Among men, significant effects were found for stresses in the domains of physical health, work situation, and finances. The strongest effect is for physical health and the weakest is for work situation. All effects other than that of physical health are constant across the age range of the sample, whereas the physical health effect is significantly stronger in midlife than in the youngest and older age groups. Among women, significant effects were found for stresses in all six domains of physical health, work situation,

TABLE 4 Relationships between Age and

Life Stresses	25–34		35–44	
	%	SE	%	SE
Men				
Physical health	8.5	(1.8)	12.7	(1.9)
Work situation	21.1	(2.6)	19.7	(2.3)
Finances	18.6	(2.4)	15.8	(2.1)
Children	0.4	(0.4)	3.8	(1.1)
Marriage	5.5	(1.4)	10.0	(1.8)
Sexuality	31.4	(3.0)	30.0	(2.6)
Women				
Physical health	15.1	(2.2)	16.1	(2.1)
Work situation	21.3	(2.5)	21.2	(2.4)
Finances	22.8	(2.6)	17.3	(2.2)
Children	1.4	(0.8)	2.3	(0.9)
Marriage	16.3	(2.3)	14.1	(2.0)
Sexuality	34.2	(3.0)	38.3	(2.8)

Note: Life stresses were entered as dichotomous variables; cutoff points were determined on the basis of prior analyses.

$^*p < .05.$ $^{**}p < .01.$ $^{***}p < .001.$

finances, sexuality, marriage, and children. The strongest consistent effect is for children and the weakest for sexuality. Unlike the situation with men, the effects of stresses in physical health, work situation, finances, and marriage become smaller for women with increasing age.

The Effects of Stress on the Relationship between Age and Depression

It is possible to quantify the joint effects of changes in roles, in stress exposure, and in stress reactivity on the relationship between age and depression by the use of demographic rate standardization (Iams and Thornton 1975). This method manipulates the slopes and means of the predictor variables in pairs of regression equations to calculate how difference in average rates of the outcomes in two subsamples would change if the means and/or slopes of the predictors were constant across the subsamples. By doing this in a systematic way for each logically possible combination of mean and slope differences, it is possible to partition the observed mean difference in the outcome into components due to age differences in roles, in exposure to stress, in the impact of stress on depression, and into a residual that is not explained by the predictor variables.

There are ten logically possible pairwise comparisons among the five age groups considered here. However, we focus on only the subset of these

Satisfaction in Seven Life Domains, by Sex

Age							
45–54		55–64		65–74			
%	SE	%	SE	%	SE	F	
11.7	(1.9)	20.1	(2.7)	13.2	(3.0)	3.4**	
19.3	(2.3)	18.7	(2.6)	14.7	(3.1)	0.7	
8.4	(1.6)	7.2	(1.8)	5.1	(1.9)	7.3***	
2.4	(0.9)	2.7	(1.1)	0.9	(0.8)	2.5*	
7.0	(1.4)	3.2	(1.3)	1.6	(1.1)	4.3**	
34.5	(2.7)	42.6	(3.3)	54.9	(4.3)	8.7***	
22.3	(2.4)	15.2	(2.2)	14.9	(3.0)	1.7	
23.3	(2.4)	20.9	(2.4)	12.9	(2.8)	1.7	
14.4	(2.0)	13.6	(2.1)	10.8	(2.6)	3.8**	
3.1	(1.0)	0.5	(0.4)	0.9	(0.8)	1.5	
8.1	(1.5)	8.0	(1.6)	4.6	(1.8)	5.7***	
44.3	(2.8)	54.8	(3.0)	60.3	(4.2)	11.4***	

ten that involves significant differences in rates of depression. There are seven of these among men and eight among women. The rationale for selecting these subsets can be seen by returning briefly to table 1. We see there that among men, the prevalence of depression is not significantly different in the three youngest age groups, but it decreases significantly in the fourth group and decreases again significantly in the oldest age group. As a result, we are interested in the pairwise comparisons among men in each of the first three groups with the fourth and in each of the first four groups with the fifth. Among women, in comparison, the prevalence of depression is not significantly different in the two youngest age groups, but it decreases significantly in the third group and again in the fourth group. The fourth and fifth groups do not differ significantly. As a result, we are interested in the pairwise comparisons among women in each of the first two groups with the third and in each of the first three groups with the fourth and fifth.

The decompositions of these significant differences are reported in table 6. We begin by considering men. The results of the seven decompositions are similar in that the smallest two components, in most cases, are the results of differences in roles or differences in stress exposure, and (in four of the seven comparisons) the largest to stress reactivity. All of these effects combined explain between 3 percent and 94 percent of the observed pairwise mean differences in depression.

TABLE 5 Multiple Linear Regression of Twelve-Month

	25–34		35–44	
	b	SE	b	SE
Men[a]				
Physical health	.02	(.07)	.18***	(.03)
Work situation	.04*	(.02)	.04*	(.02)
Finances	.07**	(.03)	.07**	(.03)
Women[b]				
Physical health	.24***	(.05)	.08**	(.03)
Work situation	.13**	(.05)	.02	(.03)
Finances	.13**	(.05)	.09**	(.03)
Sexuality	.05*	(.02)	.05*	(.02)
Marriage/relationship	.08*	(.04)	.08*	(.04)
Children	.26***	(.08)	.26***	(.08)

[a]The five subgroup regression equations for men were estimated in a single model that assessed all respondents. The model included four intercepts for the five age cohorts, two dummy variables that were constant across age for the effects of stresses in the domains of work situation and finances, and separate dummy variables for stress in the domain of physical health for those in the age ranges of 25–34, 35–54, and 55–74. We also controlled for social roles. The overall model is significant ($F_{(15,1444)} = 6.59$, $p < .001$; $R^2 = .08$), and each of the predictors is significant at the .05 level, two-tailed test, in at least one subgroup.

[b]As with men, the five subgroup regression equations for women were estimated in a single model that assessed all respondents. The model included four intercepts for the five age cohorts, two dummy variables that were constant across age for the effects of stresses in the domains of sexuality and children, and separate dummy variables for stresses in the domains of physical health, work situation, finances, and marriage. We also controlled for social roles. The overall model is significant ($F_{(21,1512)} = 7.64$, $p < .001$; $R^2 = .11$), and each of the predictors is significant at the .05 level, two-tailed test, in at least one subgroup.

*$p < .05$. **$p < .01$. ***$p < .001$.

The consistently small component due to role differences is the result of counteracting differences in roles over the age range of the sample. As shown in table 2, older men are advantaged in having lower rates of separation/divorce and of other unemployment than younger men, but they are disadvantaged in having a higher rate of widowhood. These opposite effects cancel each other out to produce the small role exposure components shown in the table, with the sign varying from one pair to the next, depending on whether the advantages are larger or smaller than the disadvantages in any particular comparison.

The somewhat larger component due to differences in stress exposure is the result of a similar balancing of opposites. As shown in table 4, older men are advantaged in having lower rates of stress in the domains of work and finances than are younger men, but they are disadvantaged in having

DSM-III-R Major Depressive Episode on Stress, by Sex

Age					
45–54		55–64		65–74	
b	SE	b	SE	b	SE
.18***	(.03)	−.04	(.04)	−.04	(.04)
.04*	(.02)	.04*	(.02)	.04*	(.02)
.07**	(.03)	.07**	(.03)	.07**	(.03)
.08**	(.03)	.08**	(.03)	.08**	(.03)
.02	(.03)	.02	(.03)	.02	(.03)
.09**	(.03)	.09**	(.03)	.09**	(.03)
.05*	(.02)	.05*	(.02)	.05*	(.02)
.00	(.05)	.00	(.05)	.00	(.05)
.26***	(.08)	.26***	(.08)	.26***	(.08)

higher rates of stress in the domains of physical health and sexuality. The balance favors younger men up through the midsixties but older men thereafter.

The consistently positive component due to stress reactivity, finally, is the result of the lower impact of physical health problems on older rather than middle-aged men. This difference alone explains on average 71 percent of the age difference in depression in the comparisons of men in the three youngest age groups with those in the age group 55–64, and between 8 percent and 36 percent of the differences of men younger than 55 with those aged 65–74. Differential stress reactivity plays no part in the comparison between men in the two oldest age groups, though, because low stress reactivity characterizes men in both these groups.

The results are somewhat different among women. As with men, older women are advantaged by having lower rates of separation/divorce and lower rates of membership in the other unemployed category than younger women have, but they are disadvantaged by having a much higher rate of widowhood and a higher rate of being homemakers than middle-aged women have. Unlike men, though, these opposite effects cancel each other out in a way that produces a consistent disadvantage for older women. The main sex difference here involves the fact that many women, but virtually no men, are homemakers. As shown in table 2, the proportion of women who are homemakers generally increases with age.

TABLE 6 Decompositions of Age Differences in Twelve-Month
DSM-III-R Major Depressive Episodes (percentage)

| Age Groups Compared[a] | | | Reasons for Depression | | |
Younger	Older	Roles	Stress Exposure	Stress Reactivity	Residual
Men					
25–34	55–64	−21.3	21.6	19.6	79.9
35–44	55–64	−5.3	2.5	96.6	6.3
45–54	55–64	−1.4	−14.0	95.8	19.7
25–34	65–74	−9.6	14.1	7.8	87.7
35–44	65–74	−1.1	11.9	35.8	53.5
45–54	65–74	0.9	4.3	34.7	60.5
55–64	65–74	2.7	0.5	0.0	96.6
Women					
25–34	45–54	−0.2	−19.5	144.9	−25.4
35–44	45–54	−5.5	−7.8	14.1	99.5
25–34	55–64	−4.4	6.1	57.0	41.5
35–44	55–64	−6.5	3.0	7.3	96.3
45–54	55–64	−7.5	14.7	0.0	92.8
25–34	65–74	−21.9	13.5	53.9	54.6
35–44	65–74	−21.6	5.2	6.4	110.0
45–54	65–74	−40.6	18.3	0.0	122.4

[a]Comparisons are limited to pairs in which the older group has a significantly lower prevalence of depression than the younger group at the .05 level (one-tailed test).

As shown in table 3, being a homemaker is associated with increased risk of depression throughout the age range of the sample.

There is a consistently positive component, in comparison, that results from differences in stress exposure. Again, this is due to counteracting forces. As shown in table 4, older women are advantaged in having lower rates of stress in the domains of work, finances, children, marriage, and, surprisingly, physical health. They are disadvantaged in only one area, sexuality. In almost all the pairwise comparisons, the advantages outweigh this one disadvantage. However, differences due to stress exposure do not account for a large part of the mean difference in depression in any of the age comparisons.

The consistently positive stress reactivity component, finally, is the result of lower impacts of a number of stresses on older as opposed to younger women. As shown in table 5, these include lower effects of stresses in the domains of physical health and work situation. The stress reactivity component in table 6 is the largest substantive component in five of the eight pairwise comparisons among women, explaining between 7 percent and 145 percent of the observed mean difference in depression between age groups.

DISCUSSION

The MIDUS survey has a lower response rate than do some other surveys that have examined the relationship between age and depression. This is potentially an important issue for the investigation of this particular association because depression might be related to age differences in response bias. An additional potential problem is that MIDUS used a CIDI screening measure of major depression rather than the full CIDI. Despite these two potential limitations, though, we still found the same negative relationship between age and twelve-month DSM-III-R major depression in the MIDUS data that has been documented in other surveys having higher response rates and using the full CIDI (e.g., Robins and Regier 1991; Blazer et al. 1994).

Our analysis suggests that differences in roles over the age range of the sample do not play an important part in the age–depression relationship among men. However, these differences appear to dampen the age gradient among women as a result of increases in depression associated with higher proportions of older women who are widowed and homemakers, more than offsetting the decreases in depression associated with lower proportions of older women who are separated/divorced or unemployed. Our results suggest that were it not for these differences in roles, the negative relationship between age and depression would be even stronger than it is.

It is important to recognize that this conclusion is based on the naive assumption that the relationship between roles and depression is recursive, that role-related experiences influence risk of depression but that depression does not influence the selection of roles. Although this assumption is routinely made in studies of sex roles and mental illness (e.g., Gore and Mangione 1983; Mirowsky and Ross 1986), there is good reason to believe that it is incorrect. Indeed, recent epidemiological surveys have shown that a variety of psychiatric disorders, depression included, influence such important role transitions as high school graduation, college entry, and college dropout (Kessler et al. 1995), marital timing and marital stability (Kessler and Forthofer 1999), teenage childbearing (Kessler et al. 1997), and employment status (Ettner, Frank, and Kessler 1997). As a result of these considerations, it is not appropriate to interpret the slopes in table 3 as representing *effects* of roles on depression. There is presumably some part of these associations that is due to

245

differences in the stresses, vulnerabilities, and resources to which people are exposed as a function of their social roles, but we have no way of separating these components from the components that are the result of selection.

We also found that there are important age-related differences in exposure to stress. Contrary to the naive view that aging is invariably associated with increases in a variety of stresses, we find that this is not the entire story. There are increases in role loss with age because of widowhood and retirement and increases in the stresses associated with sexuality. However, there are more areas of life in which stresses decrease with age, including stresses in the areas of job, finances, and personal relationships. On balance, these changes are to the advantage of older people. This is especially true among women.

It is important to appreciate, in interpreting this last result, that the measures of stress used here were based on rating scales of how things are going in various areas of life. Although the questions implied that respondents were supposed to make objective assessments rather than report emotional reactions, it is clear that standards for assigning oneself a score on a 0–10 scale from "the worst possible situation" in that area to "the best possible situation" depend critically on standards for what is possible. The latter almost certainly change over time and probably account for at least some part of the observed differences in the age gradient of reported stresses. This is the most plausible interpretation, for example, of the finding that there is a significant drop between the next to oldest and oldest age groups in the percentage of men who rated their physical health in the range we defined as indicating stress. It is unlikely that these older men are actually in better physical health. Their responses more likely reflect lowering of expectations of what is possible at their age.

If this is true, we may need a more active view of the processes involved in the decrease in stress exposure with age seen in the MIDUS data, to see people as modifying their expectations as they age in order to reduce the extent to which objective increases in stress provoke depression. Research by Brandtstadter and Renner (1990) documents that changes of this sort do, in fact, occur with age. These authors find that people increasingly adopt an accommodative mode of coping with stress as they age in which preferences and expectations are adjusted in light of increasing situational constraints. Brim (1992) advanced a similar argument in his discussion of strategies used to redefine goals with increasing age in an effort to maintain a just manageable level of difficulty that promotes continued engagement and feelings of mastery in light of the fact of objectively declining capacities.

Similar processes could be at work to explain the finding that stress reactivity decreases with age. One way in which this could occur is by people reducing their emotional investment in areas of life where they are having difficulties, a process that appears to be more common with increasing age (Brandtstadter and Rothermund 1994). Other processes are also likely at work. One set might involve greater access to objective coping resources that increase with age, such as financial assets and social networks, which have been found to buffer the impact of stress on depression (Brown and Harris 1978). Another set might involve intrapsychic resources that increase with age, such as the use of more effective coping strategies to manage stress and the ability to focus coping energies increasingly on problems that one can control (Blanchard-Fields and Irion 1988).

The MIDUS data can be used to evaluate most of these possibilities because the survey included information about a wide range of objective and intrapsychic resources and vulnerabilities. In exploring their effects on reactivity, we will have to make sense of the fact that the evidence for age-related changes is much more consistent for women than for men. We must also explain the fact that the critical age range in which decreased reactivity begins varies across the domains of stress considered here. These specifications mean that no one global resource could explain all of the age-related changes in reactivity that emerge in the data. A series of accumulating resources with stress-buffering effects that involve some sort of threshold are more likely to be involved.

An important issue that cannot be assessed in more detailed analysis of the MIDUS data concerns change versus selection. Even if we can pinpoint resources that appear to account for the decreasing depressogenic effects of stress with age among women, we will probably be unable to determine how much of their increase with age in our community sample is the result of resource accumulation in the lives of individuals over time and how much is the result of the fact that people who lack these resources are at increased risk of early death and institutionalization. The only feasible way of sorting out these possibilities is by following people through time. We are in the fortunate position of having a wide-enough age range in the MIDUS sample that this is possible. Our work with the data over the next few years will tell us whether enough provocative, targeted hypotheses of significance (either for theory or social policy) emerge from the data to warrant follow-up of the sample. If so, we will be in a position to sort out the relative contributions of resource accumulation and selection.

Acknowledgments

The authors thank Carol Ryff, Paul Griffin, Ken Texiera, Andrew Shippy, Douglas Katz, Paula Calabrese, Debbie Heiser, Kathy Jankowski, Rosie Sood, and Tonly Tonona for helpful comments on the manuscript. Support for this work was provided by National Institute of Mental Health grants K05-MH00507 and T32 MH16806.

References

Abramson, L. Y., G. L. Metalsky, and L. B. Alloy. 1989. Hopelessness depression: A theory-based subtype of depression. *Psychological Review* 96:358–72.

American Psychiatric Association (APA). 1980. *Diagnostic and statistical manual of mental disorders.* 3d ed. Washington, D.C.: American Psychiatric Press.

———. 1987. *Diagnostic and statistical manual of mental disorders.* 3d ed. rev. Washington, D.C.: American Psychiatric Press.

Aseltine, R. H., Jr., and R. C. Kessler. 1993. Marital disruption and depression in a community sample. *Journal of Health and Social Behavior* 34:237–51.

Baltes, P. B. 1993. The aging mind: Potential and limits. *Gerontologist* 33:580–94.

Baruffol, E., L. Gisle, and P. Corten. 1995. Life satisfaction as a mediator between distressing events and neurotic impairment in a general population. *Acta Psychiatrica Scandinavica* 92:56–62.

Blanchard-Fields, F., and J. C. Irion. 1988. The relation between locus of control and coping in two contexts: Age as a moderator variable. *Psychology and Aging* 3:197–203.

Blazer, D. G., R. C. Kessler, K. A. McGonagle, and M. A. Swartz. 1994. The prevalence and distribution of major depression in a national community sample: The National Comorbidity Survey. *American Journal of Psychiatry* 151:979–86.

Brandtstadter, J., and G. Renner. 1990. Tenacious goal pursuit and flexible goal adjustment: Explication and age-related analysis of assimilative and accommodative strategies of coping. *Psychology and Aging* 5:58–67.

Brandtstadter, J., and K. Rothermund. 1994. Self-percepts of control in middle and later adulthood: Buffering losses by rescaling goals. *Psychology and Aging* 9:265–73.

Brim, O. G. 1992. *Ambition: How we manage success and failure throughout our lives.* New York: Basic Books.

Brim, O. G., and D. Featherman. 1997. Surveying midlife development in the United States. Manuscript.

Bromberger, J. T., and K. A. Matthews. 1994. Employment status and depressive symptoms in middle-aged women: A longitudinal investigation. *American Journal of Public Health* 84:202–6.

Brown, G. W., and A. Bifulco. 1990. Motherhood, employment, and the development of depression: A replication of a finding? *British Journal of Psychiatry* 156:169–79.

Brown, G. W., and T. O. Harris. 1978. *Social origins of depression: A study of psychiatric disorders in women.* New York: Free Press.

Bruce, M. L., and P. J. Leaf. 1989. Psychiatric disorders and 15-month mortality in a community sample of older adults. *American Journal of Public Health* 79:727–30.

Colsher, P. L., and R. B. Wallace. 1989. Data quality and age: Health and psycho-behavioral correlates of item nonresponse and inconsistent responses. *Journal of Gerontology* 44:45–52.

Cross-National Collaborative Group. 1992. The changing rate of major depression: Cross-national comparisons. *Journal of the American Medical Association* 268:3098–3105.

Ettner, S. L., R. G. Frank, and R. C. Kessler. 1997. The impact of psychiatric disorders on labor market outcomes. *Industrial and Labor Relations Review* 51:64–81.

Giuffra, L. A., and N. Risch. 1994. Diminished recall and the cohort effect of major depression: A simulation study. *Psychological Medicine* 24:375–83.

Gore, S., and T. W. Mangione. 1983. Social roles, sex roles, and psychological distress. *Journal of Health and Social Behavior* 24:300–312.

Gove, W. R., S. T. Ortega, and C. B. Style. 1989. The maturational and role perspectives on aging and self through the adult years: An empirical evaluation. *American Journal of Sociology* 94:1117–45.

Hall, J. R., L. H. Matthews, and H. Keeler. 1984. Demographics, stress, and depression in a community health screening. *Journal of Psychology* 118:45–50.

Heithoff, K. 1995. Does the ECA underestimate the prevalence of late-life depression? *Journal of the American Geriatrics Society* 43:2–6.

Hock, E., and D. K. DeMeis. 1990. Depression in mothers of infants: The role of maternal employment. *Developmental Psychology* 26:285–91.

Iams, H. M., and A. Thornton. 1975. Decomposition of differences: A cautionary note. *Sociological Methods and Research* 3:341–50.

Jorm, A. F. 1987. Sex and age differences in depression: A quantitative synthesis of published research. *Australian and New Zealand Journal of Psychiatry* 21:46–53.

Kanowski, S. 1994. Age-dependent epidemiology of depression. *Gerontology* 40:1–4.

Kessler, R. C. 1997. The effects of stressful life events on depression. In *Annual review of psychology,* ed. J. T. Spence, J. M. Darley, and D. J. Foss, 48:191–214. Palo Alto, Calif.: Annual Reviews, Inc.

Kessler, R. C., P. A. Berglund, C. L. Foster, W. B. Saunders, P. E. Stang, and E. E. Walters. 1997. Social consequences of psychiatric disorder, II: Teenage parenthood. *American Journal of Psychiatry* 154:1405–11.

Kessler, R. C., and M. S. Forthofer. 1999. The effects of psychiatric disorders on family formation and stability. In *Conflict and cohesion in families: Causes and consequences,* ed. J. Brooks-Gunn and M. Cox, 301–20. New York: Cambridge University Press.

Kessler, R. C., C. L. Foster, W. B. Saunder, and P. E. Stang. 1995. The social consequences of psychiatric disorders. 1. Educational attainment. *American Journal of Psychiatry* 152:1026–32.

Kessler, R. C., C. Foster, P. S. Webster, and J. S. House. 1992. The relationship between age and depressive symptoms in two national surveys. *Psychology and Aging* 7:119–26.

Kessler, R. C., K. A. McGonagle, C. B. Nelson, M. Hughes, M. Swartz, and D. G. Blazer. 1994. Sex and depression in the National Comorbidity Survey. 2: Cohort effects. *Journal of Affective Disorders* 30:15–26.

Kessler, R. C., K. A. McGonagle, M. Swartz, D. G. Blazer, and C. B. Nelson. 1993. Sex and depression in the National Comorbidity Survey. 1: Lifetime prevalence, chronicity and recurrence. *Journal of Affective Disorders* 29:85–96.

Kessler, R. C., J. B. Turner, and J. S. House. 1989. Unemployment, reemployment, and emotional functioning in a community sample. *American Sociological Review* 54:648–57.

Kish, L. 1965. *Survey sampling.* New York: John Wiley.

Lennon, M. C., and S. Rosenfield. 1992. Women and mental health: The inter-action of job and family conditions. *Journal of Health and Social Behavior* 33:316–27.

Link, B. G., and F. T. Cullen. 1986. Contact with the mentally ill and perceptions of how dangerous they are. *Journal of Health and Social Behavior* 27:289–303.

McLanahan, S., and J. Adams. 1987. Parenthood and psychological well-being. *Annual Review of Sociology* 5:237–57.

Midanik, L. T., K. Soghikian, L. J. Ransom, and I. S. Tekawa. 1995. The effect of retirement on mental health and health behaviors: The Kaiser Permanente Retirement Study. *Journals of Gerontology: Psychological Sciences and Social Sciences* (ser. B) 50:S59–S61.

Mirowsky, J., and C. E. Ross. 1986. Social patterns of distress. *Annual Review of Sociology* 12:23–45.

Murphy, J. M., R. R. Monson, D. C. Olivier, A. M. Sobol, and A. H. Leighton. 1987. Affective disorders and mortality: A general population study. *Archives of General Psychiatry* 44:473–80.

Osipow, S. H., R. E. Doty, and A. R. Spokane. 1985. Occupational stress, strain, and coping across the life span. *Journal of Vocational Behavior* 27:98–108.

Pasley, K., and V. Gecas. 1984. Stresses and satisfactions of the parental role. *Personnel and Guidance Journal* 62:400–404.

Robins, L. N. 1985. Epidemiology: Reflections on testing the validity of psychiatric interviews. *Archives of General Psychiatry* 42:918–24.

Robins, L. N., J. E. Helzer, M. M. Weissman, H. Overschel, E. Gruenberg, J. Burke, and D. A. Regier. 1984. Lifetime prevalence of specific disorders in three sites. *Archives of General Psychiatry* 41:949–58.

Robins, L. N., and D. A. Regier, eds. 1991. *Psychiatric disorders in America: The Epidemiologic Catchment Area Study.* New York: Free Press.

Rosenfield, S. 1989. The effects of women's employment: Personal control and sex differences in mental health. *Journal of Health and Social Behavior* 30:77–91.

Simon, G. E., and M. R. Von Korff. 1992. Reevaluation of secular trends in depression rates. *American Journal of Epidemiology* 135:1411–22.

Staudinger, U. M., J. Smith, and P. B. Baltes. 1992. Wisdom-related knowledge in a life review task: Age differences and the role of professional specialization. *Psychology and Aging* 7:271–81.

Stoudemire, A., ed. 1995. *Psychological factors affecting medical conditions.* Washington, D.C.: American Psychiatric Press.

Umberson, D., C. B. Wortman, and R. C. Kessler. 1992. Widowhood and depression: Explaining long-term gender differences in vulnerability. *Journal of Health and Social Behavior* 33:10–24.

Wittchen, H.-U. 1994. Reliability and validity studies of the WHO Composite International Diagnostic Interview (CIDI): A critical review. *Psychiatric Research* 28:57–84.

World Health Organization (WHO). 1990. *Composite International Diagnostic Interview (CIDI)*, version 1.0. Geneva: World Health Organization.

———. 1997. *Composite International Diagnostic Interview (CIDI)*, version 2.1. Geneva: World Health Organization.

CHAPTER NINE

The Quality of American Life at the End of the Century
William Fleeson

The first part of this chapter answers two questions: What is the quality of life in the United States in the mid-1990s? and How does quality differ across age? The answer to the first question describes not only quality of life as a whole but also the quality of specific domains of life (e.g., work, health, family). The second question is in line with the central focus of MIDUS, and in answering it, I pay particular attention to the midlife period.

The second part of the chapter addresses the relative importance of the specific life domains in contributing to a life of high quality. "Importance" is not meant to refer to what individuals value or place importance on but rather to how much the domain is critical for achieving and maintaining a high-quality life. Importance in this sense is determined indirectly and empirically, by comparing the overall life quality of those who are doing well in a domain against the overall life quality of those who are not.

The current study also provides a useful twenty-five-year update to an earlier study conducted by Campbell, Converse, and Rodgers (1976) (CCR). A replication of their seminal study is needed for at least three reasons. First, many of the CCR findings were intriguing, and an entirely independent replication would add considerably to their credibility. Second, there has been large-scale social change in the intervening twenty-five years, and it seems that life quality and its determinants would be particularly sensitive to such changes; divergences from the CCR findings may indicate the impact of those changes, whereas similarities may indicate findings and principles that are resistant to such kinds of social change. Third, age-related changes in quality are ambiguous as to their origin in historical cohort or in the aging process. Two samples separated by twenty-five years can disentangle such issues by having two different sets of cohorts; as a result, any similarities in age trajectories can be somewhat confidently attributed to age. Although CCR did not believe their work was complete until at least two waves were completed, no one has had the resources to conduct the large-scale, national survey these questions require. MIDUS is the first opportunity to arise in twenty-five years.

A MODEL OF LIFE QUALITY

There is no consensus about the conceptual or operational definitions of life quality (Ryan and Deci 2001). There is continuing consideration of whether objective or subjective indicators are preferred (Kahneman 1999; Lawton et al. 1999; Schwarz and Strack 1991, 1999; Stone, Shiffman, and DeVries 1999), whether criteria are to be specified by researchers or left "blank" to be filled in by participants (Diener, Sapyta, and Suh 1998; Ryff 1989; Ryff and Singer 1998; Ryan and Deci 2001), and whether affective or cognitive judgments or both are involved. In line with previous work (Smith et al. 1999; Staudinger, Fleeson, and Baltes 1999), this chapter adapts the groundbreaking model developed by Campbell, Converse, and Rodgers (1976). The basic assumption of this model is that people know the quality of their life and, if asked directly, will honestly and accurately report it. Furthermore, in addition to knowing the quality of their life as a whole, individuals also know and can accurately report the quality of several distinct and relatively independent domains of their life (e.g., marriage, work, health). The quality of each—that is, the quality of life and the quality of the domains—is experienced as an integral whole that has personal meaning to the individual and describes how well things are going in that domain for that individual. Thus, the quality of an individual's life is defined as his or her evaluation of the quality of life overall and the evaluation of each of the several life domains.

Thus, this approach is committed to subjective, "blank," and cognitive evaluations of quality. The commitment to subjective evaluations deserves stressing from the outset. This commitment means that the concept of "quality of life" is being used and assessed in ways that other scholars, such as economists, might not. That is, in contrast to those who might argue that quality of life can refer to and be assessed by only objective criteria, this chapter is based on the assumption that individuals' subjective reports of the quality of their lives are valid indicators of this quality (Kahneman 1999; Lawton et al. 1999; Schuessler and Fisher 1985; Schwarz and Strack 1991, 1999; Stone, Shiffman, and DeVries 1999). The commitment to "blank" indicators means that the criteria for evaluation are not specified by the researchers but are left to the respondents—in contrast to taking a theoretical stand on the criteria for well-being (e.g., Carr, chap. 16, this volume; Keyes and Shafiro, chap. 12, this volume;

Ryff and Singer 1998; Ryff 1989). Finally, the commitment to cognitive evaluations is in contrast to affective evaluations (see Mroczek, chap. 7, this volume, and Almeida and Horn, chap. 15, this volume, on the affective quality of life): Although the cognitive evaluation is often called "life satisfaction," satisfaction is not to be taken in its emotional sense. In fact, Diener and Diener (1995) demonstrated that life satisfaction is only weakly related to emotion in many cultures. At the same time, and here I diverge from the CCR model, life satisfaction is not meant as a rational or mathematical calculation. Rather, it is a "cold" judgment and consideration of the overall value, worth, and completeness of one's life (99 percent of the subjects in Andrews and Withey 1976 reported experiencing such an evaluation). Furthermore, the experience of life quality is a distinct and integral entity. The model assumes that individuals do not experience life only as a series of more or less quality moments but that they also cognize (experience) life as an integral whole, with its own identifiable quality evaluation.

Diener (1984) reviewed several measures of the cognitive component. The present one is unique but highly similar to one of the original formulations, Cantril's (1965) ladder. In MIDUS, the quality of each of the domains and of overall life was assessed with the same format. The respondents used an eleven-point scale to rate the quality of a domain in their own lives, with 0 meaning the "worst possible" and 10 the "best possible." For example, quality of health was assessed with the following item: "Using a scale from 0 to 10 where 0 means 'the worst possible health' and 10 means 'the best possible health,' how would you rate your health these days?" The item assessing overall life quality was as follows: "Using a scale from 0 to 10 where 0 means 'the worst possible life overall' and 10 means 'the best possible life overall,' how would you rate your life overall these days?" Thus, this method encourages subjects to compare their lives to possible ideals and therefore should encourage similarity of standards across individuals (furthermore, subjects, unlike those in Cantril 1965, were not encouraged to define "worst" and "best possible" in idiosyncratic ways).

In dividing life into a set of domains, what is desired is that the domains jointly cover all of the important areas and events of life yet overlap minimally with each other. MIDUS assessed seven domains of life that adequately meet these criteria: marriage (or close marriage-like relationship), health, work, relationship to children, sexuality, contribution to others, and financial situation. This set overlaps largely with the CCR set, with both studies including marriage, work, health, children, and financial situation. MIDUS does not replicate CCR's inclusion of leisure, friendship, religion, savings, education, or community domains, but it extends the CCR study by adding the potentially important domains of sexuality and contribution to others.[1] The seven domain and "life over-all" ratings were distributed throughout the interview, hopefully reducing any possible correlated error. Such single items have adequate if not ideal reliability (Diener 1984).

THE QUALITY OF SEVERAL LIFE DOMAINS IN THE UNITED STATES

At least four relevant and intriguing findings emerged from the CCR study. At the broadest level, the CCR data indicated that the typical American was highly satisfied with his or her life overall and with most domains. CCR employed a 1–7 rating scale on which respondents indicated their level of satisfaction; every domain had a mean above 4, and all but two domains had means above 5.3 (savings and amount of education were the exceptions). Second, marriage and family had the highest satisfaction means, at 6.3 and 5.9, respectively. Third, the distribution of responses was strongly skewed, with most respondents close to the high end of the scale. Fourth, all but two domains showed a steady linear increase in satisfaction with age (health satisfaction declined with age, and marriage satisfaction was relatively low until about age 50, after which it increased sharply).

Although intriguing, these findings would be made more credible if they were replicated, particularly after twenty-five years of social change. MIDUS represents a rare opportunity to conduct such a replication and thus obtain definitive answers to these questions. First, a large, nationally representative sample is required to describe the quality of life in the United States. Second, MIDUS has the ideal balance of overlap with and divergence from the CCR study. It overlaps in most of the domains, in size, sampling, and age distribution, and in having cognitive evaluations of several domains and of life overall. It diverges in that it was conducted by an independent team of researchers, has some different domains, uses a 0–10 Cantril ladder rather than a 1–7 satisfaction scale, and was conducted in a different year (1971 versus 1995). The overlap is enough to count as a conceptual replication, and the divergence is enough to rule out trivial methodological explanations for common findings.

Additionally, quality of life seems to be a phenomenon particularly vulnerable to social changes (Mallard, Lance, and Michalos 1997), and MIDUS allows consideration of how social changes in the intervening twenty-five years (e.g., the end of the cold war, unparalleled prosperity,

TABLE 1 Quality of American Life

Domain	Mean	SE	SD	Skew	CCR Mean (1–7)
Life overall	7.65	.03	1.67	−1.18	5.54
Marriage	8.10	.04	2.03	−1.58	6.27
Finances	5.97	.04	2.23	−.59	5.31[a]
Children	8.60	.03	1.64	−1.96	5.92[a]
Health	7.34	.03	1.66	−.96	5.78
Work	7.22	.04	2.38	−1.21	5.67
Sexuality	5.62	.06	3.12	−.44	
Contribution to others	6.59	.04	2.23	−.70	

Notes: CCR (Campbell, Converse, and Rodgers 1976) means are presented for comparison. SE, standard error; SD, standard deviation. *N* varies from 2114 to 3015.

[a]In CCR, these categories are "standard of living" and "family life," respectively.

the shift in values from the rebellion of the 1960s to the materialism of the 1980s) have affected levels of quality of life and their interrelationships. Many of the social changes in the intervening years seem particularly relevant to the quality of specific life domains, such as the increased divorce rate, advances in medical care, improvement and spread of civil rights, increased entry of women into the workforce, and the transfer of social responsibility from governmental and corporate institutions to individuals. This replication allows discovery of how these changes have impacted life quality or, conversely, of which findings appear to be unaffected by cultural changes; any replicated findings across such divergent periods will have demonstrated a measure of resistance to historical and cultural influences. Other similar projects have been conducted in the intervening years (e.g., Andrews 1991; Davis 1988; Diener and Diener 1995); however, few have had the size, sampling, and age distribution of MIDUS. These features provide an unusual opportunity to describe the quality of American life at the close of the twentieth century.

The data are from the primary respondent sample of MIDUS, with *N* = 3032. *N*'s vary across analyses because respondents did not rate the quality of a domain not relevant to them (e.g., unmarried respondents did not rate the quality of their marriage). As shown in table 1, the first message from MIDUS is that Americans lead high-quality lives, both at the domain level and overall. The means for all domains are closer to the "best possible" than to the "worst possible," and five of the eight means are higher than 7. Three domains are of only moderate quality for the typical American: financial situation, contribution to others, and sexuality. These findings are remarkably similar to those reported in CCR, regarding both the overall averages and the relative ordering of the domains. However, the two domains MIDI added extended the range of qualities, because sexuality and contribution to others were two of the lowest-quality domains of life. In sum, it seems that the many social changes have had a very small impact on the aggregate quality of these domains or of overall life.

There was only a moderate amount of variability across Americans in the ratings of most of these domains. Table 1 also presents standard errors of the means, standard deviations, and skews for the quality ratings. The standard errors highlight a strength of MIDUS: its large size means that its estimates are highly precise and accurate, such that any means about 3 or more standard errors apart are significantly different at the $p < .001$ level. The standard deviations show (because roughly two-thirds of the sample are within one standard deviation of the corresponding mean) that not only the typical but also the vast majority of Americans report high quality in most domains of life and of life overall. The negative skews for all of the domains only strengthen this conclusion, meaning that Americans are bunched up near the top of the scales. The greatest differences between Americans are in the quality of finances, work, contribution to others, and sexuality. Financial and work-quality variability correspond to the growing economic disparity in this country: Although the mean level is reasonably high, fewer people are close to that mean level, and many people report either the highest-quality finances and work or the lowest-quality finances and work. The variability in ratings of quality of contribution to others shows that the burden of caring for others is not equally shared in this country, with individuals taking on either much of it or very little of it (see Fleeson 2001; Rossi, chap. 19, this volume, for further elaboration).

It is important to note that the limited variability does not mean that the study suffers from a lack of individuals with very low quality. Every domain had at least some individuals who reported the worst possible quality. For example, nearly a hundred individuals rated their health at 3 or worse. Thus, there are no problems with restricted range in this study, and the findings describe those with poor quality as well as those with high quality. In fact, because of their relative infrequency, those with low qualities in a domain have the greatest impact on the regression results reported later. Thus, for example, individuals with very poor health have more impact on the beta predicting overall life quality from health quality than do those with good health.

On the whole, men and women differed very little from each other in the patterns described throughout this chapter. Where they did differ, it

William Fleeson

TABLE 2 Correlations among Domain Qualities and Age

Domain	Age	Finances	Children	Health	Work	Sexuality	Contributions to Others	Life
Marriage	.16	.30	.23	.17	.23	.47	.08	.54
Finances	.22		.15	.30	.41	.21	.18	.52
Children	.08			.16	.16	.13	.19	.35
Health	−.02[a]				.30	.22	.15	.38
Work	.10					.16	.19	.41
Sexuality	−.22						.12	.37
Contributions to others	.02[a]							.22
Life overall	.15							

Notes: All correlations are significant at the $p < .001$ level, except for the two correlations marked with a superscript a. N varies from 1860 to 3015.

was typically a matter of degree rather than of overall pattern. Such an internal replication provides further confidence in the generality of the findings. However, in the following I mention gender differences where they were found. As for the level of quality of life, there were a few small differences. Women reported significantly higher-quality contribution to others (mean or $M = 6.90$) and higher-quality relationships to their children ($M = 8.74$) then did men ($M = 6.27$, 8.44, respectively), who reported higher-quality marriages ($M = 8.36$), sexuality ($M = 5.98$), and financial situations ($M = 6.11$) than did women ($M = 7.80$, 5.26, 5.85, respectively).

Does Quality across Domains Co-occur in the Same Individuals?

A second question is how much the quality of several domains tends to cluster in the same individuals. That is, do individuals with higher quality in one domain tend also to have higher quality in other domains? Table 2 shows correlations among the domains and age (age is discussed soon). Note that the intercorrelations among domains are all positive and significant. On the one hand, the fact that all of the correlations are positive shows some tendency for success (or failure) to accumulate in individuals across domains. That is, things going well in one domain for an individual makes it somewhat more likely that things are going well in all domains for that individual. Similarly, things going poorly in one domain bodes poorly for that individual's other domains. On the other hand, the correlations generally are not very large in magnitude. Only two of the correlations are larger than .30, and more than half are smaller than .20. Thus, the tendency toward accumulation is weak. Rather, most individuals have greater-than-average quality in a few domains combined with lower-than-average quality in other domains.

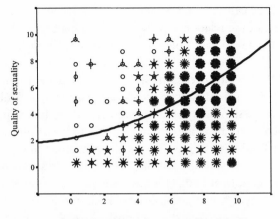

Quality of marriage or close marriage-like relationship

FIGURE 1. Relationship between quality of sexuality and quality of marriage. Because of the large number of individuals at each coordinate, each individual is represented by a circle or a spoke from the circle (thus, denser points represent more individuals). This figure shows first that quality of sexuality is highly related to quality of marriage. Second, it shows that below a marriage quality of about 4, sexuality quality is nearly uniformly poor; above 4, improvements in marriage quality are associated with increasingly larger improvements in quality of sexuality.

The pattern of correlations is consistent with the possibility that how things are going in some domains affects how things are going in other related domains. Although there isn't space in this chapter to examine each of the correlations, several stand out for particular attention. For example, the quality of work likely affects the quality of one's financial situation, and the correlation between the quality of the two domains is .41. Similarly, health likely facilitates productivity, thereby facilitating work situation quality, $r = .30$. The largest correlation, that between marriage and sexual quality, is particularly interesting. These two domains likely facilitate each other, but the data show that this facilitation is not symmetrical. Figure 1 shows the scatter plot of responses to the two items, with each circle and each spoke representing one person. The scatter plot vividly depicts the strong relationship between the two responses, as well as its curvilinear nature. When marriage quality is lower than about 4, quality of sexuality is nearly uniformly low. When a minimal level of quality in marriage (around 4) is reached, slight increases in marriage quality are associated with large and increasingly larger improvements in quality of sexuality. Thus, sexuality quality is intimately tied to quality in the rest of the relationship. Nonetheless, a substantial portion of Americans are able to have a high quality marriage despite lower quality sexuality.

Some of the lowest correlations are with the domain of contributions to others. High-quality financial situations, marriages, and jobs do not appear to increase the quality of contribution to others. It also appears that very little benefit to the quality of any domain of life results from high-quality contribution to others. Finally, the remaining low but positive correlations suggest that none of the domains appears to conflict with another. For example, although the low positive correlation of the quality of work to the quality of relationship to children suggests little positive effect of high-quality work on the relationship to children, it also suggests that there is little or no detrimental effect either.

The Quality of American Life at Different Adult Ages

Two important foci in MIDMAC are midlife and success. This section unpacks the means of quality across the adult age span to see how quality differs across age, and in particular what the quality of life is in the middle years. Quality is likely to be affected by age, as individuals learn better skills of life management (e.g., Freund and Baltes 1998; Lachman and Bertrand 2001; Staudinger 1999), as many domains have time to play themselves out (e.g., marriage and career are just getting started in early adulthood), as successes and failures accumulate, and as environmental conditions change (Diener and Suh 1998). Although MIDUS data are cross-sectional, and thus confound age with birth cohort, the ability to compare our findings with the CCR findings should allow us to determine which findings are more likely due to age and which to cohort.

Earlier, table 2 presented bivariate correlations of age with overall life quality and domain quality. Although such findings are interesting and useful, they describe only linear relationships. It is likely that age relates in a curvilinear way to quality, however, and an additional strength of MIDUS is that it has the power to detect any existing curvilinear relationship. Each domain was predicted from age, age squared, and age cubed, and the highest-order power that was significant is depicted in figure 2. Figure 2 has been split into two panels for ease of reading; on the top are five domains that show a similar positive age-related pattern, and on the bottom are three domains that differ substantially from this pattern. The five domains of children, marriage, work, financial situation, and life overall all show a general increase across age groups; where these

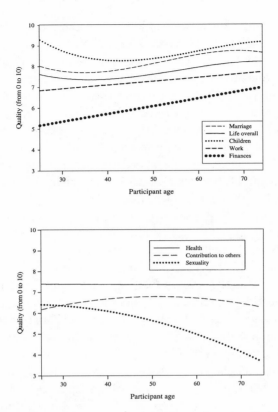

FɪɢᴜRE 2. Age-related trajectories of the seven domains and overall life quality.

domains differ is primarily in where the upward association starts. Quality of marriage, life overall, and relationship to children do not begin to improve until the age group of the late thirties or early forties, whereas quality of finances and work have a steady association with age, beginning with those in the early adult years. These domains are consistent with the notion that midlife represents the beginning or continuation of increasingly higher quality of life.

The bottom panel of figure 2 shows three domains that diverge from the basic positive pattern. Contribution to others peaks in the midlife group, as is expected from developmental theories of generativity (Erikson 1963; Fleeson 2001; see also Rossi, chap. 19, this volume, and Rossi 2001, for further elaboration of the relationship between age and contribution to others). Health surprisingly showed no relationship to age. However, it is one of only two domains that do not increase in quality across age groups. Furthermore, Cleary, Zaborski, and Ayanian (chap. 2, this volume) report an age-related decrease in self-reported health using a different item, from the telephone part of the survey. Finally, sexuality is the only domain to decrease substantially in quality across age groups.

Interactions of these age differences with gender were also tested at all powers of age (linear, quadratic, cubic), and three were found to be significant at the $p < .01$ level. First, quality of sexuality had a steeper negative association with age for women than for men. Second, women showed a more linear positive association between age and quality of marriage than did men. Finally, social responsibility showed a midlife peak for women but not for men (Fleeson 2001).

This very positive picture of aging in the United States is consistent with the findings of the CCR study. CCR also found substantial age-related increases in quality of marriage, work, family, and overall life. The only domain to decrease in their findings was health, which remained flat in our data (CCR did not assess the quality of sexuality). The two studies together provide a special opportunity to argue that these findings are the result of age rather than cohort. The fact that both samples, despite different cohorts, showed a general increase in quality across age groups suggests that age may be the factor ultimately responsible for the increase.

Given that this phenomenon of general increase may be an aging phenomenon (that is, the average individual can expect the quality of his or her life to increase as he or she grows older), the next question is why age improves quality. Some models of aging argue that older adults engage in strategic social comparison or downward adjustment of standards to enhance apparent quality (e.g., Brandtstadter, Wentura, and Rothermund 1999; Heckhausen 2001). Other models suggest that older adults get better at life management skills, accumulate success over years, or progressively improve their person–environment fit (e.g., Carstensen et al. 2000; Freund and Baltes 1998). This finding needs additional research.

WHICH DOMAINS ARE MOST IMPORTANT FOR A LIFE OF GOOD QUALITY?

The second half of this chapter addresses the issue of relative importance of the domains in predicting overall life quality. To be clear, "importance" is not meant in the sense of individuals placing importance on or valuing domains. "Importance" here is meant in the sense of influence and describes only what turns out to be a strong predictor of life quality. Perhaps it indicates what individuals ought to hold in importance, but it does not indicate what they in fact hold in importance.

Two disadvantages to this approach to importance are that (1) it does not obtain individual differences in importance but rather produces one level of importance for the entire sample, and (2) it does not describe any individuals' subjective levels of importance. In chapter 10 of this volume, Markus, Ryff, Curhan, and Palmersheim describe the rich and sophisticated beliefs about importance that individuals hold, and Cantor and Fleeson (1994) have looked at subjective importance in a motivational context. In contrast, an advantage to the approach of this chapter is that importance becomes an indirect and empirical matter; that is, the approach reveals importance to us as an aid in our own decision making about life choices rather than forcing us to rely on possibly ill-advised suppositions.

What makes an individual judge his or her life as high quality or makes him or her experience it as complete? Although much of this judgment derives from internal factors such as life tasks, traits such as extraversion and neuroticism, and coping strategies (e.g., Diener and Lucas 1999; Cantor et al. 1991; Scheier, Carver, and Bridges 2001; Fleeson, Malanos, and Achille 2002), it also likely comes from things going well in the various domains of life (e.g., in marriage, work, and so forth). For example, if a person's marriage is going well, he or she is likely to experience life overall as complete, whereas if a person's marriage is going poorly, life may seem to be missing something.

I continue to follow the CCR model in proposing that all such domains of life have an impact on life quality but that the degree of impact differs across domains. That is, some domains make more difference to life quality than do others. A domain that makes a difference is one in which life quality is greatly impacted by how things are going in that domain. If things go well in that domain, then life is experienced as high quality; if things go poorly in such a domain, then life is experienced as of poor quality, incomplete, and not satisfying. Domains that make less of a difference do not influence overall life quality as strongly: even when things go very wrong in such domains, individuals can maintain a high level of overall life quality (e.g., perhaps individuals can easily experience high-quality life even with an unsuccessful career), and things going well may not provide the individual with very much of a boost in overall quality.

Determining which domains of life are most important for achieving and maintaining a high-quality life is important for at least two reasons. First is the enduring theoretical issue of what makes a human's life complete or fully functioning (Ryan and Deci 2001; Ryff 1989). Second is the more pragmatic issue of investment of limited resources (e.g., time, effort, status). Few individuals have the resources to guarantee that all domains of life operate smoothly but rather must selectively invest in some domains in lieu of others. The best domains in which to invest resources may be those that have the greatest impact on overall life quality. If an individual has a choice between two life domains in which to invest limited resources, he or she might wisely invest in the one that has the biggest impact on overall life quality while allowing the domain that has less impact to subside. This issue of investment of limited resources applies not only to individuals but also to research priorities (we should expend research resources on domains that are important in affecting overall life quality) and at the societal level (society should invest its resources in domains that matter to its members' life quality). Thus, knowing the relative importance of various domains in terms of their impact on life quality is important.

One way to determine the importance of a domain to life quality is to start with a large enough sample so that it contains individuals who have done very well and those who have not done well at all in each of the domains. Then, for each domain, one can compare such individuals on their overall life quality. If those who did well in the domain have much greater overall life quality than those who did poorly in the domain, then this domain possibly has a big impact and is therefore very important to life quality. On the other hand, if those who did very poorly in the domain do not differ much in overall life quality from those who did well in the domain, then this domain is not likely important to overall life quality.

Rather than compare only those who have done very well in a domain against those who have done very poorly, MIDUS allows the more fine-tuned linear comparison. Specifically, the unstandardized betas from a regression predicting overall life quality from the domain qualities describe the amount of change in life quality for each point change in the quality of each domain. However, a large beta does not guarantee that the domain has a large impact on life quality, because the direction of causality is undetermined by these cross-sectional data. As Diener (1984) first noted when he contrasted bottom-up models of quality, in which quality in the domains causes overall life quality, with top-down models, in which overall life quality affects the quality in the various domains, this is an important issue. Tests of the causal direction are very difficult because large samples with at least two waves are required to adequately test the competing models. Evidence to date has been mixed, primarily because of moderate sample sizes, and has found that the causal direction may differ across domains and that family or marriage domains are

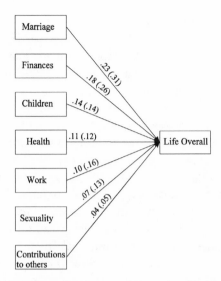

FIGURE 3. Importance of domain qualities in predicting overall life quality. Coefficients are unstandardized betas from a multiple regression predicting overall life quality from the qualities of all seven domains simultaneously. All betas are significant at the $p < .001$ level (contribution to others was significant at the $p < .01$ level) and can be interpreted as the importance of that domain to overall life quality. Standardized betas are in parentheses (and can be squared to obtain unique percentages of variance accounted for in overall life quality).

those likely to have the strongest bottom-up effects (Brief et al. 1993; Headey, Veenhoven, and Wearing 1991; Lance, Mallard, and Michalos 1995; Scherpenzeel and Saris 1996). The analyses in the current chapter assumed at least some bottom-up effects.

Figure 3 shows the results of a simultaneous multiple regression predicting overall life quality from the quality of each of the seven life domains. Each beta represents the importance of the respective domain, while qualities of the other domains are held constant; it can be interpreted as showing how many points in overall life quality are associated with a one-point change in the domain quality. Standardized betas are in parentheses; they can be squared to obtain the percentage of variance accounted for uniquely by the domain. An advantage to obtaining independent (semipartial) betas from a simultaneous multiple regression is that the associations are not the result of quality in any other domain (e.g., the predictive power of high-quality financial situation is not the result of any related advantages in work situation). Another advantage is that factors such as response bias are largely partialed out, because their effects are held constant when holding all other domains constant. Together the domains accounted for 51 percent of the variance in overall quality of life, implying that they are a reasonably comprehensive set of domains and that the quality of life and the quality of the individual domains are closely tied to each other.

The domains are listed in order of importance. At the top of the list is marriage or marriage-like close relationship. These results argue that marriage is the most important domain for a high-quality life. More than any other domain, it is difficult and rare to have a high-quality life without having a high-quality close relationship. Financial situation is close behind, and the two domains are far ahead of the remainder in degree of importance. The results for financial situation are surprising in light of the contrary findings for income level. Diener et al. (1993) showed that income (actual dollars) is highly predictive of life quality at only very low levels of income; above the threshold, additional income makes very little difference. The current findings show that the subjective evaluation of that income continues to be predictive of life quality even at high levels.

Health was much lower in importance than might be anticipated. It is fourth on the list, and the beta shows that dropping from the best to the worst health possible (while holding other domains constant) is associated with only a little more than a point change in overall life quality on average. That is, many individuals manage to lead more satisfying lives than most others despite having very poor health. Sexuality is of even less importance to overall life quality, and the least important domain in the United States (as a predictor of life quality) is contribution to others. Additionally, gender did not interact with any domain in predicting overall life quality at the $p < .01$ level.

This general pattern is again closely in accord with findings reported by CCR. Specifically, in 1971, as in the present data, financial and family matters were most important, health was not very important, and work was somewhere in between in importance to overall life quality. There are two important exceptions to this similarity: (1) in MIDUS, health was found to be second in importance to life quality but only when unpartialed and unstandardized, meaning that if health quality has a large impact on overall life quality, it works its impact through the quality of the other domains; and (2) family was divided into two aspects in MIDUS, and only the relationship-to-spouse aspect was found to be strongly predictive of life quality, whereas family as a whole was strongly

266

predictive in CCR. This strong similarity of results has two implications. First, cultural changes in the United States in the last twenty-five years have had little net impact on the quality of life in the United States and on which domains are important to a quality life. Second, the similarity of results reinforces the credibility of both studies' findings, specifically that love and money are the most important domains of life.

It is also worth comparing these findings to individuals' direct evaluations of domains as important or not. CCR had also asked respondents to rate how important each domain was to them individually. The highest average rating of importance was received by health, followed by marriage and family life. Job was in the middle, but financial situation was rated as very low in importance. Thus, what individuals hold to be important does not necessarily agree with what has a sample-wide large association to life quality. In particular, health is held to be important and does not appear to be powerfully predictive of life quality, whereas financial situation is generally not held to be important yet has a strong relationship to life quality. These disagreements underscore the need for consideration of both types of importance.

Note that individuals who did not complete all of the quality ratings because they did not have children or were not in a close relationship were not included in the above analysis. To investigate the importance of domains for these individuals, additional regressions were calculated. First, the regression was repeated but included only single individuals without children ($N = 274$). Only five domains were included as predictors, because it is not possible to assess the importance of the quality of marriage and of relationships to children in the lives of those who are single and have no children. Of the remaining five domains, health ($b = .25$) and work ($b = .22$) became of primary importance, and finances dropped in importance ($b = .12$). The regression was then repeated for only those individuals who were unmarried yet nonetheless had children ($N = 512$), using six domains as predictors. After I removed the domain of marriage, relationship to children ($b = .26$) emerged as tied with finances for most important ($b = .26$), and the other domains held their relative positions. That is, relationships to children appear to become of primary importance among those who have children but are not in a close, marriage-like relationship. It is also worth noting that married individuals reported significantly higher life quality ($M = 7.85$) than did single individuals ($M = 7.21$), $p < .001$, and that those with children reported significantly higher life quality ($M = 7.72$) than did those without children ($M = 7.36$), $p < .001$.

267

These findings described unique predictions of life quality. However, because a given domain's effects on life quality may include facilitation of other domains, which in turn affect life quality, table 2 earlier included the bivariate correlations of each domain to overall life quality. These correlations are naturally larger, but the basic pattern of associations is essentially identical.

Does Domain Importance Vary with Age?

Just as the levels of domain qualities are expected to depend on participant age, the importance levels of domains are also expected to depend on participant age. To test this possibility, I conducted regressions in which overall life quality was predicted from age, a given domain's quality, and the multiplicative product of age and the domain's quality. In addition, interactions between a domain and age-squared were tested. One domain showed a linear interaction with age, and three showed a quadratic interaction with age. The quality of sexuality became decreasingly predictive of overall life quality across participant ages, somewhat diminishing the impact of the age-related decline in the quality of sexuality. Work, finances, and contribution to others all showed quadratic interactions with age. In each case, the domain's importance was strongest in the midlife group and somewhat less strong in other age groups. Men and women did not differ in these interactions.

Perhaps what is most noticeable is the domain that did not interact with age: quality of health. Health was no more and no less important to the overall quality of life for older participants. That is, the impact of physical health on life quality appears relatively small, regardless of adult age.

IMPLICATIONS AND CONCLUSION

These findings present a broad descriptive overview of the quality of life in the United States. This big picture is useful for locating more focused and analytic explanatory studies, and in particular as a guide for hypothesis generation.

The first contribution of this chapter is a relatively definitive description of the quality of American life and of the predictive powers of the various life domains. That is, the consistency of the findings with the CCR findings from twenty-five years previous, despite different methodologies, different wording of the quality ratings, and most importantly, despite the intervening cultural and historical changes, provides great confidence in these findings. The findings that American life is of high quality and that marriage and finances are the most important predictors of that high quality appear to be relatively insensitive to the kinds of cultural and historical changes that have happened in the United States, nor do they depend on any specific methodological decisions or team of researchers. However, even though a bottom-up model was assumed in this chapter, the fact is that the causal direction of this relationship is still to be determined. It is critical to have a large-scale, national sample collect at least two waves of domain and life qualities on the same subjects, to allow the cross-lagged analyses needed to conclusively resolve this issue.

A second contribution is that marriage and financial situations were revealed as the two domains most closely linked to overall quality of life. Because CCR showed in contrast that individuals hold health to be highly important and finances to be unimportant, both sets of results point to the difference between importance as a matter of personal judgment and importance as a matter of predictive influence. Future research should address why these two domains of marriage and finances are of central importance and the implications of their importance in reshaping life priorities. It is possible that these domains foster either realization of one's true potential (Ryff and Keyes 1995; Ryff and Singer 1998) or the self-determination elements of autonomy, competence, and relatedness (Ryan and Deci 2001; see also Marks, Bumpass, and Jun, chap. 18, this volume, and Lachman and Firth, chap. 11, this volume), although it may be hard to reconcile financial concerns with self-determination and realization (Kasser and Ryan 1993). It might also be useful to include the friendship domain in future research, so that individuals who are not married have a stronger representation of their social life. Given the importance of marriage in this study, it may turn out that friendships are also highly important for those who are not married.

The third theoretical implication involves theories of adult development and aging. These data confirm that aging, at least up until the midseventies, appears to be a positive phenomenon. What needs to be explained is not how older adults manage to cope with the negativity of aging but rather how older adults are managing to get more quality out of life than are younger adults. Midlife, the focus of MIDMAC (1999), appeared to be the beginning of this upward trend with aging; future research may fruitfully address why this is so.

Acknowledgments

The author thanks colleagues in MIDMAC and those involved in producing this volume, and especially Paul B. Baltes and Ursula M. Staudinger, for helpful discussions of this material.

NOTE

1. The specific wordings of the domains were as follows: marriage, "marriage or close relationship"; finances, "financial situation"; children, "overall relationship with your children"; health, "health"; work, "work situation, whether part-time or full-time, paid or unpaid, at home or at a job"; sexuality, "the sexual aspect of your life"; contribution, "contribution to the welfare and well-being of other people. . . . Take into account all that you do, in terms of time, money or concern, on your job, and for your family, friends, and the community" (this item is significantly predicted by indicators of what people actually do; see Rossi 2001, and Rossi, chap. 19, this volume, for more details); and life, "life overall."

REFERENCES

Andrews, F. M. 1991. Stability and change in levels and structure of subjective well-being: USA 1972 and 1988. *Social Indicators Research* 25:1–30.

Andrews, F. M., and S. B. Withey. 1976. *Social indicators of well-being: America's perception of life quality.* New York: Plenum Press.

Brandtstadter, J., D. Wentura, and K. Rothermund. 1999. Intentional self-development through adulthood and later life: Tenacious pursuit and flexible adjustment of goals. In *Action and self-development: Theory and research through the life span,* ed. J. Brandtstadter and R. M. Lerner, 373–400. Thousand Oaks, Calif.: Sage.

Brief, A. P., A. H. Butcher, J. M. George, and K. E. Link. 1993. Integrating bottom-up and top-down theories of subjective well-being: The case of health. *Journal of Personality and Social Psychology* 64:646–53.

Campbell, A., P. E. Converse, and W. L. Rodgers. 1976. *The quality of American life: Perceptions, evaluations, and satisfactions.* New York: Sage.

Cantor, N., and W. Fleeson. 1994. Social intelligence and intelligent goal pursuit: A cognitive slice of motivation. In *Nebraska symposium on motivation,* vol. 41. *Integrative views of motivation, cognition, and emotion,* ed. W. D. Spaulding, 125–79. R. Dienstbier, series ed. Lincoln: University of Nebraska Press.

Cantor, N., J. Norem, C. Langston, S. Zirkel, W. Fleeson, and C. Cook-Flannagan. 1991. Life tasks and daily life experience. *Journal of Personality* 59:425–51.

Cantril, H. 1965. *The patterns of human concerns.* New Brunswick, N.J.: Rutgers University Press.

Carstensen, L. L., M. Pasupathi, U. Mayr, and J. R. Nesselroade. 2000. Emotional experience in everyday life across the adult life span. *Journal of Personality and Social Psychology* 79:644–55.

Davis, J. A. 1988. *General social surveys 1972–1988: Cumulative codebook.* Chicago: National Opinion Research Center.

Diener, E. 1984. Subjective well-being. *Psychological Bulletin* 95:542–75.

———. 1994. Assessing subjective well-being: Progress and opportunities. *Social Indicators Research* 31:103–57.

Diener, E., and M. Diener. 1995. Cross-cultural correlates of life satisfaction and self-esteem. *Journal of Personality and Social Psychology* 68:653–63.

Diener, E., and R. E. Lucas. 1999. Personality and subjective well-being. In *Handbook of midlife development,* ed. M. E. Lachman, 213–29. New York: John Wiley.

Diener, E., E. Sandvik, L. Seidlitz, and M. Diener. 1993. The relationship between income and subjective well-being: Relative or absolute? *Social Indicators Research* 28:195–223.

Diener, E., J. J. Sapyta, and E. Suh. 1998. Subjective well-being is essential to well-being. *Psychological Inquiry* 9:33–37.

Diener, E., and E. Suh. 1998. Subjective well-being and age: An international analysis. *Annual Review of Gerontology and Geriatrics* 17:304–24.

Erikson, E. 1963. *Childhood and society.* New York: W. W. Norton.

Fleeson, W. 2001. Judgments of one's own global contribution to the welfare of others: Life-course trajectories and predictors. In *Caring and doing for others: Social responsibility in the domains of family, work, and community,* ed. A. S. Rossi, 75–96. Chicago: University of Chicago Press.

Fleeson, W., A. B. Malanos, and N. M. Achille. 2002. An intra-individual process approach to the relationship between extraversion and positive affect: Is acting extraverted as "good" as being extraverted? *Journal of Personality and Social Psychology* 83:1409–22.

Freund, A. M., and P. B. Baltes. 1998. Selection, optimization, and compensation as strategies of life management: Correlations with subjective indicators of successful aging. *Psychology and Aging* 13:531–43.

Headey, B., R. Veenhoven, and A. Wearing. 1991. Top-down versus bottom-up theories of subjective well-being. *Social Indicators Research* 24:81–100.

Heckhausen, J. 2001. Adaptation and resilience in midlife. In *Handbook of midlife development,* ed. M. E. Lachman, 345–91. New York: John Wiley.

Kahneman, D. 1999. Objective happiness. In *Well-being: The foundations of hedonic psychology,* ed. D. Kahneman, E. Diener, and N. Schwarz, 3–25. New York: Russell Sage Foundation.

Kasser, T., and R. M. Ryan. 1993. A dark side of the American dream: Correlates of financial success as a central life aspiration. *Journal of Personality and Social Psychology* 65:410–22.

Lachman, M. E., and R. M. Bertrand. 2001. Personality and the self in midlife. In *Handbook of midlife development,* ed. M. E. Lachman, 279–309. New York: John Wiley.

Lance, C. E., A. G. Mallard, and A. C. Michalos. 1995. Tests of the causal directions of global-life facet satisfaction relationships. *Social Indicators Research* 34:69–92.

Lawton, M. P., L. Winter, M. H. Kleban, and K. Ruckdeschel. 1999. Affect and quality of life: Objective and subjective. *Journal of Aging and Health* 11:169–98.

Mallard, A. G. C., C. E. Lance, and A. C. Michalos. 1997. Culture as a moderator of overall life satisfaction: Life facet satisfaction relationships. *Social Indicators Research* 40:259–84.

Maslow, A. H. 1954. *Motivation and personality.* New York: Harper.

MIDMAC (John D. and Catherine T. MacArthur Foundation Research Network on Successful Midlife Development). 1999. *Annual report* (1998). Vero Beach, Fla.: Life Trends.

Rossi, A. S. 2001. *Caring and doing for others: Social responsibility in the domains of family, work, and community.* Chicago: University of Chicago Press.

Ryan, R. M., and E. L. Deci. 2001. On happiness and human potentials: A review of research on hedonic and eudaimonic well-being. *Annual Review of Psychology* 52:141–66.

Ryff, C. D. 1989. Happiness is everything, or is it? Explorations on the meaning of psychological well-being. *Journal of Personality and Social Psychology* 57:1069–81.

Ryff, C. D., and C. L. M. Keyes. 1995. The structure of psychological well-being revisited. *Journal of Personality and Social Psychology* 69:719–27.

Ryff, C. D., and B. Singer. 1998. The contours of positive human health. *Psychological Inquiry* 9:1–28.

Scheier, M. F., C. S. Carver, and M. W. Bridges. 2001. Optimism, pessimism, and psychological well-being. In *Optimism and pessimism: Implications for theory, research, and practice,* ed. E. C. Chang, 189–216. Washington, D.C.: American Psychological Association.

Scherpenzeel, A., and W. Saris. 1996. Causal direction in a model of life satisfaction: The top-down/bottom-up controversy. *Social Indicators Research* 38:275–301.

Schuessler, K. F., and G. A. Fisher. 1985. Quality of life research and sociology. In *Annual review of sociology,* ed. R. H. Turner and J. F. Short, Jr., 11:129–49. Palo Alto, Calif.: Annual Reviews.

Schwarz, N., and F. Strack. 1991. Evaluating one's life: A judgment model of subjective well-being. In *Subjective well-being: An interdisciplinary perspective,* ed. F. Strack, M. Argyle, and N. Schwarz. Oxford: Pergamon Press.

———. 1999. Reports of subjective well-being: Judgmental processes and their methodological implications. In *Well-being: The foundations of hedonic psychology,* ed. D. Kahneman, E. Diener, and N. Schwarz, 61–84. New York: Russell Sage Foundation.

Smith, J., W. Fleeson, B. Geiselmann, R. Settersten, and U. Kunzmann. 1999. Well-being in very old age: Predictions from objective life conditions and subjective experience. In *The Berlin Aging Study: Aging from 70 to 100,* ed. P. B. Baltes and K. U. Mayer, 450–71. New York: Cambridge University Press.

Staudinger, U. M. 1999. Social cognition and a psychological approach to the art of life. In *Social cognition and aging,* ed. T. M. Hess and F. Blanchard-Fields, 343–75. San Diego: Academic Press.

Staudinger, U. M., W. Fleeson, and P. B. Baltes. 1999. Predictors of subjective physical health and global well-being: Similarities and differences between the United States and Germany. *Journal of Personality and Social Psychology* 76:305–19.

Stone, A. A., S. S. Shiffman, and M. W. DeVries. 1999. Ecological momentary assessment. In *Well-being: The foundations of hedonic psychology,* ed. D. Kahneman, E. Diener, and N. Schwarz, 26–39. New York: Russell Sage Foundation.

CHAPTER TEN

In Their Own Words: Well-Being at Midlife among High School-Educated and College-Educated Adults

Hazel Rose Markus, Carol D. Ryff, Katherine B. Curhan,

and Karen A. Palmersheim

What does it mean to experience well-being at midlife in contemporary America? According to current media accounts, well-being requires being healthy, staying active, looking young, having money, and enjoying oneself. Do these popular claims have it right? Are these the open secrets to well-being? Is the path to life satisfaction and the life well lived the same for everyone, or are there a variety of ways to be well? And does the experience of well-being vary systematically by sociocultural factors such as education or gender?

In this chapter we explore the meanings and sources of well-being with a subsample of respondents from MIDUS, all of whom reported that they were reasonably happy and satisfied with their lives. On the whole, respondents in the MIDUS survey participate in much of the same media and consumer culture and live lives shaped by common legal and political systems. Thus, one would expect to find similarities in how these individuals define and experience the "good life." Although our research indeed revealed several areas of common ground, we were repeatedly struck not by the homogeneity of their lives but by the differences in the worlds we observed. Some of the most striking differences in living environments, daily routines, and typical social interactions among respondents are those associated with educational level.

Relative to the worlds of the college-educated, the worlds of the MIDUS high school–educated respondents are characterized by fewer financial resources, family members with less advanced educations, higher rates of divorce, and earlier death of parents. These respondents also report that they have more health problems, exercise less, and are three times more likely to smoke cigarettes.[1] In contrast, the worlds of the college-educated MIDUS respondents typically include family members with more advanced education, longer lives, lower rates of divorce, and almost twice the total household income than high school–educated respondents. Furthermore, the college-educated report decidedly fewer health problems, lower rates of smoking, and greater levels of participation in physical exercise. In spite of these apparent contrasts in the lives of the college-educated and the high school–educated MIDUS respondents, both groups report being reasonably well satisfied and happy with their lives. How can people faced with a different set of life circumstances and engaged in comparatively diverse everyday routines claim to experience similar levels of well-being?

We hypothesize that although Americans at midlife are likely to agree on much of what it means to have a good life, the uniqueness of their worlds (indexed here by level of education) affords and requires somewhat different ways of being a person and is associated with different ways of "being" well or experiencing well-being.[2] We suggest that well-being is intimately tied to what people are doing in their lives, that is, to their understandings of their everyday lived experience, including how they make sense of themselves, their actions, and their places in the world—and that their perception of the world is, in part, systematically determined by the opportunities and constraints associated with their level of education.

A Sociocultural Analysis

The gauge of individual well-being entails more than just a summary of previous actions and experiences. It involves an awareness of what is good, what is self, what is moral, and a sense of how one is doing with respect to these dynamic local norms. These standards are often quite diverse and specific to particular communities and periods of time. Images, ideals, and norms of the "proper" way to be, the "right" way to feel, and the "appropriate" way to think are derived primarily from the various sociocultural worlds (delineated by shared meanings and patterns of relationships among families, friends, churches, workplaces, neighborhoods, and regions of the country) in which people engage (Markus, Mullally, and Kitayama 1997; Oyserman and Markus 1993; Shweder 1990). Well-being then reflects and requires the sense that one fits in, belongs, or is a member in good standing in some set of communities, and an analysis of well-being may require some assessment of these contexts.

A representative sample of Americans like those in MIDUS can be expected to hold some understandings of the good life in common (see Markus, Plaut, and Lachman, chap. 21, this volume). We expect those understandings to derive from their engagement in institutions such as the national media and a common legal and political culture. In particular, we hypothesized that for nearly all Americans, the definition of a good life would include some concern with commitment to others and opportunity for self-expression (Bellah et al. 1985; Hewitt 1989; Rossi 2001).

The high school–educated and the college-educated may, however, be expected to diverge in their ideas of well-being because of their participation in *local* worlds in which family, health, employment, and community experiences and expectations are likely to vary. On the basis of studies that have begun to link education with well-being, and education with self-definition (Heise 1990; Herzog et al. 1998; House et al. 1994; Marmot et al. 1997, 1991; Ryff et al. 1999; Ryff and Singer 1998), we hypothesized that well-being for the college-educated would involve elements of personal accomplishment and self-fulfillment. We also anticipated that the different lives and worlds of the high school–educated respondents would be associated with somewhat different ways of being well, ways that focused more on supportive relationships with close others such as family members. We also hypothesized that the two groups would typically approach the world in different ways given their various opportunities and constraints. In other words, they would have different conceptions of how to act in the world, divergent models of agency.

Educational variation in ways of well-being and agency may help explain a set of seemingly contradictory findings that emerge from the MIDUS data. On the one hand, using scales of positive psychological functioning (Ryff and Keyes 1995) that measure six specific components of well-being (environmental mastery, self-acceptance, positive relations with others, autonomy, purpose, and personal growth), we find that the college-educated MIDUS respondents score higher on nearly every component of well-being than do the high school–educated respondents, and that they seem to have higher levels of well-being. On the other hand, when we examine those MIDUS questions that asked for general assessments of well-being—questions that required ratings of positive affect, negative affect, and satisfaction with work, children, sex life, and life overall—we find that the average scores of the high school–educated and the college-educated respondents are high and do not differ significantly from one another. What might explain these different survey data patterns? One important aim of this chapter is to suggest an explanation for this apparent inconsistency.

The Everyday Well-Being Study

This chapter draws on data collected in the Everyday Well-Being Study (EDWB), which gave a subset of MIDUS respondents an opportunity to reflect on what well-being meant to them and to describe their experiences and understandings of well-being in their own words in a relatively unconstrained format. We asked respondents open-ended questions about

275

their positive experiences and about their ideas of well-being. The respondents' own words were analyzed in two ways. First, we analyzed the content, or explicit meaning, of *what* they said in answers to questions about well-being—for instance, whether they were talking about such topics as children, physical health, faith, or a positive attitude. Second, we analyzed their open-ended narrative responses for *how* they described their own actions and experiences—for instance, whether they described their actions as occurring in reaction to some external event or as a planned manipulation of the external environment. Building on concepts in the control and coping literature (Gurin and Brim 1984; Lachman and Weaver 1998), we developed a code for the type of agency evident in their descriptions of themselves and their lives. We determined, for each sentence in their narratives, whether the respondents described themselves and their actions in terms of adjusting to the world or of taking charge and acting directly on the world.

Unlike most qualitative studies, the EDWB ($N = 83$) was done within the context a national survey sample, MIDUS ($N = 3032$). This study-within-a-study afforded us the unprecedented opportunity to gain substantial insight into the everyday meanings and accounts of well-being as well as to compare, frame, and extend the findings from the open-ended interview with the closed-ended findings from the MIDUS sample for individuals of the same education level, age, gender, and levels of positive psychological functioning ($N = 504$). Embedding the interview study within a large-scale survey meant we had all the background data provided by MIDUS on each respondent and could use these results to amplify the well-being narratives provided by the EDWB. We were also able to select respondents with particular levels of education and well-being, and thereby compare our sample with the larger MIDUS sample of respondents having similar demographic profiles. When we observe differences in responses among our groups of EDWB respondents, we can suggest that these differences will be characteristic of the MIDUS subsample as a whole. As a consequence, we can have greater confidence when generalizing our findings than is the case in most other in-depth interview studies.

The EDWB is also unique in its focus on positive human functioning. Many sociological studies have focused on the links between socioeconomic status (including level of education) and reduced well-being and increased psychological distress (stress, depression, anxiety, etc.) (Dohrenwend et al. 1992; Kessler 1982; Kessler and Cleary 1980; Kubzansky, Kawachi, and Sparrow 1999; Link, Lennon, and Dohrenwend 1993;

Marmot et al. 1997). We chose in this study to concentrate on people (40-
to 59-year-old men and women at each of two levels of education) who
reported that their lives were going reasonably well, as measured by scales
of positive psychological functioning (i.e., they were in the top two-thirds
of the distribution), but who were differentially situated in society because of their level of education. We gave them the opportunity to share
their own ideas about well-being and how to live a good life in America
today. We were interested first in the common American response to what
it means to have a good life, and then, how these responses may differ
by level of education and gender. Although this study focuses mainly on
educational variation in well-being, recent studies suggest that there is
considerable cross-national variation in some meanings and practices of
well-being (Diener and Suh 2000), and it is useful when theorizing about
the sources of well-being to identify those patterns of well-being that are
held by a majority of Americans, regardless of gender and education level.

METHODS

EDWB Sample

The EDWB included a subsample of 83 individuals who (1) participated in the MIDUS national survey, (2) were randomly selected within
the specified age, education level, and gender parameters discussed below,
and (3) agreed to be audio-recorded during a face-to-face interview. The
sample consists of 21 men with a bachelor's degree or further education,
22 women with a bachelor's degree or further education, 20 men with
a high school diploma (but no further education), and 20 women with
a high school diploma (but no further education). All respondents were
between the ages of 40 and 59, and were selected from among those in
the top two-thirds of psychological well-being as measured by Ryff's six
dimensions of positive psychological functioning (Ryff and Keyes 1995).
Within each education group, half of the respondents scored at a "moderate" level of positive psychological functioning and half scored at a "high"
level. The subsample includes residents from twenty-one states, representing a wide diversity of geographic regions in the continental United
States. The participation rate for our study was 86.5 percent.

Comparability of the EDWB Sample with the MIDUS Sample

Before beginning analyses of the well-being data, we established that
our qualitative subsample of 83 respondents was reasonably representative of MIDUS respondents of the same age (40–59), education level,

277

TABLE 1 Psychological Well-Being

| | Everday Well-Being Sample ($N = 83$) | | | | |
| | All ($N = 83$) | High School | | College | |
		Men ($N = 20$)	Women ($N = 20$)	Men ($N = 21$)	Women ($N = 22$)
Psychological well-being					
Self-acceptance[eE]	17.82	17.00	17.00	19.00	18.18
	(2.54)	(2.41)	(2.88)	(2.10)	(2.32)
Purpose in life[eE]	17.93	17.50	16.23	18.26	19.55
	(2.89)	(2.93)	(2.98)	(2.75)	(1.97)
Environmental mastery[eE]	17.36	16.90	16.30	18.60	17.55
	(2.40)	(2.27)	(2.43)	(1.89)	(2.50)
Positive relations with others[EG]	17.54	17.10	18.35	17.14	17.59
	(3.26)	(3.88)	(2.66)	(3.64)	(2.81)
Personal growth[gEX]	19.28	18.10	19.90	18.90	20.14
	(2.09)	(2.64)	(1.17)	(2.21)	(1.52)
Autonomy[X]	17.60	17.75	17.45	17.62	17.59
	(2.44)	(2.38)	(2.78)	(2.42)	(2.36)
Total psychological well-being[eEX]	107.52	104.35	105.23	109.52	110.59
	(9.14)	(11.52)	(8.90)	(7.09)	(7.61)

Notes: The superscripts indicate the significant difference within the EDWB sample (e = education effect, g = gender effect, x = interaction effect; $p < .05$) and the significant difference within the MIDUS comparable sample (E = education effect, G = gender effect, X = interaction effect; $p < .05$). The first number in each group is the mean; the second number, in parentheses, is the standard deviation.

gender, and psychological well-being ($N = 504$). Mentions of the MIDUS comparable sample throughout this chapter refer to this larger matched-age subsample. Tables 1–4 show mean scores and population proportions of a variety of sociodemographic factors as well as numerous indicators of physical and psychological well-being. The columns headed "All" represent mean values and percentages for the entire EDWB sample and the MIDUS comparable sample, respectively. Using analysis of variance (ANOVA) to compare group means, and chi-square tests for population proportions, we found that the EDWB qualitative subsample did not differ significantly from the MIDUS comparable sample, with the exception of one variable. The EDWB subjects were significantly more satisfied with their work situations than were those in the larger MIDUS comparable sample (see table 2).

Well-Being, Sociodemographic, and Health Profiles by Education Level and Gender for the MIDUS Comparable Sample

As shown in tables 1–4 (superscript E), there are significant education-related differences within the MIDUS comparable sample. The in EDWB and MIDUS Samples

	MIDUS Comparable Sample ($N = 504$)			
	High School		College	
All ($N = 504$)	Men ($N = 102$)	Women ($N = 132$)	Men ($N = 151$)	Women ($N = 119$)
17.98	17.57	16.98	18.68	18.54
(2.67)	(2.51)	(3.17)	(2.30)	(2.22)
18.02	17.56	17.55	18.53	18.38
(2.82)	(3.34)	(2.30)	(2.31)	(2.59)
17.20	17.15	16.66	17.66	17.27
(2.86)	(2.85)	(2.90)	(2.83)	(2.81)
17.53	16.92	17.42	17.33	18.43
(3.36)	(3.60)	(3.38)	(3.54)	(2.68)
19.25	19.01	18.58	19.38	20.04
(2.15)	(2.15)	(2.72)	(1.85)	(1.41)
17.44	17.87	17.24	17.20	17.61
(2.78)	(2.65)	(3.04)	(2.67)	(2.71)
107.42	105.98	104.43	108.78	110.26
(8.62)	(9.52)	(9.43)	(7.79)	(6.39)

college-educated MIDUS comparable respondents scored higher than did their high school–educated counterparts on every aspect of positive psychological functioning (positive relations with others, self-acceptance, personal growth, purpose, environmental mastery) except one (autonomy) (table 1). Nonetheless, high school–educated and college-educated respondents did not differ in scores on a number of MIDUS questions that probe for more general assessments of well-being (i.e., ratings of positive affect, negative affect, general life satisfaction, and satisfaction with work, children, and sex life) (table 2). We found, however, that the college-educated respondents were more satisfied with their financial situations and that those with a high school education reported higher levels of satisfaction with their marriage/close relationship.

Using the MIDUS data, we also examined a set of indicators typically assumed to gauge quality of life, including income, marital status, parental education, and physical health symptoms and behaviors. As evident from tables 3 and 4, there were striking differences between high school–educated and college-educated respondents: namely, high school–educated respondents earned less money, had spouses who earned less, were more likely to be divorced, had more children, had less-educated parents, and had poorer health (i.e., they reported worse physical health, more chronic conditions, more symptoms such as headaches and back pain, more smoking, higher waist–hip ratios, and

TABLE 2 Affect and Satisfaction in

	EDWB Sample ($N = 83$)				
		High School		College	
	All ($N = 83$)	Men ($N = 20$)	Women ($N = 20$)	Men ($N = 21$)	Women ($N = 22$)
Affect indicators					
Positive affect	21.76	22.60	21.50	21.48	21.50
	(3.66)	(3.46)	(2.93)	(3.56)	(4.56)
Negative affect[G]	7.63	7.55	8.05	7.19	7.76
	(2.02)	(2.06)	(1.51)	(1.40)	(2.81)
Satisfaction indicators					
Satisfaction with	6.93	6.65	6.65	7.14	7.24
finances[E]	(1.45)	(1.09)	(2.01)	(1.15)	(1.37)
Satisfaction with	8.30	8.00	8.78	8.10	8.36
work*	(1.71)	(2.50)	(1.56)	(1.04)	(1.36)
Satisfaction with	8.75	8.83	8.79	8.59	8.76
relationship w/children[G]	(1.45)	(1.42)	(1.87)	(1.33)	(1.22)
Satisfaction w/marriage/	8.70	9.00	8.87	8.53	8.36
close relatives[E]	(1.21)	(1.24)	(1.41)	(1.31)	(1.74)
Satisfaction with	6.30	6.80	6.05	5.90	6.43
sex life[G]	(2.82)	(2.50)	(3.26)	(2.95)	(2.66)
Satisfaction with life	8.37	8.55	8.30	8.29	8.33
	(0.94)	(0.83)	(1.30)	(0.78)	(0.80)

Notes: The superscripts indicate the significant difference within the EDWB sample (e = education effect, g = gender effect, x = interaction effect; $p < .05$) and the significant difference within the MIDUS comparable sample (E = education effect, G = gender effect, X = interaction effect; $p < .05$). The first number in each group is the mean; the second number, in parentheses, is the standard deviation.

*Significant difference between the EDWB sample and the MIDUS comparable sample ($p < .05$).

less exercise). We hypothesized that an analysis of respondents' narratives about well-being would help clarify (1) the high school–educated respondents' equally high scores on general assessments of well-being (e.g., life satisfaction, positive affect), in spite of their significantly lower quality-of-life indicators, and (2) the discrepancy between the general assessments of well-being results (i.e., the absence of education-level differences) and positive psychological-functioning results (i.e., the presence of education-level differences).

Although the primary focus of the present analysis is on differences associated with level of education, we also explored gender differences in well-being (whose significance is also designated in tables 1–4, superscript G). Analyses revealed that relative to women, men from the MIDUS comparable sample reported higher positive affect and greater satisfaction with their sex lives. They haded higher total household and

EDWB and MIDUS Samples

	MIDUS Comparable Sample ($N = 504$)			
	High School		College	
All	Men	Women	Men	Women
($N = 504$)	($N = 102$)	($N = 132$)	($N = 151$)	($N = 119$)
21.33	21.60	20.80	21.36	21.21
(3.73)	(4.12)	(4.01)	(3.19)	(3.70)
8.18	8.05	8.76	7.80	8.12
(2.56)	(2.71)	(2.91)	(2.25)	(2.30)
6.58	6.20	6.34	6.94	6.73
(1.90)	(1.77)	(2.12)	(1.62)	(2.01)
7.75	7.57	7.61	7.90	7.90
(1.85)	(1.84)	(2.21)	(1.72)	(1.56)
8.70	8.39	9.02	8.53	8.84
(1.37)	(1.75)	(1.27)	(1.27)	(1.09)
8.50	8.84	8.54	8.40	8.24
(1.72)	(1.43)	(1.75)	(1.77)	(1.85)
6.27	6.91	5.94	6.56	5.69
(2.81)	(2.51)	(3.23)	(2.51)	(2.82)
8.13	8.25	8.02	8.13	8.15
(1.26)	(1.10)	(1.52)	(1.07)	(1.29)

personal incomes, were more likely to be married, and were more likely to exercise vigorously. Men also reported having experienced greater levels of family abuse during childhood relative to women. Women from the MIDUS comparable sample scored higher than men on positive relations with others and reported greater satisfaction with relationships with their children. Their spouses earned more income and had higher levels of education. In addition, women reported higher levels of negative affect, more chronic health conditions, more daily symptoms of illness, more headaches, and more use of prescription medications and vitamins.

Finally, our analyses of the MIDUS comparable sample revealed a number of education by gender interaction effects on measures of psychological well-being (table 1, superscript X). Although men with a high school education scored higher than their female counterparts on personal growth, college-educated women scored higher than college men. A similar interaction was found in our measure of autonomy, with high school–educated men and college-educated women both scoring higher than high school–educated women and college-educated men, respectively. Furthermore, an interaction effect was noted in the positive psychological functioning scores in the same education by gender direction.

TABLE 3 Sociodemographics and Early Life

		EDWB Sample ($N = 83$)			
		High School		College	
	All ($N = 83$)	Men ($N = 20$)	Women ($N = 20$)	Men ($N = 21$)	Women ($N = 22$)
Sociodemographics					
Total household	$83,395	$79,700	$38,550	$127,429	$85,489
income, past year[egEG]	(65,403)	(69,738)	(19,490)	(74,325)	(57,596)
Personal earnings[egEG]	$39,650	$47,800	$7,025	$73,962	$29,840
	(39,956)	(45,570)	(9.264)	(35,855)	(26,489)
Spouse's earnings[egxEGX]	$33,547	$19,333	$30,933	$26,158	$67,042
	(27,501)	(17,010)	(17,026)	(19,777)	(32,946)
Married[gG]	78%	90%	75%	90%	59%
Ever divorced[E]	35%	45%	40%	19%	36%
Spouse's education[eEG]	3.00	2.47	2.27	3.42	3.85
	(0.92)	(0.72)	(0.80)	(0.69)	(0.36)
Number of children[eE]	2.36	2.50	2.95	1.76	2.27
	(1.44)	(1.54)	(1.54)	(1.34)	(1.20)
Early life and family background					
Mother's education[eE]	2.06	1.68	1.6	2.38	2.68
		(0.75)	(0.75)	(1.02)	(0.95)
Father's education[eE]	1.99	1.58	1.32	2.29	2.68
	(1.02)	(0.94)	(0.58)	(1.06)	(0.97)
Biological mother still alive[E]	67%	59%	56%	71%	79%
Biological father still alive[E]	41%	44%	17%	45%	58%
Total abuse[G]	1.69	1.98	1.64	1.62	1.64
	(0.569)	(0.57)	(0.47)	(0.45)	(0.74)

Notes: The superscripts indicate the significant difference within the EDWB sample (e = education effect, g = gender effect, x = interaction effect; $p < .05$) and the significant difference within the MIDUS comparable sample (E = education effect, G = gender effect, X = interaction effect; $p < .05$). The first number in each group is the mean; the second number, in parentheses, is the standard deviation.

Interviews and Procedures

In the course of the EDWB interviews, we explored the meaning of well-being and positive life events across several dimensions of time (e.g., past, present, future) and life domains (e.g., family, work, home, community) through thirty open-ended questions. Three experienced and trained interviewers conducted the interviews at either the respondents' home or a public location of their choice nearby. All interviews followed a strict protocol, and additional probes were used only to clarify meanings of terms, to elicit varied examples, or to bring the focus of the interview back to the question at hand.

Background in EDWB and MIDUS Samples

	MIDUS Comparable Sample ($N = 504$)				
		High School		College	
All ($N = 504$)	Men ($N = 102$)	Women ($N = 132$)	Men ($N = 151$)	Women ($N = 119$)
$72,853	$55,228	$48,707	$98,839	$81,772
(57,180)	(37,766)	(37,925)	(67,802)	(58,405)
$36,595	$32,666	$14,639	$58,682	$36,290
(33,514)	(19,226)	(13,895)	(42,252)	(29,033)
$30,001	$15,171	$33,497	$21,217	$57,412
(31,011)	(16,459)	(27,505)	(21,827)	(41,542)
72%	78%	70%	79%	59%
38%	47%	45%	27%	39%
2.93	2.32	2.44	3.28	3.64
(0.95)	(0.75)	(0.90)	(0.81)	(0.63)
2.58	2.89	2.98	2.31	2.20
(1.58)	(1.58)	(1.56)	(1.40)	(1.69)
1.96	1.64	1.54	2.21	2.35
(9.91)	(0.69)	(0.69)	(0.93)	(0.99)
1.98	1.45	1.43	2.39	2.44
(1.10)	(0.74)	(0.66)	(1.16)	(1.28)
64%	63%	66%	68%	65%
42%	34%	36%	46%	49%
1.66	1.72	1.65	1.70	1.57
(0.47)	(0.47)	(0.50)	(0.43)	(0.49)

This chapter focuses specifically on respondents' answers to the following questions: (1) "What does it mean to you to have a good life?" and the follow-up probe, "Do you have anything to add about what's important for well-being?"; (2) "What do you think are some of the reasons your life has gone well?"; and (3) "What are your hopes for the future?" These three questions were selected from the original thirty questions because they were the most general probes about well-being and made reference to the past, present, and future.

Multiple members of the research team read and re-read a subset of transcript excerpts representing four respondent subgroups (high school–educated women, high school–educated men, college-educated women, and college-educated men) to develop inductive coding schemes. After several iterations, a consensus of codes was developed, and the transcripts were downloaded to create a database in a qualitative software package (QSR NUD*IST). Researchers analyzed the data on a

TABLE 4 Physical Health and Health

| | EDWB Sample ($N = 83$) | | | | |
| | | High School | | College | |
	All ($N = 83$)	Men ($N = 20$)	Women ($N = 20$)	Men ($N = 21$)	Women ($N = 22$)
Physical health and health behavior					
Subjective physical health[eE]	3.65 (1.01)	3.35 (0.93)	3.25	3.95	4.00
Chronic conditions[egEG]	2.16 (2.26)	2.10 (1.25)	3.50 (3.33)	1.24 (1.00)	1.95 (2.21)
Total symptoms in the past 30 days[egEG]	7.58 (6.92)	7.00 (5.78)	12.49 (8.51)	4.91 (4.85)	6.14 (5.99)
Headaches[EG]	1.23 (1.18)	0.90 (0.97)	1.65 (1.34)	1.19 (1.21)	1.19 (1.33)
Lower back pain[E]	0.96 (1.38)	1.35 (1.57)	1.05 (1.23)	0.86 (1.46)	0.60 (1.23)
No. of prescription medications[gG]	0.80 (1.13)	0.37 (0.50)	1.65 (1.69)	0.48 (0.68)	0.71 (0.85)
Waist–hip ratio[eE]	0.94 (.06)	0.96 (.05)	0.98 (.05)	0.92 (.05)	0.91 (.05)
Regularly smokes cigarettes now[eE]	13%	30%	20%	5%	0%
Takes vitamins 2+ times/week[G]	52%	55%	70%	43%	41%
Moderate exercise (times/month)[E]	9.48 (4.85)	8.14 (5.19)	9.00 (4.81)	9.31 (4.81)	11.20 (4.36)
Vigorous exercise (times/month)[eG]	6.35 (5.40)	5.00 (4.88)	5.28 (5.58)	7.86 (5.39)	7.23 (5.54)

Notes: The superscripts indicate the significant difference within the EDWB sample (e = education effect, g = gender effect, x = interaction effect; $p < .05$) and the significant difference within the MIDUS comparable sample (E = education effect, G = gender effect, X = interaction effect; $p < .05$). The first number in each group is the mean; the second number, in parentheses, is the standard deviation.

question-by-question basis and, where appropriate, grouped questions together. The analyses began by applying the inductive consensus codes to all the data and combining or eliminating categories that did not produce high-enough frequencies (at least 10 percent of the total population). This process resulted in a number of major categories (designated in this chapter by the words in small capital letters). A number of the major categories were fairly general (e.g., FAMILY), and thus several subcategories could be identified within them, which are designated in this chapter by italic typeface (e.g., *Spouse, Offspring*). The percentages recorded here for the various subcategories represent the percentage of respondents within the major category that mentioned the subcategory.

Behavior in EDWB and MIDUS Samples

	MIDUS Comparable Sample ($N = 504$)				
	High School		College		
All ($N = 504$)	Men ($N = 102$)	Women ($N = 132$)	Men ($N = 151$)	Women ($N = 119$)	
3.62	3.31	3.43	3.83	3.84	
(0.94)	(0.90)	(1.01)	(0.86)	(0.89)	
2.05	2.13	2.79	1.45	1.94	
(2.28)	(2.36)	(2.83)	(1.56)	(2.10)	
8.21	7.67	11.03	6.38	7.88	
(6.72)	(6.91)	(7.94)	(5.04)	(5.97)	
1.27	1.16	1.63	1.03	1.30	
(1.26)	(1.27)	(1.40)	(1.08)	(1.21)	
1.27	1.48	1.48	1.09	1.07	
(1.58)	(1.66)	(1.71)	(1.46)	(1.46)	
0.73	0.57	1.10	0.37	0.93	
(1.14)	(1.16)	(1.36)	(0.66)	(1.17)	
0.95	0.98	0.97	0.94	0.94	
(.08)	(.08)	(.09)	(.05)	(.07)	
21%	34%	29%	13%	10%	
50%	37%	55%	47%	59%	
9.19	8.67	8.79	9.30	9.95	
(4.66)	(5.03)	(4.63)	(4.61)	(4.35)	
6.26	7.20	4.42	7.37	6.02	
(5.20)	(5.09)	(4.61)	(5.44)	(5.05)	

We devoted a great deal of effort to developing reliable coding categories that would consistently capture the ideas and meanings generated in the well-being narratives. Low-frequency and low-reliability categories were eliminated or merged with other categories unless they were small subcategories that held particular theoretical interest (e.g., the subcategory *Friends*). Kappa coefficients, used to assess interrater reliability, were calculated for seventy-seven categories (the total number of major categories and subcategories). For the question "What does it mean to you to have a good life?" and the follow-up probe, "Do you have anything to add about what's important for well-being?" the average reliability for the thirty-three categories (including agency categories) was .83 (range = .38–1.00), with 76 percent of categories showing reliability greater than .70 and 88 percent of categories greater than .65. For the question "What do you think are some of the reasons your life has gone well?" the average reliability for twenty-eight categories was .72 (range = .40–.92), with 61 percent of categories greater than .70 and 75 percent of categories greater than .65. For the question "What are your hopes for the future?" the average reliability for sixteen categories was .78 (range $= .51-.95$), with 56 percent of categories greater than .70 and 88 percent of categories greater than .65.

In reporting the results of our analyses, we first discuss the percentage of respondents who answered in each of the major categories. We then probe more deeply into the meanings of these frequent responses by examining subcategories within the major coding categories as well as the actual text of the responses. The overarching aim is to summarize respondents' interview responses both quantitatively (e.g., how many respondents mentioned a particular category) and qualitatively (e.g., what were the exact words and examples used by individuals within particular categories). Chi-square tests were used on our binary data to determine significant differences between gender and education subgroups. In reports of statistically significant ($p < .05$) differences in parentheses throughout the text, M stands for men, W for women, HS for high school–educated, and BA for college-educated.

Throughout this analysis we compare the narratives of the EDWB respondents with survey data from the MIDUS comparable sample. It is the premise of our study that the interview data illuminate, via respondents' self-generated thoughts, aspects of well-being not captured by current questionnaire measures.

RESULTS
Consensus in Well-Being American Style
What Does It Mean to Have a Good Life?

> *High school–educated woman:* A good life is having the things you need. Bein' happy and content. Having your health. You know, with the things you need. I mean, we always want more than what we have. I guess that's human nature. But I'm talkin' about havin' a roof over your head, a job, some kind of security. That would be to me—it's havin' a good life. Friends and family. Without them, maybe I'd be a little lonely.

> *College-educated woman:* I think a life should be challenging. So if everything goes too easily it's not a good life. So you should have some challenges, and you should be able to have to push yourself a little bit to reach some goals. I think

having a strong family and a loving relationship with your family is important. And I think that leads toward a good life. I feel having work that you enjoy leads toward a good life. And I believe in having outside activities that you find either relaxing or comforting or challenging, whether they be hobbies or sports or something you can involve yourself in. [They] all kind of blend together. Going back to that initial perception of mine that everything should be balanced in order to have a good overall feeling about yourself and what you're doing.

We began our analysis of well-being by examining EDWB respondents' answers to the question "What does it mean to you to have a good life?" as well as answers to a follow-up probe, "Do you have anything to add about what's important for well-being?" We noted the percentage of respondents who gave a particular type of answer at least once in their answers. There were no education-level or gender differences in the number of sentences used to answer the questions. In this section we report the percentage of respondents who mentioned a given category for all eighty-three respondents; differences within categories (by education and gender) are reported in the section on diversity in well-being.

In their own words, what matters most to the EDWB respondents is relationships with other people (especially family), good physical health, the opportunity to enjoy oneself, financial security, self-development, and satisfactory jobs. Figure 1 displays the most frequently mentioned categories in respondents' answers to these two questions (all major categories reported were mentioned by at least 25 percent of the respondents). Major categories and their corresponding subcategories, along with a representative example of responses, can be found in table 5. Throughout the chapter we include verbatim examples in the tables to demonstrate the breadth of the categories (the span of content each category encompasses) and to reveal that despite the seemingly personal and individual nature of well-being, there is considerable overlap among respondents in how they answer a given question, and a strong consensus is often evident even with the very words used to answer.

The highest-frequency categories that emerged in response to thinking about a good life reflected the social nature of well-being. This idea was elaborated in multiple ways. As one respondent summarized his sentiment, "You can't live in a vacuum . . . you have to build friendships

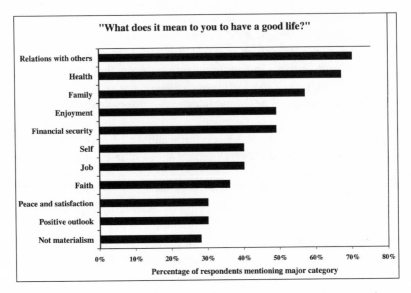

FIGURE 1. Responses to the question "What does it mean to you to have a good life?"

and relationships that are meaningful." Indeed, 70 percent of respondents agreed that RELATIONS WITH OTHERS was a major component of well-being. Most respondents who mentioned RELATIONS WITH OTHERS also mentioned FAMILY, another high-frequency category that was included in RELATIONS WITH OTHERS. The category FAMILY (57 percent of all respondents) was further differentiated into four subcategories, which are designated by italic typeface. Although respondents generating the FAMILY category most often used the general term "family," 38 percent of the respondents who mentioned FAMILY specifically mentioned their *Spouses,* 17 percent mentioned their *Offspring,* 15 percent mentioned *Parents and siblings,* and 13 percent referred to their own *Upbringing.*

What is it about social relationships that make them so important to a sense of well-being? Six specific subcategories pertaining to qualities of social relationships that emerged within RELATIONS WITH OTHERS help illuminate what it is about the company of other people that seems crucial to living a good life. The high-frequency subcategories included a *Positive evaluation of others* (49 percent of respondents mentioning RELATIONS WITH OTHERS); *Loving and caring* (37 percent), an indication that relationships with other people are important because people love, care, and support each other emotionally; *Advising and respecting*

TABLE 5 What Does It Mean to You to Have a Good Life?

Major Category and Subcategories	Verbatim Examples from Interviews
Relations with others[a] *Positive evaluation* *Loving and caring* *Advising and respecting* *Time together* *Instructions* *Financial help*	• "I also have friends that are nice and extended family that's nice." • "A good life means: being loving, peaceful, working together." • "That's part of well-being to me—making connections, finding out what other people think about things." • "We devote time when we just sit down and talk to each other, and try to be very, very open, and not keep things bottled up inside of us, from my husband on down to the kids." • "I know when I'm wrong, I'll admit it. It doesn't happen often, but it does happen." • "I'm very appreciative of the fact that I have some equity that I've been able to put money aside for my daughter's education and something toward my retirement."
Health	• "The basic thing is you have to sleep tight, and not smoke, which I keep tellin' my husband." • "If you're not healthy you don't have a very good time. Nothing is as much fun." • "Your body is God's temple, on loan, so you shouldn't abuse it with anything to excess."
Family[a] *Spouse* *Offspring* *Parents/siblings* *Upbringing*	• "Someone to share [life] with who has the same outlook on life that you do." • "My kids are a constant factor in that as long as I think that my kids are doing okay, it's pretty easy for me to be doing okay." • "Having mom making my life good too." • "You have to be nurtured as a child."
Enjoyment	• "You have to enjoy, to be able to smell the roses a little bit as well as to do a good job." • "A sense of humor is real important to me. Not taking yourself too seriously all the time." • "Taking those vacations, cross-country skiing with my wife, downhill skiing with my daughter . . . Just doing those things that are exciting and fun and memorable."
Financial security	• "To make an income where I'm not having to worry about how the bills are going to get paid, or if they're going to get paid."

(continued)

TABLE 5 *continued*

Major Category and Subcategories	Verbatim Examples from Interviews
	• "Not being wealthy by any means, it's never been particularly important to me, but being comfortable, and . . . having enough money that you don't have to take all the darn creditors' calls." • "A good life is having the things you need. But I'm talkin' about havin' a roof over your head, a job, some kind of security."

Self
  Know/love the self
  Purpose and fulfillment
    autonomy
  Seeking new learning
    Accomplishment
	• "You really need to know who you are and what works for you, what you like doing. Don't try to be a square peg in a round hole."
	
	 • "Feeling fulfilled, in general terms. That can come . . . from totally different places for different people."
	
	 • "Being able to do what I want to do, when I want to do it."
	
	 • "Not to be afraid to try different things like . . . I have so many people that I see that are afraid of the computer."
	
	 • "People have certain abilities, certain potentials, and I think you have to fulfill them."

Job	• "When you're on a job, take care of the job. Work, do what the person tells you to do on a job. A job will take care of you." • "I think it's very important to wake up in the morning and want to do what you're doing, rather than drag yourself into work." • "It means having a situation where you can feel that you are involved in meaningful activity— meaningful work, typically, though it doesn't have to be work."
Faith	• "People who haven't had that belief in God have had a lot more trouble handling problems. They just really don't have anything to turn to." • "What's most important in my life is to maintain a level of spirituality. But it comes from in here. It doesn't come at all from the belief in a particular practice, although I get very moved when I go to an Easter mass with my wife." • "See I can go sit in church, and then you can come just as peaceful as you can. I think you really need it."

(*continued*)

TABLE 5 *continued*

Major Category and Subcategories	Verbatim Examples from Interviews
Peace and satisfaction	• "A good life is a life in which I'm at peace with whatever is going on in my life. And that takes a lot of acceptance, it takes a lot of tolerance, to know that no matter what happens, that I can still have peace inside." • "To be content with your lot in life and not necessarily be happy all the time, but generally you're in a situation where the good outweighs the bad." • "I purposely try to be a calm person. And it doesn't mean I'm not passionate about ideas or things."
Positivity	• "Life can't get you down if you have that sense of humor, the playfulness, the some kind of sense of turning tragedy into something fun." • "You've got to believe in the fact that things are going to be okay, that you can prevail in the face of adversity." • "My mantra, if I have one, is instead of thinking problems, think challenges."
Not materialism	• "Having [a] certain kind of inner happiness, not something that can come from outside, from material possessions, but from just a very good feeling on the inside, having to do with people that are close to you." • "You can be poor and have a good life if you're happy; you can be rich and have a bad life if you're unhappy." • "So the tangible assets—anybody can have those. But it's the intangibles that are the most important." • "I don't need the big house and the big car, and all the money. It would be nice, but I don't need it to be happy."

^aSee table 6 for additional subcategories.

(30 percent), an indication that relationships with other people are important because people advise each other, teach each other new things, and enable each other to feel respected and worthy; and *Spend time/physical presence together* (27 percent). Lower-frequency subcategories included *Instructions for how to relate well together* (20 percent) and *Help others financially* (10 percent). (See table 6 for examples of responses included in these subcategories.)

TABLE 6 Family and Relations with Others Subcategories

Subcategories	Verbatim Examples from Interviews
Positive evaluation of others	• "To have a family that I'm proud of and happy with." • "My wife—she's nice and she's sweet. I just love her." • "I am really happy with my husband and my kids. I mean, I'm not saying that every single day is happy. We have your bad days and your good days. But I think if I was living out on an island somewhere, I would just live with them. I think I'd really be happy."
Loving and caring	• "The most important is having someone who loves you, and who you love." • "Just take each day as it comes, and try to do the best with it, and have lots of love in your heart to give to others." • "They [kids] need that loving and caring—that's the most important thing is to be cared about."
Advising and respecting	• "Respect peoples, 'cause you want respect." • "When you talk to somebody, you're sharing with your ideas, what you're thinking about different issues or yourself. The responses you get when you share reaffirm your perception of yourself. If they don't, then at least you have some input . . . mean, sharing implies that you're going to get something back, and therefore that it will either reaffirm or tell you that you're out in left field. And that's a good thing too."
Spend time/ physical presence together	• "Just being able to do something like that—relax and enjoy yourself and be with friends and relate way very satisfying." • "That your hours of work are reasonable so that you can enjoy your family, or you can enjoy other things in your life." • "I also have friends that are nice and extended family that's nice, and we have time enough to spend with them now. It's sort 'a like rediscovering them, later in life after you're done doing all the kiddy things."
Instructions for how to relate well together	• "Not to harbor hard feelings or bad feelings about people and hold grudges against people." • "Treat others as you would want others to treat you." • "So I think the whole well-being thing to me is just try to put yourself in that other person's place, and try to question a lot of what you do, not necessarily what everybody else does."
Help others financially	• "I like to buy things for people." • "I'm very appreciative of the fact that I have some equity that I've been able to put money aside for my daughter's education." • "I'd say having a good life is having a wonderful family and having the financial means to provide for them."

The importance of physical HEALTH, including health-promoting behaviors such as walking, golf, diet, and so forth, was mentioned by a
large majority (67 percent) of respondents. In addition to health and
social relationships, respondents frequently noted that ENJOYMENT (49
percent) is an important aspect of living a good life. FINANCIAL SECURITY
(49 percent) was also on the minds of many of the respondents. Topics that related to aspects of the respondents' JOB (40 percent) and the
development of the SELF (40 percent) were also found in many of the respondents' answers. Five subcategories comprised the SELF category. The
most common responses from the respondents who talked about the self
included the ability to *Know and love the self* (52 percent), a feeling of *Purpose and fulfillment* (45 percent), and a sense of *Autonomy* from others'
expectations and opinions (42 percent). Also noted was the importance
of being curious and *Seeking new learning* (18 percent). Finally, a sense of
Accomplishment (16 percent) was mentioned as one part of a good life.
(See table 7 for verbatim examples.)

Other less frequent but commonly mentioned aspects of the good life
included one's FAITH (36 percent) and feelings of PEACE AND SATISFAC-
TION (30 percent).[3] The feeling of well-being induced by maintaining a
POSITIVE OUTLOOK (30 percent) was also a major category mentioned by
some respondents. Finally, although many people mentioned the importance of having enough money to meet their needs, some respondents
pointed out that an excess of money is not important for well-being, a
sentiment captured by the major category NOT MATERIALISM (28 percent).

What Are Some of the Reasons Your Life Has Gone Well?

To explore respondents' ideas about the sources of a life well lived,
interviewers asked them, "Thinking back over your life, what do you think
are some of the reasons your life has gone well?" Twelve major categories
(each mentioned by at least 10 percent of respondents) emerged from
the resulting answers (see fig. 2). Similar to the narratives about what it
means to have a good life and well-being in the present, many of these
high-frequency categories reflect the importance of other people as a
source of well-being.

More than half of the respondents (52 percent) felt their lives had
gone well because of various experiences and relationships during their
UPBRINGING. A variety of subcategories were identified within this major
category. As might be expected, the majority of respondents (72 percent)
who gave an answer that fit within this major category made reference to
the influence their *Parents* (and grandparents) had in their lives. Some

TABLE 7 Self Subcategories

Subcategories	Verbatim Examples from Interviews
Knowing and loving the self	• "I think you have to have some sense of who you are and what satisfies you, what your needs are, and then a situation that satisfies those needs." • "That's very important, that anyone has to have some self-respect, certainly confidence in themselves." • "Love yourself . . . When you love you, then you can love people."
Purpose and fulfillment	• "Always to have a goal. I think when people stop having that, they really stop living the good life, because then they have nothing to strive for. And if you don't strive for something, if you're not working toward something, then you lose your sense of purpose. And if you have no sense of purpose, I don't think you have a very good life." • "To have some sense of purpose and goals to work toward. Some reason to get up and do what you do everyday and not just exist." • "That would come down to the question where 'Do you wander aimlessly in life?' and that would be somebody who has no spirituality at all."
Autonomy	• "I could care less what other people think." • "Question yourself and others, question your situations." • "Having the ability or living in the circumstances that allow you to be pretty much in control. It gives you a good life because you will make the choices that make it good for you."
Seeking new learning	• "Having the opportunities to do different things, to meet different people." • "You need other people around you to bring in new ideas, 'cause you can get some from books, but more so probably from talking to people." • "Sit down and figure out who you are, and then develop a healthy curiosity, and learn how to learn."
Accomplishment	• "You have to have decided that you want to do something and successfully accomplish it." • "You have to earn things. If you don't earn some things, you don't work for some things, I don't think they're gonna to be meaningful for you." • "Where you think at the end of day—that I have accomplished something. And I have learned to not be unhappy that it didn't shake the earth."

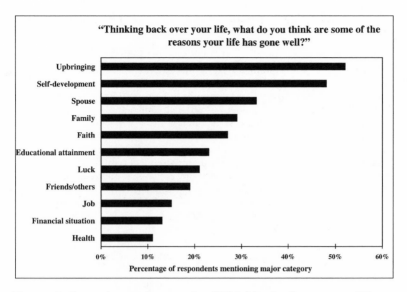

FIGURE 2. Responses to the question "Thinking back over your life, what do you think are some of the reasons your life has gone well?"

respondents discussed the benefits of their upbringing in terms of *General positive family relationships* (28 percent), such as having a loving family or perceiving a strong sense of family. Some respondents spoke of more specific aspects of their upbringing that contributed to their lives having gone well, such as learning *Values* (40 percent), feeling *Supported* (26 percent), experiencing *Normalcy* (19 percent), receiving *Attention* (9 percent), or having been *Disciplined* (7 percent). (See table 8 for verbatim examples.)

The social nature of well-being also was expressed beyond the realm of early family life. For example, SPOUSES were given credit for the role they have played in helping the lives of one-third of the respondents (33 percent) go well. A similar number of respondents (29 percent) mentioned other current FAMILY members (i.e., children and siblings). In addition, 19 percent of the respondents reported that their relationships with FRIENDS AND OTHERS had a positive impact on their lives.

The self also was given credit for causing life to go well. Almost half of the respondents (48 percent) discussed ways in which facets of their SELF-DEVELOPMENT have contributed to the positive parts of life. Within this major category, six specific subcategories emerged, including putting forth *Effort* (38 percent), being able to take *Control* (28 percent) when

TABLE 8 What Are Some of the Reasons Your Life Has Gone Well?

Major Category and Subcategories	Verbatim Examples from Interviews

Upbringing
  Parents
  Values
  Positive family
    relations
  Support
  Normalcy
  Attention
  Discipline
	• "I think he [father] was extremely honest, an extremely hard worker, and taught me that whatever, if I was going to make it I was going to have to do it on my own."
	• "My mother was very self-confident . . . and she imparted that to my sister and I."
	• "My parents showed us the importance of hard work, getting a good education, and saving money."
	• "My parents taught me a sense of right from wrong."
	• "The life that they gave me, even though it was not money-filled, in a way it was still rich."
	• "I was raised in a household with two parents, and they appeared to be loving."
	• "They encouraged us to try things, and were real supportive, and still are real supportive."
	• "You need a basic background to be a normal person."
	• "They were always very interested in what the kids were doing."
	• "When I was young, she kept me on the straight and narrow."

Self-development
  Effort Control
  Goals Compassion
  Adaptability
  Resiliency Skills
	• "None of it came on a silver platter: I worked for everything I got."
	• "You just kinda' take control of your life, and you say, well I gotta' do something about this."
	• "I set up my goals, and I followed my goals."
	• "I've always cared about other poeple and tried to put myself in their position."
	• "I've learned the ability to change and be happy about it."
	• "I've had to work through a lot of things . . . I don't give up."
	• "I was always good at what I did . . . that helped me from the start."

Spouse	• "I think our relationship is what has cemented me together." • "I've had a really good partner for most of my life."

Family
  Offspring
  Family
  Siblings
	• "I have five children . . . they filled up my life . . . watching them grow."
	• "Just by having the blessing of having family."
	• "My family—both my parents, and brothers and sisters, and my wife and kids . . . that's ninety-nine percent of it."

Faith	• "I think having a strong faith has helped us through a lot." • "The only time my life ever goes well is when I'm doing what I ought to be doing when I'm obeying God's word."

(*continued*)

Table 8 *continued*

Major Category and Subcategories	Verbatim Examples from Interviews
Educational attainment	• "Even though I'm not using my education, I'm who I am because of it." • "I was fortunate enough to go through school, and do well, and then, get to go to college, and do well."
Luck	• "Sometimes I just think I was in the right place at the right time, and maybe it was meant to be." • I have honestly always felt like that I was leading a charmed life... things have tended to fall into place."
Friends/others	• "I can count on them when I need help ... whether it's for spiritual need or I need help with at project, or whatever." • "He was more like a father to me than a boss or an employer ... he gave me some good advice."
Job	• "I've always had a job, I have a good work ethic." • "I've got a great environment to work in ... with people that I like."
Financial situation	• "I think having financial stability is important, even though I would like to say, you know, it's not that important." • "We're not rich, but we've got enough money."
Health	• "I don't have any major diseases ... I'm healthy." • "I guess I've taken care of myself, I've gotten rest, I've eaten well."

needed, and setting and achieving *Goals* (20 percent). Other aspects of SELF-DEVELOPMENT generated less frequently included *Developing compassion* (18 percent) as a social skill, being able to *Adapt* to life's circumstances (15 percent), maintaining *Resiliency* (the strength to persevere and cope with difficult situations; 15 percent), and relying on one's *Skills and abilities* (10 percent). Finally, some of the reasons listed for life going well invoked more metaphysical forces. Slightly more than one-fourth of the respondents (27 percent) felt their lives had gone well because of their FAITH. In addition, 21 percent of the respondents thought that LUCK had played a role in how their lives had turned out thus far.

Three other major categories that emerged from the respondents' discussions about why they think their lives have gone well included EDUCATIONAL ATTAINMENT (23 percent), JOB (15 percent), and FINAN-CIAL SITUATION (13 percent). The discussion in these three areas was often interrelated. For example, one woman explained, "I worked till

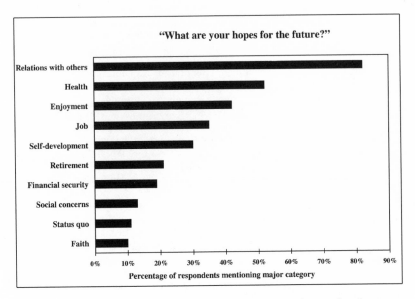

FIGURE 3. Responses to the question "What are your hopes for the future?"

midnight every night and went to school all day to achieve what I wanted." Finally, 11 percent of the sample felt that their good HEALTH had contributed to their lives going well.

What Are Your Hopes for the Future?

To explore respondents' wishes and expectations regarding well-being and the good life in the future, we asked our respondents, "What are your hopes for the future?" Their responses fell within the domains of ten major categories (answered by at least 10 percent of respondents) (see fig. 3 and table 9). Similar to answers to previous questions, the largest category to emerge in response to hopes for the future was RELATIONS WITH OTHERS. Eighty-two percent of the respondents communicated that their hopes for the future involve other people. Within the major RELA- TIONS WITH OTHERS category, a number of subcategories were identified. Seventy-four percent of the respondents who answered within this major category discussed their hopes about the future of their *Offspring* (chil- dren and grandchildren), and 29 percent expressed their aspirations in terms of continuing to share their lives with a *Spouse*. Some of the respon- dents spoke in more general terms about their futures with their *Families* (16 percent), not specifying a certain family member. Others did specify

TABLE 9 What Are Your Hopes for the Future?

Major Category and Subcategories	Verbatim Examples from Interviews
Relations with others *Offspring* *Spouse* *Others* *Family* *Parent* *Relative* *Friends*	• "That my children and my grandchildren will prosper and be happy." • "That our relationship will continue to grow and deepen." • "Try to make a difference in other peoples' lives, like through Habitat for Humanity." • "That I will continue to enjoy my family." • "That she [mother] can remain healthy and happy with her grandchildren." • "My aunt is eighty-nine . . . getting less capable . . . I hope I can help." • "To continue to be good friends."
Health *Health* *Longevity*	• "To keep good health, and for my family to have their health." • "I just want to be able to continue to do the things that I want to do, and be productive, and not be a burden." • "Hope me and my wife live for a hundred years."
Enjoyment	• "For my wife and I to be able to go out and travel, have fun." • "Just to keep on being as happy as I am now . . . wake up every morning with a smile on my face."
Job	• "To keep doing what I'm doing now . . . I may just go on until I drop." • "I just hope that the difficulties that I'm going through right now in my business get resolved."
Self-development *Goals* *Active* *Education*	• "My eventual goal is to have my own court reporting firm." • "To stay active and doing things with and for other people as long as we can." • "I would really like to go back to school and finish my master's."
Retirement	• "I hope everything goes fine, as far as the job, and my future, and my family, and if everything goes well, in a few years I'll have enough money to retire." • "We're like a lot of baby boomers, we're going to get hosed when it comes to retiring."
Financial security	• "To live another thirty, forty years, and be able to live on our farm, have enough money to pay the taxes so I won't have to give it up." • "We're not asking to be wealthy, but at the same time, financially in a position where we can enjoy life instead of having to work all the time."

(continued)

TABLE 9 *continued*

Major Category and Subcategories	Verbatim Examples from Interviews
Social concerns	• "I hope our country gets its act together in terms of morality." • "I hope that we're able to protect and take care of this planet of ours."
Status quo	• "Just kind 'a keep goin' the way things are, in a lot 'a ways." • "That there are no unexpected glitches down the road."
Faith	• "As far as the world is concerned, I wish that they would come to their senses and come back to the Lord." • "And I ask the Lord, use me, use me in any way he sees fit . . . whether it's preaching your word, whether it's singing your word, whether it's helping people."

that their hopes for the future involved *Parents* (6 percent), their *Relatives* (3 percent), or *Friends* (2 percent). Eighteen percent of the respondents who answered within the RELATIONS WITH OTHERS category spoke more broadly about interacting with unspecified *Others* in the future.

HEALTH was also very much on the minds of our respondents (52 percent) as they looked to their future. Most respondents who mentioned HEALTH did so in general terms, although 28 percent of the respondents explicitly discussed their hope for *Longevity*.

Themes involving life ENJOYMENT were reflected in the answers of 45 percent of the respondents, including comments about continuing or developing new hobbies and enjoying leisure-time activities. Thirty-five percent of the respondents cited ways in which their hopes for the future included aspects of their JOB, either continuing in a current position or aspirations for a new line of work. Thoughts directed at impending RETIREMENT (20 percent) and FINANCIAL SECURITY (19 percent) reveal that these issues also are expected to play a relatively important role in the future of these midlife respondents. These two categories were often interrelated; respondents hoped to have enough money to be able to retire.

Slightly more than one-third of the respondents (35 percent) noted that their hopes for the future included various aspects of continuing SELF-DEVELOPMENT. Within this category, 59 percent of respondents mentioned *Goals* that they had hopes of attaining. Specific goals were also mentioned, including remaining physically fit or psychologically *Active* (28 percent) and furthering their *Education* (17 percent).

Thirteen percent of the interviews generated discussion directed at broader SOCIAL CONCERNS. Here their narratives included concern over morality and family values, environmental issues, and world peace. In addition, 11 percent of all the respondents felt comfortable with the STATUS QUO and hoped that things would remain pretty much the same. Finally, 10 percent of all respondents shared their hopes for the future in terms of their FAITH (hoping that their own faith would continue to grow and that others would find faith).

Summary

The preceding analyses reveal a consensus among Americans at midlife as to one major element that constitutes the good life—relations with others. Whether defining the good life, identifying the causes of life going well, or expressing hopes for the future, respondents mentioned relationships with other people (especially with one's parents, spouse, and offspring) most often in their narratives. The importance of good health was also frequently mentioned, especially when describing what is necessary for a good midlife and future life. Across the questions, two additional concepts were also central and important: developing aspects of the self (loving the self, pursuing goals, experiencing autonomy, etc.) and enjoying life as it progresses.

Lower-frequency categories that consistently appeared in answers to each question included the need to have financial security (enough money to meet one's needs) as well as a steady and enjoyable job, and the opportunity to comfortably retire. For about a third of the respondents, faith and a positive outlook were important parts of well-being. Finally, many respondents described a feeling of contentment comprised of peacefulness, satisfaction with the status quo, and adaption to and acceptance of what life presents.

It is interesting to note the relative lack of responses regarding civic engagement, community service, or volunteer activities. The low frequency of these types of answers might imply a focus on local instead of public worlds (see Markus et al. 2001). It also leads one to ask whether the pursuit of individual well-being is good for society as a whole.

Diversity in Well-Being American Style: Variation by Education and Gender

Meaning of a Good Life

> *College-educated woman:* Always to have a goal. I think when people stop having that, they really stop living the good life,

because they have nothing to strive for, and if you don't strive for something, if you're not working towards something, then you lose your sense of purpose, and if you have no sense of purpose, I mean, I don't think you have a very good life.

High school–educated man: A good wife. How she takes care of me. She's nice and she's sweet. I just love her. And each day God blesses me to see her. It seems like I grow more in love with her. It's just, she's just a sweet person.

Although we were not surprised to find considerable consensus among Americans at midlife about what constitutes a good life, we anticipated differences in explanations and experiences of well-being among sub-groups of respondents who are engaged in local worlds that differ from one another. Specifically, we expected variation among respondents with respect to gender and education level. For example, RELATIONS WITH OTHERS is an apparent key to a good life, but do college-educated and high school–educated respondents have similar understandings of the role of others in their lives? Similarly, many respondents mentioned that purpose and fulfillment are essential elements for a life well lived. Is this a view shared by college-educated and high school–educated respondents, and if so, is it realized in similar ways? Although gender differences did exist and are reported when significant, most of the variation found in the answers related to respondents' level of education.

The MIDUS comparable sample results show that the high school–educated and the college-educated respondents are living in quite different structural and social worlds (see tables 3 and 4), and we explored whether these differences are reflected in their narratives about well-being. Looking first at the major categories of well-being displayed in figure 1 (RELATIONS WITH OTHERS, HEALTH, FAMILY, ENJOYMENT, FINANCIAL SECURITY, SELF, JOB, and so forth), generated in answer to the question "What does it mean to you to have a good life?" and the follow-up probe "Do you have anything to add about what's important for well-being?" some significant differences according to gender and education level are evident. First, more college-educated respondents (60 percent) than high school–educated respondents (38 percent) mentioned ENJOYMENT. This difference may reflect the fact that college-educated respondents had more of their basic needs met (job security, health care, and so forth), as well as more disposable income, and thus they had the means to expend time and energy on leisure activities, hobbies, and "fun." Men (59 percent) mentioned JOB more than women (21 percent), which is understandable given that almost half of the high school–educated women in the EDWB sample did not work for pay. Within the FAMILY category, men specifically mentioned their *Spouses* (M = 32 percent; W = 20 percent) and *Parents and siblings* (M = 15 percent; W = 2 percent) more than women did. Women, on the other hand, mentioned FINANCI AL SECURITY more than men did (W = 62 percent; M = 37 percent).

We also calculated the relative emphasis our respondents placed on each category. These percentages reflect the *proportion* of each respondent's answer to "What does it mean to you to have a good life?" and its follow-up probe that was dedicated to a specific category. For example, RELATIONS WITH OTHERS was more likely to be emphasized by high school–educated women. In fact, the largest proportion (more than one-third) of answers by high school–educated women concerning what it means to have a good life were responses in which other people are focal—RELATIONS WITH OTHERS and FAMILY. This proportional analysis also clarifies two gender differences that appeared in the earlier analysis of what it means to have a good life. FINANCIAL SECURITY, noted earlier to be a category mentioned by more women, is shown here to be a particularly salient issue for high school–educated women. Almost half of these women did not work outside the home. Perhaps the high school–educated women emphasize the importance of having basic needs met because they were more likely to have had times when their own needs were not met or they knew others who did not have them met. Similarly, JOB was a category of response generated more by men in the previous analysis and can be seen here to be one of the major features of the good life for high school–educated men specifically.

More variation among education groups appeared in the subcategories within the major categories than in the major categories themselves. For instance, with respect to the major category RELATIONS WITH OTHERS, there were two subcategories that reflected different ways of relating to others: *Advising and respecting* and *Loving and caring* (see table 6 for verbatim examples). Although most respondents reported both types of interactions and did not differ in the number of sentences generated in their narratives, the ratio of sentences involving *Loving and caring* to sentences involving *Advising and respecting* (BA = 1.55, HS = 1.11; p = .08) reveals that relatively more of the college-educated respondents' explanations (especially those of college-educated men) about *how* others are important for the good life reflected the idea that others are important because of the knowledge they can impart and the self-confidence they can engender.

Thus, the broad cultural mandate to work on oneself and develop oneself is for some college-educated respondents realized in relations with others. Relationships are not just about support or connection; they are about developing the self and affirming and praising each other. For example, a college-educated woman said, "I think it is very helpful if you have some stalwart persons in your corner. They'll string your confidence [along] in saying positive things." These divergent ways of thinking about the role of others in one's life is more than just a difference in how people with different educational levels "talk" about other people. Instead it is related, we suggest, to the conditions of life experienced by these two groups of respondents and a reflection of the general nature of their social interaction with other people. The context of the high school–educated respondents does not require them to experience themselves as agents influencing and being influenced by other agents. Instead, other people are interpreted as affording connection and relationship.

Subcategories within the major SELF category also reflected educational variation. First, the college-educated respondents elaborated the general category SELF more frequently. That is, they mentioned significantly more SELF subcategories than did the high school–educated respondents (BA = 2.1; HS = 1.5). Specifically, the college-educated respondents were decidedly more likely to mention *Fulfillment* (BA = 28 percent; HS = 0 percent), *Accomplishment* (BA = 33 percent; HS = 0 percent), and *Seeking new learning* (BA = 28 percent; HS = 7 percent) as aspects of the good life (see fig. 4 and table 7). These are some of the aspects of well-being that have been central in well-being theories and measures.

Although the high school–educated respondents were just as likely as the college-educated respondents to mention at least one aspect of the self and its development as important for living a good life, they seemed to mean something different by it. For example, there were no high school–educated respondents, men or women, who mentioned feeling good about oneself because of *Accomplishment* or *Fulfillment*. Moreover, although a few high school–educated men mentioned *Seeking new learning* as important for the good life, no high school–educated women generated any responses that fit this subcategory. Instead, the high school–educated respondents were somewhat more likely (although not statistically significant) to say that it is important to *Know and love the self* and to have *Autonomy* from others' expectations and opinions. For the

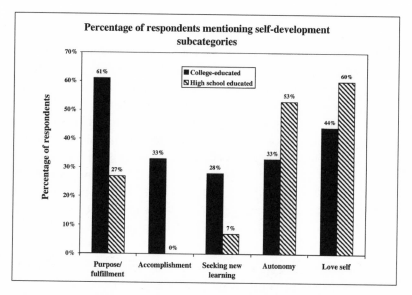

FIGURE 4. Percentage of respondents mentioning self-development subcategories.

high school–educated, self-development is more about liking the self and protecting it from imposition by others than about being a fulfilled and accomplished self. Again, we suggest these differences go beyond styles of answering questions and reflect the different lives and the activities afforded and required by these lives.

Reasons Why Life Has Gone Well

There are only a few differences by education level or gender in responses to the question "Thinking back over your life, what do you think are some of the reasons your life has gone well?" Forty percent of the college-educated respondents cited EDUCATION as a reason their lives had gone well, compared with only 5 percent of those with a high school education. In addition, the FRIENDS AND OTHERS category revealed a significant difference between gender groups. Twenty-nine percent of the male respondents believe their lives have gone well partly because of their relationships with friends and other people, whereas only 10 percent of the women gave answers that fit in this category.

Analyses within the major categories resulted in a number of significant gender and educational differences between subcategories. Within the UPBRINGING category, 28 percent of those with a college education identified *General positive family relationships* as a reason their lives have gone well, but no high school–educated respondents mentioned this subcategory. Two significant subcategory differences are noted within the major category FRIENDS AND OTHERS. A gender difference can be seen in that 20 percent of the men in this study mentioned unspecified *Others* who have in some way benefited their lives, whereas only 2 percent of the women did. In addition, more college-educated respondents (14 percent) than high school–educated respondents (3 percent) mention *Friends* as a reason their lives have gone well ($p < .06$). Finally, within the SELF-DEVELOPMENT category, 9 percent of the college-educated respondents cited their *Skills and abilities* as a reason their lives have gone well, but none of the high school–educated respondents gave this answer.

Hopes for the Future

A few significant gender and educational differences in answers to "What are your hopes for the future?" were evident in analysis of subcategories. Within the RELATIONS WITH OTHERS major category, 23 percent of the high school–educated respondents made reference to their *Family* in general terms when discussing their hopes for the future compared with only 5 percent of those respondents with a college education. A gender difference is also noted within this major category. Women are more likely (71 percent) to discuss their *Offspring* (children and grandchildren) as part of their hopes for the future than are men (49 percent).

Agency Analyses

College-educated woman: To be able to make choices. To have circumstances and the ability to make choices in your life. Not to be in a position where you have to do something because you have no choice. Like going to work, for instance. I can either work or stay home.

High school–educated man: God has helped me out a lot too, to reinforce my feelings. . . . Just gives me an inner-self confident feeling that no matter how bad things get they can always get worse. That if they get bad enough that God feels I can't handle it, then he'll help me out of it. If things get bad, I just feel that maybe God is testing me to see what I am capable of. . . . Yeah, probably the self-confidence, endurance, not giving up, just hang in there, hang tough, things are going to get around to here real eventually.

Respondents' answers to the three questions organizing this chapter give us a sense of what they care about and hope for at midlife and how they characterize themselves, but their answers can also provide a view of the respondents' implicit theories of action as well as additional indirect insight into how they think about themselves and their roles in their diverse worlds. To gain a more complete picture of the nature of the self and its relation to being and well-being, we developed a code that was designed to reflect respondents' sense of agency, by which we mean how these respondents described what they were doing in their lives or how they understood their way of interacting with the world.

Most Americans generally have an optimistic view of the future and show a belief in their ability to do what they have set their minds to. Thus they score high on MIDUS items designed to assess plans and control (e.g., "I can do just about anything I really set my mind to" and "When things don't go according to my plans, my motto is 'where there's a will there's a way'"). However, the college-educated respondents were decidedly more likely to agree with MIDUS statements reflecting a sense of control, including a feeling of mastery and freedom from constraint (Lachman and Weaver 1998), planning for the future, and making sense of the past. They gave significantly stronger endorsements to 25 of 42 such items from MIDUS than did the high school–educated respondents. In addition, they scored higher on the purpose and environmental mastery components of positive psychological functioning. In contrast, the high school–educated were significantly more likely than the college-educated to endorse statements that imply adjustment and adaptation. They appear to be focused more on the present than the future, implying that the future may not be able to be controlled or predicted.

Overall, looking across the answers given to the EDWB questions, we found that when talking about themselves and their lives in their own terms, people sometimes characterized themselves as *influencing* the world by proactively taking charge and acting directly on the world; at other times they characterized themselves as *adjusting* to the world's circumstances. When describing their behavior in proactive terms or themselves as instrumental agents, respondents talked about the ways in which they create, manage, rearrange, change, initiate, stick to agendas, plan actions in advance, set long-term goals, and prevent future nega-tivity. For example, a college-educated woman's answer to why her life has gone well illustrates this proactive sense of self: "All the good things in my life? Yeah, I think I made them myself. I mean, I think I created the situations, and I think everybody has that ability, I think. Whatever happened, you know, it was a result of whatever I did or said, or good or bad, or otherwise."

When describing themselves as adjusting, respondents did not report themselves to be influencing or rearranging their circumstances. Still they characterize themselves active; they neither give in nor give up. They frame, interpret, regulate thought, control emotions, focus on the present, avoid bad circumstances, respond to luck, and generally "hang tough." A high school–educated man illustrated this active adjustment when talking about what it means to him to have a good life: "I've got limitations, physical limitations right now with, um . . . I can't go off, and take a one-mile walk without getting distinctly out of breath. But I've learned to work within the limitations. I'm happy with it."

We hypothesized that it would be the college-educated respondents who would most often characterize themselves as agents who influence the world, while the high school–educated would be more likely to describe themselves and their behavior as adjusting to the world. Every sentence given in answer to the EDWB questions presented in this chapter was coded as ADJUSTING, INFLUENCING, or neither. (See table 10 for category definitions and examples.) In general, all respondents showed more sentences involving themes of ADJUSTING than themes of INFLUENCING. Across answers to the three questions, the average respondent had 14.5 ADJUSTING sentences that characterize the respondent as actively adapting to the world and 10.5 INFLUENCING sentences that characterize the respondent in terms of acting directly on the world.

Although respondents more often used the language of ADJUSTING than the language of INFLUENCING, when INFLUENCING language was used, the college-educated respondents used it significantly more often (see fig. 5). College-educated respondents had significantly more sentences that fall into the INFLUENCING category (BA = 17.8; HS = 11.6). Within this major category we could identify three subcategories: *Internal attributions,* in which the self is responsible for life going well; *Proactive hopes,* which reflects hopes for future events on which the respondent will have a direct effect; and *Influencing language,* which included sentences with active verbs (i.e., verbs related to influencing, controlling, choosing, and planning) as opposed to passive verbs (i.e., sentences in which the respondent was the object, not the subject, of the sentence). Why might the college-educated have used more influencing language? We assume that a sense of one's self as an influencing agent is in some important part afforded by the particular circumstances (e.g., income level, particular types of employment, physical health) in one's life in which it is

TABLE 10 Agency Categories

Major Category and Subcategories	Verbatim Examples from Interviews
Influencing *Internal* *attributions* *Proactive hopes* *Influencing* *language*	• "I think I created the situations and I think everybody has that ability." • "Probably the main reason I think is I've always accepted responsibility for making my own way through life, not look for excuses. • "I set up my goals, and I followed my goals. The goals I have set, that's the reason that I guess I'm fairly well-off." • "When I get . . . older . . . get myself a pair of bib overalls and straw hat, move to the Gulf Coast of Florida, and mow lawns for people." • "I'm going to have a second career." • "That we're [husband and self] both still around where we can really just do things for ourselves." • "You have to have decided that you wanna do somethin' and successfully accomplish it." • "To kind of plan out my life, and to be able to achieve some of my . . . objectives . . . whether it be for myself or with other people." • "To have circumstances and the ability to make choices in your life; not to be in a position where you have to do something because you have no choice."
Adjusting	• "[Take] one day a time; get in there and do what needs to be done and tomorrow will take care of itself." • "There's just some things that you can't have control over. I could die of cancer in two years, and everything I'm telling you would probably change." • "Try to look at the positive aspect of every situation."

possible to exercise some direct influence over the world. We know from the MIDUS comparable sample data that the college-educated are more likely to experience such circumstances.

DISCUSSION AND CONCLUSION

Returning to the questions that motivated this chapter, we again ask what does it mean to experience well-being in America at midlife, and does it differ by education and gender? We focused on a subsample of MIDUS respondents (half high school–educated, half college-educated; half men, half women) who reported that they were currently experiencing moderate to high well-being. In terms of frequency of mention across respondents and the proportion of any one respondent's reflections to general open-ended questions about well-being, one answer stands out

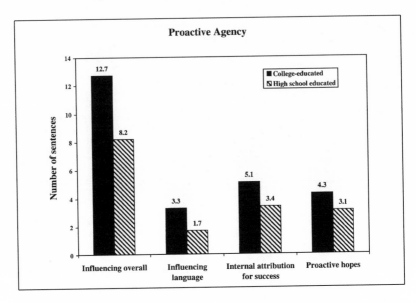

FIGURE 5. Proactive agency.

from the others. For American respondents 40–59 years old, across educational level and gender, there is a clear consensus that relations with others is the most important key to well-being. This answer emerges as the common answer in response to questions about what a good life is, why life has gone well, and what hopes respondents have for the future. Most often respondents talk about people who are part of their local, everyday worlds—parents, spouses, children, other family members, co-workers, and friends—rather than general others or the wider community. Other studies have also noted the importance of interpersonal aspects of well-being (Dowd 1990; Myers 2000; Ryff 1989b). These qualitative findings emphasizing the social nature of well-being are interesting in light of existing quantitative measures of well-being that give relatively little emphasis to the interpersonal realm (Diener et al. 1999; Ryff 1989a; Ryff and Keyes 1995).

The EDWB respondents also agree that well-being is strongly affected by having physical health, being able to enjoy oneself, and developing the self (feeling autonomous, feeling good about oneself, being open to new experience, feeling a sense of accomplishment, feeling fulfilled, and so forth). The American midlife well-being prescription includes a capacity to look on life events with peaceful and positive attitudes, in some cases with a faith in God. Finally, many respondents point out the importance of having a good job, financial security, and the chance to retire as part of the definition of a good life.

Although the respondents were basically in agreement about some aspects of what is desirable and important in life, the relative importance of key elements of well-being and the existence of distinct elements depend on level of education (which may be a proxy for socioeconomic class) and to some extent gender. The largest differences are that the college-educated more often mention the desire for enjoyment, and men are more likely than women to focus on job-related issues while women are more likely than men to be concerned with financial security and having basic needs met.

Further differences found in subcategories help to clarify why Americans with different levels of education report equally high levels of global life satisfaction despite marked differences in quality-of-life measures such as income, health, and early childhood experience. Detailed analysis of the form and content of their narratives reveals that respondents with different sociodemographic profiles take somewhat different routes to life satisfaction and well-being. These varying approaches to well-being are related to differences in the primary and extended social and structural worlds of respondents and, in turn, to differences in the sense of agency that develops as individuals engage in their relevant communities and societies. In other words, respondents whose worlds diverge from one another according to education or gender are realizing similar life satisfaction and positive affect (general assessments of overall well-being) in different ways.

Those with a college education engage others and their social environments in ways that diverge systematically from those with a high school education; members of these different groups have a different stance toward their worlds and their places within them. The well-being of those with a college education (feelings of positive affect and satisfaction with the various domains of life) reflects the nature of their "being," which includes a sense that one is influencing, choosing, planning, changing, or in some respects in charge or in control. Feelings of well-being among the high school–educated respondents are more likely associated with a sense of having adjusted, or having managed to do the "right" thing, or having survived and not given up.

Respondents with a college education emphasize that having a purpose, accomplishing their goals, seeking new opportunities, and enjoying themselves are the foundations of well-being and the life well-lived. They stress that their educational attainment and their own skills and abilities have contributed to their lives having gone relatively well. The narratives of their lives reflect a self that is structured by purpose and goals. They describe themselves as acting directly on the world and as being responsible for their lives having gone well. Relations with others are central, but they often emphasize the role of friends and characterize these relationships in terms of influencing, advising, and respecting one another.

The MIDUS sociodemographic variables such as health, income, and family relations provide insight into the lives of these college-educated respondents and suggest that the nature of their selves and well-being can be linked to the specific nature and extent of their connections to others. Compared with the high school–educated, the college-educated are in some senses "freer" from others and can focus on themselves. They are likely to have fewer demands made on them by family members who need immediate support, and they are more likely then to have both more time and resources to act on their own individual needs and preferences. In many cases, a college education may require an initial move away from home and may create the beginning of an extended social network in which friends become central and one encounters more diverse expectations and requirements from others. Moreover, the tasks and requirements of both a college education and the jobs and careers that are linked to them likely involve a relatively high degree of choice, planning, and decision-making, which in turn fosters a sense of self as relatively separate from others and a sense of agency as influencing, exercising control, and taking charge. As might be expected, the comparable college-educated MIDUS respondents scored higher than did the high school–educated respondents on those components of well-being that assess self-acceptance, personal growth, purpose, and environment mastery. Presumably, their social worlds afford them this way of being well.

Those with a high school education, in contrast, are more likely to be engaged in worlds where relatively more people are confronting serious illnesses, unemployment, and a variety of complex financial and family problems, either of their own or of their significant others. Moreover, these respondents have fewer resources of every type with which to confront these difficulties. The high school–educated respondents are aware of these difficulties and their relative positions in society. In the MIDUS survey, the high school–educated compared with the college-educated were significantly more likely to report not having had as many work opportunities as others, not being able to live in as nice a home or neighborhood as others, and feeling when they were growing up that "they were worse off financially than the average family." One high school–educated man said in his narrative about well-being,

> My quality 'a life is good. And it's simple. I mean, we don't go out a lot. . . . Couldn't afford it. . . . We do play a lot 'a board games at home. We have video games that we play. Or go out and rent movies instead of going to the movie theater at seven, eight bucks a pop. . . . So you don't see it right away, but in six months to a year they're all out anyway. So we do things like that. And that's a pretty good life . . . considering some of the people, what they go through, and they keep on going.

When characterizing their lives and their well-being, the high school–educated respondents do not focus on personal accomplishments, do not explain the course of their lives in terms of their own skills and abilities, and do not focus on enjoyment as key to the good life as often as college-educated respondents do. Instead, they tend to focus more on the role of their families, on financial security, and on jobs. Some suggest that Americans with less education are more concerned with religion and spirituality (Idler and George 1998), although this trend did not surface in the current analysis. The immediate contingencies associated with lives involving health-related physical limitations, financial constraints, and fewer opportunities for self-development (Dowd 1990) may well preclude the opportunity to focus on one's own interests and enjoyment. Instead, the needs and requirements of others are what seem to structure everyday life. Consistent with this suggestion is the observation that the high school–educated respondents are more likely to describe themselves as adjusting to the world, and they appear to experience themselves primarily as incorporating these expectations and obligations.

Given the social worlds of the high school–educated respondents, it is not surprising that they scored lower than the college-educated on scales of self-acceptance, personal growth, purpose, and environmental mastery.[4] Their social worlds do not afford or encourage a self-focused and influential way of being. Yet despite the self-reported difficult circumstances of their lives, these respondents also reported relatively high levels of well-being as indicated by general measures of life satisfaction and positive affect. Apparently they have found alternate paths to well-being. They have developed somewhat different means of maintaining relations with others and of attending to and understanding the self and one's actions in the world. It is a way of being well that is intimately tied to what these high school–educated respondents are doing in their lives and to the local norms for the "appropriate" or "good" way to be. In particular, well-being in high school–educated contexts involves being a good person, fulfilling duties, upholding responsibilities, and caring for others. For example, a high school–educated man said, "I'm not looking to be rewarded for what I do. I just think that . . . there are certain things in life everybody has to fulfill, and one thing is . . . to be able to take care of themselves and take care of others and be helpful and kind and generous and do it all with a moral attitude."

As we looked more closely at how these high school–educated respondents discussed their well-being, we found that their evaluations of their own well-being commonly appeared to be rooted in the standard set in one's immediate community—specifically, the community's expectations for the respondent, the respondent's own expectations for himself or herself, and the way one compares with others in a relevant community. Many respondents seemed to gauge their own well-being on the local expectations about educational attainment, financial status, positive family relationships, religious devotion, and other such keys to well-being. As one high school–educated woman offered, "I didn't have to deal with a lot of bad things during our kids' teenage years. Sometimes I think I just had it really well. I listen to other people, things that have happened to them and with their kids." A further analysis of these high school–educated respondents' ways of being well may provide some insight into how and why some people are more resilient in the face of challenge than others.

Which Way of Well-Being Is Best?

The observation of different pathways to well-being leads to a number of challenging questions. For instance, overall our respondents agree about the important aspects of well-being (positive relationships, opportunities to develop and enjoy oneself, physical health, financial security, job satisfaction), but does a sense of well-being for each individual require all of them, and if so, at what level? Our findings suggest, for example, that many people can develop a sense of well-being with only moderate financial resources, but it is clear that some minimal level of security is essential. As one woman explained, "having enough money that I don't have to eat potato skins any more, and that's not that much money."

Many other questions about diversity in well-being also remain to be answered. Can our high school–educated respondents' ways of being well afford them some measure of psychological or even physical resilience and the means for adjusting to the limitations imposed by their health and financial status? In contrast, will proactive college-educated Americans who suffer from an unexpected financial or physical loss be less resilient in the face of sudden and unfamiliar dependency (see Elder 1996)? Are the different ways of being well equally "good"? MIDUS and other studies reveal that high school–educated respondents are significantly more likely to have compromised health, finances, and opportunities to make their own choices (Heise 1990; Herzog et al. 1998; House et al. 1994; Marmot et al. 1997; Ryff et al. 1999; Ryff and Singer 1998). If the well-being style of the high school–educated respondents is not associated with an active healthy life, with longevity, with financial prosperity, with opportunities for choice and self-development, is it in some sense less "good"?

What criteria should be used to determine which is the "best" type of well-being? Level of physical health and longevity? Career and financial success? Number of daily opportunities for self-determination, freedom of choice, and personal development? Number of acts of social responsibility, extent of close relationships, or extent of recognition by one's community? Goodness of fit with the surrounding community's values, norms, and expectations? And what implications do these criteria have for social policy and social justice within American society?

Informing Current Measures of Well-Being

Finally, a major advantage of embedding the EDWB within the MIDUS is that we can ask how the results from each study compare with one another and how they both can inform existing well-being theories and measures. Specifically, how do these open-ended responses to "What does it mean to you to have a good life?" "What do you think are some of the reasons your life has gone well?" and "What are your hopes for the future?" compare with what we know about existing understandings of well-being from the MIDUS questionnaire measures of well-being? Overall, when using their own words, respondents generated most of the domains that have been identified and elaborated in various theories of well-being (relations with others, especially family, self-development, physical health, financial security, job satisfaction, enjoyment, and so forth). But their responses also suggest ways to expand current theories by incorporating newly recognized components of well-being. For instance, the self and its development surfaced frequently in answers to the questions about well-being. The scales of psychological well-being seem to capture most of what it is about the self that is important for well-being for the college-educated (purpose in life, personal growth, environmental mastery, self-acceptance); they are somewhat less good at capturing what it is for the high school–educated.

The narratives indicate that some previously identified domains merit further exploration and emphasis. For instance, the interview results indicated that relations with others (whether the other is a spouse, children, friend, or co-worker) is not just one category among others but instead the major source of the good life for nearly everyone at midlife. The role of other people in one's sense of well-being is the number one most frequently mentioned topic for every interview question discussed. Parents and spouses seem to be major causes of life going well, current family (especially one's spouse) is key to well-being in the present state of midlife, and hopes for one's offspring is a major focus for future well-being. Friends are emphasized more often by the college-educated, perhaps because they replace some of the roles typically played by family in lives that are less mobile or less distant. Because relations with others is such a salient feature of well-being and because it takes different forms, depending on the questions and respondent, perhaps additional scales involving relations with others warrant development for use in large surveys.

Several other domains that have not received much emphasis in existing scales of well-being, but that were frequently mentioned by these respondents, include faith, peace and satisfaction, a positive outlook, and a recognition that money does not guarantee a good life. Future well-being measures might consider adding such previously unidentified components of well-being. Weighting at least some of the different scales of well-being according to the norms, values, and expectations of the respondents' communities might also be explored. In addition, although these findings confirm observations that Americans are a determined, purposeful, and optimistic lot, it is also evident that a solid sense of well-being can be realized through active adjustment to others and to one's world, and without the feeling that one is always directly in control of one's actions.

Well-being is a dynamic and personal state, yet by examining respondents' own words along with their sociodemographic profiles, we begin to see the ways in which an individual's well-being is given form and substance by the prevalent meanings, practices, and institutions that configure the contexts in which people participate. Our analyses reveal that among Americans at midlife there exists considerable consensus about what it means to live a good life, which, presumably, reflects joint participation in national media and consumer culture. Further, our comparison between the college-educated and the high school–educated respondents reveals some systematic differences in ways of well-being that appear to reflect divergent understandings of what is good, what is self, and how individual action, or agency, is experienced. Additional research on how well-being varies according to education level as well as other such sociocultural parameters will continue to sharpen theories and measures of positive human functioning.

ACKNOWLEDGMENTS

Special thanks to undergraduate research assistants Christine Celio and Eno Sarris.

NOTES

1. All education levels and gender differences reported have *p* values less than or equal to .05 unless otherwise stated.

2. The terms "well-being," "being well," and "living a good life" are used interchangeably in this chapter. Although most of the interview discussions revolved around the term "well-being," some respondents were more comfortable with the less abstract phrase "living a good life." These different but related terms were designed to focus the interview on the positive aspects of life.

3. PEACE AND SATISFACTION included reports of feeling "calm" and "content," different from the more intense, elated emotions like "happy" and "having fun," which were coded as ENJOYMENT.

4. The high school–educated MIDUS comparable sample also scored lower on positive relations with others, yet the EDWB high school–educated respondents spoke often about how important relations with others are to well-being. The statements included in the scale asked specifically about the ease with which long-term, meaningful relationships are maintained. The high school–educated respondents may have scored lower on the scale because they indeed have had more difficulties with long-term relationships (e.g., they are significantly more likely to have been divorced and to have experienced health problems), or because "meaningful relationships" may imply spouse-like relationships that are "chosen" rather than relationships with kin and co-workers.

REFERENCES

Bellah, R. N., R. Madsen, W. M. Sullivan, A. Swidler, and S. M. Tipton. 1985. *Habits of the heart: Individualism and commitment in American life*. New York: Harper and Row.

Diener, E., and E. M. Suh, eds. 2000. *Culture and subjective well-being*. Cambridge: MIT Press.

Diener, E., E. Suh, R. Lucas, and H. Smith. 1999. Subjective well-being: Three decades of progress. *Psychological Bulletin* 125:276–302.

Dohrenwend, B. P., I. Levav, P. E. Shrout, S. Schwartz, G. Naveh, B. G. Link, A. E. Skodol, and A. Stueve. 1992. Socioeconomic status and psychiatric disorders: The causation–selection issue. *Science* 255:946–51.

Dowd, J. J. 1990. Ever since Durkheim: The socialization of human development. *Human Development* 33:138–59.

Elder, G. H. 1996. Human lives in changing societies: Life course and developmental insights. In *Developmental science*, ed. R. B. Cairns and G. H. Elder, 31–62. New York: Cambridge University Press.

George, L. K. 1992. Economic status and subjective well-being: A review of the literature and an agenda for future research. In *Aging, money, and life satisfaction: Aspects of financial gerontology*, ed. N. E. Cutler, D. W. Gregg, and M. P. Lawton, 69–99. New York: Springer-Verlag.

Gurin, P., and O. G. Brim, Jr. 1984. Change in self in adulthood: The example of sense of control. In *Life-span development and behavior*, ed. P. B. Baltes and O. G. Brim, Jr., 218–334. New York: Academic Press.

Heise, D. R. 1990. Careers, career trajectories, and the self. In *Self-directedness: Cause and effects through the life course*, ed. J. Rodin and C. Schooler, 59–84. Hillsdale, N.J.: Lawrence Erlbaum Associates.

Herzog, A. R., M. M. Franks, H. R. Markus, and D. Holmberg. 1998. Activities and well-being in older age: Effects of self-concept and education attainment. *Psychology and Aging* 13 (2): 179–85.

Hewitt, J. P. 1989. *Dilemmas of the American self*. Philadelphia: Temple University Press.

House, J. S., J. M. Lepkowski, A. M. Kinney, R. P. Mero, R. C. Kessler, and A. R. Herzog. 1994. The social stratification of aging and health. *Journal of Health and Social Behavior* 35:213–34.

Kessler, R. C. 1982. A disaggregation of the relationship between socioeconomic status and psychological distress. *American Sociological Review* 47:752–64.

Kessler, R. C., and P. D. Cleary. 1980. Social class and psychological distress. *American Sociological Review* 45:463–78.

Kohn, M. L., and C. Schooler. 1983. *Work and personality: An inquiry into the impact of social stratification*. Norwood, N.J.: Ablex.

Kubzansky, L., I. Kawachi, and D. Sparrow. 1999. Socioeconomic status, hostility, and risk factor clustering in the normative aging study: Any help from the concept of allostatic load? *Annals of Behavioral Medicine* 21 (4): 330–38.

Lachman, M., and S. Weaver. 1998. The sense of control as a moderator of social class differences in health and well-being. *Journal of Personality and Social Psychology* 74:763–73.

Link, B. G., M. C. Lennon, and B. P. Dohrenwend. 1993. Socioeconomic status and depression: The role of occupations involving direction, control, and planning. *American Journal of Sociology* 98:1351–87.

Markus, H. R., P. R. Mullally, and S. Kitayama. 1997. Selfways: Diversity in modes of cultural participation. In *The conceptual self in context: Culture, experience, self-understanding*, ed. U. Neisser and D. Jopling, 13–61. New York: Cambridge University Press.

Markus, H., C. Ryff, A. Conner, E. Pudberry, and K. Barnett. 2001. Themes and variations in American understandings of responsibility. In *Caring and doing for others*, ed. A. Rossi, 349–99. Chicago: University of Chicago Press.

Marmot, M., C. D. Ryff, L. L. Bumpass, M. Shipley, and N. F. Marks. 1997. Social inequalities in health: Converging evidence and next questions. *Social Science and Medicine* 44:901–10.

Marmot, M. G., G. D. Smith, S. Stansfeld, C. Patel, F. North, J. Head, I. White, E. Brunner, and A. Feeney. 1991. Health inequalities among British civil servants: The Whitehall II study. *Lancet* 337:1387–93.

Myers, D. G. 2000. The funds, friends, and faith of happy people. *American Psychologist* 55:56–67.

Oyserman, D., and H. R. Markus. 1993. The sociocultural self. In *The self in social perspective*, ed. J. Suls, 187–220. Hillsdale, N.J.: Lawrence Erlbaum Associates.

Rossi, A. S. 2001. Contemporary dialogue on civil society and social responsibility. In *Caring and doing for others: Social responsibility in the domains of family, work, and community*, ed. A. S. Rossi, 3–72. Chicago: University of Chicago Press.

Ryff, C. D. 1989a. Happiness is everything, or is it? Explorations on the meaning of psychological well-being. *Journal of Personality and Social Psychology* 57:1069–81.

———. 1989b. In the eye of the beholder: Views of psychological well-being among middle and old-aged adults. *Psychology and Aging* 4:195–210.

Ryff, C. D., and C. L. M. Keyes. 1995. The structure of psychological well-being revisited. *Journal of Personality and Social Psychology* 69:719–27.

Ryff, C. D., W. J. Magee, K. C. Kling, and E. H. Wing. 1999. Forging macro-micro linkages in the study of psychological well-being. In *The self and society in aging processes*, ed. C. D. Ryff and V. W. Marshall, 247–78. New York: Springer-Verlag.

Ryff, C. D., and B. Singer. 1998. The contours of positive human health. *Psychological Inquiry* 9:1–28.

Shweder, R. A. 1990. Cultural psychology: What is it? In *Cultural psychology: Essays on comparative human development*, ed. J. W. Stigler, R. A. Shweder, and G. Herdt, 1–46. Cambridge: Cambridge University Press.

CHAPTER ELEVEN

The Adaptive Value of Feeling in Control during Midlife

Margie E. Lachman and Kimberly M. Prenda Firth

Sense of control has been identified repeatedly as an important aspect of the self: "Sense of control is a pivotal contributor to a wide variety of behaviors and to both mental and physical well-being, which are essential elements of quality of life" (Abeles 1991, 297). Much of the previous research has focused on control in childhood and old age, with little attention paid to the period of midlife (Lachman 1986; Rodin, Timko, and Harris 1985; Skinner 1996). In this chapter we adopt a life-span developmental perspective and explore the manifestations and effects of control in middle adulthood relative to early and later adulthood. First, we present a brief overview of the sense of control as operationalized in MIDUS by using a multidimensional, multidomain conception. The findings we report from multiple studies consider control in relation to age, gender, and socioeconomic status as well as in relation to adaptive functioning and outcomes, including psychological and physical well-being, social relationships, and management processes. Across studies, control is examined as an outcome, an antecedent or predictor, a moderator, and a mediator variable. The findings consistently show that many aspects of control are maintained throughout the middle years and into old age. Moreover, the evidence demonstrates that having a sense of control over outcomes in key life domains helps one to negotiate challenges and demands and to minimize the negative consequences of declines and losses associated with aging.

There is consistent evidence that believing one has some degree of control over outcomes has powerful consequences (Rodin, Timko, and Harris 1985). Moreover, there are negative effects under circumstances when control is assumed to be lacking (Rodin 1986; Seligman 1991). The benefits of control have been identified across the life span (Bandura 1997; Skinner 1997), and control beliefs appear to play a particularly important role during later adulthood when losses begin to increase relative to gains (Baltes and Baltes 1986; Brandtstadter and Renner 1990; Brim 1992; Lachman 1986; Langer and Rodin 1976; Rodin 1986; Rodin, Timko, and Harris 1985; Rowe and Kahn 1987, 1997; Schulz, Heckhausen, and Locher 1991). Sense of control has been widely studied and operationalized in numerous ways (Abeles 1991; Rodin 1990; Skinner 1996). From the general, unidimensional conceptions of control (Rotter 1966) to multidimensional, dual-process operationalizations (Heckhausen and Schulz 1995; Levenson 1981), from global assessments (Rotter 1966) to domain-specific conceptualizations (Bandura 1997; Lachman 1986; Wallston and Wallston 1981), and from objective outcome expectancies (Weisz 1983) to phenomenological subjective perceptions (Skinner 1996), the definition of control has multiple variations.

This chapter presents an overview and integration of the MIDMAC findings on the sense of control by using several sources of data: pilot studies, the MIDUS survey, the Boston In-Depth Study of Management, and the Whitehall II study. In so doing, we address the following questions: How is the sense of control defined and assessed? What are the varied manifestations of the sense of control in midlife? How is a sense of control related to adaptive outcomes in midlife?

Definition and Measurement of Control Beliefs

Our conceptualization and measurement perspective focus on *perceived* control rather than on objective assessments of control. The sense of control, that is, the perception that one can influence what happens in one's life, includes beliefs or expectations about the extent to which one's actions can bring about desired outcomes. Two main sources of control can be distinguished: one's own efficacy (internal control or personal mastery), and the responsiveness of the environment or other people (external control or perceived constraints; Bandura 1997). Consistent with Skinner's (1996) twofold conceptualization of control in terms of competence and contingency, we included two control subscales referred to as personal mastery and perceived constraints (Lachman and Weaver 1998b). Personal mastery is defined as one's sense of efficacy or effectiveness in carrying out goals. Perceived constraints indicates to what extent one believes there are obstacles or factors beyond one's control that interfere with reaching goals. In the MIDUS survey, we included multiple measures of perceived control that were both generalized and domain-specific. The general control measure includes twelve items, seven of which are from Pearlin and Schooler's (1978) personal mastery scale. When we factor analyzed the personal mastery scale in our pilot work, we found two factors rather than one. Because one of the subscales had only two items, we developed and tested additional items to increase the reliability. The final version of the personal mastery subscale includes four items with a coefficient alpha of .70; the perceived constraints subscale includes eight items with a coefficient alpha of .86. The scales are moderately correlated in the negative direction (r (2998) $= -.40$, $p < .001$). In some cases, when there are no theoretically guided or empirically driven predictions about differential results for testing the two subscales separately, or when it is necessary for parsimony and data reduction, it is possible to combine the two subscales by recoding items in the same direction and creating a generalized, twelve-item control beliefs scale. This combined scale had a coefficient alpha of .85 in the MIDUS sample. Other conceptual distinctions have guided alternate ways to parcel the items. For example, it is possible to separate perceived constraints items into internal and external constraints subscales (Andreoletti, Zebrowitz, and Lachman 2001). In addition to personal mastery and perceived constraints, we assessed general control of life overall with one item (0–10 point scale).

The MIDUS battery also includes single-item assessments of control in six domains (work, finances, marriage, sex life, health, contribution to others) (McAvay, Seeman, and Rodin 1996; Lachman and Weaver 1998a). These domains were selected for MIDUS because they were considered key areas relevant to successful midlife development. Because of time and space constraints, we were unable to include multiple control items for each domain. Thus, the domain-specific assessments of control do not follow the same two-pronged conceptual framework just described. Instead they provide a unidimensional assessment of control for each domain. The question asks: "Using a 0–10 scale where 0 means no control at all and 10 means very much control, how would you rate the amount of control you have over your——these days?" For two of the domains, health and work, we also included more detailed assessments of control. Four additional health control items were included. For the health domain we asked participants to rate four statements on a seven-point scale, from strongly disagree to strongly agree: (a) Keeping healthy depends on things that I can do; (b) When I am sick, getting better is in the doctor's hands; (c) There are certain things I can do for myself to reduce the risk of a heart attack; and (d) There are certain things I can do for myself to reduce the risk of getting cancer. These items were not intended to comprise a subscale and were analyzed separately.

A work control scale was composed of items from the decision authority and skill discretion scales (Karasek and Theorell 1990). The scale for decision authority was computed from the following items: Please indicate how often each of the following is true of your job: (a) On your job, how often do you have to initiate things such as coming up with your own ideas, or figuring out on your own what needs to be done? (b) How often do you have a choice in deciding how you do your tasks at work? (c) How often do you have a choice in deciding what tasks you do at work? (d) How often do you have a say in decisions about your work? (e) How often do you have a say in planning your work environment, that is, how your workplace is arranged or how things are organized? and (f) In the past year, how often has the following occurred at your job? You control the amount of time you spend on tasks. We computed the scale for skill discretion from the following items: Please indicate how often each of the following is true of your job: (a) How often do you learn new things at work? (b) How often does your work demand a high level of skill or expertise? (c) How often does your job provide you with a variety of things that interest you? The decision/skills work control scale was computed as the mean for the skill discretion and decision authority scales (see Dauber and Lachman 2001).

AGE DIFFERENCES IN CONTROL BELIEFS

Previous studies investigating control beliefs in adulthood have concentrated on comparing young and older adults, with little consideration of the middle years; for the most part, these studies have used small, nonrepresentative samples. In the few studies that have included middle-aged adults, findings have been inconsistent. Some studies reveal no differences in control beliefs in middle age (e.g., Andrisani 1977; Brandtstadter and Rothermund 1994; Gatz and Siegler 1981), while others report an increased sense of internal control as one moves from young adulthood to middle age (Staats 1974), and sometimes more internal control is shown for elderly adults when compared with middle-aged adults (Lachman 1985).

Previous research on age differences in control beliefs suggests different outcomes as a function of domain (Bradley and Webb 1976; Brandtstadter and Rothermund 1994; Clark-Plaskie and Lachman 1999; Heise 1990; Huyck 1991; Lachman 1991). Domains that are more salient for a particular age group may take on a greater sense of importance and therefore have greater influence (beneficial or detrimental) on the perceived sense of control for that particular domain at different points in the life span (Lachman and Bertrand 2001)). For instance, previous research suggests that the importance of the work domain typically increases in midlife, especially for men (Clark-Plaskie and Lachman 1999;

TABLE 1 Means and Standard Deviations for Control

Control Dimension	Age Group			Gender	
	Young	Middle	Old	Men	Women
Personal mastery					
Mean	5.93	5.81	5.75	5.94	5.74
SD	.89	1.08	1.08	.94	1.09
Perceived constraints					
Mean	2.62	2.72	2.93	2.60	2.85
SD	1.13	1.31	1.43	1.22	1.33
Life overall					
Mean	7.68	7.75	8.16	7.84	7.79
SD	1.78	1.91	1.94	1.75	2.00
General control (unidimensional)					
Mean	5.56	5.46	5.29	5.57	5.34
SD	.93	1.07	1.13	.99	1.08
Finances					
Mean	6.29	6.64	7.08	6.70	6.51
SD	2.49	2.40	2.67	2.38	2.60
Sex					
Mean	7.21	6.68	5.67	6.39	6.95
SD	2.51	2.92	3.63	2.84	3.10
Contribute					
Mean	6.94	7.15	7.08	6.99	7.14
SD	2.47	2.43	2.79	2.55	2.48
Child					
Mean	8.44	7.44	6.93	7.52	7.65
SD	1.86	2.39	2.98	2.46	2.49
Marriage					
Mean	7.66	7.78	8.11	7.98	7.61
SD	2.16	2.14	2.13	1.96	2.33
Health overall					
Mean	7.81	7.58	7.53	7.69	7.61
SD	1.86	1.88	1.91	1.74	2.01
Do things to stay healthy					
Mean	6.41	6.41	6.21	6.40	6.34
SD	.98	.92	1.25	.99	1.05
Do things to reduce heart attack					
Mean	6.64	6.63	6.40	6.59	6.59
SD	.84	.81	1.15	.89	.92
Do things to reduce cancer					
Mean	5.89	5.92	5.72	5.85	5.89
SD	1.31	1.29	1.39	1.29	1.35
Getting better in doctor's hands					
Mean	3.41	3.85	4.66	3.76	3.98
SD	1.87	1.98	1.92	1.95	2.00
Work overall					
Mean	6.94	6.90	7.72	7.11	7.02
SD	2.38	2.71	2.91	2.61	2.70
Skill discretion and authority at work					
Mean	3.61	3.66	3.67	3.71	3.56
SD	.65	.68	.75	.68	.66

Dimensions, by Age Group, Gender, and Education

| | Education | | |
Less than High School	High School	Some College	Bachelor's or More
5.73	5.85	5.78	5.92
1.16	1.00	1.07	.94
3.43	2.89	2.72	2.36
1.57	1.29	1.24	1.07
7.74	7.92	7.69	7.87
2.28	1.94	1.91	1.64
4.95	5.35	5.45	5.73
1.21	1.02	1.04	.92
6.35	6.65	6.41	6.83
3.02	2.46	2.52	2.32
6.35	6.79	6.69	6.65
3.50	2.99	3.07	2.70
6.53	6.89	6.98	7.48
2.98	2.60	2.54	2.17
7.48	7.76	7.45	7.60
2.82	2.47	2.60	2.17
7.76	7.90	7.66	7.87
2.49	2.10	2.26	1.96
7.18	7.67	7.59	7.84
2.35	1.90	1.96	1.58
6.13	6.36	6.38	6.44
1.34	1.06	1.01	.86
6.22	6.61	6.58	6.70
1.38	.84	.90	.73
5.53	5.83	5.91	5.97
1.65	1.33	1.30	1.19
4.39	4.18	3.85	3.44
2.10	1.97	1.97	1.87
6.60	7.07	6.90	7.38
3.24	2.77	2.66	2.28
3.44	3.51	3.62	3.81
.78	.70	.67	.59

Howard and Bray 1988; Ryff 1989). Heise (1990) additionally contends that differences in sense of control within the work domain exist between young and middle-aged adults as a function of progress along the career path at different stages of the life course. Middle-aged workers, with their more developed networks and experiences on the job, may possess a greater sense of control over the work environment than do younger, less-seasoned workers. The MIDUS survey has allowed us to examine the sense of perceived control within specific domains of functioning and to shed light on some of the gaps in past research by investigating mechanisms that lead to more adaptive outcomes across the adult life course.

One advantage of MIDUS was that it enabled us to examine perceived control among middle-aged adults in comparison with that of younger and older adults by use of a large representative sample (Lachman and Weaver 1998a). Our findings revealed that although there were no age differences in a general sense of mastery, there were age-related increments in beliefs about external constraints; that is, older adults indicated facing more constraints than did members of the other age groups (see table 1). Interestingly, however, older adults reported greater perceived control for life overall than did the younger and middle-aged adults, despite the perception of increased perceived constraints.

MIDUS also provided an opportunity to examine perceived control within specific domains at various stages in the life span. When we compared young, middle-aged, and older adults, the findings revealed an upward age trajectory for work, finances, and marriage and a downward age trajectory for children and sex life (see table 1). With regard to the underresearched middle-aged group, we found that overall, middle-aged adults did not differ from younger adults in control over work, marriage, and life; however, they reported less control over their relationships with children and their sex life. Less control over sex life was associated with lower frequency of sexual relations. Control over children was associated with children's age. The older the children, the less control parents perceived. In the health domain, older adults generally had a lower sense of control than did the younger and middle-aged adults. Older adults reported less control over keeping healthy, avoiding a heart attack, and preventing cancer. Older adults also were more likely to believe that getting better is in the doctor's hands. The only domain in which middle-aged adults had higher control than younger adults was in the area of finances. For the domains that showed age-related increases in control, the middle-aged looked more like the younger adults than the older adults, with the exception of finances, for which they differed from both younger and older adults. For the relationships with children and sex life domains, which showed age-related decreases over the adult age span, the middle-aged had lower control than the younger adults but higher control than the older adults. Although older adults had the highest reported level of overall control in some domains, diminished control is acknowledged. The results could indicate that the domains included in the study were more appropriate and relevant to the lives of those in midlife. Perhaps older adults are able to maintain higher levels of general control by selecting compatible domains of functioning (e.g., leisure), which were not included in the MIDUS battery. MIDUS has allowed us to examine trajectories of perceived control for young, middle, and old-aged adults, indicating that with aging, adults are able to find ways to achieve an overall balance of control in their lives, despite perceptions of increased constraints.

Control Beliefs in Relation to Education and Gender

In addition to variations in control by age differences, we found variations in control by sex and education, although there were no interactions with age (Lachman and Weaver 1998a). In the MIDUS sample, we found that men had higher general control, with higher mastery and lower perceived constraints than women did (see table 1). This finding is consistent with past work in which men typically report an advantage regarding control (Feingold 1994). However, when looking within specific domains, we found that both men and women felt the least amount of control over their sex life and their finances and the most control over their marriage and life overall. Although women reported a higher sense of control over their sex life than did men, men reported a higher sense of perceived control over their marriage than did women. As for health, women were more likely to believe that getting better is in the doctor's hands, but there were no differences between genders in regard to the other health control variables.

When examining the influence of education on participants' perceived control, we found that higher levels of education were associated with fewer perceived constraints and greater control over health, work, finances, and making a contribution to the welfare of others. Those with more education also reported greater authority and use of skills at work. Results showed no differences in perceived control, among participants with different education levels, over sex life, children, marriage, personal mastery, or life overall. Those with more education experienced greater control over instrumental resources, which may account for the fewer constraints that they report. However, those with less education did not report less control in interpersonal relations. The feeling of control over interpersonal resources may contribute to an overall feeling of mastery, which did not differ by education. Educational differences were found in the health domain. Those with a college education were more likely to feel that they were in control of their health and were less likely to believe that getting better is in the doctor's hands. This is consistent with findings that individuals with higher socioeconomic status are more likely to take charge of their health and to engage in more health-promoting behaviors (Lachman, Ziff, and Spiro 1994). It is not possible, given the cross-sectional data, to determine whether a person's educational level leads to a greater sense of control because of more opportunities and resources or whether those who have a greater sense of control were the ones more likely to seek advanced education. Further work is needed to explore the association between control beliefs and education.

One of the challenges of midlife and the later years is to maintain a sense of control over life in the midst of the changing balance of gains and losses (Baltes and Baltes 1990). These beliefs may play a protective role in the face of such decrements. Maintaining a sense of control may help prevent or minimize declines associated with the aging process. Moreover, these beliefs may facilitate adaptive responses to declines. These findings led us to examine how control beliefs are related to physical and mental health and the mediational processes involved.

Control Beliefs and Well-Being

There has been much interest in examining well-being and control (e.g., Abeles 1991; Lachman and Weaver 1998b; Rodin 1986; Smits, Deeg, and Bosscher 1995). The findings consistently show a positive association between a sense of control and well-being (e.g., Bandura 1997; Brim 1992; Lachman 1986; Rowe and Kahn 1987, 1997; Schulz, Heckhausen, and Locker 1991; Skinner 1995). Examining the mechanisms and contexts in which multiple dimensions of control are related to adaptive or maladaptive outcomes can lead to a clearer picture of the nature of these associations. The MIDUS data set provided a rich set of biopsychosocial variables for testing hypotheses about the adaptive value of control beliefs.

A conceptual model is presented in figure 1 as a heuristic for examining the processes linking control beliefs and adaptive functioning during adulthood and old age. The model shows that sense of control has positive

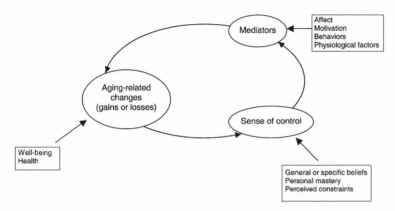

FIGURE 1. Conceptual model of the relationship between control beliefs and well-being.

effects on well-being and health through various mechanisms. These mediators can include affective, behavioral, and physiological factors. For example, control may lead to positive psychological states, such as high self-esteem and positive affect. Feeling in control may also lead to favorable neuroendocrine responses (e.g., low levels of stress hormones) as well as participation in health-promoting behaviors (e.g., exercise, healthy diet), which can minimize aging-related declines in health and promote psychological well-being. Those who believe they do not have control over outcomes would be less likely to experience positive feelings or to engage in adaptive behaviors. Consequently, health and well-being may suffer. The model is cyclical (Skinner 1997), suggesting that not only do control beliefs affect well-being but that feeling or doing well can also lead to an increased sense of control. The deterioration of a person's health could lead to further reductions in perceived control.

Recently, there has been some debate about the limits of the adaptive value of internal control beliefs (Colvin and Block 1994). Under some circumstances it is possible that control beliefs are detrimental. For example, having control may be a disadvantage if it is ultimately removed (Schulz and Hanusa 1978). In stressful situations, those with a view of the world as highly controllable and predictable may be particularly vulnerable when faced with an uncontrollable event such as widowhood (Wortman et al. 1992). However, there is also evidence that the sense of control is ultimately adaptive because it provides the motivation to cope and take action even in the face of great adversity (Taylor and Brown 1988), leading, ultimately, to greater well-being.

Given the unique qualities of the MIDUS data set, we were able to examine, across the adult life span, control beliefs in relation to a number of measures of well-being, including overall life satisfaction and depression. As expected, we found that those who had a higher sense of control had higher life satisfaction and lower depression (Lachman and Weaver 1998b).

Epidemiological studies have shown that sense of control along with social support are among the most important psychosocial predictors of morbidity, mortality, and psychological well-being in later adulthood (House, Landis, and Umberson 1988; Rodin 1986; Rowe and Kahn 1987, 1997). Less is known, however, about the relationship between control beliefs and subjective well-being during early and middle adulthood (Lachman and Weaver 1998b). Research investigations have shown a small but significant relationship between subjective well-being and health, especially in later life (Diener and Suh 1998). Education has been associated with subjective well-being (Marmot et al. 1997; Ryff and Singer 1998), but age and gender have typically shown little relationship with it (Myers and Diener 1995). Personality dispositions (e.g., neuroticism; Costa and McCrae 1994) as well as self-regulatory characteristics (e.g., control beliefs; Lachman and Weaver 1998b) have been found to show stronger relationships with subjective well-being than with sociodemographic characteristics (e.g., Staudinger, Fleeson, and Baltes 1999). However, little is known about whether these same factors are related to changes in subjective well-being.

Although, given the cross-sectional MIDUS design, we could not examine change directly, we were able to examine perceived trajectories of subjective well-being, that is, the direction of anticipated change in well-being over time (whether things are expected to get better, get worse, or stay the same). Using data from MIDUS and the pilot data collected in Germany ($N = 1000$; see Lachman, Staudinger, and Walen 2001) for a full description of the sample), we found evidence that control beliefs were related not only to subjective well-being but also to perceived trajectories of change in subjective well-being (Lachman, Staudinger, and Walen, forthcoming). This pattern was found in both the U.S. and German samples. A cluster analysis of life satisfaction that rated the past, present, and future revealed four perceived trajectories of change in subjective well-being for both samples: high stable, incremental, decremental, and present low. In the high-stable group, life satisfaction was relatively high and was expected to remain high. The incremental group saw life satisfaction as increasing from the past to the present to the future. The decremental group was characterized by lower life satisfaction in the present relative to the past and expected decline in the future. The present low group showed lower perceived satisfaction in the present relative to the past but expected improvement in the future. An examination of demographic and psychosocial predictors revealed control beliefs to account for the most variance in well-being trajectories for both the U.S. and German samples. Those adults who had a greater sense of control were more likely to have a high level of life satisfaction and to expect it to remain high or to assume that things would get better in the future. In contrast, those who had a lower level of control had a pattern associated with perceived decline or low present level relative to the past and future.

There has been some suggestion of nation-based differences in self-reports of subjective well-being (Cantril 1965; Diener and Suh 1998). Conceptions of both global and domain-specific control have also been suggested to vary across cultures in their importance as predictors of subjective well-being (Antonovsky 1979; Little et al. 1995; Staudinger, Fleeson, and Baltes 1999). For example, Staudinger, Fleeson, and Baltes (1999) found that perceived control over work and health was more strongly related to subjective well-being in Germany than in the United States.

Our results from both the U.S. and German samples show there are individual differences in expected trajectories of perceived subjective well-being. The typologies identified by use of cluster analysis represent variations from what would have been observed by examining only group means at each time perspective. Although the largest percentages were found in the high-stable group for both samples, 32 percent of the U.S. sample and 63 percent of the German sample fell into other typologies,

TABLE 2 Correlations for Sense of Control and Health Variables

	Health Variables			
Control Variables	Acute Symptoms	Chronic Problems	Functional Limitations	Health Rating
Personal mastery	−.18	−.16	−.15	.13
Perceived constraints	.36	.30	.30	−.31
Health control	−.32	−.33	−.35	.41
Can keep healthy	−.12	−.11	−.20	.16
Doctor control	.05	.09	.12	.13
Heart attack control	−.07	−.08	−.14	.08
Cancer control	−.08	−.08	−.13	.10

Note: All correlations are significant at $p < .01$.

TABLE 3 Correlations for Sense of Control,

Variable	1	2	3
1. Age	—	−.04	.18**
2. Education	−.19**	—	−.10**
3. Waist–hip ratio	.18**	−.25**	—
4. Body mass index	.15**	−.14**	.44**
5. Can keep healthy	−.03	.12**	−.08**
6. Heart attack control	−.10**	.17**	−.10**
7. Beyond my control	.19**	−.15**	.05
8. Exercise	−.30**	.17**	−.14**

Note: Correlations for men ($N = 1257$) are presented on the top half of diagonal; for women ($N = 1273$) on the bottom half.
*$p < .05$. **$p < .01$.

TABLE 4 Correlations for Sense of Control, Health

Variable	1	2	3
1. Age	—	−.09**	.20**
2. Grade	.29**	—	.10**
3. Waist–hip ratio	.23**	.19**	—
4. Body mass index	.14**	.16**	.55**
5. Can keep healthy	.02	.05*	−.07**
6. Heart attack control	−.06**	−.02	−.07**
7. Beyond my control	.16**	.19**	.05*
8. Exercise	−.21**	−.15**	−.14**
9. Diet	.04	.27**	.11**

Note: Correlations for men ($N = 5149$) are presented on the top half of diagonal; for women ($N = 2246$) on the bottom half.
*$p < .05$. **$p < .01$.

indicating that perceived changes in subjective well-being are prevalent. The findings also shed light on psychosocial, health, and demographic factors that are associated with the different portraits of subjective well-being in adulthood. Nonpsychological predictors were more important with regard to trajectory type than usually is the case when predicting current subjective well-being. Cluster membership was associated with health, age, and education. Those in the stable or incremental subjective well-being trajectories were healthier, younger, and more educated.

These findings suggest that general control beliefs are strongly related to evaluative temporal patterns of the self in both Americans and Germans. Although past studies have found a robust relationship between control beliefs and concurrent well-being, the present study expands these findings to demonstrate how control relates to expected trajectories of well-being during adulthood. Having a sense of control may lead to positive affect, which helps one to appraise and respond to stress in a more

Health Behavior, and Health in the MIDUS Sample

4	5	6	7	8
.10**	.07*	−.05	.06*	−.21**
−.05	.02	.07*	−.10**	.12**
.41**	−.04	.00	.07*	−.08**
—	.03	.02	−.03	.01
−.07*	—	.60**	−.10**	.07*
−.05	.62**	—	−.08**	.09**
.05	−.13**	−.12**	—	−.09**
−.14**	.10**	.09**	−.10**	—

Behaviors, and Health in the Whitehall II Sample

4	5	6	7	8	9
.06**	.03*	.01	.01	−.08**	−.07**
.04**	−.01	−.04**	.15**	−.12**	.24**
.63**	−.02	−.05**	.001	−.13**	.09**
—	−.01	−.03	−.01	−.05**	.06**
−.04*	—	.49**	−.10**	.12**	−.09**
−.03	.48**	—	−.08**	.11**	−.15**
.04*	.01	.03	—	−.05**	.08**
−.12**	.09**	.11**	−.08**	—	−.09**
.03	−.10**	−.14**	.10**	−.09**	—

positive proactive way. Feeling in control of outcomes also gives one increased hope about the future and motivation to remain active.

CONTROL BELIEFS AND PHYSICAL HEALTH

Sense of control has also commonly been associated with positive physical health outcomes (e.g., Baltes and Baltes 1986; Cohen 1990; Menec and Chipperfield 1997) and adjustment to health problems (e.g., Reed, Taylor, and Kemeny 1993; Thompson et al. 1993). However, contradictory findings suggest that an overemphasis on seeking control can have detrimental effects on physical and mental health (Lachman and Burack 1993; Thompson, Cheek, and Graham 1988). For instance, type A personality behavior patterns and coronary heart disease have been shown to be related to a strong need for control (Strickland 1978).

In previous research, sense of control has been primarily studied in relation to subjective ratings of health. With MIDUS, however, we were able to investigate its relationship with perceived health as well as with more objective measures of health, such as number of chronic and acute symptoms and functional limitations (Lachman and Weaver 1998b). Beliefs about control were associated with health status (see table 2, above on p. 331). Those who had a greater sense of control had fewer acute and chronic illnesses and had higher functional status.

In addition, we examined waist–hip ratio and body mass index, which have been shown to be related to cardiovascular health (Lachman et al. 2000; see above, tables 3 and 4). We used data from MIDUS and Whitehall II to test a mediational model and examined differences by gender. We expected control beliefs to affect health outcomes through their influence on health-promoting behaviors, including frequency and intensity of exercise (in both data sets) and dietary behavior (Whitehall II data). We found that control beliefs were related to waist–hip ratio in MIDUS and Whitehall samples. When a mediational model was tested, there was support for the prediction that control beliefs are related to health because of their influence on exercise and healthy diet. Those women who reported a greater sense of perceived control over general health and specifically over heart disease were more likely to engage in regular vigorous exercise. This relationship between control and waist–hip ratio was mediated by exercise behavior. For men, those who felt there were many factors beyond their control were less likely to exercise and had lower waist–hip ratios.

In Whitehall, similar results were found. Among women the belief that there are things they can do to keep healthy and among men the belief that they can control a heart attack were associated with engaging in more exercise and healthier diet. In turn, this was related to a lower waist–hip ratio. Although body mass index showed a small relationship with control beliefs, this relationship was not mediated by health behaviors. The results suggest that those who feel more in control of their health are more likely to engage in health-promoting behaviors such as exercise, which in turn affects health in terms of the waist–hip ratio. Further research is needed to articulate the mediational processes involved.

Control Beliefs, Social Class, and Health

Previous research examining the effects of social class on sense of control suggests that those with less education and lower income have a lower sense of control, both in terms of their own personal efficacy and the belief that powerful others control their destiny (e.g., Gurin and Brim 1984; Lachman 1985). Fewer opportunities to experience the relationship between self-motivated actions and positive outcomes may have a detrimental effect on sense of control for people within lower social classes (Lachman and Weaver 1998b). Using the MIDUS data set, we were able to examine this relationship. Consistent with previous research (e.g., Gurin and Brim 1984; Lachman 1985), we found evidence that those who had lower incomes had a lower sense of personal mastery and a higher level of perceived constraints than did those with higher incomes (Lachman and Weaver 1998b). Nevertheless, the variability within income groups was high, and the distributions were overlapping. We were interested to examine whether these differences in control within groups would be associated with positive adaptation in terms of psychological and physical health.

Social class differences in physical health have been widely recognized. The social class gradient exists at all levels of the socioeconomic status hierarchy (Adler et al. 1994; Marmot et al. 1991), and more recent attention has been focused on the implications of psychosocial variables for social class (Adler et al 1994; Mirowsky, Ross, and Van Willigen 1996). Using data from MIDUS and two nationally representative samples selected for MIDUS pilot studies, we were able to examine the interacting and moderating influences of sense of control on social class differences in physical health and well-being (Lachman and Weaver 1998b). Although there are social class differences in control, some persons in lower social class groups show a relatively high sense of control. We found evidence to support our prediction that those in the lower social class groups who had a higher sense of control would have physical health comparable to those in the higher social classes. Control beliefs had a moderate relationship to health in the higher social class groups but a stronger relationship in the lower class groups.

There were convergent findings from the three national samples regarding social class differences in the sense of control, the relationship between control and health, and the moderating role of control beliefs. Those in lower-income groups indeed had lower levels of perceived mastery and stronger beliefs in the existence of external constraints in their lives. To some extent these differences may be realistic and reflective of the actual variations in life situations among social class groups. Just as important as these differences between groups, however, were the large within-group differences. The variability within groups was comparable, as evidenced by the standard deviations, and the group distributions were overlapping. Thus, there are some with lower incomes who have high levels of mastery beliefs and low levels of perceived constraints. At the same time, some in the higher-income groups have a low sense of control. One interesting focus for future work is to look at the possible antecedents of control beliefs in these different social class groups. It will be interesting to investigate how some in the lower social class groups come to develop and maintain a strong sense of control, both in terms of personal mastery and low perceived constraints, in the face of economic adversity.

What about the adaptive value of the sense of control? Does it vary by social class group? Overall, the findings suggest that a high sense of mastery and a belief in low external constraints are beneficial for all social class groups. Those with higher mastery and lower perceived constraints had better health. These relationships varied somewhat by social class. There was no evidence, however, that high mastery and low perceived constraints were detrimental for the lower-income groups. Of particular interest, control was found to play a moderating role, with even greater benefit for lower-income groups. For the higher social class groups, health and well-being were generally high and showed less variation as a function of level of control than they did in the other social class groups. In contrast, for lower social class groups, level of control mattered. The results demonstrated that those in the lower social class groups who managed to maintain a high sense of control resembled their higher social class counterparts more than they did others in their own income group. Thus, control beliefs appear to serve as a buffer for the negative ramifications of low social class in regard to health and well-being. Those with a greater sense of control may be more likely to engage in health-promoting behaviors and seek medical attention or social support to prevent or alleviate health problems. Of course, it is also important to recognize that health can have an impact on control beliefs. Given that the MIDUS data are cross-sectional, we were not able to test a longitudinal or reciprocal model. Nevertheless, it is likely that those who experience health problems in midlife may as a result feel less in control of their life.

SOCIAL RELATIONSHIPS AND CONTROL BELIEFS

Recent findings, both longitudinal (e.g., Berkman 1984; Seeman et al. 1995) and cross-sectional (e.g., Cohen and Wills 1985; Rodin and Timko 1992; Taylor 1995), suggest that positive social networks increase both psychological well-being and physical health. Lachman, Ziff, and Spiro (1994) found that people reporting high levels of control had more positive health outcomes regardless of their level of social support. However, of the individuals who reported lower levels of control, those reporting higher levels of social support evidenced more positive outcomes, which suggests a buffering effect of social support for people with lower perceived control.

Recent research has begun to examine the negative aspects of social relationships such as social strain (e.g., Ingersoll-Dayton, Morgan, and Antonucci 1997; Rook 1992). Social strain has been found to be more strongly predictive of chronic physical health problems than is social support (Ewart et al. 1991; Keicolt-Glaser et al. 1984), even when controlling for prior depression and personality traits such as neuroticism and extraversion (Walen and Lachman 2000). Using the adults who were married or cohabitating in the MIDUS sample, Walen and Lachman (2000) examined the relationship between social exchanges, and well-being and health. Social support and strain were examined for the following relationships: family, friends, and spouse/partner. Each relationship domain was assessed by four questions, on the basis of a four-point scale (ranging from "not at all" to "a lot"). Items included "How much does your spouse or partner (friends, family members) really care about you?" and "How much can you rely on them for help if you have a serious problem?" The findings indicated that the partner relationship was an important predictor of well-being for both genders and that family relationships had more of an effect for women than for men. The younger and middle-aged adults were more adversely affected by strained friendship networks than were the old. Partner and family strain were the most important predictors of poor health, especially for middle-aged women (Walen and Lachman 2000). When the "big five" personality traits were included in the model, the effects of social support on health were reduced but still remained significant.

In a follow-up study, Walen (forthcoming) examined personal control beliefs in relation to social exchanges and well-being across the adult life span. Previous research has found that social support and control beliefs are consistent as key psychosocial variables predicting health in adulthood (House, Landis, and Umberson 1988; Rodin, Timko, and Harris 1985). Although social support and control beliefs are related, there has been little attempt to understand the nature of the relationship or the way in which these two variables affect health. Walen (2001) found that control beliefs mediated the relationship between social exchanges and health. The nature of the relationship varied by age and gender as well as by type of relations. The mediational model was supported for the young and middle-aged adults but not for the older adults. For middle-aged adults, partner strain, friend support, and family strain and support were related to subjective well-being and health through their effects on sense of control. The effects of friend support on subjective well-being were mediated by control for both men and women. The effects of family support and strain on subjective well-being were mediated by control for women but not men. The effects of partner strain on subjective well-being and health were also mediated by control for women. These results show that the nature of social relationships can affect feelings of control, which in turn affect health and well-being. The effects of strain from family and partner had a particularly damaging effect on health for women, in part because stressful relationships diminish their sense of control.

CONTROL BELIEFS AND MANAGEMENT PROCESSES

Planning, as a life management process, and its relationship to perceived control have rarely been investigated (for exceptions, see Aspinwell 1997; Lachman and Burack 1993; Scholnick and Friedman 1993; Skinner 1997). Although planning can be seen as one way in which people control and manage their lives, it is not considered a necessary condition for control (Lachman and Burack 1993); in fact, it has even been suggested that too much planning can have a detrimental effect on control (Lachman and Burack 1993; Thompson, Cheek, and Graham 1988). Even so, effective planning has been shown to have positive implications for control and life satisfaction (e.g., Aspinwell 1997; Lachman and Burack 1993; Macan 1994; Skinner 1997), and previous research investigating planning and well-being, a significant correlate of control, generally supports a positive, reciprocal relationship between the two (Brandtstadter and Baltes-Gotz 1990; Burack and Lachman 1995; Eronen, Nurmi and Salmela-Aro 1997; Macan et al. 1990). Much of the past work, however, has been done with children, and few studies have considered multiple antecedents simultaneously. Therefore, MIDUS provided an ideal opportunity to advance our understanding of the relationship between planning, perceived control, and life satisfaction across adulthood, using a nationally representative sample.

Existing process models suggest antecedents and outcomes for the life-planning domain (Little 1983; Nurmi 1989; Cantor 1990). Friedman and Scholnick (1997) present a theoretical model illustrating how antecedent variables such as environment (social support, predictability), cognition (working memory, reasoning), and personality/motivation (individual personality variables, stress) impact an individual's ability to plan and the effectiveness of their planning. We investigated (a) multiple antecedents of planning styles and (b) the relationship of planning to perceived control and life satisfaction during adulthood. Further, we investigated a mediational model of planning, control, and life satisfaction (Prenda and Lachman 2001). We also examined the effect that planning had on

338

perceived control in midlife, when work and family roles are most demanding (Barnett 1997; Lachman and James 1997).

To enable replication and extension of results, we used two separate samples. Participants of study 1 were from the MIDUS sample. The participants of study 2 were 302 adults from the MIDUS oversample in the greater Boston area (see Prenda and Lachman 2001 for a full description of the samples).

Using the Friedman and Scholnick (1997) model as a guide, we investigated antecedents of planning from the environmental, personality, motivation, and cognitive domains. We also investigated age, sex, education, and income as predictors of future planning. These variables were controlled when testing a mediational model of control and planning in predicting life satisfaction. Environmental measures included social support (from family, friends, and spouse/partner) and predictability ("good at predicting what is going to happen to me"). Personality/motivational measures included personality dimensions and stress. Personality was assessed by use of self-description scales for the big five (McCrae and Costa 1985) personality constructs of agreeableness, conscientiousness, extraversion, openness, and neuroticism (Lachman and Weaver 1997). Stress was measured using a multidimensional measure assessing stressful events for significant others and self-stress from the domains of health, work, and family. Cognitive measures (available for study 2 only) included working memory span, assessed using the WAIS Forward and Backward Digit Span (Wechsler 1981) and a counting backward task, and reasoning, measured by the Advanced Progressive Matrices (Raven, Court, and Raven 1994) and the Schaie-Thurstone Letter Series test (Schaie 1985).

Planning was defined as the extent to which participants self-reported that they "planned for the future" as opposed to "living for today." A five-item, continuous scale (from "a lot" to "not at all") assessing planning was developed using the following items from the MIDI mail questionnaire: (1) "I like to make plans for the future"; (2) "I find it helpful to set goals for the near future"; (3) "I live one day at a time"; (4) "I have too many things to think about today to think about tomorrow"; and (5) "I believe there is no sense planning too far ahead because so many things can change." Perceived control was measured with the twelve-item scale assessing participants' perceived control (personal mastery, perceived constraints) over their current life. To assess life satisfaction, we constructed a four-item scale that assessed satisfaction with life overall, work, health, and family relationships (see Prenda and Lachman 2001 for a full description of all measures).

Multiple regression was used to assess the relationship between the identified precursor variables and future planning. Results revealed variations in planning by demographic, environmental, and personality indicators. Stressful events and cognitive factors were not significantly related to planning. Our findings revealed that sex, education, and income were positively predictive of planning for both studies. Men reported more future-oriented planning than did women, supporting findings by Burack and Lachman (1995) that women tend to be more short-term, or "list-making," planners than men. Future research considering men's and women's work and gender roles (Boswell 1981; Bouffard, Bastin, and Lapierre 1996; Mintz and Mahalik 1996; Weitz 1977) may shed some light on this finding. Work and family roles could influence men to take a more long-term, generalized planning approach, whereas women may focus more on the day-to-day logistics of raising a family and find short-term planning strategies more effective (Gilbert 1985). Those with higher education and income were more likely to plan for the future, which is consistent with past research (Nurmi 1992; Teahan 1958). Nurmi (1992) has found that more highly educated people expect negative (e.g., poor health) outcomes to be realized further off in the future. Thus, they may be more optimistic about what their future holds, which is likely to be reflected in increased future planning.

Predictability was also significantly related to future-oriented planning strategies, suggesting that uncertainty of future events may lead to decreased planning or a lack of effective planning strategies (Friedman and Lackey 1991). Personality also was found to play a role in planning. For example, those who were more conscientious and open to experience were more likely to report planning behavior. Finally, those who reported receiving more social support from friends and family were more likely to plan for the future. It is possible that significant others in their network are included in their future plans. In future research it will be interesting to examine the specific content of plans.

Another goal of the study was to examine the relationship between planning, control beliefs, and life satisfaction. Life satisfaction (a composite of well-being ratings for work, spouse, children, and in general) was positively associated with age, income, and personality. In addition, those who reported more future planning had higher life satisfaction. Moreover, an interaction between age and planning was found. Although older adults reported less future planning overall compared with that of younger age groups, the effects of planning on life satisfaction were most pronounced for older adults. Middle-aged participants, although feeling the pressures of the more day-to-day responsibilities placed on them in their roles as parents, spouses, bosses, and children of aging parents, among others (Lachman and James 1997), behave more like the young with respect to future planning; that is, they may still see the future as open to different possibilities for which they can and do plan. Moreover, planning may be an essential management strategy in the context of increased demands and responsibilities. Older participants, who reported the least amount of future planning, may do so as a compensatory mechanism in the process of maintaining well-being. By selectively focusing on the positive and possible realities of today, elderly respondents optimize their perceptions of well-being in spite of the reality of a more limited future (Baltes and Baltes 1990; Carstensen, Isaacowitz, and Charles 1999). Nevertheless, among the elderly, those who focused on planning for the future seem to maintain the highest levels of life satisfaction. The fact that age was positively predictive of life satisfaction—that is, the older the respondent, the higher the life satisfaction—lends support for the contention that older adults who are able to balance their focus on present and future are most successful.

Finally, we investigated the mediational effects of perceived control for planning when predicting life satisfaction. As expected, those who were future-oriented planners had a higher sense of control, and those with a higher sense of control had higher life satisfaction. We also found support for the mediational model in that the effects of planning and the planning–age interaction were no longer significant predictors of life satisfaction when control beliefs were included in the model. Thus, it appears that those who plan for the future may have greater well-being because it gives them a greater sense of control over their lives. Of course, given the cross-sectional nature of the data, we could not rule out alternate directional hypotheses. Nevertheless, the results are consistent with the interpretation that planning fosters a greater sense of control, which in turn increases well-being.

The findings of this study lend support to the Friedman and Scholnick (1997) model of planning, which suggests, among other things, a significant impact of environmental and personality antecedents on planning. Perhaps most importantly, however, these results indicate that future planning is related to life satisfaction and that the nature of this relationship varies by age. Those who were more future-oriented had greater life satisfaction, and this relationship was more pronounced for older adults, as evidenced by a significant age–planning interaction. If age-related patterns of future-time perspective can be altered (Carstensen, Isaacowitz, and Charles 1999), these findings could be useful in designing interventions to enhance outcomes for older adults. Encouraging older adults to continue to plan for the future, even in the face of its diminished temporality, may lead to a greater sense of control as well as greater life satisfaction.

These results not only lend further support for the idea that a greater sense of control is positively related to well-being but they begin to address the processes involved in planning and life management. The use of a multi-item, multidomain measure of planning may facilitate a more in-depth understanding of the planning process. Additionally, a closer examination of future planning by domain may reveal differences in planning strategies and outcomes between the middle-aged and younger participants. Although generally these data suggested no significant differences in the prevalence of future planning between the young and middle-aged groups, the domains in which they plan for the future may prove to be quite different and worthy of more thorough examination.

CONCLUSION

The MIDUS survey provided an opportunity to examine the sense of control in adulthood by using a multidimensional approach to assessment with a nationally representative sample. The sense of control has typically been studied with more highly selective volunteer samples. The MIDUS sample enabled comparisons by age, education, sex, and income. In addition, given the interdisciplinary nature of the data set, it was possible to investigate the relationship of control beliefs to other variables such as health and well-being. It was also possible to begin exploring the processes linking control to a wide range of outcomes. Control beliefs were considered as a mediator of the relationship between planning and well-being in the study of management processes. Control beliefs were found to be a moderating variable of the relationship between social class and health.

Although we were able to compare the results from the United States with those of two other Western countries, Germany and Great Britain, it is important to examine these relationships in other cultures, especially Eastern cultures. This may require inclusion of additional aspects of control such as primary and secondary control, which have been found to vary by culture. Having a strong sense of control may be less desirable and less adaptive for individuals in collective cultures such as Japan compared with those in westernized cultures (Markus and Kitayama 1991).

The present study found consistent evidence for the adaptive value of believing one is in control. Control was associated with better health and well-being for adults of all ages. There may be situations where believing one has control could have detrimental effects. For example, when circumstances are such that one cannot influence the outcome, accepting the lack of control may prove to be more adaptive. Nevertheless, we found clear patterns indicating the importance of control beliefs for well-being and health throughout adulthood. Although control beliefs may show declines in some areas during the course of aging, one indicator of successful adaptation may be the ability to select domains of functioning in which it is possible to maximize one's ability to control outcomes (Baltes and Baltes 1990). This strategic selection of life domains in itself may be a clear manifestation of one's ability to take control of the aging process.

ACKNOWLEDGMENTS

We appreciate the support from the National Institute on Aging, grant number AG17920, and the John D. and Catherine T. MacArthur Foundation, which enabled us to conduct the research and to write the chapter.

REFERENCES

Abeles, R. 1991. Sense of control, quality of life, and frail older people. In *The concept and measure of quality of life in the frail elderly*, ed. J. Birren, J. Rowe, and D. Deutschman, 297–314. San Diego: Academic Press.

Adler, N. E., T. Boyce, M. A. Chesney, S. Cohen, S. Folkman, R. Kahn, and L. Syme. 1994. Socioeconomic status and health: The challenge of the gradient. *American Psychologist* 49:15–24.

Andreoletti, C., L. Zebrowitz, and M. E. Lachman. 2001. Physical appearance and control beliefs in young, middle aged and older adults. *Personality and Social Psychology Bulletin* 27:969–81.

Andrisani, P. J., 1977. Internal–external attitudes, personal initiatives, and the labor market experience of black and white men. *Journal of Human Resources* 12:309–28.

Antonovsky, A. 1979. *Health, stress, and coping.* San Francisco: Jossey-Bass.

Antonucci, T. C., and J. S. Jackson. 1990. The role of reciprocity in social support. In *Social support: An interactional view,* ed. B. P. Sarason, I. G. Sarason, and G. R. Pierce, 173–98. New York: John Wiley.

Aspinwell, L. G. 1997. Planning and perceived control. In *The developmental psychology of planning: Why, how, and when do we plan?* ed. S. L. Friedman and E. K. Scholnick, 285–320. Mahwah, N.J.: Lawrence Erlbaum Associates.

Baltes, M. M. and P. B. Baltes. 1986. *The psychology of control and aging.* Hillsdale, N.J.: Lawrence Erlbaum Associates.

Baltes, P. B., and M. M. Baltes. 1990. Psychological perspectives on successful aging: The model of selective optimism with compensation. In *Successful aging: Perspectives from the behavioral sciences,* ed. P. B. Baltes and M. M. Baltes, 1–34. Cambridge: Cambridge University Press.

Bandura, A. 1997. *Self-efficacy: The exercise of control.* New York: Freeman.

Barnett, R. C. 1997. Gender, employment, and psychological well-being: Historical and life course perspectives. In *Multiple paths of midlife,* ed. M. E. Lachman and J. B. James, 325–43. Chicago: University of Chicago Press.

Berkman, L. S. 1984. Assessing the physical health effects of social networks and social support. *Annual Review of Public Health* 5:413–32.

Boswell, J. 1981. The dual-career family: A model for egalitarian family politics. *Elementary School Guidance and Counseling* 15 (3): 262–68.

Bouffard, L., E. Bastin, and S. Lapierre. 1996. Future time perspective according to women's age and social role during adulthood. *Sex Roles* 34:253–85.

Bradley, R. E., and R. Webb. 1976. Age-related differences in locus of control orientation in three behavior domains. *Human Development* 19:49–55.

Brandtstadter, J., and B. Baltes-Gotz. 1990. Personal control over development and quality of life perspectives in adulthood. In *Successful aging,* ed. P. Baltes and M. Baltes, 197–221. Cambridge: Cambridge University Press.

Brandtstadter, J., and Renner, G. 1990. Tenacious goal pursuit and flexible goal adjustment. Explication and age-related analysis of assimilative and accommodative strategies of coping. *Psychology and Aging* 5:58–67.

Brandtstadter, J., and K. Rothermund. 1994. Self-percepts of control in middle and later adulthood: Buffering losses by rescaling goals. *Psychology and Aging* 9:265–73.

Brim, O. G., Jr. 1992. *Ambition: How we manage success and failure throughout our lives.* New York: Basic Books.

Burack, O. R., and M. E. Lachman. 1995. The use and benefits of time management strategies in adulthood. Poster presented at the annual meeting of the American Psychological Association, New York.

Cantor, N. 1990. From thought to behavior: "Having" and "doing" in the study of personality and cognition. *American Psychologist* 45:735–50.

Cantril, H. 1965. *The pattern of human concerns.* New Brunswick, N.J.: Rutgers University Press.

Carstensen, L. L., D. M. Isaacowitz, and S. T. Charles. 1999. Taking time seriously: A theory of socioemotional selectivity. *American Psychologist* 54:165–81.

Clark-Plaskie, M., and M. E. Lachman. 1999. The sense of control in midlife. In *Life in the middle,* ed. S. L. Willis and J. D. Reed, 181–208. New York: Academic Press.

Cohen, S. 1990. Control and the epidemiology of physical health: Where do we go from here? In *Self-directedness: Cause and effects throughout the life course,* ed. J. Rodin, C. Schooler, and K. W. Schaie, 231–40. Hillsdale, N.J.: Lawrence Erlbaum Associates.

Cohen, S., and T. A. Willis. 1985. Stress, social support, and the buffering hypothesis. *Psychological Bulletin* 982:310–57.

Collins, N. L., C. Dunkel-Schetter, M. Lobel, and S. C. Scrimshaw. 1993. Social support and pregnancy: Psychosocial correlates of birth outcomes and postpartum depression. *Journal of Personality and Social Psychology* 65 (6): 1243–58.

Colvin, C. R., and J. Block. 1994. Do positive illusions foster mental health? An examination of the Taylor and Brown formulation. *Psychological Bulletin* 116 (1): 3–20.

Costa, P. T., Jr., and R. R. McCrae. 1994. Set like plaster? Evidence for the stability of adult personality. In *Can personality change?* ed. T. F. Heatherton and S. L. Weinberger, 21–40. Washington, D.C.: American Psychological Association.

Das, J. P., B. C. Kar, and R. K. Parilla. 1996. *Cognitive planning: The psychological basis of intelligent behavior.* New Deli: Sage Publications India.

Dauber, S. G., and M. E. Lachman. 2001. Physical appearance and perceived control over work. Manuscript. Brandeis University.

Diener, E., and M. E. Suh. 1998. Subjective well-being and age: An international analysis. In *Annual review of gerontology and geriatrics,* ed. K. W. Schaie and M. P. Lawton, 11:304–24. New York: Springer-Verlag.

Eronen, S., J. Nurmi, and K. Salmela-Aro. 1997. Planning oriented, avoidant, and impulsive social reaction styles: A person-oriented approach. *Journal of Research in Personality* 31:34–57.

Ewart, C. K., C. B. Taylor, H. C. Kraemer, and W. S. Agras. 1991. High blood pressure and marital discord: Not being nasty matters more than being nice. *Health Psychology* 10:155–63.

Feingold, A. 1994. Gender differences in personality: A meta-analysis. *Psychological Bulletin* 116:429–56.

Friedman, M. I., and G. H. Lackey. 1991. *The psychology of human control: A general theory of purposeful behavior.* New York: Praeger.

Friedman, S. L., and E. K. Scholnick. 1997. An evolving "blueprint" for planning: Psychological requirements, task characteristics, and social-cultural influences. In *The developmental psychology of planning: Why, how, and when do we plan?* ed. S. Friedman and E. K. Scholnick, 3–22. Mahwah, N.J.: Lawrence Erlbaum Associates.

Gatz, M., and I. C. Siegler. 1981. Locus of control: A retrospective. Paper presented at the American Psychological Association Convention, Los Angeles.

Gilbert, L. A. 1985. *Men in dual-career families: Current realities and future prospects.* Hillsdale, N.J.: Lawrence Erlbaum Associates.

Gurin, P., and O. G. Brim, Jr. 1984. Change in self in adulthood: The example of sense of control. In *Life-span development and behavior,* ed. P. B. Baltes and O. G. Brim, Jr., 6:218–334. New York: Academic Press.

Gurin, G., and P. Gurin. 1970. Expectancy theory in the study of poverty. *Journal of Social Issues* 26:83–104.

Hayes-Roth, B., and F. Hayes-Roth. 1979. A cognitive model of planning. *Cognitive Science* 3:275–310.

Heckhausen, J. and R. Schulz. 1995. A life-span theory of control. *Psychological Review* 102:284–304.

Heise, D. R. 1990. Careers, career trajectories, and the self. In *Self-directedness: Cause and effects throughout the life course,* ed. J. Rodin, 59–84. Hillsdale, N.J.: Lawrence Erlbaum Associates.

House, J. S., K. R. Landis, and D. Umberson. 1988. Social relationships and health. *Science* 241:540–45.

Howard, A., and D. W. Bray. 1988. *Managerial lives in transition: Advancing age and changing times.* New York: Guilford Press.

Hudson, J. A., B. B. Sosa, and L. R. Shapiro. 1997. Scripts and plans: The development of preschool children's event knowledge and event planning. In *The developmental psychology of planning: Why, how, and when do we plan?* ed. S. L. Friedman and E. K. Scholnick, 77–102. Mahwah, N.J.: Lawrence Erlbaum Associates.

Huyck, M. H. 1991. Predicates of personal control among middle-aged and young-old men and women in middle America. *International Journal of Aging and Human Development* 324:261–75.

Ingersoll-Dayton, B., D. Morgan, and T. C. Antonucci. 1997. The effects of positive and negative social exchanges on aging adults. *Journal of Gerontology* 524:S190–S199.

Karasek, R. A., and T. Theorell. 1990. *Healthy work: Stress, productivity, and the reconstruction of working life.* New York: Basic Books.

Keicolt-Glaser, J. K., W. Garber, C. Speicher, G. M. Penn, J. Holliday, and R. Glaser. 1984. Psychosocial modifiers of immunocompetence in medical students. *Psychosomatic Medicine* 461:7–14.

Lachman, M. E. 1985. Personal efficacy in middle and old age: Differential and normative patterns of change. In *Life-course dynamics: Trajectories and transitions, 1968–1985,* ed. G. H. Elder Jr. Ithaca, N.Y.: Cornell University Press.

———. 1986. Locus of control in aging research: A case for multidimensional and domain-specific assessment. *Psychology and Aging* 1:34–40.

———. 1991. Perceived control over memory aging: Developmental and intervention perspectives. *Journal of Social Issues* 47 (4): 159–75.

Lachman, M. E., and R. M. Bertrand. 2001. Personality and self in midlife. In *Handbook of midlife development,* ed. M. W. Lachman, 279–309. New York: John Wiley.

Lachman, M. E., and O. R. Burack. 1993. Planning and control processes across the life span: An overview. *International Journal of Behavioral Development* 162:131–43.

Lachman, M. E., and J. B. James. 1997. *Multiple paths of midlife.* Chicago: University of Chicago Press.

Lachman, M. E., M. Marmot, M. Shipley, and H. Walen. 2000. Control beliefs and health: Exercise and diet as mediators. Manuscript, Brandeis University.

Lachman, M. E., U. M. Staudinger, and H. Walen. 2001. Sense of control and perceived trajectories of subjective well-being in American and German adults. Manuscript, Brandeis University.

Lachman, M. E., and S. L. Weaver. 1997. The Midlife Development Inventory (MIDI) personality scales: Scale construction and scoring. Technical report. Brandeis University, Waltham, Mass.

———. 1998a. Sociodemographic variations in the sense of control by domain: Findings from the MacArthur studies of midlife. *Psychology and Aging* 13 (4): 553–62.

———. 1998b. The sense of control as a moderator of social class differences in health and well-being. *Journal of Personality and Social Psychology* 74:763–73.

Lachman, M. E., M. Ziff, and A. Spiro. 1994. Maintaining a sense of control in later life. In *Aging and quality of life,* ed. R. Abeles, H. Gift, and M. Ory, 6–132. New York: Sage.

Langer, E. J., and J. Rodin. 1976. The effects of choice and enhanced personal responsibility for the aged: A field experiment in an institutional setting. *Journal of Personality and Social Psychology* 34:191–98.

Levensen, H. 1981. Differing among internality, powerful others, and chance. In *Research with the locus of control construct,* vol. 1.*Assessment methods,* ed. H. M. Lefcourt, 15–63. New York: Academic Press.

Little, B. R. 1983. Personal projects: A rationale and method for investigation. *Environment and Behavior* 15:273–309.

Little, T. D., G. Oettinger, A. Stentsenko, and P. B. Baltes. 1995. Children's action control beliefs about school performance: How do American children compare with German and Russian children? *Journal of Personality and Social Psychology* 69:686–700.

Macan, T. H. 1994. Time management: Test of a process model. *Journal of Applied Psychology* 79:381–91.

Macan, T. H., C. Shahani, R. L. Dipboye, and A. P. Phillips. 1990. College students' time management: Correlations with academic performance and stress. *Journal of Educational Psychology* 82:760–68.

Markus, H., and S. Kitayama. 1991. Culture and the self: Implications for cognition, emotion, and motivation. *Psychological Review* 98:224–53.

Marmot, M. G., C. Ryff, L. Bumpass, M. J. Shipley, and N. F. Marks. 1997. Social inequalities in health: Next questions and converging evidence. *Social Science and Medicine* 44:901–10.

Marmot, M. G., G. D. Smith, S. Stansfeld, C. Patel, F. North, J. Head, I. White, E. Brunner, and A. Feeney. 1991. Health inequalities among British civil servants: The Whitehall II study. *Lancet* 337:1387–93.

McAvay, G. J., T. E. Seeman, and J. Rodin. 1996. A longitudinal study of change in domain-specific self-efficacy among older adults. *Journal of Gerontology: Psychological Sciences* 51B:243–53.

McCrae, R. R., and P. T. Costa. 1985. Comparison of EPI and psychoticism scales with measures of the five-factor model of personality. *Personality and Individual Differences* 6 (5): 587–97.

Menec, V. H., and J. G. Chipperfield. 1997. The interactive effect of perceived control and functional status on health and mortality among young–old and old–old adults. *Journal of Gerontology: Psychological Sciences* 52B:118–26.

Miller, G. A., E. Galanter, and K. H. Pribram. 1960. *Plans and the structure of behavior.* New York: Holt, Rinehart, and Winston.

Mintz, R. D., and J. R. Mahalik. 1996. Gender role orientation and conflict as predictors of family roles for men. *Sex Roles* 34:805–21.

Mirowsky, J., C. E. Ross, and M. Van Willigen. 1996. Instrumentalism in the land of opportunity: Socioeconomic causes and emotional consequences. *Social Psychology Quarterly* 594 (December): 322–37.

Myers, D. G., and E. Diener. 1995. Who is happy? *Psychological Science* 6:10–19.

Nurmi, J. E. 1989. Development of orientation to the future during early adolescence: A four-year longitudinal study and two cross-sectional comparisons. *International Journal of Psychology* 24:195–214.

———. 1992. Age differences in adult life goals, concerns, and their temporal extension: A life course approach to future-oriented motivation. *International Journal of Behavioral Development* 15:487–508.

Pearlin, L., and C. Schooler. 1978. The structure of coping. *Journal of Health and Social Behavior* 19:2–21.

Prenda, K. M., and M. E. Lachman. 2001. Planning as a life management strategy in adulthood: Implications for perceived control and life satisfaction. *Psychology and Aging* 16:206–16.

Raven, J. C., J. H. Court, and J. Raven. 1994. *Raven manual.* Section 4. *Advanced progressive matrices.* 4th ed. Oxford: Oxford Psychologist Press.

Reed, G. M., S. E. Taylor, and M. E. Kemeny. 1993. Perceived control and psychological adjustment in gay men with AIDS. *Journal of Applied Social Psychology* 23:791–824.

Rodin, J. 1986. Health, control, and aging. In *The psychology of control and aging,* ed. M. M. Baltes and P. B. Baltes, 139–66. Hillsdale, N.J.: Lawrence Erlbaum Associates.

————. 1990. Control by any other name: Definitions, concepts, and processes. In *Self-directedness: Cause and effect throughout the life course,* ed. J. Rodin, C. Schooler, and K. W. Schaie, 1015. Hillsdale, N.J.: Lawrence Erlbaum Associates.

Rodin, J., and C. Timko. 1992. Sense of control, aging, and health. In *Aging, health, and behavior,* ed. M. E. Ory and R. P. Abeles, 172–206. Newbury Park, Calif.: Sage.

Rodin, J., C. Timko, and S. Harris. 1985. The construct of control: Biological and psychosocial correlates. In *Annual review of gerontology and geriatrics,* ed. C. Eisdorfr, M. P. Lawton, and G. L. Maddox, 3–55. New York: Springer-Verlag.

Rook, K. 1992. Detrimental aspects of social relationships: Taking stock of an emerging literature. In *The meaning and measurement of social support,* ed. H. O. Veiel and U. Baumann, 157–69. New York: Hemisphere.

Rothbaum, F., J. R. Weisz, and S. S. Snyder. 1982. Changing the world and changing the self. *Journal of Personality and Social Psychology* 42:5–37.

Rotter, J. B. 1966. Generalized expectancies for internal versus external control of reinforcement. *Psychological Monographs* 80, whole no. 609.

Rowe, J. W., and R. L. Kahn. 1987. Human aging: Usual and successful. *Science* 237:143–49.

————. 1997. Successful aging. *Gerontologist* 37 (4): 433–40.

Ryff, C. D. 1989. In the eyes of the beholder: Views of psychological well-being among middle-aged and older adults. *Psychology and Aging* 4 (2): 195–210.

Ryff, C. D., and B. H. Singer. 1998. Middle age and well-being. In *Encyclopedia of mental health,* ed. H. S. Friedman, 707–19. San Diego: Academic Press.

Schaie, K. W. 1985. *Manual for the Schaie-Thurstone Adult Mental Abilities Test STAMAT.* Palo Alto, Calif.: Consulting Psychologists Press.

Scholnick, E. K., and S. L. Friedman. 1993. Planning in context: Developmental and situational considerations. In *Planning and control processes across the life span,* ed. M. E. Lachman, 145–67. East Sussex, U.K.: Lawrence Erlbaum Associates.

Schulz, R., and B. H. Hanusa. 1978. Long-term effects of control and predictability-enhancing interventions: Findings and ethical issues. *Journal of Personality and Social Psychology* 36 (11): 1194–1201.

Schulz, R., J. Heckhausen, and J. L. Locher. 1991. Adult development, control, and adaptive functioning. *Journal of Social Issues* 47:177–96.

Seeman, T. E., L. F. Berkman, P. A. Charpentier, D. G. Blazer, M. S. Albert, and M. E. Tinetti. 1995. Behavioral and psychosocial predictors of physical performance: MacArthur studies of successful aging. *Journal of Gerontology* 504:M177–M183.

Seligman, M. E. P. 1991. *Learned optimism.* New York: Knopf.

Skinner, E. A. 1995. *Perceived control, motivation, and coping.* Thousand Oaks, Calif.: Sage.

————. 1996. A guide to constructs of control. *Journal of Personality and Social Psychology* 17:549–70.

————. 1997. Planning and perceived control. In *The developmental psychology of planning: Why, how, and when do we plan?* ed. S. L. Friedman and E. K. Scholnick, 263–84. Mahwah, N.J.: Lawrence Erlbaum Associates.

Smits, C. H., D. J. Deeg, and R. J. Bosscher. 1995. Well-being and control in older persons: The prediction of well-being from control measures. *International Journal of Aging and Human Development* 40 (3): 237–51.

Staats, S. 1974. Internal versus external locus of control for three age groups. *International Journal of Aging and Human Development* 5:7–10.

Staudinger, U. M., W. Fleeson, and P. B. Baltes. 1999. Predictors of subjective physical health and global well-being during midlife: Similarities and differences between the U.S. and Germany. *Journal of Personality and Social Psychology* 76 (2): 305–19.

Strickland, B. R. 1978. Internal–external expectancies and health-related behaviors. *Journal of Consulting and Clinical Psychology* 46:1192–11.

Taylor, S. E. 1995. *Health psychology.* 3d ed. New York: McGraw Hill.

Taylor, S. E., and J. D. Brown. 1988. Illusion and well-being: A social psychological perspective on mental health. *Psychological Bulletin* 103 (2): 193–210.

Teahan, J. E. 1958. Future time perspective, optimism, and academic achievement. *Journal of Abnormal and Social Psychology* 57:379–80.

Thompson, S. C., P. R. Cheek, and M. A. Graham. 1988. The other side of perceived control: Disadvantages and negative effects. In *The social psychology of health,* ed. S. Spacapan and S. Oskamp, 69–93. Newbury Park, Calif.: Sage.

Thompson, S. C., A. Sobolew-Shubin, M. E. Galbrith, L. Schwankovsky, and D. Cruzen. 1993. Maintaining perceptions of control: Finding perceived control in low-control circumstances. *Journal of Personality and Social Psychology* 64:293–304.

Walen, H. Forthcoming. Social exchange, control beliefs, and health in adulthood: A test of factorial invariance and an examination of a mediational model.

Walen, H., and M. E. Lachman. 2000. Social support and strain from partner, family, and friends: Costs and benefits for men and women. *Journal of Social and Personal Relationships* 17:5–30.

Wallston, K. A., and B. S. Wallston. 1981. Health-related locus of control scales. In *Research with the locus of control construct,* vol. 1. *Assessment methods,* ed. H. M. Lefcourt, 189–243. New York: Academic Press.

Wechsler, D. 1981. *Wechsler adult intelligence scale, revised.* New York: Psychological Corporation.

Weisz, J. R. 1983. Can I control it? The pursuit of veridical answers across the life span. In *Life-span development and behavior,* ed. P. B. Baltes and O. G. Brim, 5:233–300. New York: Academic Press.

Weitz, S. 1977. *Sex roles: Biological, psychological, and social foundations.* New York: Oxford University Press.

Wortman, C. B., C. Sheedy, V. Gluhoski, and R. Kessler. 1992. Stress, coping, and health: Conceptual issues and directions for future research. In *Hostility, coping and health,* ed. H. S. Friedman, 227–56. Washington, D.C.: American Psychological Association.

CHAPTER TWELVE

Social Well-Being in the United States: A Descriptive Epidemiology

Corey L. M. Keyes and Adam D. Shapiro

This chapter investigates the prevalence and the epidemiology of social well-being in the United States using the 1995 MIDUS data. Social well-being is defined as an individual's self-report of the quality of his or her relationship with other people, the neighborhood, and the community (Keyes 1998; Larson 1993). What is unique to the MIDUS study is that social well-being is operationalized as an individual's perceptions of his or her integration into society, of his/her acceptance of other people, of the coherence of society and social events, of a sense of contribution to society, and of the potential and growth of society.

In 1948, the World Health Organization identified social well-being as one of several facets of an individual's overall health. However, the construct of social well-being is often equated with social indicators that are operationalized by economic measures (e.g., the Gross Domestic Product, the poverty rate) that reflect the "health" of narrow sectors of society (see, e.g., Andrews and Withey 1976; Bell and Olson 1969). According to Larson (1996, 186), "The key to deciding whether a measure of social well-being is part of an individual's health is whether the measure reflects *internal* responses to stimuli—feelings, thoughts and behaviors reflecting satisfaction or lack of satisfaction with the social environment." From this standard, the MIDUS social well-being scales are measures of a notable but understudied facet of an *individual's* health.

This chapter therefore investigates two descriptive research questions. First, what proportion of adults in the United States is healthy versus unhealthy from the perspective of social well-being? Toward that end, we situate the study of subjective well-being in the literature on perspectives on individual health, particularly mental health, and review the concept of social well-being as a facet of the overall domain of subjective well-being. Second, is social well-being unequally distributed in the population? Toward that end, this chapter focuses on the variables of age, sex, martial status, and socioeconomic status, which have been shown to structure the distribution of cases of mental illness (e.g., depression) as well as levels of facets of emotional (e.g., happiness) and psychological (e.g., personal growth) well-being.

Models of Functioning in Life

Two models characterize research approaches to discerning whether or how well individuals are functioning in their daily lives. The *illness model* depicts health as a state in which there is a relative or complete absence of significant symptoms or diagnoses of illness (i.e., physical or psychological). The *health model,* however, conceives of health as the presence of a high level of well-being (i.e., physical or psychological). Thus, for example, an individual would be considered healthy from the illness perspective if she had been free of major depression during the past year; from the health perspective, an individual would be considered healthy if he had high levels of social well-being, for example, if he felt very integrated into his community. There are valid reasons for employing both models to the study of human functioning.

The lion's share of health research has focused on the presence or absence of illnesses for several reasons. First, numerous studies reveal that acute and chronic cases of major depression, for example, reduce an individual's productivity and cost society billions of dollars each year through sick days, disability insurance claims, and increased health-care costs (Greenberg et al. 1993; Mrazek and Haggerty 1994; Murray and Lopez 1997). Second, mental illnesses (e.g., major depression) often cause secondary illnesses and social problems such as cardiovascular disease and suicide (Rebellon, Brown, and Keyes 2001; U.S. Department of Health and Human Services 1998). Third, mental illnesses are prevalent whether viewed annually or over an individual's lifetime (Kessler et al. 1994; Robins and Regier 1991; U.S. Department of Health and Human Services 1999).

Are those adults who remain free of mental illness each year and over their lifetimes necessarily healthy? This is a key question for proponents of the health model, especially those who investigate mental health via the presence and absence of subjective well-being (Keyes 2002). Mental health is, according to the surgeon general (U.S. Department of Health and Human Services 1999, 4), "a state of successful performance of mental function, resulting in productive activities, fulfilling relationships with people, and the ability to adapt to change and to cope with adversity."

This definition of mental health goes beyond the absence of mental illness to include indicators of positive feeling and functioning. Data also support the proposed independence of symptoms of mental illness and symptoms of mental health. In particular, Keyes and Lopez's (2002) review indicates that measures of depressive symptoms (e.g., CESD scale) and subjective well-being correlate, on average, between −.40 and −.50. Factor analyses of measures of mental illness and mental health symptoms (Keyes and Ryff, in press) also reveal that a two-factor theory provides a superior fit to the data than does a single-factor theory of mental health. As such, mental health may be best conceived of as a complete state consisting of the presence and absence of mental illness and the presence and absence of subjective well-being (Keyes and Lopez 2002).

During the thirty years of empirical research on the topic of subjective well-being, most research has equated subjective well-being with emotional well-being, which consists of avowed happiness and satisfaction with life as well as the balance of positive to negative affect (see Diener et al. 1999). The model of psychological well-being proposed by Ryff (1989), however, expanded the scope of well-being to include dimensions of positive psychological functioning. These dimensions include self-acceptance, personal growth, positive relations with others, environmental mastery, purpose in life, and autonomy. Studies have shown that measures of psychological well-being are modestly and positively correlated with measures of emotional well-being (Ryff and Keyes 1995; Keyes, Shmotkin, and Ryff 2002).

Social Well-Being: An Individual-Level Perspective

What has been missing in the subjective well-being literature, according to Keyes (1998), is the recognition that individuals may evaluate the quality of their lives and personal functioning against social criteria. Social well-being consists of several elements that, together, indicate whether and to what degree individuals are functioning well in their social lives—for example, as neighbors, as co-workers, and as citizens (Keyes 1998).

Table 1 provides a useful organization of the various ways that the construct of social well-being has been measured. Theoretically, social well-being originates in the sociological literature on anomie and alienation (Durkheim 1951; Mirowsky and Ross 1989; Seeman 1959, 1983). However, and consistent with the mental illness model, the absence of feelings of anomie or alienation may not reflect the presence of feelings of social well-being. The measures of social well-being developed in the MIDUS study (Keyes 1998) belong to a positive continuum and reflect individuals' assessments of their experiences in society. These new

TABLE 1 Social Well-Being Constructs by Level of Analysis and Continuum of Measurement

| Continuum | Level of Analysis | | |
	Individual	Interpersonal	Societal
Negative	Alienation, anomie	Aggression, incivility	Rates of poverty, suicide, or crime
Positive	Social well-being dimensions	Exchange of types of social support, trust	Social capital, collective efficacy

measures are distinct from extant measures of social well-being that reflect the interpersonal (e.g., aggression, social support) and the societal (e.g., poverty, social capital) levels of analysis.

Guided by the health model, Keyes (1998) proposed five dimensions of social well-being operationalized at the level of the individual. *Social integration* is the evaluation of the quality of one's relationship to society and community. People must try to cultivate a genuine sense of belonging in a world where they do not live their entire lives basking in the unconditional love of family or friends. Healthy individuals feel that they are a part of society. Integration is therefore the extent to which people feel they have something in common with others who constitute their social reality (e.g., their neighborhood) as well as the degree to which they feel they belong to their communities and society. *Social contribution* is the evaluation of one's value to society. It includes the belief that one is a vital member of society, with something of value to give to the world. Adults struggle to feel like and be valuable contributors to a world that does not value them equally or value them merely for being human.

Social coherence is the perception of the quality, organization, and operation of the social world, and it includes a concern for knowing about the world. Innumerable events occur daily, some positive and others negative, some inexplicable and others predictable, some personal and others more distal. As such, another challenge is for people to strive to make sense of a busy, complex world. Socially healthy individuals care about the machinations of society and feel they can understand what is happening around them. Such people do not delude themselves that they live in a perfect world; they have maintained or promoted the desire to make sense of life. Social coherence is the analogous opposite of meaninglessness in life (Mirowsky and Ross 1989; Seeman 1959, 1983) and involves appraisals that society is discernable, sensible, and predictable.

Social actualization is the evaluation of the potential and the trajectory of society. This is the belief in the evolution of society and the sense that society has potential that is being realized through its institutions and citizens. It is a challenge, however, to perceive growth and positive development in a world that does not automatically change or improve for all people. Healthier people are hopeful about the condition and future of society, can recognize the potential that resides in a collective, and believe the world can improve for people like themselves. *Social acceptance* is the construal of society through the character and qualities of other people as a generalized category. Society consists of a diversity of people, most of whom we will never know personally. Individuals must function in a public arena that consists primarily of strangers. Individuals who illustrate social acceptance trust others, think that others are capable of kindness, and believe that people can be industrious. Socially accepting people hold favorable views of human nature and feel comfortable with others.

A study employing a random sample of adults in Dane County, Wisconsin, and the MIDUS sample have supported the measurement theory of social well-being. In both samples, confirmatory factor models have revealed that the proposed five-factor theory of social well-being is the best-fitting model (Keyes 1998). Moreover, elements of social and psychological well-being are empirically distinct. The scales of social and psychological well-being correlated as high as .44, and exploratory factor analysis revealed two correlated ($r = .34$) factors, with the scales of social well-being loading on a separate factor from the items measuring happiness, satisfaction, and the overall scale of psychological well-being (Keyes 1996).

Given its independence from traditional measures of subjective well-being, social well-being is an important marker of the quality of life in this country. Although there have been numerous studies of the distribution of emotional and psychological well-being in the U.S. population, there are literally no studies of social well-being. Moreover, although sociologists have monitored the social well-being of the United States in terms of perceived alienation and anomie (Mirowsky and Ross 1989), Keyes (1998) has shown that measures of anomie correlated modestly with only two of the five measures of social well-being ($r = -.55$ with social actualization, and $r = -.49$ with social acceptance).

Indeed, the MIDUS scales of social well-being have exhibited strong linkages with various indicators of civic engagement and prosocial behavior. Levels of social well-being, but notably social integration and social contribution, were highest among adults who had worked with others in their neighborhoods to solve a problem, compared with adults who had been involved in their neighborhood over a year ago and those who had never engaged in such activities (Keyes 1998). All measures of social well-being, especially social integration, increased as levels of the perceived safety of one's neighborhood and trustworthiness of neighbors increased (Keyes 1998). Moreover, in multivariate regressions that controlled for numerous sociodemographic variables, Keyes and Ryff (1998) found that five of seven measures of civic engagement and prosocial behavior predicted positive levels of overall social well-being (i.e., all five scales of social well-being summed together). That is, the level of overall social well-being increased as perceived civic responsibilities increased, as level of concern for others' welfare and well-being increased, as perceptions of being caring, wise, and knowledgeable increased, as perceived generativity toward others increased, and as the provision of emotional support and assistance increased. Although it is unclear whether it is a cause or consequence of civic engagement, social well-being is intimately linked to measures of civic health and social capital (see Putnam 2000). Yet little is known about the distribution of social well-being in the U.S. population.

Toward an Epidemiology of Social Well-Being

This chapter begins with a descriptive epidemiology of social well-being by focusing on the distribution of the various dimensions of social well-being by key demographic groups. We limit this chapter to the variables of age, sex, marital status, and socioeconomic status. Studies have revealed a somewhat consistent pattern of relationships of these four demographic variables with measures of mental illness (namely, depressive symptoms and caseness), and with emotional and psychological well-being. Thus, we ask, is social well-being distributed in the population in ways that correspond with other measures of mental illness and health?

Focusing on mood disorders among adults aged 18 or older, research has shown that depression diagnosis is most likely and that the number of depression symptoms are highest among younger adults (although it may rise again among the oldest adults). Studies also reveal that unipolar depression is more likely to occur among women, among the previously or never married, and among adults with lower socioeconomic status (less education, lower income, and lower occupational status) (see Horwitz and Scheid 1999; Turner, Wheaton, and Lloyd 1995).

Research also has indicated that emotional well-being tends to be lower among younger adults, among the previously or never married, and among adults with lower socioeconomic standing. However, there does not appear to be a gender gap in happiness, life satisfaction, or affect balance (Andrews and Withey 1976; Diener et al. 1999; Myers 2000). Psychological well-being also increases as socioeconomic status increases. Overall psychological well-being (all scales summed together) increases as years of educational attainment increases (Keyes and Ryff 1998), and each dimension of psychological well-being increases as education increases (Marmot et al. 1997).

The portrait of psychological well-being becomes more complex when viewed by age, sex, and marital status. Levels of purpose in life and personal growth are higher among younger adults (ages 18–39) than among midlife and older adults. Levels of environmental mastery and autonomy, however, are usually higher among older (ages 60 and older) than midlife and younger adults. Levels of self-acceptance and positive relations with others tend to be the same at all ages. Studies also consistently reveal that females report higher levels of positive relations with others (i.e., warm, trusting relations) than do males. In all other respects, men and women report similar levels of psychological well-being (Keyes and Ryff 1998, 1999; Ryff 1989; Ryff and Keyes 1995; Marmot et al. 1997).

In sum, although men are more likely to be free of depression, they are not more likely to appear healthier than women from the criterion of emotional well-being or psychological well-being.[1] Similarly, age and gender show diverse patterns of relationships with measures of mental illness and mental health. For instance, younger adults are more likely than older adults to report depression, but younger adults report higher levels of personal growth and purpose in life than do older adults. Females, too, are more likely than men to be diagnosed with unipolar depression; however, females report similar levels of happiness, and they report higher levels of positive relations with others than do men. Socioeconomic status is the sole variable that shows a consistent pattern with both sets of measures. Adults with low socioeconomic status are more likely than high-status adults to have depression, to report lower life satisfaction and happiness, and to report lower levels of psychological well-being.

In this chapter, we focus on the distribution of the five dimensions of social well-being by age cohort, sex, marital status, and socioeconomic status. We investigate two descriptive questions. First, what is the prevalence of high-level and low-level social well-being in the United States? We operationalize high-level social well-being as the number of dimensions on which a respondent scores in the upper tertile of the scale distribution. Similarly, we operationalize low-level social well-being as the number of dimensions on which a respondent scores in the bottom tertile of the scale distribution.

Second, we explore whether high-level and low-level social well-being, as well as scores on each scale, are randomly distributed in the population of adults between the ages of 25 and 74. The relationships of the variables of age, sex, marital status, and socioeconomic status with other dimensions of mental illness (e.g., depression) and mental health (e.g., emotional and psychological well-being) suggest that social well-being will not be randomly distributed. However, an important empirical question is whether the pattern of social well-being in the population coincides with previous findings obtained using other measures of mental health.

METHODS
Measures

Social Well-being

Table 2 presents the operational definition of the high scorers and the items used to operationalize each dimension of social well-being. The social well-being items were embedded in a self-administered questionnaire and within a section of measures of social networks and social responsibility. Respondents were asked to react to each item by evaluating the degree to which the statement represented how they typically feel, think, or behave. The response consisted of the options of agree or disagree "strongly," "somewhat," or "a little" (a middle response option was "don't know"). The items are summed to form scales with modest-to-acceptable internal consistency for scales with few items (see Keyes 1998).[2] Moreover, the social well-being scales demonstrated construct validity, correlating modestly with measures of the number of dysphoric symptoms and global well-being (happiness and satisfaction), and correlating minimally with self-reported physical health and perceived sense of optimism. The scales of social wellness correlate strongly with measures of social health and functioning such as self-reported anomie, perceived external control, and perceived neighborhood quality (see Keyes 1998).

To determine the extent of high or low levels of well-being across dimensions, we computed two variables. *High-level* social well-being is a count (0–5) of the number of dimensions on which respondents' reports are in the upper tertile of each scale. Similarly, *low-level* social well-being is a count (0–5) of the number of dimensions on which respondents' reports are in the bottom tertile of each scale. The internal reliability of the overall social well-being scale is .81.

TABLE 2 Operational Definitions of High Scorers and Items Measuring Dimensions of Social Well-Being in the MacArthur Foundation's Successful Midlife National Study

Social Actualization: Care about and believe society is evolving positively, think society has potential to grow positively; think society is realizing potential

- The world is becoming a better place for everyone.
- Society has stopped making progress. $(-)$
- Society isn't improved for people like me. $(-)$

Social Acceptance: Have positive attitudes toward people; acknowledge others and generally accept people, despite others' sometimes complex and perplexing behavior.

- People who do a favor expect nothing in return.
- People do not care about other people's problems. $(-)$
- I believe that people are kind.

Social Coherence: See a social world that is intelligible, logical, and predictable, care about and are interested in society and contexts.

- The world is too complex for me. $(-)$
- I cannot make sense of what's going on in the world. $(-)$

Social Integration: Feel part of community; think they belong, feel supported, and share commonalities with community.

- I don't feel I belong to anything I'd call a community. $(-)$
- I feel close to other people in my community.
- My community is a source of comfort.

Social Contribution: Feel they have something valuable to give to society; think their daily activities are valued by their community.

- I have something valuable to give to the world.
- May daily activities do not create anything worthwhile for my community.
- I have nothing important to contribute to society. $(-)$

Note: $(-)$ means item is reverse-coded.

Social Demographics Variables

In multivariate analyses, we employ four primary independent variables: age cohort (25–34, 35–44, 45–54, 55–64, and 65–74), marital status, sex, and occupational status. Marital status was measured as a trichotomous variable including previously married, never-married, and currently married persons (currently married is the omitted category in regression models). Occupational status was measured by the revised

TABLE 3 Distribution of the Number of Dimensions on Which Respondents Were in the Top and Bottom Tertiles of Social Well-Being

Number of Dimensions	Top Tertile (%)	Bottom Tertile (%)
0	15.9	45.1
1	21.2	27.9
2	24.5	16.0
3	18.1	7.5
4	12.0	2.8
5	8.3	.7
N	2976	2976

version (Hauser and Warren 1996) of the socioeconomic index (SEI). Originally conceived by Duncan (1961), the SEI is a weighted average of occupational education and income that corresponds to occupational prestige ratings in the 1980 Census.[3] The range of scores for SEI varies between 0 and 100. The SEI score assigned for each respondent was the higher of his or her own job or the job of his or her spouse, whichever was higher. We believe this operationalization to be most reflective of respondents' socioeconomic class given that marital partners' earnings may be highly discrepant. In the event that the spouse was unemployed, the respondent's SEI score from his or her previous job was used (see also Turner, Wheaton, and Lloyd 1995).

RESULTS

Table 3 presents the distribution of high and low social well-being in the MIDUS sample. Overall, the results suggest that respondents report a relatively high degree of wellness. Only about 16 percent (15.9 percent) of respondents did not report being in the top tertile of any dimension of social well-being. More than 20 percent (20.3 percent) of the respondents' reports were in the top tertile on at least four or five dimensions of social well-being. Nearly 40 percent (38.4 percent) of adults in MIDUS scored in the top tertile on at least three or more of the scales of social well-being. Thus, the MIDUS estimates that between one-fifth (using the four or more dimension rule) to two-fifths (using the three or more dimension rule) of the U.S. population between the ages of 25 and 74 has high-level social well-being.

When examining the extent of low social well-being, we found that almost half (45.1 percent) of respondents did not score in the bottom

TABLE 4 Ordinary Least Squares Regression Coefficients Predicting the
Number of Dimensions in the Top and Bottom Tertiles of Social Well-Being

	Top Tertile		Bottom Tertile	
	Bivariate	Multivariate	Bivariate	Multivariate
Age	−.034	—	.019	—
35–44	—	−.088	—	.068
45–54	—	.044	—	−.025
55–64	—	.016	—	.015
65–74	—	−.209*	—	.069
Male	.181***	.139**	−.140***	−.089*
Never married	−.115	−.069	.062	.025
Previously married	−.185**	−.011	.225***	.082
SEI	.019***	.018***	−.016***	−.015***
R^2		.049		.041
N		2923		2923

Notes: Age cohort 25–34 is omitted category; married is omitted category.
$^*p < .05$. $^{**}p < .01$. $^{***}p < .001$ (two-tailed).

tertile on any of the dimensions of social well-being. Fewer than 4 percent (3.6 percent) of the respondents' reports were in the bottom tertile on four or five dimensions of well-being. However, one-tenth (10.0 percent) scored in the lower tertile on at least three or more of the dimensions of social well-being. In sum, our data suggest that many adults are feeling socially healthy. However, about 16 percent of adults in this sample did not report high-level well-being on any dimension of social well-being, and 10 percent are functioning very poorly on at least three or more dimensions (Keyes and Shapiro 2001).

To determine how high and low social well-being is distributed across the population, we estimated a series of regression models. Table 4 presents the results of ordinary least squares regression analyses that predict the number of dimensions on which respondents report high and low social well-being. We present both bivariate and multivariate coefficients that allowed us to determine which of the predictors were most robust after the addition of controls.[4] In the bivariate model, all predictors with the exception of age and being never married were significantly associated with high social well-being. However, in the full multivariate model, only being male and occupational status remained significant and positive. Similarly, when age is decomposed, the results show that respondents between the ages of 65 and 74 scored in the highest tertile of well-being significantly less frequently than did 25- to 34-year-olds. The effect of gender was reduced by 23 percent, while the effect of occupational status was reduced by only 5 percent. On the other hand, the effect of being never married was reduced by 40 percent and being previously married by 94 percent. Thus, the most robust predictor of high well-being is occupational status followed by being male.

The bivariate coefficients for low social well-being suggest that being female and previously married are positively and significantly associated with the number of dimensions of low social well-being. In contrast, occupational status is negatively predictive of low social well-being. In the full multivariate model, the significance of the previously married effect was eliminated, and its size was reduced by 64 percent. Effect sizes for other variables were similarly reduced. For example, the effect of being never married was reduced by 60 percent. Meanwhile, the effects for sex and occupational status remained highly robust and statistically significant as the effects were reduced by 36 percent and 6 percent, respectively.[5]

In sum, high occupational status and, to a lesser extent, being male were highly indicative of placing in the highest category, and avoiding the lowest category, on a number of dimensions of social well-being, even when controlling for respondents' age and marital status. Findings therefore indicate that males and adults with higher socioeconomic status are more likely to have high-level social well-being. Moreover, currently married adults are also more likely than previously married adults to have high-level social well-being, partially because married adults have higher socioeconomic status than do adults who have been divorced.

Although the preceding analysis has been able to discern the influence of sociodemographic characteristics on the prevalence of "compound" social well-being, the possibility of interdimensional variation of social well-being may exist. Table 5 presents the results of each dimension of social well-being regressed on the sociodemographic variables. The analysis strategy is the same as that used in table 4, where each dependent variable is regressed on each of the sociodemographic variables separately and then in a full multivariate model.

The first general finding from table 5 was the overall consistent and strong positive impact of occupational status on each of the five dimensions of social well-being. Furthermore, the bivariate effect of occupational status was not reduced by more than 8 percent in any of the full multivariate models. None of the other sociodemographic variables was as robust, nor did the variables consistently maintain the direction of their effects across dimensions.

Respondents' age was also a strong predictor of social well-being in both bivariate and multivariate models, although the direction and

TABLE 5 Ordinary Least Squares Regression Coefficients

	Social Acceptance		Social Coherence	
	Bivariate	Multivariate	Bivariate	Multivariate
Age	.133***	—	−.166***	—
35–44	—	.127*	—	−.274***
45–54	—	.322***	—	−.195*
55–64	—	.440***	—	−.366***
65–74	—	.545***	—	−.768***
Male	−.103*	−.126**	.555***	.522***
Never married	−.200**	−.035	.195*	.143
Previously married	−.074	−.052	−.084	.235**
SEI	.010***	.010***	.023***	.022***
R^2		.041		.084
N		2928		2924

Notes: Age cohort 25–34 is omitted category; married is omitted category.
*$p < .05$. **$p < .01$. ***$p < .001$ (two-tailed).

linearity of the effects of age varied across dimensions. For example, age was linearly associated with social acceptance and social integration in a positive direction but with social coherence in a negative direction in the multivariate model. Examining the age effect in the multivariate model predicting social contribution, we found that well-being for those aged 65–74 was significantly less than for those aged 25–34. Thus, the findings for social coherence and social contribution may suggest a pattern of cumulative disadvantage. However, it is premature to imply that age is uniformly negative with respect to social well-being because the findings for social acceptance and social integration suggest a pattern of cumulative advantage over the life course. Similarly, because of the cross-sectional design of the present study, it is difficult to discern whether the age effects indeed reflect effects of cumulative advantage or cohort differences.

Although sex was a strong predictor of high overall social well-being in table 4, its effect is less consistent when analyzed separately within each dimension of social well-being. Sex is significant in only two of the multivariate models in table 5. Females reported higher social acceptance than males, but males reported a greater sense of social coherence than females. Although sex is statistically significant in bivariate models predicting social actualization and social contribution, these effects are reduced by 36 percent and 67 percent, respectively, in the multivariate models. Sex is insignificant in both bivariate and multivariate models predicting social integration (Keyes and Shapiro 2001).

Predicting Each Dimension of Social Well-Being

Social Actualization		Social Contribution		Social Integration	
Bivariate	Multivariate	Bivariate	Multivariate	Bivariate	Multivariate
−.020	—	−.117***		.168***	—
—	.064	—	−.016	—	.032
—	.222**	—	.001	—	.294***
—	.134	—	−.100	—	.500***
—	−.138	—	−.487***	—	.617***
.140**	.089	.120*	.039	−.054	−.086
−.072	.010	.122	.174*	−.396***	−.241**
−.157*	−.013	−.248***	−.093	−.247***	−.228***
.014***	.013***	.026***	.025***	.010***	.010***
	.029		.099		.042
	2928		2925		2923

The effect of marital status on social well-being was, at best, inconsistent. One strong finding, however, was that married persons report significantly higher social integration than their nonmarried counterparts. In particular, being previously married appears to have a very robust negative effect on social integration, being reduced by only 8 percent in the multivariate model. Comparably, the bivariate effect for never-married persons on social integration was reduced by 39 percent in the multivariate model (though it maintained statistical significance). Nonmarried persons also fared better than the married on two dimensions of social well-being. Never-married persons reported significantly higher social contribution and previously married persons reported significantly higher social coherence than the married. Although several significant bivariate effects for the nonmarried were observed, these effects were drastically reduced in the multivariate models.

Because of the strong effects of occupational status on social well-being, we estimated interaction models for occupational status on each dimension of social well-being. The statistically significant interaction coefficients are plotted against predicted values of the dependent variables from regression models in figures 1–3. The dependent variables in these figures were transformed into *z-scores* to permit standard comparisons across each of the dependent variables.

The most consistent interaction effects were found between occupational status and sex (fig. 1). These interaction coefficients were significant in models for each dimension except social actualization. Overall,

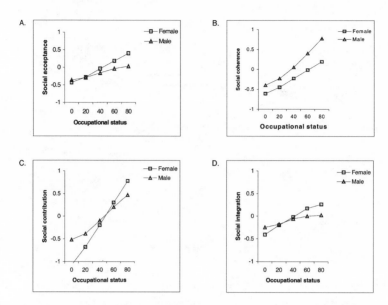

FIGURE 1. (A) Social acceptance, (B) social coherence, (C) social contribution, and (D) social integration, by sex and occupational status.

occupational status was more important to the social well-being of women than of men. As seen in figures 1A, 1C, and 1D, women of lower occupational status report lower levels of social well-being than do men of the same status. However, the rate of change in social well-being increases more for women than men as occupational status increases. On the other hand, males report more social coherence than do females, and the advantage of men over women in social coherence increases as occupational status increases (see fig. 1B).

Another consistent interaction was between occupational status and age. As seen in figure 2, being poor and older are especially negative indicators of low social well-being. Thus, the importance of occupational status to social well-being increases with age. As seen in figure 2, adults between the ages of 65 and 74 who are at the bottom of the occupational status scale reported social coherence and social contribution (figs. 2A and 2B) of roughly 1.5 standard deviations below the mean. The slope for adults aged 65–74 is steeper than that of other age cohorts; thus, age cohort differences in social coherence and social contribution are eliminated toward the higher end of the occupational status scale. Examining the interactions for social integration (fig. 2C), we find that adults between the ages of 65 and 74 at lower occupational status levels did

A.

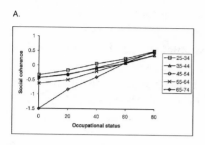

B.

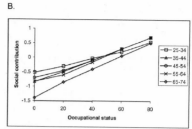

C.

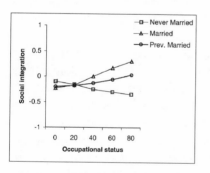

FIGURE 2. (A) Social coherence, (B) social contribution, and (C) social integration, by age and occupational status.

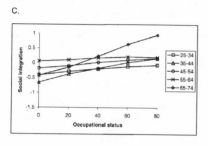

FIGURE 3. Marital status differences in social integration, by occupational status.

not report significantly lower social integration. However, the slope of the interaction for adults aged 65–74 is steeper than that for any other age cohort, actually producing an advantage for adults in the age cohort of 65–74 in the upper levels of occupational status relative to other age cohorts.

Finally, most interactions of marital status by occupational status were not statistically significant. However, the relationship of marital status with social integration depends on the individual's occupational status. As seen in figure 3, there are no definitive marital status differences in social integration at lower occupational status levels. From the middle to upper range of occupational status, the trajectory for married and previously married persons is upward, but downward for never-married persons. Thus, never-married adults do not appear to receive the "benefits" of high occupational status. As occupational status increases, however, the differences between never-married persons and their counterparts widen, with never-married persons at a significant disadvantage, particularly relative to married persons (see Keyes and Shapiro 2001; Shapiro and Keyes 2001).

DISCUSSION

Social well-being has been identified as a key component of mental health (World Health Organization 1948; U.S. Department of Health and Human Services 1999). However, because of the absence of reliable and valid measures, social well-being has remained a topic of policy debates (see Larson 1996) rather than epidemiological study. The MacArthur Foundation's 1995 MIDUS study represents the first opportunity to examine the epidemiology of social well-being in the United States. The MIDUS measures of social well-being reflect the mental health model of human functioning and complement the customary approach to studying individual health as the absence of illness. We therefore investigated two descriptive questions: What is the prevalence of high- and low-level social well-being? and How is social well-being distributed in the adult population by age, sex, marital status, and occupational status?

Results suggest that nearly 40 percent of adults between the ages of 25 and 74 scored in the upper tertile on at least three of the social well-being scales. However, as many as 16 percent of adults did not score in the upper tertile on any of the scales, and 10 percent scored in the lower tertile on at least three or more of the social well-being scales. Thus, the MIDUS data suggest that a majority of adults in the United States have moderate to high levels of social well-being. However, a substantial portion of the population has very low levels of social well-being and would be considered socially unhealthy from the mental health perspective.

Levels of social well-being are clearly distributed unequally in the United States. Levels of social integration are highest among older persons (i.e., 65–74), married persons, and females with high occupational status. Social integration is at its lowest among younger and previously or never-married adults with low occupational status. A sense of social contribution is highest among never-married females with high occupational status, but it is at its lowest among older (i.e., 65–74) males with low social status. Social actualization is highest among adults in early (ages 45–54) midlife and who have high occupational status; social actualization is low among adults not in the peak of midlife and who have low social status.

Social coherence is highest among high-status males who were previously married, while it is lowest among older (ages 65–74) females with low occupational status who have never married or are married. Last, social acceptance is highest among older females with high occupational status, but acceptance of others is lowest among younger males with low social status.

Although our findings point to the clear advantage of high occupational status, all other demographics show distinct advantages and disadvantages in terms of specific outcomes of social well-being. However, when high-level and low-level (overall) social well-being are the outcome variables, the results paint a clear and unambiguous picture. Social well-being is highest among high-status persons, males, and those who are married or never married. In contrast, females, those who are previously married, and those who have low occupational status have the lowest level of overall social well-being. Our findings complement the literature on the risk factors for unipolar depression, which suggests that divorced females with low occupational status are at a high risk for distress and mental illness.

Theoretically, the interactions of sex and of age by occupational status converge with the theoretical perspectives of cumulative advantage and double jeopardies to health from possession of multiple disadvantaged social statuses (Allison, Long, and Krause 1982; Dowd and Bengtson 1978; Ferraro 1987; Ferraro and Farmer 1996). According to these perspectives, social inequalities in health worsen throughout life, because disadvantages can accumulate and have a compounding effect on health outcomes with time or with the addition of disadvantaged statuses (multiple roles with low social status).[6]

Most studies employing the cumulative advantage and the double jeopardy perspectives focus on physical health and mortality outcomes of the interactive effects of age and socioeconomic status (cf. Keyes and Ryff 1998). Moreover, most earlier studies of cumulative disadvantage have employed cross-sectional data (cf. Ross and Wu 1996) and therefore had to assume that observed health disparities by age reflected processes of change (i.e., time) rather than cohort differences. The present study, in that it employed the cross-sectional MIDUS data, rests on the same assumption that age difference reflects, at least in part, change rather than solely cohort effects. Several earlier studies—both cross-sectional and longitudinal—have shown that disparities in physical health and functioning between adults with different levels of educational attainment diverge with age, and that the physical health gap by education increases as age increases (Ross and Wu 1996; Smith and Waitzman 1994).[7] Cumulative disadvantage (as well as advantage) may explain the distribution of aspects of social well-being by occupational status. In particular, social coherence and social contribution are lowest among older adults, and the age gap in coherence and contribution increases as occupational status decreases.

Women may accumulate specific advantages to men as occupational status increases. Our study found small gender differences in social acceptance, social contribution, and social integration at low levels of occupational status. However, as occupational status increases, women report increasingly higher levels of social acceptance, social contribution, and social integration than men. The exception to the rule of cumulative advantage for females is the criterion of social coherence.

Males report higher levels of social coherence at all levels of occupational status. However, as occupational status increases, the gender gap in social coherence increases. Thus, high-status males see their social world as much more coherent than do high-status females. In contrast, high-status females are more accepting of others, feel more integrated into their communities, and feel a greater sense of contribution to society than do high-status males. In short, high occupational status may provide more "returns" in social well-being for females than for males.

Marital status appears to play a relatively small but important role in social well-being. Like Marks and Lambert (1998), who found that single adults had higher levels of some measures of psychological well-being (autonomy and personal growth) than married adults, we found that previously married adults report higher levels of social coherence and never-married adults report higher levels of social contribution than do married adults. However, married adults show a clear advantage over single adults in terms of social integration. In fact, as occupational status increases, the social integration of married adults increases while the sense of integration decreases among never-married adults. This finding supports a great deal of research in social epidemiology linking marriage to social, psychological, and physical health (Berkman and Syme 1979; Marks and Lambert 1998).

Last, in the multivariate models of overall (high- and low-level) social well-being, the effect of being previously married on social well-being is mitigated with controls for occupational status. This finding strongly suggests that being previously married is related to low-level social well-being through the mechanism of low occupational status (either because low social status increases the risk for being previously married or this status interrupts employment and lowers one's occupational status). This finding compliments Shapiro's (1996) national study that suggested that economic status mitigates the association between divorce and depression. Whether low-level social well-being is a cause or an effect of being previously married remains an empirical question for future longitudinal research.

The MIDUS study affords numerous opportunities for further research at the intersection of social well-being and health and human functioning. First, MIDUS, which included DSM-III-R structured diagnoses of depression, generalized anxiety, panic disorder, and substance abuse, permits the study of the intersection of measures of positive mental health with mental illness (see Keyes 2002, 2003; Keyes and Lopez 2002). Second, MIDUS included the most comprehensive assessment of subjective well-being of any national study to date and thereby permits the taxonomic assessment of the well-being concept (emotional, psychological, and social well-being; see Keyes, Shmotkin, and Ryff 2001). Third, MIDUS includes a comprehensive assessment of physical health morbidity and risk factors, and permits the assessment of the intersection of social well-being and physical health as adults age. Fourth, the MIDUS data from twins permit the assessment of the shared and non-shared variance components of social well-being and its linkages with a host of variables. Fifth, MIDUS included daily time-diary assessments, which permits the cross-referencing of daily stressors and life events with measures of social, psychological, and physical well-being. Sixth, the potential for a second wave of MIDUS data is important in answering many questions that require a longitudinal examination. It would permit a better assessment of life-course trajectories in inequalities of social, psychological, and physical well-being. In sum, the MIDUS study includes assessments of physical, mental, and social health that permit the study of many of the most pressing questions facing the field of human development and aging (see Ryff and Singer 2001).

NOTES

1. Although the prevalence of depression is higher among females, the prevalence of behavioral disorders (e.g., substance abuse, violence) is higher among males (Kessler et al. 1994). Whether this gender pattern of mental illness suggests that males and females are equally depressed but express it in different ways remains an empirical question.

2. Alpha reliabilities presented in Keyes 1998 ranged between .60 and .73, with the exception of the scale of social coherence (alpha = .41), which is a two-item scale (the third item reduced the internal consistency and had to be omitted).

369

3. The 1980 SEI is used because few changes were made in occupational classifications between the 1980 and 1990 Census.

4. We included race and education as additional controls in ancillary analyses. Race was not a significant predictor of well-being in any model, and education was highly correlated ($r = .56$) with SEI. Thus, the models include only the primary predictors.

5. Regression models including interactions between occupational status and the other variables were fitted in ancillary analyses. None of the interaction coefficients achieved statistical significance, and thus they were not displayed in the table.

6. The original sampled middle-aged and older blacks, Mexican Americans, and whites in Los Angeles but received mixed empirical support; it was challenged by later national studies (Ferraro 1987; Ferraro and Farmer 1996).

7. Some research suggests that educational disparities in physical health may diverge throughout younger and middle adulthood, and then convergence during older adulthood (i.e., after the ages of 60–65) (House et al. 1994, 1990).

References

Allison, P. D., J. S. Long, and T. K. Krauze. 1982. Cumulative advantage and inequality in science. *American Sociological Review* 47:615–25.

Andrews, F. M., and S. B. Withey. 1976. *Social indicators of well-being: Americans' perceptions of life quality.* New York: Plenum Press.

Bell, D., and M. Olson. 1969. Toward a social report, I. The idea of a social report, II. The purpose and plan of a social report. *Public Interest* 15:72–97.

Berkman, L. F., and S. L. Syme. 1979. Social networks, host resistance and mortality: A nine-year follow-up study of Alameda County residents. *American Journal of Epidemiology* 109:186–204.

Diener, E., E. M. Suh, R. E. Lucas, and R. E. Lucas. 1999. Subjective well-being: Three decades of progress. *Psychological Bulletin* 125:276–302.

Dowd, J. J., and V. L. Bengtson. 1978. Aging in minority populations: An examination of the double jeopardy hypothesis. *Journal of Gerontology* 33:427–36.

Duncan, O. D. 1961. A socioeconomic index for all occupations. In *Occupations and social status,* ed. A. L. Reiss, Jr., 109–38. New York: Free Press.

Durkheim, E. 1951. *Suicide.* New York: Free Press. First published in 1897.

Ferraro, K. F. 1987. Double jeopardy to health for black older adults? *Journal of Gerontology* 42:528–33.

Ferraro, K. F., and M. M. Farmer. 1996. Double jeopardy to health hypothesis for African Americans: Analysis and critique. *Journal of Health and Social Behavior* 37:27–43.

Greenberg, P. E., L. E. Stiglin, S. N. Finkelstein, and E. R. Brendt. 1993. The economic burden of depression in 1990. *Journal of Clinical Psychiatry* 54:405–26.

Hauser, R. M., and J. R. Warren. 1996. A socioeconomic index for occupations in the 1990 census. Working paper 96-01. Center for Demography and Ecology, University of Wisconsin, Madison.

Horwitz, A. V., and T. L. Scheid, eds. 1999. *A handbook for the study of mental health: Social contexts, theories, and systems.* New York: Cambridge University Press.

House, J. S., R. C. Kessler, A. R. Herzog, R. P. Mero, A. M. Kinney, and M. J. Breslow. 1990. Age, socioeconomic status, and health. *Milbank Quarterly* 68:383–411.

House, J. S., J. M. Lepkowski, A. M. Kinney, R. P. Mero, R C. Kessler, and A. R. Herzog. 1994. The social stratification of aging and health. *Journal of Health and Social Behavior* 35:213–34.

Kessler, R. C., K. A. McGonagle, S. Zhao, C. B. Nelson, M. Hughes, S. Eshleman, H. U. Wittchen, and K. S. Kendler. 1994. Lifetime and 12-month prevalence of DSM-III-R psychiatric disorders in the United States: Results from the National Comorbidity Survey. *Archives of General Psychiatry* 51:8–19.

Keyes, C. L. M. 1996. Social functioning and social well-being: Studies of the social nature of personal wellness. *Dissertation Abstracts International: Sciences and Engineering*, vol. 5612-B.

———. 1998. Social well-being. *Social Psychology Quarterly* 61:121–40.

———. 2002. The mental health continuum: From languishing to flourishing in life. *Journal of Health and Social Behavior* 43:207–22.

———. 2003. Complete mental health: An agenda for the 21st century. In *Flourishing: Positive psychology and the life well lived*, ed. C. L. M. Keyes and J. Haidt, 293–312. Washington, D.C.: American Psychological Association.

Keyes, C. L. M., and S. J. Lopez. 2002. Toward a science of mental health: Positive directions in diagnosis and interventions. In *Handbook of positive psychology*, ed. C. R. Snyder and S. J. Lopez, 45–59. New York: Oxford University Press.

Keyes, C. L. M., and C. D. Ryff. 1998. Generativity in adult lives: Social structural contours and quality of life consequences. In *Generativity and adult development: Perspectives on caring for and contributing to the next generation*, ed. D. McAdams and E. de St. Aubin, 227–63. Washington, D.C.: American Psychological Association.

———. 1999. Psychological well-being in midlife. In *Middle aging: Development in the third quarter of life*, ed. S. L. Willis and J. D. Reid, 161–80. Orlando, Fla.: Academic Press.

Keyes, C. L. M., and C. D. Ryff. In press. Somatization and mental health: A comparative study of the idiom of distress hypothesis. *Social Science and Medicine* (forthcoming).

Keyes, C. L. M., and A. D. Shapiro. 2001. Cumulative advantage and disadvantage in social well-being: Profiles by sex, age, and socioeconomic index. Manuscript. Emory University.

Keyes, C. L. M., D. Shmotkin, and C. D. Ryff. 2002. Optimizing well-being: The empirical encounter of two traditions. *Journal of Personality and Social Psychology* 82 (6): 1007–22.

Larson, J. S. 1993. The measurement of social well-being. *Social Indicators Research* 28:285–96.

———. 1996. The World Health Organization's definition of health: Social versus spiritual health. *Social Indicators Research* 38:181–92.

Marks, N. F., and J. D. Lambert. 1998. Marital status continuity and change among young and midlife adults: Longitudinal effects on psychological well-being. *Journal of Family Issues* 19:652–86.

Marmot, M., C. D. Ryff, L. L. Bumpass, M. Shipley, and N. F. Marks. 1997. Social inequalities in health: Next questions and converging evidence. *Social Science and Medicine* 44:901–10.

Mirowsky, J., and C. E. Ross. 1989. *Social causes of psychological distress.* New York: Aldine de Gruyter.

Mrazek, P. J., and R. J. Haggerty, eds. 1994. *Reducing risks for mental disorders.* Washington, D.C.: National Academy Press.

Murray C. J., and A. D. Lopez. 1997. Global mortality, disability, and the contribution of risk factors: Global Burden of Disease Study. *Lancet* 349:1436–42.

Myers, D. C. 2000. The funds, friends, and faith of happy people. *American Psychologist* 55:56–67.

Putnam, R. D. 2000. *Bowling alone: The collapse and revival of American community.* New York: Simon and Schuster.

Rebellon, C., J. Brown, and C. L. M. Keyes. 2001. Suicide and mental illness. In *The encyclopedia of criminology and deviant behavior,* vol. 4, *Self destructive behavior and disvalued identity,* ed. C. E. Faupel and P. M. Roman, 426–29. London: Taylor and Francis.

Robins, L. N., and D. A. Regier, eds. 1991. *Psychiatric disorders in America: The Epidemiological Catchment Area study.* New York: Free Press.

Ross, C. E., and C.-L. Wu. 1996. Education, age, and the cumulative advantage in health. *Journal of Health and Social Behavior* 37:104–20.

Ryff, C. D. 1989. Happiness is everything, or is it? Explorations on the meaning of psychological well-being. *Journal of Personality and Social Psychology* 57:1069–81.

Ryff, C. D., and C. L. M. Keyes. 1995. The structure of psychological well-being revisited. *Journal of Personality and Social Psychology* 69:719–27.

Ryff, C. D., and B. H. Singer, eds. 2001. *New horizons in health: An integrative approach.* Washington, D.C.: National Academy Press.

Seeman, M. 1959. On the meaning of alienation. *American Sociological Review* 24:783–91.

———. 1983. Alienation motifs in contemporary theorizing: The hidden continuity of the classic themes. *Social Psychology Quarterly* 463:171–84.

Shapiro, A. D. 1996. Explaining psychological distress in a sample of remarried and divorced persons: The influence of economic distress. *Journal of Family Issues* 17:186–203.

Shapiro, A. D., and C. L. M. Keyes. 2001. Marriage and social well-being over the life-course. Manuscript. University of North Florida.

Smith, K. R., and N. J. Waitzman. 1994. Double jeopardy: Interaction effects of marital and poverty status on the risks of mortality. *Demography* 31:487–507.

Turner, R. J., B. Wheaton, and D. A. Lloyd. 1995. The epidemiology of social stress. *American Sociological Review* 60:104–25.

U.S. Department of Health and Human Services. 1998. *Suicide: A report of the Surgeon General.* Rockville, Md.: U.S. Government Printing Office.

———. 1999. *Mental health: A report of the surgeon general.* Rockville, MD: U.S. Government Printing Office.

World Health Organization. 1948. World Health Organization constitution. In *Basic documents.* Geneva.

CHAPTER THIRTEEN

Ethnic Conservatism, Psychological Well-Being, and the Downside of Mainstreaming: Generational Differences

Randall Horton and Richard A. Shweder

"The longer your family stays in this country the worse it gets" is a rather shocking message for those of us who would like to believe that the Unites States is still a land of opportunity for poor or persecuted peoples from around the world. Nevertheless, in so many words, that is the major conclusion of a recent review of the literature on the well-being of Hispanic and Asian immigrant families, conducted by the National Research Council's Institute of Medicine (Hernandez and Charney 1998). The NRC report drew attention to the "paradoxical finding" that "despite their overall lower socioeconomic levels, higher poverty rates, and racial or ethnic minority status," (1) "children in [first-generation] immigrant families have better health than U.S. born children in U.S. born families on most available measures" (1998, 108), and (2) there is a link between declining physical and mental health in immigrant families and the length of time their families have resided in the United States (1998, 24). In other words, the aggregate amount of suffering in a Hispanic or Asian immigrant family's descent line seems to rise from generation to generation, and typically, it is the first generation that does the best (also see Suarez-Orozco and Suarez-Orozco 1995 on the problem of generational decline and some of the hazards of "assimilation").

The "paradoxical finding" that first-generation Hispanic and Asian immigrants to the United States are both more physically fit and relatively sane or happy compared with their own descendants (and sometimes even when compared with members of long-settled majority groups) begs for explanation. The authors of the NRC report suggest that there must be "protective factors" that favor first-generation immigrants, and they point to strong family bonds that "act to sustain cultural orientations leading to healthful behavior." They also allude to "other unknown social or cultural factors" that "may serve to protect them" (108). In this chapter we examine the extent to which behaviors that sustain the distinctive cultural orientations of Mexican and Puerto Rican immigrants (e.g., continued Spanish language use, ethnic pride communicated to one's children, and a preference for in-group affiliation) are associated with higher levels of self-reported psychological well-being. The results of our study lead us to point a finger, however tentatively, in the direction of "ethnic conservatism" as either an index or component of the "protective factors" imagined in the NRC report.

By *ethnic conservatism* we mean an inclination to resist the ideal of rapid and full assimilation to the meanings, values, and practices (including linguistic practices) of mainstream Anglo-American culture. In this study, ethnic conservatism is indexed by a variable we call weak acculturation ideals, by a disposition to communicate feelings of distinctive ethnic pride to one's children, and by continued use of the Spanish language in thinking. The study examines the impact of resistance to assimilation on the psychological well-being of first- and second-generation midlife adults from Mexican and Puerto Rican immigrant populations in the cities of Chicago and New York. We discover that for first-generation immigrants from both ethnic groups, ethnic conservatism predicts higher levels of self-reported psychological well-being (Ryff 1989) in the domains of autonomy, quality of relationships, and sense of purpose in life. These associations between aspects of ethnic conservatism and aspects of psychological well-being remain positive and significant even after controlling for demographic and socioeconomic status (SES) variables. Nevertheless, as anticipated by the NRC report, the longer an immigrant family stays in the United States the worse it gets, at least with regard to the effectiveness of ethnic conservatism as a protective strategy. We discover that ethnic conservatism diminishes in its effectiveness in promoting psychological well-being as one moves from generation to generation in these Hispanic communities. Stated more cautiously, ethnic conservatism can be a useful index of psychological well-being, but it seems to predict happiness and mental health best for the generation that has most recently arrived.

METHODS
Participants

The participants in this study consisted of individuals from three sample groups. All respondents were adults aged 25 or older at the time of the survey. The first group, the first-generation Mexican American sample, consisted of 176 adult residents (80 female, 96 male) from the urban Chicago area (mean age = 40.1 years). All were born in Mexico of Mexican parents and had immigrated to the United States after their fifteenth birthday. The second group, the first-generation Puerto Rican

TABLE 1 Selected Demographic Characteristics for Respondents from All Sample Groups

Variables	First-Generation Mexican Americans ($N = 176$)		First-Generation Puerto Rican Americans ($N = 144$)		Second-Generation Puerto Rican Americans ($N = 242$)	
Generation variables	*n*	%	*n*	%	*n*	%
Gender						
Male	96	55.1	73	50.7	123	50.8
Female	80	44.9	71	49.3	119	49.2
Education						
Up to high school	124	74.4	82	62.1	80	33.2
Finished high school	24	14.9	35	26.5	81	33.6
Some college/2 years college	16	9.5	14	10.6	64	26.6
Bachelor's or more	2	1.2	1	0.8	16	6.6
Marital status						
Currently married	135	76.7	64	44.4	113	46.7
Been married	15	8.5	53	36.8	54	22.3
Never married	26	14.8	27	18.8	75	31.0
Additional variables	Mean	SD	Mean	SD	Mean	SD
Respondent age	40.1	(11.3)	51.9	(14.4)	39.6	(12.5)
Years in United States	16.5	(9.6)	27.9	(14.4)	na	na
Median family income	$22,000		$18,300		$28,500	

Note: na, not applicable.

sample, was comprised of 144 adult residents (71 female, 73 male) from the urban Chicago and New York City areas (mean age = 51.9 years). All were born in Puerto Rico of Puerto Rican parents and had immigrated to the United States after their fifteenth birthday.[1] The final group, the second-generation Puerto Rican sample, consisted of 242 adult residents (119 female, 123 male) from the urban Chicago and New York City areas (mean age = 39.6 years). All were born in the United States of Puerto Rican parents or had immigrated to the United States with their families before their fifth birthday. Additional demographic and background information on all three sample groups is presented in table 1.

Sampling Procedures

Participants were selected and contacted through a two-stage randomized sampling design. The sample was stratified to reach equal numbers of individuals living in both low- and high-density ethnic communities, defined as census block groups with 10 percent to 20 percent and 50 percent to 70 percent Latino concentration. A smaller number of additional participants ($n = 40$) were recruited in the Chicago area from two very high density ethnic neighborhoods in which more than 70 percent of the population were Latino. The sample was further stratified to reach equal numbers of individuals living in low and high SES communities, as defined by a 1990 Census–based cutoff value of $24,000 per year median family income. Surveyors canvassed randomly assigned census tracts and census block groups, going door to door and following procedures to ensure a balanced representation of working and nonworking adult men and women. Respondents completed a two-hour face-to-face survey in their choice of either Spanish or English and received a small sum of money in compensation. English- and Spanish-language versions of the survey and all measures for this study were developed through a translation and focus-group feedback procedure and piloted ($n = 80$) to assess comparability of versions.

Measures

We conceptualize ethnic conservatism as an inclination to resist the ideal of full assimilation into the meanings, values, and practices (including linguistic practices) of the "mainstream" of some dominant culture. Assimilation or "acculturation" measures typically assess individuals across several related domains. Questions designed to assess socialization and leisure preferences, language use and competence, degree of identification with one's ethnic group, and participation in culture-specific activities and organizations have all been used to operationalize and test assimilation or acculturation status. (See Dana 1996 for a review of measures for use with Hispanic adults.) Acknowledging the growing interest in bicultural models of acculturation (LaFramboise, Coleman, and Gerton 1993; Rogler, Cortes, and Malgady 1991), we ideally would have liked to be able to assess assimilation or acculturation along a two-dimensional continuum. This would have involved separately estimating orientation toward both the individual's host culture and her culture of origin. Such measures, however, were not available for the data with which we were working. Hence, within this study we have employed a somewhat unidimensional set of measures of ethnic conservatism, which we have operationalized using three variables.

Weak assimilation ideals. The first variable, weak assimilation ideals, was derived from responses to two questions: (1) "How closely do you identify with being Mexican American [or Puerto Rican American]?" and (2) "How much do you prefer to be with other people who are Mexican American [or Puerto Rican American]?" Responses to these questions could assume four values: "not at all," "a little," "some," or "a lot." Item responses correlated at roughly $r = .40$ and were averaged. Within the terms of our conceptualization, higher scorers were endorsing more ethnically conservative attitudes and weaker assimilation ideals than their peers.

Ethnic pride. Ethnic pride as communicated to one's children (sometimes shortened to ethnic pride) was our second variable for indexing ethnic conservatism. Data for this measure derive from a set of questions asking how often in the past year interviewees with children under the age of 18 had engaged in the following activities: (a) encouraged their children to be proud of their ethnic heritage, (b) did things with their children to commemorate events in their ethnic group's history, or (c) read to their children from books by authors from their ethnic group or about the history of their ethnic group. Responses could assume six values ranging from "never" to "very often." A scale variable (Cronbach's alpha $= .85$) was generated as the arithmetic mean of the three responses.

Language of thought. The language in which respondents thought was the third index of ethnic conservatism used in this study. For reasons to be discussed, we coded this measure as a pair of binary contrast variables (language contrast 1 and language contrast 2). These variables represented subjects' responses to the question "When you are thinking to yourself, what language do you usually think in?" Questions assessing relative language use and competence have proven to be the most reliable anchor points for the assessment of assimilation or acculturation (Dawson, Crano, and Burgoon 1996). Data derived from such variables correlate most centrally and strongly with a wide range of behavioral, social, and attitudinal indices (Dana 1996). Although it is far from ideal to work from a one-item assessment of linguistic use and competence, questions such as "What language do you think in?" have been shown to be fairly strong predictors of other acculturation variables and of the results of broader scales of acculturation (Epstein et al. 1996).

Within the present survey, answers to this question could assume five values: "Spanish only," "more Spanish than English," "both equally," "more English than Spanish," or "English only." Within both first-generation samples, "Spanish only" was the modal response, with 70 percent of Mexican American and 47 percent of Puerto Rican adult immigrants choosing this response. Few first-generation individuals reported thinking in both languages equally, and almost none said that they favored English.[2] For analytic purposes, these responses were treated as categorical data and entered into regression models as a dummy coded pair of contrast variables. In the analyses of first-generation data, language contrast 1 (first generation) was the contrast of "Spanish only" with "more Spanish than English." Language contrast 2 (first generation) was the contrast between "more Spanish than English" and the combined categories "both Spanish and English equally," "more English," and "English only."

In sharp distinction to data from our first-generation samples, responses from members of our second-generation sample were distributed quite normally across the five possible categories. For this group, mental bilingualism was the norm.[3] For test purposes with this data, the first two Spanish-dominant response categories, "Spanish only" and "more Spanish than English," were grouped together and contrasted with the modal bilingual response group, "both Spanish and English equally." This was language contrast 1 (second generation). For language contrast 2 (second generation), the modal bilingual group was contrasted with the two English-dominant response categories, "more English" and "English only." Constructing contrasts in this way made it possible to look for nonlinearity and disjunction in the relationship of this language variable to measures of psychological well-being.[4]

These three ethnic conservatism indices were significantly and positively correlated in the range of $.20 < r < .50$ in the first-generation samples. These correlations were lower in the second-generation sample. In addition, among members of the first-generation samples, these measures correlated mildly and positively with total years an individual had lived in the United States.

Within our first-generation Mexican American sample, two ethnic conservatism measures, weak assimilation ideals and ethnic pride, also correlated significantly ($r = .36$ and $.22$, respectively) with the ethnic density of communities in which our participants lived. Adults from higher-density ethnic communities tended to score higher on ethnic conservatism measures. The density of communities in which interviewees from all three samples lived varied from 10 percent to 95 percent Latino population, with an average ethnic density of 43 percent. Our ethnic conservatism measures were not significantly correlated with ethnic density in our two Puerto Rican American samples.[5] Across all three samples, the ethnic conservatism measures with which we worked show disjunction from variables on the community level such as ethnic density. Individual and community-level processes were linked but not reducible to one another.

Methodological Note

In deciding not to use the language in which the survey was administered as one of our ethnic conservatism variables, we weighed several considerations. First and foremost, although field surveyors in both cities were technically bilingual Spanish-English speakers, the data from several interviewers showed a strong bias toward administration in one language or the other. In other words, the language of administration sometimes seemed to reflect the surveyor's language preference as much as the subject's. This was particularly the case with the bilingual second-generation sample. This was less of an issue with first-generation respondents, the vast majority of whom (84 percent) chose to be interviewed in Spanish.

To check for method-variance effects that may have resulted from the language in which the interview was administered, we conducted a series of t-tests for systematic differences in our outcome measures based on language of administration. These tests showed no significant differences across language of administration.

Psychological Well-Being Measures

Psychological well-being was assessed using the eighteen-item version of Ryff's Well-Being Inventory (Ryff and Keyes 1995). Six core domains of positive human health were measured: (1) enjoying a strong sense of purpose in life, or being engaged in ongoing meaningful activity, such as creating, parenting, loving, and learning; (2) forging and sustaining positive relations with others; (3) possessing a sense of self-acceptance and regard; (4) valuing and striving for personal growth; (5) engaging with and enjoying a sense of mastery in one's environment; and finally, (6) possessing and exercising a sense of self-guidance and self-determination in life, which Ryff labels autonomy. In the longer version of her well-being inventory, each domain is assessed by a set of twenty questions (Ryff 1989). In the consolidated version of the instrument used here, a factor score for each well-being domain is typically established as the sum of responses to a set of three questions. (See Ryff and Keyes 1995 for a validation study.)

We approached the use of this instrument with members of our immigrant samples with particular care. Because we were concerned about the cultural and language differences between our samples and those upon which the Ryff scales had been piloted, we tested the proposed a priori six-factor solution by using a path-modeling procedure. This test did not confirm the full a priori six-factor structure within our sample. We thus conducted a further set of exploratory factor analyses (principal component analyses with varimax rotation, accepting eigenvalues > 1.0). Those analyses were run first for subjects from our separate immigrant samples and then for our combined subject pool. Both sets of tests yielded a similar set of unforced five-factor solutions. The five-factor solution from the pooled subject response data possessed strong face validity. Because we wished to obtain maximum distinctiveness for the factors to be used in this study, we used this solution as the basis for the psychological well-being factors.

The adopted five-factor model accounted for 54 percent of the variance in psychological well-being responses. The first two factors, autonomy and positive relations with others, are identical to Ryff's original factors. Many of the negatively cast items in the inventory clustered together and formed two additional factors. One might be called lack of purpose in life, and the second lack of self-acceptance. Because two of the three items for each of these factors derived from Ryff's original factors of the same name, and in order to avoid the confusion of double-negative references, we retained the labels "purpose in life" and "self-acceptance" for these two factors. A fifth, and final, factor accounted for the greatest amount of variance in the model. This was a combination of five items from Ryff's Personal Growth and Environmental Mastery factors. We labeled this last factor "growth and mastery" in our analyses. All items loaded at greater than $r = .35$ on their final assigned factors. One item that did not load strongly on any factors was discarded, and two items that had double-factor loadings (r's > .35) were restored to their a priori Ryff factors. (See the appendix for a list of survey items with their loadings on assigned factors.)

Responses to well-being questions were on a seven-point Likert formatted scale with values ranging from "strongly disagree" to "strongly agree." Final factor scores were derived as the arithmetic mean of summed item scores, with higher values reflecting reports of greater well-being.

PROCEDURES

To explore and test for possible relationships of ethnic conservatism to psychological well-being, we conducted a series of two-stage tests. In an initial test we looked at simple zero-order correlations between the ethnic conservatism variables and the factors of psychological well-being. At this first stage, we used a Bonferroni correction procedure for a test of twenty possible relationships in each sample (four ethnic conservatism variables, including two ways of assessing language of thought × five well-being factors). We required a value of $p \leq .0025$ (.05 / 20) to accept a result as significant. Associations that met this first-stage criterion were passed on to a second test.

Each significant ethnic conservatism/psychological well-being relationship from the first-stage analyses was tested again. This was done by entering it at the second stage as a predictor variable into a hierarchical linear regression equation (least unweighted squares procedure) after a control block of six demographic and SES variables had been entered. The psychological well-being factor was the dependent variable in this equation. The control variables consisted of age, education, gender, total family income, marital status, and city of residence (New York or Chicago). SES variables are well-documented confounds and correlates of both ethnic conservatism and psychological well-being. The aim of our analysis was to determine the degree of association between ethnic conservatism and psychological well-being independent of the influence of age, education, family income, and so forth.

We conducted a final set of analyses to contrast the relative strength of the association of ethnic conservatism and psychological well-being across the first- and second-generation Puerto Rican American samples. To test for a formal moderating effect of generational status on the relationship of ethnic conservatism and psychological well-being, we conducted a comparison test of unstandardized b coefficients (Baron and Kenny 1985; Cohen and Cohen 1975).

RESULTS
Overall Observations

Mean psychological well-being factor scores and standard deviations broken down by sample group are provided in table 2. Responses to many of the well-being items stacked toward the higher end of the scales, with most individuals endorsing relatively high levels of agreement for the positively cast questions in the inventory. Unlike the second-generation children in many of the studies reviewed in the NRC report, the second-generation Puerto Rican midlife adults in our sample were not significantly worse off in their psychological well-being than were first-generation Puerto Rican midlife adults. A series of t-tests showed no overall differences in levels of well-being based on generation. The decline with time ("from generation to generation") that we shall point to is, instead, a decline with time in the apparent effectiveness of ethnic conservatism as a positive protective factor in support of psychological well-being.

TABLE 2 Mean Well-Being Factor Scores for All Sample Groups

		Ryff Well-Being Factors			
Ethnic Sample Group	Autonomy	Growth and Mastery	Positive Relations	Purpose in Life	Self-Acceptance
Mexican American first generation ($n = 176$)					
Mean	5.34	6.30	5.37	5.17	5.35
SD	1.14	0.72	1.24	1.53	1.36
Puerto Rican American first generation ($n = 144$)					
Mean	5.80	6.32	5.44	5.00	5.13
SD	1.22	0.84	1.24	1.65	1.44
Puerto Rican American second generation ($n = 242$)					
Mean	5.70	6.44	5.31	5.09	4.93
SD	1.29	0.76	1.38	1.74	1.56

First-Generation Mexican American Sample

Zero-order associations. For the first-generation Mexican sample, an initial test of zero-order association between the four ethnic conservatism measures (weak assimilation ideals, ethnic pride, language contrast 1, language contrast 2) and the five Ryff psychological well-being factors showed eight significant associations. Weak assimilation ideals correlated positively with higher levels of autonomy. For language contrast 1 (the contrast between "Spanish only" and "more Spanish than English"), endorsement of thinking in "Spanish only" was associated with higher levels of autonomy, positive relations, and purpose in life. Ethnic pride correlated significantly and positively with higher levels of autonomy, growth and mastery, positive relations, and purpose in life. Overall, ethnic pride displayed the strongest relationship to psychological well-being factors. These results are presented in table 3, where coefficients of significant correlations are flagged and displayed in boldface.[6]

Demographic and SES controls. To assess the robustness of the significant associations between ethnic conservatism variables and factors of psychological well-being, we entered each of the eight first-stage significant associations into a multiple regression model (unweighted least squares procedure) after the six demographic and SES variables had been entered as a block. All ethnic conservatism variables retained a minimum significance level of $p \leq .01$ (F of entry) in these tests. Figure 1 presents in a simple visual format the proportion of the variance in each psychological well-being factor that was explained by particular ethnic conservatism variables after all demographic and SES variables had been controlled.

Table 4 presents the R^2 changes and beta and F values for the entry of the ethnic conservatism variables. For weak assimilation ideals and

TABLE 3 First-Generation Mexican American Immigrant Sample: Correlations between Acculturation Measures and Well-Being Factors

		Ryff Well-Being Factors			
Variables	Autonomy	Growth and Mastery	Positive Relations	Purpose in Life	Self-Acceptance
Weak assimilation ideals ($n = 176$)	**.29*****	−.12	−.10	−.11	−.10
Ethnic pride communicated to one's children ($n = 96$)	**.55*****	**.34*****	**.43*****	**.36*****	.23*
Language of thought					
Language contrast 1 Spanish only vs. more Spanish ($n = 163$)	**.29*****	.22**	**.29*****	**.32*****	.18*
Language contrast 2 More Spanish vs. equal bilingual or English dominant ($n = 53$)	−.36**	−.28*	−.21	−.21	−.15

Notes: Values are zero-order Pearson correlation coefficients. Using a two-tailed test with Bonferroni correction procedures applied for multiple hypothesis testing, correlations attain significance when $p \leq$ .0025. Associations significant at this p value are displayed in the table in boldface and were passed on for a second-stage test in regression analyses.
*$p < .05$. **$p < .01$. ***$p \leq .0025$.

language contrast 1, the boost in the model R^2 values associated with entry of the significant ethnic conservatism variables ranged from .06 to .10. In this particular case, this was comparable with the combined explanatory effect of the six demographic and SES control variables. Ethnic pride was even more strongly predictive of its associated psychological well-being factors, with R^2 changes ranging from .07 for growth and mastery to .31 for autonomy. All beta coefficients retained the same valence as in the original set of zero-order correlations. Higher scores on ethnic conservatism measures predicted higher scores on psychological well-being. Among the demographic and SES variables, total family income was the strongest and most consistent predictor of better psychological well-being, with its beta values averaging from .20 to .28 for those equations in which it was significant.

First-Generation Puerto Rican American Sample

Zero-order associations. Seven associations met the first-round criteria of significance in the first-generation Puerto Rican sample. In this sample as well, all significant associations were in the direction of a

1st Generation Mexican Sample

Increase in R square --the percentage of variance in well-being explained--
with entry of each Ethnic Conservatism Variable after
demographic control variables have been entered (all p's < .01)

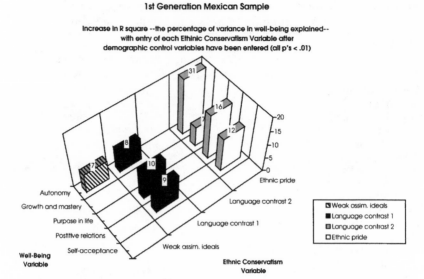

FIGURE 1. The first-generation Mexican sample shows an increase in R^2—the percentage of variance in well-being explained—with entry of each ethnic conservatism variable after demographic control variables have been entered (all p's < .01).

positive association between greater ethnic conservatism and greater psychological well-being. Ethnic pride once again showed the strongest relationship to psychological well-being factors. Weak assimilation ideals correlated positively with autonomy, positive relations, and purpose in life. Language contrast 1, the contrast between "Spanish only" and "more Spanish than English," revealed that those who indicated "Spanish only" reported higher levels of autonomy. Ethnic pride communicated to one's children correlated positively with autonomy, growth and mastery, and purpose in life. The full correlation matrix is presented in table 5.

Demographic and SES controls. When the associations reported earlier were tested with multiple regression analyses, six of the seven relationships retained significance at the level of $p \leq .01$. The association between ethnic pride and purpose in life dropped out in these controlled analyses. Figure 2 presents the proportion of the variance in each psychological well-being factor that was explained by ethnic conservatism variables beyond that which was accounted for by the demographic and SES control block.

The R^2 changes and beta and F values for entry of the ethnic conservatism variables are presented in table 6. For weak assimilation ideals and language contrast 1, the boost in model R^2 values ranges from .05 to .07. Ethnic pride was even more strongly predictive of its associated psychological well-being factors, accounting for an additional 19 percent of the variance in growth and mastery scores and 23 percent of the variance in autonomy-factor scores.

Second-Generation Puerto Rican Sample

Zero-order associations. The zero-order correlation matrix for the second-generation sample revealed only two significant associations between ethnic conservatism variables and psychological well-being factors. Ethnic pride correlated positively with both autonomy and growth and mastery. Correlations across all the indices of ethnic conservatism and the psychological well-being factors were substantially lower than in either of the first-generation immigrant samples. Table 5 presents these results alongside those for the first-generation Puerto Rican sample.

Demographic and SES controls. In the second-stage test of these associations, ethnic pride retained its significance with both autonomy ($F(1, 89)$ $= 4.35,^* \Delta > R^2 = .04, \beta = .21$) and growth and mastery ($F(1, 90) =$ $6.15,^{**} \Delta R^2 = .05, \beta = .23$), after all demographic and SES variables had been controlled.

Generational Status as a Moderator of the Relationship of Ethnic Conservatism to Psychological Well-Being

In testing this moderating relationship, we followed procedures outlined by Baron and Kenny (1985) and Cohen and Cohen (1975), generating a test of differences between unstandardized b coefficients. We conducted tests for the two predictor variables, weak acculturation ideals and ethnic pride communicated to children, across all five of the well-being factors.[7] Moderator variable tests were not conducted for language of thought (contrasts 1 and 2) because these variables were differently comprised in the two generational sample groups. The tests confirmed significant differences in the relationship of ethnic conservatism to psychological well-being factors on the basis of generational status in fully half of the ten possible relations. Results of these tests are reported in table 7.

In a comparison across generations, weaker assimilation ideals showed a significantly stronger and, in all cases, a consistently more positive association with psychological well-being scores in the domains of autonomy, positive relations, and purpose in life for adults from our first-generation

Table 4 First-Generation Mexican American Sample: Regression
Demographic Variables

	Autonomy		Growth and Mastery	
Acculturation Variables	ΔR^2	β	ΔR^2	β
Weak assimilation ideals	.07	.27	—	—
$F(1, 135) =$		10.66***		
Ethnic pride	.31	.57	.07	.26
$F(1, 72) =$		11.97***		6.23**
Language contrast 1	.08	.28	—	—
$F(1, 135) =$		11.97***		

Notes: Probability values reflect F of entry for acculturation variables at the second step in hierarchical multiple regression equation (unweighted least squares) after prior entry of demographic variables. Demographic control variables consisted of age, gender, marital status, total family income, and education level.
*$p < .05$. **$p < .01$. ***$p < .001$.

sample. Ethnic pride showed a similar stronger positive association with purpose, and growth and mastery in the first-generation sample than in the second.

Discussion
General Findings

Rather than trying, point by point, to explain every association between a predictor and criterion variable, we focus instead on identifying trends in association and discussing some of the patterns that appear most salient across different indices of ethnic conservatism in our sample groups. On the most global level, the findings that emerge from these analyses can be summarized by saying that for our first-generation adult Mexican American and Puerto Rican immigrants, an ethnically conservative set of attitudes and approaches to acculturation was associated with better psychological well-being. This was the case across several domains of psychological well-being. Most notably and strongly, our results suggest, individuals who are ethnically conservative may experience an enhanced sense of autonomy and purpose in their lives, and enjoy more positive experiences in their relationships with others.

Autonomy

Ryff's autonomy factor showed the most distinct and persistent association with our measures of ethnic conservatism in both first-generation ethnic samples. The statement "I have confidence in my own opinions,

Coefficients for Entry of Significant Acculturation Variables after
Have Been Entered

| Ryff Well-Being Factors | | | | | |
| Purpose in Life | | Positive Relations | | Self-Acceptance | |
ΔR^2	β	ΔR^2	β	ΔR^2	β
—	—	—	—	—	—
.16	.29	.12	.36	—	—
	17.67**		11.56***		
.10	.33	.09	.30	—	—
	17.68***		15.23***		

even if they are different from the way most other people think" captures the flavor of this factor. In interpreting our findings, we note that a stronger sense of independence of judgment and action is reported by those adult Latino immigrants who do not try to aggressively acculturate by adopting English-language use and seeking social ties with out-group members. This independence of temper could easily be regarded as both arising from and contributing to a desire to actively conserve and maintain a distinct ethnic identity in the face of pressures by the dominant culture to assimilate.

This prominent association of attitudes of autonomy with ethnic conservatism is intriguing, not the least because ideals of autonomy, and independence of temper and judgment, are generally held to be hallmark traits in American national character. Ryff, Lee, and Na (forthcoming) have remarked that autonomy is perhaps the most distinctively American psychological construct to be represented as a cardinal domain of well-being in their model of psychological well-being. The emphasis on autonomy in our own culture is often explained as having arisen in response to the hardships and demands of the immigration process, and of life on the national frontiers. In the life cycle and establishment of ethnic communities, the early stages of settlement present the members of a new immigrant group with a social frontier and a similar set of challenges. There may be a historically similar blending of intense familial and ethnic social ties with a strong insistence on cultural autonomy among members of these modern immigrant communities.

Positive Relations with Others

Ethnic conservatism was also associated with reports of deeper and more intimate social ties with others and more satisfying interpersonal

TABLE 5 First- and Second-Generation Puerto Rican American Immigrant Samples: Correlations between Acculturation Variables and Well-Being Factors

Acculturation Variables		Ryff Well-Being Factors			
	Autonomy	Growth and Mastery	Positive Relations	Purpose in Life	Self-Acceptance
Weak assimilation ideals					
First generation ($n = 144$)	**.39*****	.16	**.27*****	**.25*****	−.08
Second generation ($n = 242$)	.11	.10	.00	−.03	−.08
Ethnic pride communicated to one's children					
First generation ($n = 41$)	**.50*****	**.51*****	.33*	**.47*****	.15
Second generation ($n = 110$)	**.28*****	**.36*****	.18	.25**	.06
Language of thought					
Language contrast 1[a]					
First generation ($n = 108$)	**.29*****	.09	.16	.27**	−.04
Second generation ($n = 132$)	.06	−.07	.01	−.14	−.02
Language contrast 2[b]					
First generation ($n = 75$)	−.06	−.02	.04	−.09	.08
Second generation ($n = 198$)	.00	.02	.04	−.02	−.04

Notes: Values are zero-order Pearson correlation coefficients. Using a two-tailed test with Bonferroni correction procedures applied for multiple hypothesis testing, correlations attain significance when $p \leq$ .0025. Associations significant at this p value are displayed in boldface and were passed on for a second-stage test in regression analyses.

[a] In first-generation sample, this variable is the contrast between endorsing Spanish only vs. more Spanish than English. In second-generation sample, it is the contrast between Spanish dominant vs. equal bilingual.

[b] In first-generation sample, this contrast is between endorsing more Spanish than English vs. equal bilingual thinking. In second-generation sample, it is the contrast between equal bilingual vs. English dominant.

*$p < .05$. **$p < .01$. ***$p \leq .0025$.

relationships. There are many reasons to infer that in these first-generation groups, the deeper sense of relatedness that ethnically conservative individuals are reporting is arising from ties within their ethnic groups and in their home communities. Making use of additional data from the MIDUS survey, we analyzed the composition of social networks of the immigrants within our sample. We discovered that a very small percentage of our first-generation immigrant groups, only 9 percent of Mexican American and 16 percent of Puerto Rican American adults, named *even one* person of non-Latino ethnic descent as an important helper within their social networks. At least for the first-generation immigrants within this study, the experience of forming deep social ties with individuals outside of one's cultural or linguistic group of origin seemed to be far more the exception than the rule.

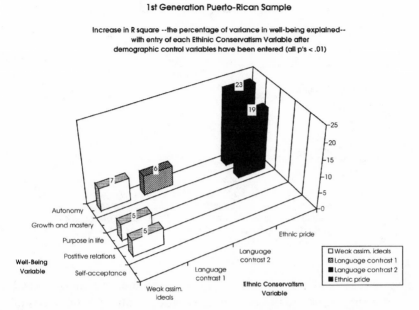

1st Generation Puerto-Rican Sample

Increase in R square --the percentage of variance in well-being explained-- with entry of each Ethinic Conservatism Variable after demographic control variables have been entered (all p's < .01)

FIGURE 2. The first-generation Puerto Rican sample shows an increase in R^2—the percentage of variance in well-being explained—with entry of each ethnic conservatism variable after demographic control variables have been entered (all p's < .01).

The positive association of ethnic conservatism to psychological well-being is primarily a phenomenon of the first-generation immigrant experience. We speculate that given this generational effect, these findings may reflect crucial developmental experiences of socialization to basic cultural roles, scripts for intimacy, and modes of relating to others. As a consequence of such early socialization, in-group relationships may be experienced as richer and more deeply satisfying than out-group relations. Under such conditions, those individuals with ethnically conservative views may simply be living in deeper consonance with this principle, and enjoying real benefits from doing so.

Parenting and Ethnic Identity

Among the most surprising findings of this study was the powerful association between ethnic pride (and cultural identity) communicated to one's children and psychological well-being. As a scale variable, ethnic pride is probably an index of both parenting resources and self-esteem

TABLE 6 First-Generation Puerto Rican Sample: Regression Coefficients for
Have Been

	Autonomy		Growth and Mastery	
Acculturation Variables	ΔR^2	β	ΔR^2	β
Weak assimilation ideals	.07	.24	—	—
$F(1, 117) =$		10.49**		
Ethnic pride	.23	.57	.19	.47
$F(1, 28) =$		16.62***		9.56**
Language contrast 1	.06	.24	—	—
$F(1, 93) =$		6.81**		

Notes: Probability values reflect F of entry for acculturation variables at the second step in a hierarchical multiple regression equation (unweighted least squares) after prior entry of demographic variables. Demographic control variables consisted of age, gender, marital status, total family income, city of residence, and education level.
*$p < .05.$ **$p < .01.$ ***$p < .001.$

as well as an index of ethnically conservative attitudes.[8] Although it was not surprising to find this measure correlating positively with aspects of general psychological well-being, the magnitude of the associations of this parenting variable to diverse aspects of well-being was quite unexpected. This effect was by far the most marked among our first-generation immigrant parents. For these individuals, the level of communication of ethnic pride, history, and customs to their children related to four out of five factors of psychological well-being almost as strongly as these factors related to each other. In fact, if we wanted to know how well the first-generation immigrants in this survey who were parents were doing psychologically, of the hundreds of variables available in the MIDUS survey, we could scarcely have done better than by asking them the series of three questions that began, "How often do you do things with your child to remember the history of his or her ethnic group?"

The issue of direction of causality deserves special attention with this finding. Immigrant parents who are flourishing and psychologically strong may be more likely to report higher levels of ethnic pride–related activities with their children. In this respect there is clear reason to acknowledge the possibility of a backward causal influence of psychological well-being on this index of ethnic conservatism. Nonetheless, we believe there remains an important potential finding here about ethnic identity, acculturation, and the centrality of parent–child ties for members of these Hispanic immigrant communities.[9] The suggestion of these analyses is that for first-generation immigrants, a desire to communicate and

Entry of Significant Acculturation Variables after Demographic Variables Entered

Ryff Well-Being Factors					
Purpose in Life		Positive Relations		Self-Acceptance	
ΔR^2	β	ΔR^2	β	ΔR^2	β
.05	.25	.05	.17	—	—
	8.18**		6.78**		
.10	.34	—	—	—	—
	3.89				
—	—	—	—	—	—

pass along key aspects of one's cultural identity is deeply indicative and reflective of broader psychological health.

A corollary to this observation perhaps deserves attention as well. It may be that for adult immigrants, movement away from or denial of one's ethnic identity and background *during the process of parenting* is indicative of and associated with a diminished experience of psychological well-being.

Low scores on this particular index of ethnic conservatism could be explained in other terms was well. Individuals suffering from a general sense of demoralization, of the kind associated with substance abuse or depression, for instance, might show up as low on ethnic pride in the realm of parenting.

Contrasting the Meaning and Correlates of Ethnic Conservatism across First- and Second-Generation Samples

As we have alluded to at many points in this discussion, data from both parts of this study support the notion that the effects of ethnic conservatism are strongly moderated by generational status. The attitudes and practices of ethnic conservatism that were associated with better psychological well-being across all domains for first-generation adult immigrants, both Mexican and Puerto Rican, were not found to be as predictive of enhanced psychological well-being for members of our second-generation sample. The differences appeared systematic and far-reaching. Although ethnic pride and communication of ethnic identity to one's children remained positively associated with psychological well-being for second-generation immigrant parents, even here the strength of this relationship to psychological well-being was attenuated.

TABLE 7 Tests of the Moderating Influence of Generational Status on the Relationship of Acculturation Variables to Well-Being Factors: T-Test Comparison of Unstandardized Regression Coefficients

Variables	df	b Value		$_tb$
		First Generation	Second Generation	
For Assimilation ideals				
Autonomy	(380)	.38	.13	6.18***
Growth and mastery	(380)	.10	.07	1.42
Purpose in life	(380)	.33	−.05	6.81***
Positive relations	(377)	.27	.00	6.15***
Self-acceptance	(377)	−.09	−.10	0.21
For Ethnic pride				
Autonomy	(147)	.45	.28	1.75
Growth and mastery	(147)	.27	.15	3.13**
Purpose in life	(147)	.42	.29	1.92*
Positive relations	(147)	.25	.14	1.47
Self-acceptance	(147)	.09	.09	−.01

Notes: Tests for mediation in language contrast variables were not performed. Differences in response distributions to the question about language of thought, across the first- and second-generation samples, rendered the test statistically unfeasible.

*$p < .05$. **$p < .01$. ***$p < .001$.

Context and Limitations of the Study

The most serious limitations of this study without doubt arise from the somewhat piecemeal nature of the ethnic conservatism measures that were used and the absence of a second-generation Mexican American sample. Also, aspects of the sampling design of the study may have resulted in our samples underrepresenting the most highly assimilated or acculturated portion of the Mexican and Puerto Rican American populations. By the nature of its survey frame, the MIDUS urban ethnic oversample pulled randomly from a subset of census tracts in the Chicago and New York metropolitan areas. These were tracts and block groups whose ethnic Hispanic populations were at least 10 percent. The most acculturated individuals, and among them, perhaps the most affluent, may tend to live or move outside of these neighborhoods, or outside the city limits entirely. These are the individuals for whom real benefits of acculturation, often argued to consist of socioeconomic advancement, might be expected to accrue. Thus the results we have reported here may reflect, in part, a design-specific finding.

The generalizability of these findings should be qualified on other grounds as well. For ethnic conservatism to be a successful adaptive strategy, many social factors may need to be in place. Ethnic conservatism may become viable and associated with psychological well-being only where relatively strong immigrant communities have been established. Although the adults in our study lived in neighborhoods of varying Latino ethnic density, all enjoy certain social advantages that accrue from living in a large, well-settled urban immigrant environment. In New York City and Chicago, it is possible for Mexican and Puerto Rican immigrants to negotiate many aspects of daily life in Spanish, with the social support of other individuals from similar cultural backgrounds. Both cities boast a profusion of Spanish-based media outlets, specialized immigrant services in law and medicine, Latino churches, and at least limited bilingual educational and social services. Although the strain on these services is often severe, their presence may nonetheless buffer against some of the hardest aspects of resettlement and make it easier for Latino immigrants to remain rooted in a sense of their own culture.

Berry (1997) and other theorists have described a host of additional economic and political factors that might also militate for or against success of this acculturative strategy in different locales. Whether it will prove possible to formulate valid general theories relating acculturation practices to psychological health remains to be seen. Certainly researchers should entertain the alternate possibility that the effects of acculturation choices will be mediated in complex ways by the exigencies of local social and cultural settings. Entrance into the American mainstream, or more recently, the development of "bicultural competence," has sometimes been held out to immigrants as a necessary condition for the enjoyment of psychological health. With due respect to such general formulations, the suggestion of the present study is that for many first-generation Hispanic immigrants, and perhaps other resettled adults, "it ain't necessarily so."

APPENDIX

Well-Being Factors Derived from Ryff's Shorter Well-Being Inventory	Factor Loading Scores[a]
Autonomy	
I tend to be influenced by people with strong opinions.	−.76
I judge myself by what I think is important, not by the values of what others think is important.	.67
I have confidence in my own opinions, even if they are different from the way most other people think.	.39

(continued)

Well-Being Factors Derived from Ryff's Shorter Well-Being Inventory	Factor Loading Scores[a]
Positive relations with others	
I have not experienced many warm and trusting relationships with others.	−.75
Maintaining close relationships has been difficult and frustrating for me.	−.51
People would describe me as a giving person, willing to share my time with others.	.37
Purpose in life	
I sometimes feel as if I've done all there is to do in life.	−.75
I live one day at a time and don't really think about the future.	−.68
I gave up trying to make big improvements or changes in my life a long time ago. (Personal growth)	−.60
Self-acceptance	
In many ways I feel disappointed about my achievements in life.	−.72
When I look at the story of my life, I am pleased with how things have turned out so far.	.68
The demands of everyday life often get me down. (Environmental mastery)	−.66
Personal growth and environmental mastery	
I think it is important to have new experiences that challenge how I think about myself and the world. (Personal growth)	.68
For me, life has been a continuous process of learning, changing, and growth. (Personal growth)	.62
I like most parts of my personality. (Self-acceptance)	.54
In general, I feel I am in charge of the situation in which I live. (Environmental mastery)	.52
I am good at managing the responsibilities of daily life. (Environmental mastery)	.50
Dropped item	
Some people wander aimlessly through life, but I am not one of them. (Purpose)	

Note: An item's original assignment in Ryff's factor structure is indicated in parentheses if the item has been moved.

[a] Factor loading values for Varimax rotation with Kaiser normalization. All eigenvalues ≥ 1.0.

ACKNOWLEDGMENTS

We are grateful to all members of the MacArthur research team.

NOTES

1. In defining our first-generation samples in this way, we have broken slightly with the practice of some acculturation researchers. We have chosen to look at individuals who immigrated to the United States as adults or young adults. In doing so we are working from the assumption that early socialization and immersion in the way of life of a different culture (coupled usually with a voluntary decision to resettle) are the experiences that distinguish first-generation from second-generation immigrants. To include as first-generation immigrants individuals who were brought to this country as young children and socialized through American schooling to English-language use and mainstream American cultural norms may confound the potentially useful distinction between first and later generations of immigrants.

2. For both the Mexican and Puerto Rican subsets of our data, individuals who arrived after age 12 only infrequently endorsed balanced bilingual thinking or, even more rarely, reported English dominance in thinking. This seemed to hold despite the number of years that resettled individuals had lived in the United States.

3. Here is an instance in which the endorsement of identical answers to a question on an acculturation instrument by first- and second-generation immigrants probably reflected vastly different underlying acculturative attitudes and experiences. A report of bilingual thinking or English dominance by an adult first-generation immigrant would reflect a far more active effort to acculturate and gain competence in the host-culture practices than would be true for a second-generation individual. This suggests a need for caution in assuming comparability of acculturation measures across the first- and second-generation divide.

4. In the second-generation sample, it also provided the opportunity to make a small test of the relative effectiveness of a bicultural strategy of acculturation. Using terms proposed by Berry (1997), we checked whether endorsement of balanced bilingual thinking (reflecting an "integrative," bicultural strategy to acculturation) would be associated with better or worse psychological well-being than either a culturally more "assimilationist" (English-dominant) or "separationist" (Spanish-dominant) response. We found no differences across these groupings. In designing this test, we followed a procedure outlined by Magana et al. (1996). We can only speculate, however, whether many of the individuals in this second-generation sample, even those answering "more Spanish" or "Spanish only" to this language question, may have been bilingually competent.

5. Although the ethnic density of the communities in which our first-generation Mexican American adults live proved a predictor in its own right of two facets of psychological well-being, it was not a predictor of the same magnitude as the individual-level measures of ethnic conservatism upon which we focus in this study.

6. We also noticed, however, a slight contrary trend in the data. Within this sample, the variable language contrast 2 showed a trend toward a negative association with some of our well-being indices. This was the single place in our

Randall Horton and Richard A. Shweder

data where ethnic conservatism, in this case endorsement of "more Spanish" as opposed to equal bilingual or English-dominant thinking, was at least marginally associated with lower well-being. These correlations approached but did not attain the level of significance.

7. We did not restrict these tests to those variable combinations that correlated significantly. Even if a set of predictor variables is not significantly correlated with their criteria variables, the moderating influence of a third variable on their relationship can be demonstrated statistically (Cohen and Cohen 1975).

8. One might also have expected this variable to correlate positively with advancing socioeconomic markers, most notably with higher levels of education and family income. In fact, in both of our first-generation samples, acculturation measures correlated only mildly and nonsignificantly with education and total family income. Ethnic pride behaved more like a true acculturation measure than a marker or index of social class. Even among second-generation immigrants, greater acculturation (that is, low ethnic conservatism) was not found to be significantly correlated with greater family income.

9. A vast body of sociological literature has discussed "familialism" as a root organizing structure of life within Hispanic-American immigrant communities.

REFERENCES

Baron, R., and D. Kenny. 1986. The moderator-mediator variable distinction in social psychological research: Conceptual, strategic, and statistical considerations. *Journal of Personality and Social Psychology* 516:1173–82.

Berry, J. W. 1994. Acculturation and psychological adaptation: An overview. In *Journeys into cross-cultural psychology,* ed. A. M. Bouvy, P. Boski, and P. Schmitz, 129–41. Berwyn, Pa.: Swets and Zeitlinger.

———. 1997. Immigration, acculturation, and adaptation. *Applied Psychology: An International Review* 461:5–68.

Cohen, J., and P. Cohen. 1975. *Applied multiple regression/correlation analysis for the behavioral sciences.* Hillside, N.J.: Lawrence Erlbaum Associates.

Dana, R. H. 1996. Assessment of acculturation in Hispanic populations. *Hispanic Journal of Behavioral Sciences* 183:317–28.

Dawson, E. J., W. D. Crano, and M. Burgoon. 1996. Refining the meaning and measurement of acculturation: Revisiting a novel methodological approach. *International Journal of Intercultural Relations* 201:97–114.

Epstein, J. A., G. J. Botvin, L. Dusenbury, and T. Daiz. 1996. Validation of an acculturation measure for Hispanic adolescents. *Psychological Reports* 79:1075–79.

Hernandez, D. J., and E. Charney. 1998. *From generation To generation: The health and well-being of children in immigrant families.* Washington, D.C.: National Academy Press.

Holmbeck, G. N. 1997. Toward terminological, conceptual, and statistical clarity in the study of mediators and moderators. *Journal of Consulting and Clinical Psychology* 654:599–610.

LaFramboise, T., H. L. Coleman, and J. Gerton. 1993. The psychological impact of biculturalism: Evidence and theory. *Psychological Bulletin* 114:395–412.

Magana, J., O. De La Rocha, H. Magana, M. Fernandez, and S. Rulnick. 1996.

Revisiting the dimensions of acculturation: Cultural theory and psychometric practice. *Hispanic Journal of Behavioral Sciences* 18 (4): 444–68.

Rogler, L. H., D. E. Cortez, and R. G. Malgady. 1991. Acculturation and mental health status among Hispanics. *American Psychologist* 46:585–97.

Ryff, C. D. 1989. Happiness is everything, or is it? Explorations on the meaning of well-being. *Journal of Personality and Social Psychology* 57 (6): 1069–81.

Ryff, C. D., and C. M. Keyes. 1995. The structure of psychological well-being revisited. *Journal of Personality and Social Psychology* 69 (4): 719–27.

Ryff, C. D., Y.-H. Lee, and K. C. Na. Forthcoming. Through the lens of culture: Psychological well-being at midlife.

Suarez-Orozco, C., and M. Suarez-Orozco. 1995. *Transformations: Immigration, family life and achievement motivation among latino adolescents.* Stanford: Stanford University Press.

CHAPTER FOURTEEN

Psychological Well-Being in MIDUS: Profiles of Ethnic/Racial Diversity and Life-Course Uniformity

Carol D. Ryff, Corey L. M. Keyes, and Diane L. Hughes

This study provides a descriptive overview of psychological well-being among multiple subgroups, differentiated by age, gender, and ethnic/racial status, in the MIDUS survey. The work extends previous studies of subjective well-being in America by the use of a theory-guided conception of positive psychological functioning, thereby offering a unique look at the psychological strengths of adults located at different positions in American social structure. This inquiry is timely in the context of minority research, which has been described as suffering from myopic attention to the problems and inadequacies, rather than strengths, of people in racially oppressed groups (Jackson and Neighbors 1996).

Quality of Life in America: Beyond Happiness and Life Satisfaction

A large body of research over the last few decades has probed who in the U.S. population is happy or satisfied with life (Campbell, Converse, and Rodgers 1976; Andrews 1991; Campbell 1981; Diener 1984; Veroff, Douvan, and Kulka 1981). These large descriptive studies map differences in avowed well-being linked with major sociodemographic factors (e.g., gender, age, race, marital status, income, education, religious orientation, and geographic location). Known initially as the "social indicators" movement, this work challenged earlier efforts to characterize quality of life in America in strictly economic terms (e.g., standard of living, GNP). Not surprisingly, the findings documented that more disadvantaged social groups (including racial subgroups) tended to report lower levels of subjective well-being.

Others, however, have argued that "most people are happy," including disadvantaged groups, such as those who are poor, disabled, or of minority status (Diener and Diener 1996; Diener et al. 1993; Myers and Diener 1995). Scholars of this persuasion suggest that the more important question is *why* most people are happy (i.e., is it socialization? is it evolutionary priming?). Many such investigations suffer from limited, nonrepresentative samples, which undermines the evidential basis for concluding that happiness is pervasive. Beyond the need for substantiating such claims with better samples, it is relevant to ask whether questions about happiness or life satisfaction are adequate to capture the full meaning of human well-being. Despite their prominence in studies of subjective well-being, neither happiness nor life satisfaction emerged from well-articulated conceptions of positive functioning (see Ryff 1989a).

The absence of theory is puzzling given the large literature in developmental and clinical psychology and the mental health arena that addresses the meaning of psychological well-being (see Ryff 1985). Points of convergence in these numerous accounts comprise core constructs in a multidimensional model of well-being (Ryff 1989b, 1995; Ryff and Keyes 1995). The distinct components are autonomy, environmental mastery, personal growth, positive relations with others, purpose in life, and self-acceptance. As a group, they encompass a breadth of wellness that includes positive evaluations of one's self and one's past life, a sense of continued growth and development, the belief that one's life is purposeful and meaningful, the possession of quality relations with others, the capacity to manage effectively one's surrounding world, and the possession of a sense of self-determination. The constructs have been operationalized with structured, self-report scales.

Previous evidence indicates that perceived happiness and life satisfaction, the ubiquitous indicators of quality of life, are not strongly related to most of these theory-based dimensions of positive functioning (Keyes, Shmotkin, and Ryff 2002; Ryff and Keyes 1995). Thus, continued reliance on the prior indicators of quality of life neglects key aspects of positive psychological functioning. The objective of this study was to investigate age, gender, and ethnic/racial variations in well-being in a national survey using the six components of well-being listed earlier.

Replicable patterns of age and gender differences have been found in previous studies based on both community and national samples (Ryff 1989b, 1991; Ryff and Keyes 1995). Women, for example, consistently score higher than men on positive relations with others and have sometimes shown higher profiles on personal growth. The life-course trajectory of psychological well-being is diverse. Some aspects of well-being (e.g., environmental mastery) show increments with age, others show decrements (e.g., purpose in life, personal growth), and others show little variation with age (self-acceptance). For two dimensions (autonomy, positive relations with others), previous patterns have varied between showing stable or incremental age profiles. These patterns could reflect age changes or cohort differences (or both), although recent longitudinal evidence documents that psychological well-being shows significant change over the course of a major life transition among aging women (Kling, Seltzer, and Ryff 1997).

Diversity and Well-Being: Racial/Ethnic Contrasts

Racial differences in subjective well-being have been a part of earlier national surveys. Veroff, Douvan, and Kulka (1981), for example, found that blacks reported less happiness compared with whites, but the differences are qualified by age, being most pronounced in young adulthood and generally nonexistent in old age. Blacks also reported worrying more than whites. Other research between 1972 and 1988 provided little evidence of differences between blacks and whites in well-being (Andrews 1991); both groups showed notable increases over this time period in their evaluations of personal self-efficacy, health, and standard of living. In specific life domains, however, blacks reported lower levels of well-being than did whites (e.g., income, marriage, neighborhood/community, national government) but also rated themselves higher than whites on two of three self-efficacy items. Summarizing work spanning nearly three decades (1972–96), Hughes and Thomas (1998) found that African Americans report consistently lower levels of quality of life (measured in terms of happiness, life satisfaction, marital happiness, mistrust, anomie, and so forth) than do whites.

In a separate literature, the mental health of minority populations has been investigated. Consistent with the imbalance pervading the mental "health" field, this work is primarily concerned with mental *illness*. Multiple studies show, for example, that African Americans are at high risk for the development of mental health problems (Jackson and Neighbors 1989). Recent findings from the National Survey of Black Americans (Jackson and Neighbors 1996) revealed a largely negative pattern over a recent thirteen-year period. From 1979 to 1992, black respondents reported significant increases in environmental problems, personal problems, and doctor-reported blood pressure, and significant declines in health satisfaction, self-esteem, and happiness. Interestingly, reports of life satisfaction *increased* over this period, which the authors suggest may reflect a kind of adjustment mechanism against more serious mental disorders in the face of declining resources and mounting stresses. A problem with the earlier literature has been the difficulty of disentangling whether the findings are about race or about the consequences of economic and educational disadvantage. Numerous studies suggest that the initially higher levels of distress among blacks were attenuated when controls for social class were introduced (Kessler and Neighbors 1986), thus implying that elevated profiles of psychological distress were partly a social-class, not a racial, phenomenon. Kessler and Neighbors (1986) challenged the exclusively social-class view and argued for an *interactive* model of race and class. Using data from eight epidemiological surveys, they showed that race has a substantial effect on psychological functioning, but that these effects are most pronounced at the *lower* levels of income. More recent studies (Kessler et al. 1994; Williams and Harris-Reid 1999) have not found that African Americans were more likely than whites to have psychiatric disorders (affective disturbances, distress, substance-abuse problems, multiple disorders).

Few studies have compared multiple ethnic and racial groups. An exception is the gerontological research on the "double jeopardy hypothesis" (Dowd and Bengtson 1978), which emphasized the combined disadvantages experienced by aged members of minority groups. The original test of the hypothesis, conducted with middle-aged and older blacks, Mexican Americans, and whites in Los Angeles, received mixed empirical support, and it was challenged by later national studies (Markides 1985). Nonetheless, this work illustrates explicit concern with variation among diverse ethnic/racial groups, and further, it attends to the cultural contexts of such groups, such as the importance of family values and authority relations among Mexican Americans, and a strong support and kinship system in African American families (Mindel 1985). More recent studies addressing mental health differences among multiple ethnic/minorities (Shrout et al. 1992) suggest that Mexican American immigrants had the fewest mental health problems of the groups considered.

In summary, earlier ethnic/racial studies have tended to underscore the compromised quality of life of minorities compared with that of members of majority groups but have shown more mixed findings regarding mental health problems. Cross-time analyses reveal notably negative patterns of change in health and quality of life from the late 1970s to the early 1990s among African Americans. An important message from earlier investigations is the need to examine race interactively with other major sociodemographic variables (e.g., social class, age). A further recurrent theme is the need to investigate possible strengths, not just weaknesses, vis-à-vis the adversity confronted by ethnic/racial minorities. Scientific pursuit of the latter requires empirical indicators of positive psychological characteristics.

Aims of the Present Study

Using data from MIDUS, the present investigation describes multiple aspects of psychological well-being in the white majority population and three ethnic/racial subgroups: African Americans in the survey, a subsample of Mexican Americans from Chicago, and another subsample of African Americans from New York City. Together, the groups provide a window through which to begin viewing profiles of positive mental health in diverse segments of American society. We chose these particular subgroups to underscore the heterogeneity among African Americans and to explore the finding from earlier work that Mexican Americans have more favored mental health status among multiple minority subgroups.

Of major interest was whether earlier findings of gender and age differences would be replicated in a national sample of whites as well as ethnic/racial subgroups. We had no major a priori predictions about how the groups might differ more generally, although the earlier literature on individualism versus collectivism, independence versus interdependence (Markus and Kitayama 1991, 1994), suggested a possible framework for examining majority–minority contrasts. That is, higher profiles on more individualistic qualities of well-being (e.g., self-acceptance, personal growth) might be evident in the majority context, whereas more interpersonal, others-oriented dimensions (e.g., positive relations with others) could have prominence in the minority context.

A final goal was to investigate in a multivariate framework the predictive influence of key sociodemographic variables (age, gender, race) on psychological well-being. Drawing on the class and health literature (Adler et al. 1994; Marmot et al. 1997), we were also interested in the influence of standing in the class hierarchy, possibly in interaction with race, on positive mental health. Following other MIDUS analyses (see chap. 3 in this volume by Marmot and Fuhrer), we chose education as our key measure of social class. Beyond the sociodemographic factors, our regression models included one psychosocial variable, which speaks to the growing interest in racism and health (Jackson et al. 1996; Williams 1999; Williams and Chung 1997), showing that poor treatment as a result of race is inversely related to mental and physical health. To pursue this question, our multivariate models included an assessment of perceived discrimination. Previous findings with the MIDUS sample have shown that perceived discrimination is common in the total population and is more prevalent among individuals with disadvantaged social status (Kessler, Mickelson, and Williams 1999).

METHODS

Sample

Our analyses are based on a subsample of 2455 white respondents aged 25–74 (1077 men, 1378 women) and a subsample of 333 blacks, from the MIDUS national survey, in the same age range (125 men, 208 women). In addition, we use city-specific subsamples of minority respondents. These ethnic/racial subsamples consisted of 345 African Americans (170 men, 165 women) drawn from New York City and 235 Mexican Americans (121 men, 111 women) drawn from Chicago. The latter studies used home interviews with quota samples of ethnic/racial minorities in Chicago and New York City. The sampling design employed census block groups as the primary sampling unit. Respondents completed about 65 percent of the material used in the national survey along with detailed descriptions of community, family, and kinship membership and stress in the workplace.

With regard to demographic characteristics, the Chicago sample of Mexican Americans was younger and less well educated than the remaining three groups (whites, national survey blacks, New York blacks). African American males in the national sample were more highly educated than males in the black New York sample. The majority of respondents were married, with the exception of black women in both the national and New York samples and black men in the New York sample. The New York sample (both men and women) had higher rates of unemployment compared with those of the other groups except Mexican American women from Chicago, of whom approximately half were not employed. These sociodemographic differences across the minority samples complicate the interpretation of findings when minority profiles are not uniform. However, they also increase the heterogeneity of the minority samples, which is the central rationale for including them in the analyses that follow.

Measures

Psychological well-being. In the original validation study (Ryff 1989b), each of six dimensions of well-being was operationalized with a twenty-item scale that showed high internal consistency and test-retest reliability as well as convergent and discriminant validity with other measures. For the national survey, only three of the original twenty items were used to measure each construct. Items were selected from the subfactors within each longer scale to maximize conceptual breadth of the shortened scales.

The shortened scales were shown to correlate from .70 to .89 with parent scales (Ryff and Keyes 1995). The alpha coefficients for the scales across the various subsamples ranged from .35 to .62. The lower coefficients are the result of an a priori decision to represent the multifactorial structure of each parent scale in selecting items for the dramatically reduced subscales (rather than selecting only to maximize internal consistency). Intercorrelations among the scales ranged from moderate to high, although previous analyses supported the six-factor model of well-being (Ryff and Keyes 1995).

Discrimination. In both studies, discrimination was measured as the perception of discriminatory experiences on a daily basis. These data were collected in the self-administered questionnaire in the national survey but by use of in-person interviews with the ethnic/racial subsamples. Instructions between the two were slightly different, with discrimination explicitly mentioned in the former but not the latter. Nine examples of discriminatory experience were listed: how often the respondent was treated with less courtesy than other people, treated with less respect than other people, received poorer service than other people at restaurants or stores, was called names or insulted, was threatened or harassed; and how often other people acted as if they thought the respondent was not smart, was dishonest, was not as good as they were, and as if they were afraid of the respondent. Response categories for the national survey were "often," "sometimes," "rarely," or "never" on a daily basis. In the ethnic/racial study, response categories were "very often," "often," "occasionally," "rarely," or "never" on a daily basis. To make the scales equivalent, the categories "very often" and "often" in the latter were combined, while all other categories were treated as roughly equivalent across the studies. Internal consistency (coefficient alpha) of the discrimination scale was .90.

RESULTS
Age and Gender Differences in Psychological Well-Being

As stated earlier, a primary objective of the study was to determine whether previously noted empirical patterns of age and gender differences in psychological well-being would be replicated with a national sample and ethnic/racial subsamples. Life-span developmental theories, which provided the basis for key dimensions of well-being, have emphasized patterns of change associated with the transitions from young adulthood to midlife to old age. Thus, we investigated mean-level differences in psychological well-being associated with these age periods.

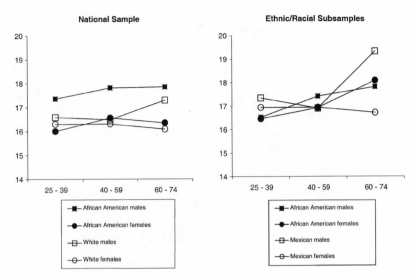

FIGURE 1. Self-acceptance: Age, gender, and ethnic/racial differences.

A limitation of these analyses was that older age groups in the ethnic racial subsamples contained only limited cases ($n = 54$ African Americans in the national sample; $n = 51$ in the New York African American sample; $n = 20$ in the Chicago Mexican American sample). Cell sizes for the remaining age groups in the minority sample sizes ranged from 94 to 228. Using ANOVA models, we investigated separately, for the national survey and the Chicago/New York subsamples, mean-level differences by age, gender, and ethnic/racial group. The primary reason for separate analyses at this point is to facilitate graphic representation to compare age and gender profiles in the four ethnic/racial subgroups. Subsequent multivariate analyses combine all samples.

Self-acceptance. In the national sample (see fig. 1), men were found to have significantly higher scores than women ($F (1, 2748) = 14.33$, $p < .001$). However, an age by gender interaction ($F (2, 2748) = 4.31$; $p < .01$) revealed that these differences occurred only among oldest respondents.

Findings for the Chicago/New York subsamples revealed no significant differences, although there was a trend toward a main effect of age ($F (2, 544) = 2.59$, $p < .07$), with young adults scoring lower than middle-aged adults, who in turn scored lower than older-aged adults.

Environmental mastery. The national sample (see fig. 2) showed a main effect of age ($F (1, 2748) = 15.07$, $p < .001$). Older respondents,

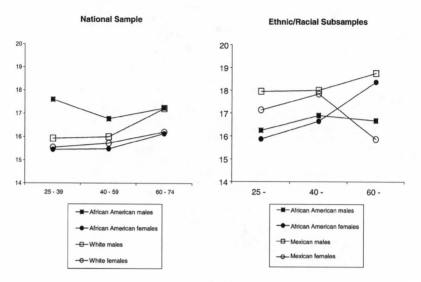

FIGURE 2. Environmental mastery: Age, gender, and ethnic/racial differences.

both black and white, had significantly higher scores on mastery than did young adult or middle-aged respondents. A main effect of gender was also obtained (F (1, 2748) = 16.95, $p < .001$), which was further qualified by a gender–race interaction (F (1, 1, 2748) = 4.77, $p < .05$). As figure 2 demonstrates, gender differences among African Americans are greater than among whites.

For the Chicago/New York subsamples, there was a trend toward ethnic differences (F (1, 534) = 3.45, $p < .06$), with African Americans scoring lower than Mexican Americans. There was also a significant gender–ethnicity interaction (F, (1, 534) = 3.89, $p < .05$), which revealed that the previous African American women, particularly in old age, scored significantly higher on environmental mastery than did the Mexican American women, whereas among men, the differences across all age groups revealed higher profiles for Mexican American than African American males.

Purpose in life. A main effect of age (F, (1, 2740) = 31.73, $p < .001$) showed that older adults had significantly lower scores on purpose in life than did middle-aged or younger adults (see fig. 3). A significant gender–age interaction was also found (F, (2, 2740) = 4.69, $p < .01$), which showed that men had significantly higher scores than women only in young adulthood.

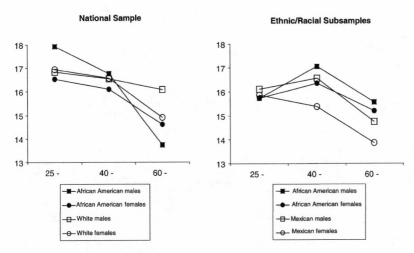

FIGURE 3. Purpose in life: Age, gender, and ethnic/racial differences.

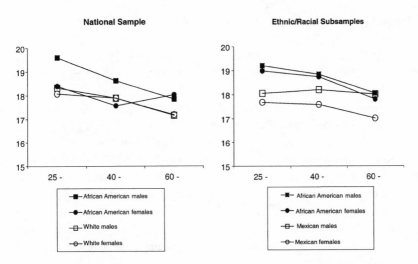

FIGURE 4. Personal growth: Age, gender, and ethnic/racial differences.

Findings for the Chicago/New York subsamples revealed a trend toward a main effect of age (F (2, 544) = 2.58, $p < .08$), indicating that older adults scored lower than young adults, who in turn scored lower than middle-aged adults.

Personal growth. The national sample (see fig. 4) revealed a main effect of age (F (2, 2740) = 18.29, $p < .001$), with each of the age groups significantly different from each other in a downward direction. Approaching

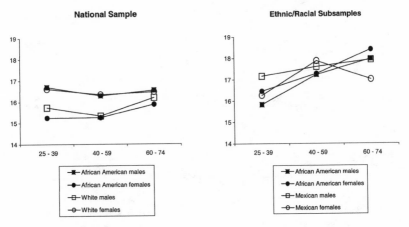

National Sample

Ethnic/Racial Subsamples

—■—African American males
—●—African American females
—□—White males
—⊖—White females

—■—African American males
—●—African American females
—□—Mexican males
—⊖—Mexican females

FIGURE 5. Positive relations with others: Age, gender, and ethnic/racial differences.

significance was a main effect of race (F $(1, 2740) = 3.41$, $p < .07$) in which blacks scored higher than whites.

Analyses for the Chicago/New York subsamples did not reveal an age effect, although ethnic differences were present (F $(1, 544) = 7.23$, $p < .01$), with African Americans scoring higher than Mexican Americans.

Positive relations with others. A main effect of gender was found for positive relations with others in the national sample (F $(1, 2748) = 19.95$, $p < .001$), with women scoring higher than men, but it was qualified by a gender–race interaction (F, $(1, 2748) = 9.47$, $p < .002$). As illustrated in figure 5, among whites, women had significantly higher scores on positive relations with others than did men. Among blacks, the reverse pattern was found: men scored significantly higher than women. A significant age effect was also found (F $(2, 2748) = 3.27$, $p < .05$). Older adults had significantly higher reports of positive relations with others than did middle-aged adults.

Interestingly, no main effects of gender were found in the ethnic/racial subsamples, although a main effect of age was evident (F $(2, 544) = 6.14$, $p < .01$), with young adults scoring significantly lower than middle-aged adults, who in turn scored significantly lower than older adults.

Autonomy. Age emerged as a key factor in the national survey as well (F, $(2, 2740) = 16.84$, $p < .001$), with young adults scoring significantly lower than middle-aged or older adults. However, a main effect of gender was also obtained (F, $(1, 2740) = 16.62$, $p < .001$), which is further qualified by a gender–age interaction (F $(2, 2740) = 3.55$, $p < .05$). As

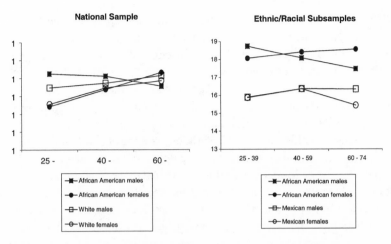

FIGURE 6. Autonomy: Age, gender, and ethnic/racial differences.

figure 6 illustrates, all age groups except African American males showed upward patterns with age on autonomy. Black males, however, revealed a decremental age pattern.

For the Chicago/New York subsamples, age was not a key differentiating factor. Rather, ethnicity was the important variable (F (1, 534) = 33.30, p < .001), with African Americans scoring notably higher than Mexican Americans.

The Prediction of Well-Being: Sociodemographic Influences and Discrimination

For the multivariate analysis, data from the national sample and ethnic/racial subsamples were combined to allow for assessment of possible differences among the three minority samples as well as between each of these samples and the white majority group, after controlling for differences in employment status and marital status. Separate regression models were run for each of the six scales of psychological well-being. Results were largely the same, using weighted or unweighted data. The tables show only unweighted sample results.

Model 1 for each analysis included major sociodemographic variables of age, gender, and race and controlled for employment status and marital status. Because of prior theory and empirical results, we checked for interactions of race with age (double jeopardy) as well as race with gender. Race was coded to maximize the majority/minority contrast; thus the contrast category is whites. Age was coded categorically (young, middle, old) to continue with the earlier analyses and literature on well-being (young is the contrast category). Model 2 for each analysis added education to the model as well as allowed for entrance into the equation of significant interactions of education with other variables (to explore, in particular, the claim that race and class have an interactive relationship). Model 3 added the psychosocial variable of perception of discrimination. Findings from these analyses are summarized in tables 1–6. Only interactions having a significant predictive influence on the dependent measure are included in the tables (exceptions are noted and explained later).

Self-acceptance. Model 1 (see table 1) revealed that self-acceptance was significantly predicted by race (blacks, from both the national survey and New York subsample, and Mexican Americans had more positive scores than whites); gender (women had more negative scores than men); age (older adults had higher scores compared with young adults); marital status (married persons had higher scores than unmarried persons); and

TABLE 1 Prediction of Self-Acceptance (unstandardized coefficients)

Predictors	Models		
	1	2	3
Control variables			
Not married	—	—	—
Married	1.1**	1.1**	1.0**
Unemployed	—	—	—
Employed	.75**	.60**	.58**
Key sociodemographics			
Whites, national sample	—	—	—
Blacks, national sample	.76**	2.1**	2.6**
Blacks, New York	1.2**	1.4**	1.2**
Mexicans, Chicago	.81**	1.6**	1.3**
Males	—	—	—
Females	−.27*	−.21	−.25*
Adults aged 25–39	—	—	—
Adults aged 40–59	.02	.01	−.06
Adults aged 60–74	.78**	.86**	.61**
Social class (education)			
Education		.51**	.51**
Blacks, national sample × Education		−.46*	−.30
Psychosocial			
Perceived discrimination			−.14**
Intercept	15.2	13.7	14.4
R^2	.05	.06	.09

Notes: $N = 3200$. Ordinary least squares estimation. All regression models estimated on the unweighted sample.
*$p < .05$. **$p < .01$ (two-tailed).

TABLE 2 Prediction of Environmental Mastery
(unstandardized coefficients)

Predictors	Models		
	1	2	3
Control variables			
Not married	—	—	—
Married	.35**	.37**	.27*
Unemployed	—	—	—
Employed	.52**	.43**	.42**
Key sociodemographics			
Whites, national sample	—	—	—
Blacks, national sample	.52**	.58**	1.5**
Blacks, New York	.95**	1.1**	.83**
Mexicans, Chicago	1.9**	2.3**	1.9**
Males	—	—	—
Females	−.42**	−.39**	−.43**
Adults aged 25–39	—	—	—
Adults aged 40–59	.17	.16	.08
Adults aged 60–74	1.3**	1.3**	1.0**
Social class (education)			
Education		.27**	.28**
Psychosocial			
Perceived discrimination			−.14**
Intercept	15.2	14.5	15.1
R^2	.04	.05	.08

Notes: $N = 3199$. Ordinary least squares estimation. All regression models estimated on the unweighted sample.
$*p < .05$. $**p < .01$ (two-tailed).

employment status (employed persons had higher scores than unemployed persons). There were no significant interactions among any of these sociodemographic variables. Model 2 showed that education also has significant positive influence on self-acceptance ratings, although it did not reduce or explain the influence of any of the previous sociodemographic variables. A significant race–education interaction was also found: blacks (in the national sample) compared with whites showed less boost in self-acceptance with increments in education. Thus, the greatest difference in self-acceptance is at the lowest levels of education, with blacks showing higher levels than whites; at higher educational levels, there is no racial difference.

Model 3 revealed the continuing influence of all prior factors (except one) when the discrimination variable was added to the model. Perceived discrimination was also a strong negative influence on self-acceptance. The race–education interaction dropped to nonsignificance

TABLE 3 Prediction of Purpose in Life (unstandardized coefficients)

Predictors	Models		
	1	2	3
Control variables			
Not married	—	—	—
Married	.82**	.84**	.75**
Unemployed	—	—	—
Employed	.73**	.50**	.48**
Key sociodemographics			
Whites, national sample	—	—	—
Blacks, national sample	.22	−1.3	−.94
Blacks, New York	−.04	.08	−.29
Mexicans, Chicago	−.70**	.23	.07
Males	—	—	—
Females	−.09	−.01	−.05
Adults aged 25–39	—	—	—
Adults aged 40–59	−.27	−.29	−.36*
Adults aged 60–74	−.94**	−.83**	−1.0**
Blacks, New York × adults aged 40–59	.99*	1.1*	1.1*
Social class (education)			
Education		.61**	.61**
Blacks, national sample × education		.60**	.74**
Psychosocial			
Perceived discrimination			−.12**
Intercept	15.6	14.0	14.6
R^2	.04	.07	.09

Notes: $N = 3202$. Ordinary least squares estimation. All regression models estimated on the unweighted sample.
*$p < .05$. **$p < .01$ (two-tailed).

once discrimination was added to the model. What this suggests is that the reason blacks in the national sample do not benefit from more education is discrimination. Once accounted for, blacks and whites experience the psychological benefits of greater education.

Environmental mastery. Model 1 (see table 2) revealed that nearly all sociodemographic variables were significant predictors of this aspect of well-being. Minority group status (for all three groups) was a significant positive predictor of environmental mastery compared with majority white status. Being married, employed, and older (compared with being a young adult) were also significant positive influences. Being female was a significant negative influence. Model 2 showed that in addition to these variables, education is a significant positive predictor of mastery, and there were no interactions with other variables. Model 3 added the significant negative influence of discrimination experiences. All other

TABLE 4 Prediction of Personal Growth (unstandardized coefficients)

	Models		
Predictors	1	2	3
Control variables			
Not married	—	—	—
Married	.15	.17	.14
Unemployed	—	—	—
Employed	.74**	.56**	.56**
Key sociodemographics			
Whites, national sample	—	—	—
Blacks, national sample	.60**	.72**	.96**
Blacks, New York	1.2**	1.4**	1.3**
Mexicans, Chicago	−.06	.74**	.65**
Males	—	—	—
Females	−.08	.01	.02
Adults aged 25–39	—	—	—
Adults aged 40–59	−.31**	−.32**	−.34**
Adults aged 60–74	−.55**	−.46**	−.53**
Social class (education)			
Education		.53**	.54**
Psychosocial			
Perceived discrimination			−.04**
Intercept	17.5	16.0	16.2
R^2	.03	.07	.07

Notes: $N = 3196$. Ordinary least squares estimation. All regression models estimated on the unweighted sample.

$^*p < .05.$ $^{**}p < .01$ (two-tailed).

variables remained significant negative predictors, even after the effects of perceived discrimination were added to the model.

Purpose in life. Model 1 (see table 3) revealed significant positive influences on purpose in life associated with being married and employed, and significant negative influences associated with being Mexican (compared with being white) and being older (compared with being a young adult). There was also a significant interaction of race by age, with midlife whites having higher levels of purpose in life than midlife blacks in the national sample.

Model 2 showed that being educated was a significant positive influence on purpose in life. In addition, the effects of education worked differently for various racial groups. Blacks in the national sample received a greater boost in purpose for each increment in education compared with the other racial/ethnic groups. The significant negative effect that was evident for Mexican Americans dropped out once educational interactions were added to the equation.

TABLE 5 Prediction of Positive Relations with Others
(unstandardized coefficients)

Predictors	Models		
	1	2	3
Control variables			
Not married	—	—	—
Married	1.5**	1.5**	1.4**
Unemployed			
Employed	.54**	.42**	.39**
Key sociodemographics			
Whites, national sample	—	—	—
Blacks, national sample	1.3**	1.4**	2.8**
Blacks, New York	.78*	.92*	.61
Mexicans, Chicago	1.3**	1.8**	1.4**
Males	—	—	—
Females	.99**	1.0**	1.0**
Mexicans × females	−1.6**	−1.6**	−1.7**
Blacks, national sample × females	−1.9**	−1.9**	−2.3**
Adults aged 25–39	—	—	—
Adults aged 40–59	−.34*	−.36*	−.47**
Adults aged 60–74	.41	.46*	.14
Blacks, New York × adults aged 60–74	1.8**	1.7*	1.9**
Blacks, New York × adults aged 40–59	1.2*	1.3*	1.3*
Mexicans × adults aged 40–59	1.2*	1.3*	1.4*
Social class (education)			
Education		.35**	.35**
Psychosocial			
Perceived discrimination			−.17**
Intercept	14.2	13.3	14.1
R^2	.05	.06	.09

Notes: $N = 3197$. Ordinary least squares estimation. All regression models estimated on the unweighted sample.
$*p < .05.$ $**p < .01$ (two-tailed).

Model 3, the final equation, revealed the same pattern of effects established in previous models, once reports of discrimination, which were significant negative influences on purpose in life, were taken into account.

Personal growth. Model 1 (see table 4) revealed that personal growth was positively predicted by being employed and being black (both the national sample and New York subsample) compared with being white. Personal growth was negatively predicted by age (both middle-aged and older adults differing significantly from young adults). All of these effects remained in model 2, which also showed that education was a significant positive predictor of personal growth. Model 3 showed the persistence of these predictor variables as well as the negative effects associated with reports of discrimination.

Positive relations with others. Model 1 (see table 5) revealed that positive relations with others was significantly predicted by being married, employed, and a member of a minority (all three subgroups had positive effects compared with whites). Women also had higher scores than men, and midlife adults had lower scores than young adults. However, numerous interaction effects were also obtained. A race–gender interaction showed that the scores for positive relations with others for two groups of minority women (Mexican Americans, blacks in the national survey) were lower than those of their male counterparts. Further, a race–age interaction revealed that older blacks (both from the national sample and the New York sample) reported higher positive relations with others compared with younger blacks, which is in contrast to white adults, who

TABLE 6 Prediction of Autonomy (unstandardized coefficients)

	Models		
Predictors	1	2	3
Control variables			
Not married	—	—	—
Married	−.05	−.04	−.07
Unemployed	—	—	—
Employed	.26	.25	.25
Key sociodemographics			
Whites, national sample	—	—	—
Blacks, national sample	.19	.19	.53*
Blacks, New York	2.1**	2.1**	2.0**
Mexicans, Chicago	−.27	−1.1*	−1.2**
Males	—	—	—
Females	−.42**	−.40**	−.43**
Adults aged 25–39	—	—	—
Adults aged 40–59	.53**	.54**	.51**
Adults aged 60–74	1.1**	1.1**	1.0**
Blacks, New York × adults aged 60–74	−1.1*	−1.1*	−1.1*
Social class (education)			
Education		.01	.01
Mexicans × education		.60*	.61*
Psychosocial			
Perceived discrimination			−.05**
Intercept	16.1	16.0	16.3
R^2	.04	.04	.05

Notes: $N = 3190$. Ordinary least squares estimation. All regression models estimated on the unweighted sample.

*$p < .05$. **$p < .01$ (two-tailed).

showed little age variation. Education was a strong positive predictor, and there were no significant interactions with education. All variables remained in the final model (model 3), and perceived discrimination was also a strong negative predictor of positive relations with others.

Autonomy. Model 1 (see table 6) revealed that autonomy is positively predicted by being an African American in New York, male, and middle-aged or old-aged. A significant race–age interaction indicated, however, that older blacks in New York did not have higher profiles on autonomy than did the two younger age groups, as was evident for the three other racial/ethnic groups. Model 2 showed that the preceding variables remained significant predictors, when education was added to the model, even though education itself was not a significant predictor of autonomy. A race–education interaction revealed that Mexican Americans in Chicago showed notable gains in autonomy with additional levels of education, whereas no such gains were evident for the other three racial/ethnic groups. Model 3 revealed a significant negative influence of perceived discrimination, with all other previous influences remaining in the model.

Discussion

A major objective of the present study was to investigate the consistency of previously established patterns of age and gender differences on six different dimensions of psychological well-being (Ryff 1989b, 1991; Ryff and Keyes 1995). The merits of these descriptive questions were underscored by the nationally representative nature of the sample plus the added sampling of diverse ethnic/racial subgroups. The life-course patterns, assessed by mean-level analyses, revealed considerable convergence with earlier findings on community samples. Specifically, age decrements were replicated for purpose in life in all ethnic/racial groups. Personal growth also replicated patterns of decrement with age for all groups, although these effects were statistically significant only for blacks and whites in the national sample. With regard to age increments, blacks and whites in the national sample replicated earlier findings of older adults scoring higher than young adult or middle-aged respondents on environmental mastery, although no such effect was evident in the Chicago and New York subsamples. Similarly, middle- and older-aged adults in the national sample showed significantly higher scores on autonomy than did young adults (for all groups except African American males), but age was not a differentiating factor for the city-specific subsamples. For positive relations with others, the older age groups scored higher than did the group of young adults, but only for the Chicago Mexican Americans and New York African Americans. Finally, as evident in earlier research, self-acceptance showed little significant variation by age across all groups.

This collective portrait of psychological well-being across the adult life course thus shows notable consistency across multiple samples, differing not only in their size and representativeness but also with regard to depth of measurement in assessing well-being (i.e., twenty-item versus three-item scales). The findings leave unanswered whether aging or cohort processes (or both) explain such patterns, but even in the absence of such understanding, the results document important diversity in life-course trajectories. As previously argued (Ryff 1989b; Ryff and Keyes 1995), the panoply of age profiles underscores the need for a multidimensional conception of positive functioning, because it suggests gains in some areas, losses in others, and stability in still others. Longitudinal analysis will, of course, be necessary to determine the actual nature of these dynamics.

Gender differences were generally stronger in the present study than has been previously documented (Ryff 1989b, 1991; Ryff and Keyes 1995). Positive relations with others has consistently shown higher scores among women compared with men, and this pattern was upheld with the MIDUS data, but in a qualified fashion. For white women in the national sample, scores were, as expected, higher than those of their male counterparts, but for blacks in the national sample, men actually scored higher than women. In addition, disadvantage for women relative to men was further evident for self-acceptance (only among older respondents in the national sample), environmental mastery (more strongly for blacks than whites in the national sample, for Mexican Americans in Chicago), purpose in life (only among young adults in national sample), and autonomy (only among young adults in national sample). Taken together, the findings underscore a wider expanse of compromised well-being among ethnic/minority women of differing ages.

The multivariate prediction of psychological well-being, which incorporated controls for employment and marital status, revealed the most novel findings of this investigation. Across numerous outcomes (self-acceptance, environmental mastery, personal growth), racial minority status was a significant *positive* predictor of well-being, an effect evident for all three minority subgroups. These positive effects also remained in the model once other factors (education, perceived discrimination) were accounted for. Minority advantage was also evident for autonomy, but only for African Americans (both national sample and New York subsample). Being Mexican American was, however, a negative predictor of autonomy and purpose in life relative to whites. On the other hand, purpose in life was positively predicted by being African American, but this effect held true only for better-educated blacks in the national sample.

Overall, these findings provide a novel portrayal of psychological strengths of ethnic/racial minorities on numerous aspects of well-being. Viewed in the context of prior research, some of which documents the higher profiles of psychological distress among racial minorities (Jackson and Neighbors 1989, 1996; Kessler and Neighbors 1986), and compromised quality of life (Hughes and Thomas 1998), the present findings draw attention to a frequently neglected phenomenon, namely, that the presence of the negative in the lives of oppressed groups does not automatically imply an absence of the positive. That is, advantage in well-being may sometimes exist concomitantly with negative outcomes (Keyes, Shmotkin, and Ryff 2002; Singer et al. 1998). In fact, some might argue that certain aspects of well-being, such as having a high sense of self-regard, mastery, and personal growth, may actually be honed by challenge, applied in this case to the difficulties of minority life. Such thinking is evident in Frankl's work (1992), which views adversity, particularly when meaning is attached to it, as a possible contributor to human strength (Ryff and Singer 1998). Similarly, others have emphasized the growth that sometimes follows in the aftermath of suffering or trauma (Tedeschi and Calhoun 1995). Our analyses offer no insight on *how* such strength building may come about but instead call for future research not only to assess the consistency of minority advantage in well-being but also to explore possible socialization practices and supportive social environments that may nurture it.

Education was also found to be a strong positive predictor of all aspects of psychological well-being (except autonomy). But importantly, educational differences did not account for the above racial effects. If anything, once education was in the model, the positive effects of minority group status were more strongly evident. Only for purpose in life did the findings show support for the argument that class and race interact to account for mental health effects (Kessler and Neighbors 1986). But the nature of the interaction was that blacks in the national sample showed greater boosts in purpose with additional increments in education, as compared with whites. Our analyses also revealed little support for the double jeopardy hypothesis (Dowd and Bengtson 1978), which predicts diminished well-being among those who are both old and members of a racial minority. Older blacks (both the national sample and New York sample) revealed higher scores on positive relations with others relative to younger blacks. Only for African Americans in the New York sample, and only for one outcome (autonomy), was the combination of age and race a negative predictor of well-being. The nature of the interaction, however, showed that age effects were diminished, rather than exacerbated, for New York blacks compared with whites.

The psychosocial variable of perceived discrimination emerged as a significant negative predictor of every dimension of psychological well-being, net of all other sociodemographic variables in the model. The juxtaposition of this subjective rating, along with the objective social structural factors (e.g., education, race), underscores the need for combined consideration of both internal and external influences on psychological well-being. Previous MIDUS findings on perceived discrimination (Kessler, Mickelson, and Williams 1999) revealed links between the perception that one has been treated unfairly by others and mental problems (depression, anxiety). Our findings show that in addition, perceived discrimination diminishes the likelihood of psychological well-being. In fact, were it not for the negative effects of such perceptions, the previously described minority advantage in psychological well-being would have been even greater.

How these strengths develop and what protective roles they serve are important items on the agenda for future research. Pursuit of such questions is usefully framed in the context of long-term, life history approaches that speak to the cumulation of adversity in people's lives (Singer et al. 1998), while simultaneously keeping track of compensating psychosocial advantages that foster resilience (Singer and Ryff 1997; Singer et al. 1998). Psychological resilience in the face of life stresses, including experiences of racism and discrimination, may also have protective effects at the physiological level, with implications for unfolding physical health trajectories (Singer and Ryff 1999; Ryff and Singer 2000). Thus, the present findings point to numerous future directions for sharpening understanding of how, in the face of difficult life circumstances, some individuals are able to lead healthy, productive, and fulfilling lives.

References

Adler, N. E., T. Boyce, M. A. Chesney, S. Cohen, S. Folkman, R. L. Kahn, and S. L. Syme. 1994. Socioeconomic status and health: The challenge of the gradient. *American Psychologist* 49:15–24.

Andrews, F. M. 1991. Stability and change in levels and structure of subjective well-being. *Social Indicators Research* 25:1–30.

Campbell, A. 1981. *The sense of well-being in America: Recent patterns and trends.* New York: McGraw-Hill.

Campbell, A., P. E. Converse, and W. L. Rodgers. 1976. *The quality of life in America.* New York: Russell Sage Foundation.

Crocker, J. and B. Major. 1989. Social stigma and self-esteem: The self-protective properties of stigma. *Psychological Review* 96:608–30.

Diener, E. 1984. Subjective well-being. *Psychological Bulletin* 95:542–75.

Diener, E., and C. Diener. 1996. Most people are happy. *Psychological Science* 7:181–85.

Diener, E., E. Sandvik, L. Seidlitz, and M. Diener. 1993. The relationship between income and subjective well-being: Relative or absolute. *Social Indicators Research* 28:195–223.

Dowd, J. J., and V. L. Bengtson. 1978. Aging in minority populations: An examination of the double jeopardy hypothesis. *Journal of Gerontology* 33:427–36.

Frankl, V. E. 1992. *Man's search for meaning.* 4th ed. Boston: Beacon Press.

Hughes, M., and M. E. Thomas. 1998. The continuing significance of race revisited: A study of race, class, and quality of life in America, 1972 to 1996. *American Journal of Sociology* 63:785–95.

Jackson, J. S., T. N. Brown, D. R. Williams, M. Torres, S. L. Sellers, and K. Brown. 1996. Racism and the physical and mental health status of African Americans: A thirteen-year national panel study. *Ethnicity and Disease* 6:132–47.

Jackson, J. S., and H. W. Neighbors. 1989. Sociodemographic predictors of psychological distress in black adults. In *Proceedings from the eleventh conference on empirical research in black psychology,* ed. A. O. Harrison, 120–28. Rockville, Md.: National Institute of Mental Health.

———. 1996. Changes in African American resources and mental health: 1979 to 1992. In *Mental health in black America,* ed. H. W. Neighbors and J. S. Jackson, 189–212. Thousand Oaks, Calif.: Sage.

Kessler, R. C., S. Z. McGonagle, B. N. Christopher, M. Hughes, S. Eshleman, H. U. Wittchen, and K. S. Kendler. 1994. Lifetime and 12-month prevalence of DSM-III-R psychiatric disorders in the United States. *Archives of General Psychiatry* 51:8–19.

Kessler, R. C., K. D. Mickelson, and D. R. Williams. 1999. The prevalence, distribution, and mental health correlates of perceived discrimination in the United States. *Journal of Health and Social Behavior* 40:208–30.

Kessler, R.C., and H. W. Neighbors. 1986. A new perspective on the relationships among race, social class, and psychological distress. *Journal of Health and Social Behavior* 27:107–15.

Keyes, C. L., D. Shmotkin, and C. D. Ryff. 2002. Optimizing well-being: The empirical encounter of two traditions. *Journal of Personality and Social Psychology* 87:1007–22.

Kling, K. C., M. M. Seltzer, and C. D. Ryff. 1997. Distinctive late life challenges: Implications for coping and well-being. *Psychology and Aging* 12:288–95.

Markides, K. S. 1985. Minority aging. In *Growing old in America: New perspectives on old age,* 3d ed., ed. B. B. Hess and E. W. Markson, 113–35. New Brunswick, N.J.: Transaction Books.

Markus, H. R., and S. Kitayama. 1991. Culture and the self: Implications for cognition, emotion, and motivation. *Psychological Review* 98:224–53.

———. 1994. The cultural construction of self and emotion: Implications for social behavior. In *Emotion and culture: Empirical studies of mutual influence,* ed. S. Kitayama and H. R. Markus. Washington, D.C.: American Psychological Association.

Marmot, M., C. D. Ryff, L. L. Bumpass, M. Shipley, and N. F. Marks. 1997. Social inequalities in health: Next questions and converging evidence. *Social Science and Medicine* 44:901–10.

Mindel, C. H. 1985. The elderly in minority families. In *Growing old in America: New perspectives on old age,* 3d ed., ed. B. B. Hess and E. W. Markson, 369–86. New Brunswick, N.J.:Transaction Books.

Myers, D. G., and E. Diener. 1995. Who is happy? *Psychological Science* 6:10–19.

Neighbors, H. W., and J. S. Jackson. 1996. Mental health in black America: Psychosocial problems and help-seeking behavior. In *Mental health in black America,* ed. H. W. Neighbors and J. S. Jackson, 1–13. Thousand Oaks, Calif.: Sage.

Ryff, C. D. 1985. Adult personality development and the motivation for personal growth. In *Advances in motivation and achievement: Motivation and adulthood,* ed. D. Kleiber and M. Maehr, 4:55–92. Greenwich, Conn.: JAI Press.

———. 1989a. Beyond Ponce de Leon and life satisfaction: New directions in quest of successful aging. *International Journal of Behavioral Development* 12:35–55.

———. 1989b. Happiness is everything, or is it? Explorations on the meaning of psychological well-being. *Journal of Personality and Social Psychology* 57:1069–81.

———. 1991. Possible selves in adulthood and old age: A tale of shifting horizons. *Psychology and Aging* 6:286–95.

———. 1995. Psychological well-being in adult life. *Current Directions in Psychological Science* 4:99–104.

Ryff, C. D., and C. L. M. Keyes. 1995. The structure of psychological well-being revisited. *Journal of Personality and Social Psychology* 69:719–27.

Ryff, C. D., and B. Singer. 1998. The role of purpose in life and personal growth in positive human Health. In *The human quest for meaning: A handbook of psychological research and clinical applications,* ed. P. T. P. Wong and P. S. Fry, 213–35. Mahwah, N.J.: Lawrence Erlbaum Associates.

———. 2000. Biopsychosocial challenges of the new millennium. *Psychotherapy and Psychosomatics* 4:30–44.

Shrout, P. E., G. J. Canino, H. R. Bird, M. Rubio-Stipec, M. Bravo, and M. A. Burnam. 1992. Mental health status among Puerto Ricans, Mexican Americans, and non-Hispanic whites. *American Journal of Community Psychology* 20:729–52.

Singer, B., and C. D. Ryff. 1997. Racial and ethnic inequalities in health: Environmental, psychosocial, and physiological pathways. In *Intelligence, genes, and success: Scientists respond to the bell curve,* ed. B. Devlin, S. E. Feinberg, D. Resnick, and K. Roeder, 89–122. New York: Springer-Verlag.

———. 1999. Hierarchies of life histories and associated health risks. *Annals of the New York Academy of Sciences* 896:96–115.

Singer, B., C. D. Ryff, D. Carr, and W. J. Magee. 1998. Life histories and mental health: A person-centered strategy. In *Sociological methodology 1998,* ed. A. Raftery, 1–51. Washington, D.C.: American Sociological Association.

Tedeschi, R. G., and L. G. Calhoun. 1995. *Trauma and transformation: Growing in the aftermath of suffering.* Thousand Oaks, Calif.: Sage.

Veroff, J., E. Douvan, and R. A. Kulka. 1981. *The inner American: A self-portrait from 1957 to 1976.* New York: Basic Books.

Williams, D. R. 1999. Race, socioeconomic status, and health: The added effects of racism and discrimination. *Annals of the New York Academy of Sciences* 89 (6):173–88.

Williams, D. R., and A. M. Chung. 1997. Racism and health. In *Health in black America,* ed. R. C. Gibson and J. S. Jackson. Thousand Oaks, Calif.: Sage.

Williams, D. R., and M. Harris-Reid. 1999. Race and mental health: Emerging patterns and Promising approaches. In *A handbook for the study of mental health: Social contexts, theories, and systems,* ed. A. V. Horwitz and T. L. Scheid, 295–314. New York: Cambridge University Press.

III Contexts of Midlife: Work and Family Experience, Neighborhood, and Geographic Region

Is Daily Life More Stressful during Middle Adulthood?

David M. Almeida and Melanie C. Horn

Despite increased attention to the understanding of middle adulthood over the past two decades, there exists great variability in how midlife is portrayed. Some portraits depict midlife as a time of "crisis" (e.g., Levinson 1978; Vaillant 1977), whereas others characterize it as the "prime of life" (e.g., Baruch 1984; Costa et al. 1986; Mitchell and Helson 1990; Neugarten 1968; Ryff 1989). We believe that one way to enhance our understanding of midlife is to explore the day-to-day stressors that middle-aged adults experience. In this chapter, we examine age and gender differences in the frequency and patterns of daily stressful experiences throughout adulthood. We focus primarily on stressors that distinguish middle adulthood from earlier and later periods of adulthood.

Midlife may best be characterized by change or adaptation in multiple arenas or life domains (Lachman and James 1997). These paths of adaptation may include changes in the social world (e.g., caring for sick parents), the physical realm (e.g., increased risk of chronic diseases), and the work world (e.g., returning to work, or beginning or changing careers). One way to chart these multiple paths is to examine the day-to-day stressors that coincide with such changes during adulthood. Using the patterns of developmental changes identified by Lachman et al. (1994) as our compass, we examine four types of age-related patterns of daily stressors: *linear paths,* where midlife is either the continual increase or decrease in frequency of daily stressors occurring from young to late adulthood; *midlife plateaus,* where midlife is marked by either the end or continuation of a particular aspect of daily stress; *midlife peaks* or *valleys,* where midlife is a time differentiated from both young and late adulthood; and *stability,* where there is no age change.

Age Differences in Life Events

Researchers interested in the association between age and stressors have typically focused on major life events, those experiences that are disruptive to customary behavior patterns (e.g., Brown and Harris 1978;

Datan and Ginsberg 1975; Dohrenwend and Dohrenwend 1974; Holmes and Rahe 1967). These events, including marriage, birth of a child, divorce, and death of a family member or loved one, have often been used as markers of adult developmental transitions. Life-course theorists have argued that age or life stage is associated with the likelihood of certain events taking place (Brim and Ryff 1980; Hultsch and Plemons 1979). Age-related norms and expectations specify appropriate social timing for certain life events such as leaving the family home and getting married. In addition, biological changes such as menopause and musculoskeletal diseases have also been linked to life events, for example, completion of the childbearing years and retirement (Bond 1992; Fogel and Woods 1995; Gallant and Derry 1995; Older Women's League 1988).

Support for this life-course theory comes from research highlighting age differences in the frequency and nature of stressful life events across adulthood. Several investigators have shown that younger adults take on a number of roles within a short period of time (e.g., marriage, parenthood, work), while middle-aged and older adults typically experience other role changes, including departure of children, caretaking of parents, illness and death of parents, and retirement (Lowenthal, Thurner, and Chiriboga 1975; Rossi 1980). Younger persons, as compared with older ones, experience more events related to school, work, finances, and changes in personal relationships and living conditions. Older persons, on the other hand, report more stressors in environmental and social issues (Henderson, Byrne, and Duncan-Jones 1981; Hultsch and Plemons 1979). These findings support the notion that changes in social roles have implications for the types of life stressors that one experiences across the adult life span.

These age differences in life stressors can also be characterized through Lachman's patterns of developmental changes. For example, compared with older adults, younger people are more often involved in the formation and dissolution of marriages and re-marriage (Lazarus and De-Longis 1983). The likelihood of first-time marriage can thus be depicted as occurring on a young-to-midlife plateau. The likelihood of other life events, such as retiring or experiencing the death of a loved one, may best be defined by a linear increase across adulthood. Many major life events are more prevalent during middle adulthood, such as having one's children leave home, becoming a grandparent, and experiencing the death of one's parents. Thus the likelihood of these events represents midlife peaks.

Daily Stressors

In addition to examining the relationship between age and major life events, stress researchers have begun to consider the stressors and hassles of everyday life (Almeida, Wethington, and Kessler 2002; Almeida and Kessler 1998; Banez and Compas 1990; Bolger et al. 1989; Evans and Nies 1997; Lazarus and DeLongis 1983; Stone, Kessler, and Haythornthwaite 1991; Grzywacz et al., in press). Although studying life events is critical to understanding adult development, we believe that daily stressors tap into those more frequent experiences that often go unrecognized by researchers but are still meaningful to individuals. Although daily stressors may be less severe than life events, they nevertheless serve as personally significant and distinct events that represent attention-getting experiences in the ongoing lives of people.

An emerging literature has shown that daily stressors, such as spousal conflicts, home overloads, and work deadlines, play an important part in health and emotional adjustment (for a review, see Stone 1992). Minor daily stressors function not only by exerting their separate, direct effects but by piling up over a series of days to create persistent irritations, frustrations, and overloads, which may result in more serious stress reactions, such as anxiety and depression (Lazarus and DeLongis 1983; Lazarus and Folkman 1984; Pearlin et al. 1981; Pearlin and Schooler 1978; Serido, Almeida, and Wethington, in press). Daily stressors have also been found to be associated with negative mood (Bolger et al. 1989), daily distress (Almeida and Kessler 1998), and physical health problems (Horn and Almeida 2000; Grzywacz et al., in press; Larsen and Kasimatis 1991).

Age Differences in Daily Stressors

As stated earlier, midlife may be a time of change in stressful experiences as a result of the type of roles that individuals take on during this period, including role changes in the family and work domains (Sales 1978). These role changes may be precipitated by one's grown children leaving home (Lowenthal and Chiriboga 1972), career transitions, such as reentry into the occupational domain or declining career opportunities (Ackerman 1990; Etaugh 1993), and renegotiating of family relationships (Blatter and Jacobsen 1993; Rollins 1989). In addition, Lachman and James (1997) point out that "being in the middle" often entails expanding and managing multiple responsibilities, such as caretaking for one's aging parents and children. Such roles should expose midlife adults not only to specific types of major life events but also to unique daily stressors.

As is the case with major life events, some research has shown that the frequency and type of daily stressors are also age-graded. For example, older adults tend to have fewer desirable and undesirable daily events (Zautra et al. 1991). This decreased exposure may be the result of a reduction in social roles and time commitments across the life course. Gruber-Baldini and Verbrugge (1993) point out that with increasing age, individuals spend more time on personal and physical care, sleep, and personal activities, while spending less time on work and participation in sports. Further, Kanner et al. (1981) found that younger individuals experience more academic or social problems associated with their time of life and school attendance (e.g., wasting time, meeting school expectations and demands), whereas older individuals experience more economic concerns, such as stress about rising prices, investments, and taxes. These findings are consistent with other researchers' observations of age-related sources of role strain (Pearlin 1983).

Not only do we expect that the frequency or source of stressors will differ across the life span, but we also predict age-related differences in the personal meaning of daily stressors. Lazarus and DeLongis (1983) point out that how individuals appraise significance of a stressor is critical to how salient or disruptive that stressor will be. They argue that this may be the result of one's values, beliefs, commitments, and expectations that change across the life course. For example, health expectations decline among people as they age because they have more realistic concerns (Costa et al. 1986), as compared with many young adults who have unrealistic, overly optimistic beliefs about future health risks. Thus, how individuals cope or struggle with a disease or physical problem is in part influenced by their perceptions of its potential impact. Researchers looking at coping behavior have found age-related trends in people's appraisals of significant events such as cancer (Cohen 1980) and death or separations (Horowitz and Wilner 1980).

These findings suggest that daily stressful events hold varying significance at different developmental periods. Little is known, however, about age differences in the meaning and nature of day-to-day stressors themselves. One way to better understand the significance that daily stressors play in the lives of individuals is to explore the characteristics that make stressors unique, to take a detailed look at the types and dimensions of stressors that people experience. In this chapter, we consider the nature of daily stressors in two ways. First, we assess specific characteristics of stressors by use of an investigator-based approach (e.g., Brown and Harris 1978; Wethington et al. 2002). Trained coders rated open-ended descriptions of daily stressors into type of stressors (e.g., arguments, overloads); they also looked at who was involved in the stressor. Second, the appraised meaning of stressors was assessed through respondents' descriptions and ratings of severity of stressors and what was at stake for them as a result of daily stressors. We believe that combining investigator-rated characteristics with respondents' subjective meaning provides a rich account of daily stressors that individuals experience at different points along the adult life course.

Gender and Daily Stressors

Although the primary focus of this chapter is on age differences in daily stressors, we recognize the importance of considering the role of gender in the frequency and nature of stressful experiences across adulthood. According to the social role perspective, men and women experience different levels and types of stressors because of the nature of the roles they enact (Gove 1972; Gove and Tudor 1973). Women's gender roles tend to be more nurturing, whereas men's roles are more instrumental (Gove and Tudor 1973). Thus, women's social roles require them to provide support to others, to be more empathetic, and to extend their concern to a wider network. Men's social roles, on the other hand, tend to expose them to more stressors related to work and finances. Using this gender social-role perspective and applying it to the experience of daily stressors, we expect that women will report more home- and network-related stressors and that men will report more stressors related to work tasks and overloads.

However, the question remains as to how age and gender interact to predict the frequency of daily stressful events. For example, although women may have more home-related stressors overall, such as tensions related to children, this may not be true for older women whose children are no longer living at home. Compared with women, men may report more overall frequent work stressors. This, however, may be true only for younger men who are starting a new job, or who have less control or less respect. Thus, to fully capture the nature of daily stressor across adulthood, we recognize age and gender as two important predictors of daily stressors.

METHODS

Data for the present analyses are from the National Study of Daily Experiences (NSDE), one of the in-depth studies that are part of the

National Survey of Midlife in the United States (MIDUS) performed under the auspices of the John D. and Catherine T. MacArthur Foundation Research Network on Successful Midlife Development (Orville Gilbert Brim, director). Respondents were 1031 adults (562 women, 469 men), all of whom had participated in the phone and questionnaire portions of the MIDUS (see Brim, Ryff, and Kessler, chap. 1 of this volume, for a description of the MIDUS project). Respondents in the NSDE were randomly selected from the MIDUS sample and received twenty dollars for their participation in the project. Of the 1242 MIDUS respondents we attempted to contact, 1031 agreed to participate, yielding a response rate of 83 percent. Respondents completed an average of seven of the eight interviews, resulting in a total of 7221 daily interviews.

Over the course of eight consecutive evenings, respondents completed short telephone interviews about their daily experiences. On the final evening of interviewing, respondents also answered several questions about their previous week. Data collection spanned an entire year (March 1996 to March 1997) and consisted of forty separate "flights" of interviews, with each flight representing the eight-day sequence of interviews from approximately 38 respondents. The initiation of interview flights was staggered across the day of the week to control for the possible confounding between day of study and day of week.

Table 1 compares characteristics of the NSDE subsample with the MIDUS sample from which it was drawn. The two samples had very similar distributions for age, marital status, and parenting status. The NSDE had slightly more females and better-educated and fewer minority respondents than did the MIDUS sample. Respondents for the present analyses were on average 47 years old. Seventy-seven percent of the women and 85 percent of the men were married at the time of the study. Forty-seven percent of the households reported having at least one child living in the home. The average family income was between $50,000 and $55,000. Men were slightly older than women and had similar levels of education.

Daily stressors were assessed through a semi-structured Daily Inventory of Stressful Events (DISE; Almeida 1998; Almeida, Wethington, and Kessler 2002). The inventory consisted of a series of stem questions asking whether certain types of daily stressors had occurred in the past twenty-four hours, along with a set of interviewer guidelines for probing affirmative responses and a series of structured questions that measured respondents' appraisal of the stressors. The stem questions, examples

TABLE 1 Demographic Comparison of the MIDUS Sample and the NSDE Subsample

Demographic Variable	MIDUS[a] (%)	NSDE[b] (%)
Age		
Young adults, 25–39	33.2	33.5
Midlife adults, 40–59	46.0	45.0
Older adults, 60–74	20.8	21.5
Gender		
Males	48.5	45.5
Females	51.5	54.5
Education		
≤12 years	39.2	37.7
≥13 years	60.8	62.3
Marital status		
Married	64.1	65.4
All others	35.9	34.6
Children in household[c]		
Yes	39.0	37.8
No	61.0	62.2
Race		
Caucasian	87.8	90.3
African American	6.8	5.9
All other races	4.4	3.8

[a] Respondents in the MIDUS survey who participated in the initial telephone interview and returned the two self-administered questionnaire booklets after the interview ($N = 3032$).

[b] Respondents in the NSDE study all of whom had previously participated in the MIDUS initial telephone interview and returned the two self-administered questionnaire booklets after the interview ($N = 1031$).

[c] Whether respondent had at least one child age 18 or younger living in the house.

of the probe questions, and appraisal questions are provided in the appendix. The stem questions were created by combining several items from existing daily-stressor checklists (Bolger et al. 1989; Ekenrode and Bolger 1995). Our strategy was to elicit reports of broad types of stressors (e.g., interpersonal tension, work stressors) and to code for more specific characteristics of these stressors on the basis of the respondents' open-ended descriptions of what occurred.

The aim of the interviewing technique was to acquire a short narrative of each stressor that included descriptive information (e.g., topic or content of the stress, who was involved, how long the stressor lasted) as well as what was at stake for the respondent. Open-ended information for each reported stressor was tape-recorded, transcribed, and coded for several

TABLE 2 Description and Interrater Coding Reliability of Daily Inventory of Stressful Events Measures

Coding Category	Description	Codes	Interrater Reliability
Content classification	Stressful events are categorized into one of seven broad classifications organized by interpersonal tensions, life domains, network events, and miscellaneous events. Next they are placed in one of 54 specific classifications. Broad classifications are listed at right, followed by the number of specific classifications associated with each heading.	Interpersonal tensions (21) Work/education (9) Home (9) Finances (3) Health/accident (5) Network (7) Miscellaneous (9)	Broad classification .90 Specific classification .66
Focus of involvement	Focus of involvement refers to who was involved in the event.	Respondent Other Joint	.88
Threat dimensions	The threat dimension describes the implications of the event for the respondent. Loss is the occurrence of a deficit. Danger is the risk of a future negative occurrence. Disappointment occurs when something does not turn out as the respondent had expected. Frustration occurs when the respondent has little or no control over the events. Opportunity is a chance for positive outcome.	Loss Danger Disappointment Frustration Opportunity	.74

TABLE 2 *continued*

Coding Category	Description	Codes	Interrater Reliability
Investigator-rated severity	The objective assessment of the severity of an event refers to the degree and duration of disruption and/or unpleasantness created for the respondent. Ratings range from 1, a minor or trivial annoyance, to 4, a severely disruptive event.	Low-severity events Medium-severity events High-severity events Extreme-severity events	.75
Subjective severity	The subjective assessment of severity is the respondent's assessment of the degree of stressfulness involved in the event.	Not at all stressful Not very stressful Somewhat stressful Very stressful	Not coded by raters
Primary appraisal domains	Primary appraisal domains refer to the respondent's report of how much the following areas were at risk or at stake in the situation: (1) disruption routine; (2) finances; (3) how respondent feels about self; (4) how others feel about respondent; (5) health or safety; (6) well-being of one close to respondent; (7) future plans.	Not at all A little Some A lot	Not coded by raters

characteristics. This investigator-based approach allowed us to distinguish between a stressful event (e.g., conflict with spouse) and the affective response to the stressor (e.g., crying or feeling sad). Another benefit of this approach was our ability to identify overlapping reports of stressors. In the present study, approximately 5 percent of the reported stressors were discarded because either they were solely affective responses or they were identical to a stressor that was previously described on that day.

Table 2 presents the description and interrater reliability of the DISE measures. For each stressor, expert coders rated (a) content classification of the stressor (e.g., work overload, argument with spouse, traffic problem); (b) focus of who was involved in event; (c) dimensions of appraised threat (loss, danger, disappointment, frustration, opportunity); and (d) severity of stress. In addition, respondents provided reports of (e) degree of severity and (f) primary appraisal domains (i.e., areas of life that were at risk because of the stressor).

The first two measures in table 2 assess the objective nature of the stressor. Each stressor was initially placed into a *content classification* that combined the broad classification (e.g., argument) with specific content or topic of the stressor (e.g., housework). A pilot study of a national sample of 1006 adults was initially conducted to generate the content classification list of daily stressors common to adults in the United States. The initial list included eight broad classifications and thirty-nine specific classifications. This list was then lengthened to incorporate ten additional specific classifications of arguments and tensions and five other miscellaneous classifications. In the present analyses, we examined three of the broad-content classifications: interpersonal tensions, network events, and work and home overloads. Interpersonal tensions included stressors involving disagreements and verbal arguments as well as nonconflictual but tense interactions with others. Network stressors were events that happened to close friends or relatives that were stressful for the respondent (e.g., sick friend). Overloads referred to stressors that involved having too much work at home or the workplace. In this preliminary examination, we choose these three classifications because of their prevalence and their purported links to the experience of middle adulthood. Interpersonal tensions, network events, and overloads accounted for 78 percent of all of the reported stressors. Another characteristic of daily stressors we measured was *focus of involvement,* which assessed whether other individuals were involved in the stressors, and if so, what their relation was to the respondent (Brown and Harris 1978).

The remaining measures in table 2 assess the meaning of the stressor for the respondent. *Threat dimensions* were the rated stressful implications for the respondent. These dimensions are similar to Lazarus and Folkman's (1984) dimensions of primary appraisal, with the addition of disappointment (an expected positive experience that did not occur) and frustration (stressors in which the respondent has little or no control). *Investigator-rated severity ratings* are similar to Brown and Harris's (1978) short-term contextual threat and are based on the degree of disruptiveness and unpleasantness associated with the stressor. The final two DISE measures were obtained from the respondents' own ratings (see appendix for the items). These included the respondents' perceived or subjective severity of stressor and reports on seven primary appraisal domains (i.e., the degree of risk the stressor posed in various areas of life). Approximately 20 percent (800 events) of the stressors were rated by two coders. Using Kappa, we found that the interrater reliability ranged from .66 to .95 across all of the codes.

The documentation and guidelines for all of these ratings are provided in an interview and coding manual (Almeida 1998). In addition, all of the transcribed descriptions of daily stressors and their corresponding ratings are contained in an "electronic dictionary" stored in a computer spreadsheet. This dictionary consists of more than four thousand rated daily stressors and can be searched and cross-referenced by any of the DISE measures. Table 3 presents dictionary entries for six of these stressors. The first column shows the respondent's verbatim description of the stressor. The second and third columns list the broad-content classifications used in the present analysis as well as the specific classification. The fourth column shows the ratings for the focus of involvement and the relationship of the person if others were involved in the stressor. The fifth column lists the investigator's and respondent's severity ratings of the stressors, and the last column shows the respondent's primary appraisal ratings. Higher numbers in these final columns represent higher severity and greater perceived disruption.

RESULTS
Frequency of Daily Stressors

The first goal of our analyses was to examine age differences in how often respondents experienced daily stressors. Across the eight study days, we calculated the percentage of days that respondents reported any daily stressors (i.e., an affirmative response to any of the stressor stem questions) and multiple daily stressors (i.e., an affirmative response to two or more of the stressor stem questions). On average, respondents reported experiencing at least one daily stressor on 39.4 percent of the study days and multiple stressors on 10.4 percent of the study days. According to these figures, people in our sample experienced at least one daily stressor three days each week and multiple stressors three days each month. Compared with men, women had more frequent days in which they reported any stressors (37.5 percent of study days versus 40.9 percent of study days; $t = 5.1$, $p < .01$) but had similar number of days involving multiple stressors (9.4 percent of study days versus 11.2 percent of study days).

	Content	Specific
Transcription	Classification	Classification

TABLE 3 Examples of Daily Stressors and Coding

Transcription	Content Classification	Specific Classification
"I work on a number of different projects. I work in the finance department and today we have taxdeadline. We had quarterly income that I had todue, I had three wire transfers that I had to do . . . had people calling me . . . many phone calls coming in that I had juggle all at once. Timely filed. Co-worker was gone so I was in charge of all of the banking and cash management for the day. We were short handed. And it was a Monday. I'm assistant to the chief financial officer. It took more time. I got through it all."	Overload	Time pressure
"I was helping open and close the store so I had to get up this morning, get my son ready, drag him to work, pick up somebody who didn't have a car, pick them up, take them to work, open the store, make sure they were okay, take him back for kindergarien, drop him off at the bus, go back to work, pick him up from the bus, run to swimming lessons for 45 minutes and then go back to work to close the store. I think that's a little bit stressful." (R had to open and close the store because the manager who usually does it was on jury duty.) "I feel good about myself for being able to get it all done today."	Overload	Time pressure
"I had a problem with an employee. And also today she called and had cancelled something I had ordered three months ago and now I have to start running and searching and waiting for something. It was a big disappointment. It wasn't an argument, it was her fear that she had ordered the wrong thing and she didn't want to go through the stress and stuff. Nor did I obviously. Both of us. Since she had doubts that she had done the right thing, she cancelled the order. So, it was very stressful for me."	Interpersonal tension	Job procedures
"I had a phone conversation with my mother about visiting my grandmother who's in the hospital. And the reasons why she would not go. It wasn't worth the argument. There's a girl who's living with her that my mother doesn't care for. Living with my grandmother. And she will not visit her because of this girl that is living with her. She'll visit at the hospital but not the home." (R's uncle is going to marry this girl, she's very young and he's quite a bit older.) "My grandmother being in the hospital I just don't think it's something we should be worrying about. I'm the only one who feels this way."	Interpersonal tension	Family responsibility
"It was regarding my mom. It's just that she was supposed to be picked up by a family member, and they didn't pick her up and didn't bother to call me. My mother is 86, so that's why it was was stressful for me."	Network	Family responsibility
"I have a close friend who has emotional problems. My friend also suffers from migraine headaches. I spent quite a bit if time with her today. I tried to comfort her. Yah, it interrupted my routine because I could not be at home to do things."	Network	Health/well-being

Using the DISE Instrument

Focus/ Who Involved	Severity	Stake Dimensions
Self	Investigator rating 2 Subjective rating 2	Disrupting daily routine 1 Finances 1 Way feel about self 1 Way others feel about you 1 Physical health/safety 1 Health/well-being of close other 1 Plans for future 1
Self	Investigator rating 2 Subjective rating 2	Disrupting daily routine 3 Finances 3 Way feel about self 1 Way others feel about you 1 Physical health/safety 1 Health/well-being of close other 3 Plans for future 1
oint/co-worker	Investigator rating 3 Subjective rating 1	Disrupting daily routine 4 Finances 4 Way feel about self 4 Way others feel about you 3 Physical health/safety 4 Health/well-being of close other 1 Plans for future 4
oint/parent	Investigator rating 3 Subjective rating 2	Disrupting daily routine 2 Finance 1 Way feel about self 1 Way others feel about you 2 Physical health/safety Health/well-being of close other 1 Plans for future 1
Other/parent	Investigator rating 2 Subjective rating 4	Disrupting daily routine 3 Finances 1 Way feel about self 3 Way others feel about you 3 Physical health/safety 1 Health/well-being of close other 4 Plans for future 3
oint/friend	Investigator rating 2 Subjective rating 3	Disrupting daily routine 4 Finances 1 Way feel about self 2 Way others feel about you 2 Physical health/safety 1 Health/well-being of close other 3 Plans for future 2

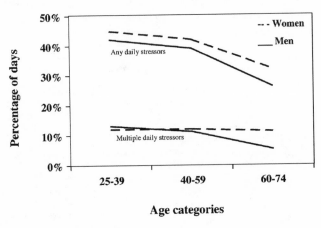

FIGURE 1. Frequency of daily stressors, by age and sex.

Figure 1 shows the pattern of age and gender differences in how often respondents reported any daily stressors and multiple daily stressors. We assessed these group differences using 2 × 3 (gender × age) ANOVAs with Tukey multiple comparison tests. The results revealed that age was negatively related to the frequency of experiencing any daily stressors ($F(2, 1025) = 22.6$, $p < .01$) and multiple daily stressors ($F(2, 1025) = 9.8$, $p < .01$). The results of the Tukey tests suggested a young to midlife plateau. Young and midlife adults reported more frequent days of any stressors and multiple stressors than did older adults. Younger women reported experiencing any daily stressors most frequently (44 percent of the study days), whereas older men reported having daily stressors on the fewest days (25 percent of the study days). A slightly different way to examine the frequency of daily stressors is to assess who was most likely to have limited stress in their daily lives. We found that 12 percent of our participants experienced no daily stressors across the entire study period. Although these respondents did not differ by gender, they did differ by age. Only 8 percent of the young adults reported no daily stressors compared with 12 percent of the midlife adults and 19 percent of the older group ($\chi^2 = 15.3$, $p < .001$). Taken together, these results suggest that overall, younger adults are more likely to experience daily stressors than their older counterparts.

Content and Focus of Daily Stressors

The next set of analyses examined the types of daily stressors that respondents were most likely to experience according to the content classifications and focus categories taken from the DISE. First, we assessed the *frequency* of each of the content classifications and focus categories by calculating the percentage of study days during which respondents experienced each of these types of stressors. Second, we calculated the *proportion* of stressors that fell into each specific type of stressor category for each respondent. This strategy was employed to control for the fact that younger and midlife adults reported a larger absolute number of daily stressors than did older adults (see fig. 1). The numbers in table 4 represent the average frequency and proportions of each of the measures across the total sample and within each of the age groups.

The first column of table 4 shows the percentage of study days that the entire sample experienced each type of stressor. In terms of stressor content, the most frequent type of daily stressors was interpersonal tension, occurring on almost 24 percent of the study days. Overload and network stressors were much less common (occurring on 5.6 percent and 8 percent of the study days, respectively). The frequency of stressors, broken down by the focus of involvement, shows that stressors involving the respondent and another person (i.e., joint focus) occurred more frequently than did both types of stressors involving either the respondent only or other individuals. When stressors included other individuals, they most likely involved a spouse or partner.

Table 5 provides a summary of results from a series of 3 × 2 ANOVAs with Tukey multiple comparisons that tested age and gender differences in content and focus of daily stressors. Consistent with our findings reported in figure 1, age was negatively related to a majority of subtypes of daily stressors. These analyses show a linear decrease across adulthood in the daily frequency of interpersonal tensions, stressors that involve only the respondent and someone else (self and joint focused), and stressors that involve a co-worker. Compared with older adults, younger and midlife adults also experienced more frequent overload stressors and stressors that involved children.

A somewhat different pattern emerged when we assessed age differences in these stressor characteristics as a proportion of all of their daily stressors. As with the frequency measure, age was negatively related to the proportion of overload stressors. Of the specific types of stressors that respondents experienced, younger and midlife adults reported a higher proportion of overloads than did older adults. However, older adults reported the highest proportion of network stressors and stressors that primarily involved another person (i.e., other focused). In terms of who else was involved in the stressors, older adults had the highest proportion

TABLE 4 Content and Focus of Dail

		Frequency of Daily Stressors[a]					
		Men			Women		
Measure	Total Sample	25–39	40–59	60–74	25–39	40–59	60–7
Content classification							
Argument/ tension	23.7	26.4	23.1	15.7	29.8	24.1	17.8
Overload	5.6	6.6	5.1	1.3	7.0	6.5	4.C
Network	8.0	6.7	6.3	4.7	9.0	9.8	9.8
Focus of involvement							
Self	12.7	16.3	14.0	6.2	13.1	13.8	6.8
Joint	26.5	29.0	25.1	16.9	33.3	27.4	2.5
Other	5.3	4.0	4.7	3.6	4.9	6.4	6.5
Others involved							
Spouse	8.2	9.6	7.7	7.0	10.3	7.1	8.6
Child	6.7	4.8	5.5	1.9	9.3	9.0	4.6
Co-worker	7.2	11.9	9.0	2.7	6.6	7.4	2.8

[a]Percentage of study days that respondents reported for each category of stressor.
[b]Propotion of stressors that fell into each category.

of spouse-related events, midlife adults had the highest proportion of child-related events, and younger adults had the highest proportion of co-worker-related events.

The age-related patterns of the content and focus of daily stressors can be interpreted through the social roles that our respondents were likely to inhabit (Pearlin 1983). These results suggest that overloads and demands are a greater source of daily stressors for young and midlife adults, although the source of the demands might differ. Younger men's daily stressors were more likely than respondents in the other groups to revolve around overloads and co-workers. Midlife women reported the same percentage of overloads as did younger women but had a greater proportion of stressors that involved other people. Although overloads were not a common type of stressor for older adults, these respondents had the greatest proportion of network and spouse-related events.

Findings for gender differences revealed that women reported more frequent overload, network, and child-related stressors than did men. Men had more frequent stressors that involved a co-worker. Women also had a higher proportion of network stressors than did men. In fact, network stressors were more common than overloads for women of all age categories. More than 25 percent of stressors reported by older women were network stressors, compared with only 8 percent of the stressors for

Stressors, by Age and Gender

| | Proportion of Daily Stressors[b] | | | | | |
| | Men | | | Women | | |
Total Sample	25–39	40–59	60–74	25–39	40–59	60–74
52.5	52.3	51.1	52.3	58.2	51.6	47.7
9.9	12.1	10.0	5.3	9.5	10.7	7.4
15.1	8.5	12.7	18.0	12.9	17.5	25.2
25.7	32.7	29.8	24.1	20.6	25.2	19.4
63.3	63.5	60.1	60.7	70.9	62.3	60.4
10.8	5.6	10.0	15.1	7.8	12.3	19.9
17.7	15.7	16.5	27.3	17.4	15.2	21.8
12.4	7.6	9.8	7.9	17.7	18.3	10.1
15.9	25.6	18.2	8.4	13.6	15.9	8.0

younger men. Indeed, men were more likely to experience self-focused stressors, whereas women's stressors included other people. These findings are consistent with research that shows women are more sensitive than men to social interactions and develop closer and more extensive social networks (Kessler, McLeod, and Wethington 1985).

Appraised Meaning of Stressors

As part of the DISE interview, respondents answered a series of structured and semi-structured questions that pertained to the appraised meaning of the stressor. These included dimensions of threat, the investigator and subjective rating of stressor severity, and primary appraisal domains (i.e., areas of life that were at risk because of the stressor). Table 6 provides a summary of the appraisal measures of daily stressors broken down by age and gender. The figures for the threat dimensions reflect the percentage of stressors that fell into each of five threat categories. Of the stressors experienced by the total sample, roughly 30 percent involved some sort of loss, nearly 37 percent posed danger, and 27 percent were frustrating or out of the control of the respondent. Table 6 also presents the mean levels of severity ratings. The total sample, on average, subjectively rated stressors as having medium severity, whereas objective coders rated, on average, that stressors posed low severity. Figures for the primary appraisal domains represent the amount of risk that stressors were

TABLE 5 Age and Gender Differences in Content and Focus of Daily Stressors

	Frequency of Stressors		Proportion of Stressors	
Measure	Age	Gender	Age	Gender
Content classification				
Overload	10.9** [Yg+Mid>Old]	4.7** [Women>Men]	4.5** [Yg+Mid>Old]	—
Interpersonal tension	20.5** [Yg>Mid>Old]	—	—	—
Network	—	17.4** [Women>Men]	11.1* [Old>Mid>Yg]	9.6** [Women>Men]
Focus of involvement				
Self	14.5** [Yg>Mid>Old]	—	—	10.4** [Men>Women]
Other	—	8.2** [Women>Men]	15.7** [Old>Mid>Yg]	4.8* [Women>Men]
Joint	20.6** [Yg>Mid>Old]	7.4** [Women>Men]	4.2** [Yg>Mid+Old]	—
Others involved				
Spouse	—	—	2.9* [Old>Yg>Mid]	—
Child	9.3** [Mid>Yg>Old]	25.7** [Women>Men]	4.5** [Mid>Yg>Old]	18.4 [Women>Men]
Co-worker	17.5** [Yg>Mid>Old]	7.4** [Women>Men]	9.3** [Yg>Mid>Old]	9.0** [Men>Women]

Notes: Figures in the table are significant F values. $N = 1031$.
$*p < .05.$ $**p < .01.$

perceived to have on seven areas of life. Daily stressors posed the most risk to disrupting the respondent's daily routine.

Next we examined age and gender differences in the appraisal measures of daily stressors. Table 7 provides results from a series of 3×2 ANOVAs with Tukey multiple comparisons that tested for differences in threat dimensions, objective and subjective severity ratings, and primary appraisal domains. Significant age differences were observed in two of the threat dimensions–danger and frustration. Middle-aged and older individuals reported a greater proportion of dangerous stressors (stressors that pose the possibility of a future negative occurrence) than did younger adults. Middle-aged respondents reported having the least proportion of stressors that were frustrating compared with younger and older respondents.

Age and gender differences were also observed in subjective ratings of stressor severity. Younger and middle-aged respondents rated stressors as more disruptive and unpleasant than did older respondents, and women

TABLE 6 Appraisal Measures of Daily Stressors, by Age and Gender

Measures	Total Sample	Men			Women		
		25–39	40–59	60–74	25–39	40–59	60–74
Threat dimensions (% of stressors)[a]							
Loss	29.7	33.5	29.4	22.0	29.8	28.7	27.9
Danger	36.5	33.7	37.2	37.5	32.2	40.4	37.9
Disappointment	4.2	4.3	4.3	2.7	5.4	4.4	4.0
Frustration	27.4	26.2	26.2	36.4	28.9	24.4	28.3
Opportunity	2.3	2.4	2.2	1.3	3.6	2.0	1.9
Severity (mean level)[b]							
Investigator rating	1.81	1.80	1.74	1.66	1.78	1.86	1.96
Subjective rating	2.69	2.62	2.50	2.27	2.88	2.87	2.75
Primary appraisal domains (mean level)[c]							
Disrupting daily routine	2.30	2.46	2.30	2.03	2.37	2.31	2.07
Financial situation	1.30	1.41	1.33	1.40	1.29	1.21	1.17
Way feel about self	1.46	1.38	1.48	1.32	1.46	1.50	1.59
Way others feel about you	1.41	1.57	1.53	1.26	1.42	1.31	1.31
Physical health of safety	1.27	1.27	1.33	1.26	1.21	1.29	1.22
Health/well-being of others	1.49	1.38	1.52	1.70	1.50	1.50	1.50
Plans for the future	1.36	1.45	1.35	1.43	1.37	1.34	1.23

[a] Percentage of stressors that were placed into each of the categories.
[b] Average severity rating across all stressors ranging from 1 (not at all stressful) to 4 (very stressful).
[c] Average rating across all stressors of how much risk each stressor posed ranging from 1 (none) to 4 (a lot).

overall rated stressors as more severe than did men. Interestingly, there were no significant age or gender differences in the investigator ratings of stressor severity. This suggests that one's age or gender does not necessarily expose one to stressors that are inherently more severe, at least according to our trained coders. However, one's own perception of stressor severity may be age- and gender-graded, possibly because younger and middle-aged adults perceive events as relatively more dramatic than do older adults, or that older adults downplay the significance of stressors. Perhaps older individuals have learned to cope better with daily stressors and thus interpret stressors as less severe than do younger adults.

Significant age patterns were observed in the degree that stressors were perceived to disrupt daily routines and risk the way others felt about the respondent. Young and middle-aged respondents reported that stressors were more likely to pose greater risks in these areas than did older respondents. Middle-aged respondents also perceived their stressors as posing

TABLE 7 Age and Gender Differences in Appraisal Measure of
Daily Stressors

Measures	Age	Gender
Threat dimensions		
Loss	—	—
Danger	3.0 [Mid+Old>Yg]	—
Disappointment	—	—
Frustration	2.9* [Yg+Old>Mid]	—
Opportunity	—	—
Severity		
Investigator rating	—	—
Subjective rating	7.3** [Yg+Mid>Old]	29.7** [Women>Men]
Primary appraisal domains		
Disrupting daily routine	7.7** [Yg+Mid>Old]	—
Financial situation	3.5* [Mid>Yg+Old]	11.9 [Men>Women]
Way feel about self	—	—
Way others feel about you	4.4* [Yg+Mid>Old]	12.8** [Women>Men]
Physical health or saftey	—	—
Health/well-being of others	—	—
Plans for the future	—	—

Notes: Figures in the table are significant F values. $N = 1031$.
*$p < .05$. **$p < .01$.

more financial risk than did both the younger and older groups. Finally, gender differences showed that men appraised their stressors as posing a higher level of financial risk, whereas women appraised their stressors as posing more risk to the way others felt about them. These findings are consistent with the gender-role perspective that contends that women's roles involve interpersonal interactions and men's roles involve instrumental activities (Gove and Tudor 1973).

CONCLUSION

We hope this chapter has provided a glimpse into the characteristics and qualities of daily life during middle adulthood. By assessing multiple dimensions of daily stressors, we gain a more comprehensive and accurate portrait of this unique period of development. Our findings reveal that various patterns and contours mark the frequency and nature of daily stressors across the adult life course. Although there was not one clear and consistent pattern distinguishing midlife from other periods of life, a picture may emerge when we consider each of these patterns in turn.

First, young-to-midlife plateaus marked many characteristics of daily stressors. The initial set of analyses revealed that young and middle-aged individuals experienced a greater daily frequency of any stressors and multiple stressors than did older individuals. Such results are consistent with previous research documenting that older adults tend to experience fewer life events and daily stressors (Chiriboga 1997). Midlife and younger adults also perceived their stressors as more severe than did older adults. Midlife adults were also similar to younger adults in the amount of overloads they experienced as well as in the amount of disruption that stressors caused to their daily routines and to how others felt about them. Midlife and younger adults experienced a greater proportion of these types of stressors than older adults did.

However, the experience of daily stressors during midlife is not only patterned by plateaus but can also be characterized as a period distinct from younger and later adulthood, and represented by midlife peaks or valleys. Compared with both young adulthood and later life, midlife is a time during which there are significant increases in the proportion of stressors posing financial risk and in stressors involving children. On the other hand, midlife adults reported fewer frustrating stressors during which they felt little or no control. Such findings are consistent with previous work showing that although midlife is a time of increased responsibilities, it is also a peak period for competence and a sense of mastery (Lachman et al. 1994). Thus, midlife is also a unique period of the life course, one that can be differentiated from young and old adulthood.

Finally, many aspects of daily stressors characterize midlife as a time marking linear transitions from early adulthood through late adulthood. The frequency of interpersonal tensions decreases from young through midlife to older adulthood. On the other hand, the proportion of network and other focused stressors increases from young adulthood to midlife and continues to climb into older adulthood. Getting older exposes one to a greater proportion of stressors involving a close friend or relative. These findings point to the fact that midlife is also a time of being in the "middle" of the adult life course, where characteristics and processes that started in younger years continue through midlife toward older adulthood.

In this chapter we have attempted to address the question "Is daily life more stressful during middle adulthood?" The answer obviously depends on the group with which midlife adults are being compared and which aspect of daily stress is being considered. The quantity and quality of daily experiences certainly vary according to a person's position in the adult life course. Midlife adults encounter more frequent daily stressors than do older adults, and they experience different types of stressors than younger adults. Furthermore, the nature and meaning of the stressors also differ with age. Such descriptive findings set the stage for more important questions, such as how aspects of daily life explain age-related differences in physical health, social responsibility, and psychological well-being. This line of research would move us beyond documenting age differences in day-to-day life experiences to understanding how such experiences contribute to health and well-being during the middle adult years.

Appendix

The Daily Inventory of Stressful Events (DISE) is a semi-structured instrument consisting of three components: (1) a list of seven "stem" questions that pertain to occurrences of stressful events in various life domains; (2) a series of open-ended "probe" questions that ascertain a description of the stressful event; (3) a question regarding the perceived severity of the stressor; and (4) a list of structured "stake" questions inquiring about aspects of the respondent's life that were at risk because of the event. An affirmative response to the stem questions prompts the interviewer to probe for a detailed description of the event, which is followed by questions pertaining to "what was at stake" for the respondent as a result of the event.

Stem Questions

1. Did you have an *argument or disagreement* with anyone since this time yesterday?

   No   Yes

2. Since (this time/we spoke) yesterday, did anything happen that you *could have argued* about but you decided to let pass in order to avoid a disagreement?

   No   Yes

3. Since (this time/we spoke) yesterday, did anything happen at *work or school* (other than what you've already mentioned) that most people would consider stressful?

   No   Yes

4. Since (this time/we spoke) yesterday, did anything happen at *home* (other than what you've already mentioned) that most people would consider stressful?

   No   Yes

5. Many people experience *discrimination* on the basis of such things as race, sex, or age. Did anything like this happen to you since (this time/we spoke) yesterday?

     No   Yes

6. Since (this time/we spoke) yesterday, did anything happen to a *close friend or relative* (other than what you've already mentioned) that turned out to be stressful for you?

     No   Yes

7. Did *anything else* happen to you since (this time/we spoke) yesterday that most people would consider stressful?

     No   Yes

Examples of Probes for Description

Ask only if "yes" for the following stem questions [question numbers are in brackets]:

1. Think of the most stressful disagreement or argument you had since (this time/we spoke) yesterday. Who was that with? [1]
2. Think of the most stressful incident of this sort. Who was the person you decided not to argue with? [2]
3. What happened and why did you decide not to get into an argument about it? [2]
4. Think of the most stressful incident of this sort. What was the basis for the discrimination you experienced—your race, sex, age, or something else? [5]
5. Think of the most stressful incident of this sort. Who did this happen to? [6]
6. How does this affect your job? [3]
7. What kinds of things were said? [1, 2]
8. When did that happen? Was that some time yesterday or today? [All]
9. What happened and what about it would most people consider stressful? [All]
10. Have you had any problems with this in the past? [All]
11. How long has this been going on? [All]
12. Does this happen often? [All]
13. Was there anything out of the ordinary in this? [All]

Subjective Severity Question

1. How stressful was this for you—very, somewhat, not very, or not at all?

1. Not at all → Go to next stem question
2. Not very → Go to next stem question
3. Somewhat → Go to primary appraisal questions
4. Very → Go to primary appraisal questions

Primary Appraisal Domains Questions

Rated on a scale of 1 to 4, 1 = Not at all; 2 = A little; 3 = Some; and 4 = A lot.

1. How much were the following things at risk in this situation: First, how much did it risk disrupting your daily routine—a lot, some, a little, or not at all?

    1   2   3   4

2. How much did it risk your financial situation?

    1   2   3   4

3. How much did it risk the way you feel about yourself?

    1   2   3   4

4. How much did it risk the way other people feel about you?

    1   2   3   4

5. How much did it risk your physical health or safety?

    1   2   3   4

6. How much did it risk the health or well-being of someone you care about?

    1   2   3   4

7. How much did it risk your plans for the future?

    1   2   3   4

REFERENCES

Ackerman, R. J. 1990. Career developments and transitions of middle-aged women. *Psychology of Women Quarterly* 14:513–30.

Almeida, D. M. 1998. Daily inventory of stressful events: Interview and coding manual. Manuscript. University of Arizona.

Almeida, D. M., and R. C. Kessler. 1998. Everyday stressors and gender differences in daily distress. *Journal of Personality and Social Psychology* 75:1–11.

Almeida, D. M., E. Wethington, and R. C. Kessler. 2002. The Daily Inventory of Stressful Experiences (DISE): An interview-based approach for measuring daily stressors. *Assessment* 9:41–55.

Banez, G. A., and B. E. Compas. 1990. Children's and parents' daily stressful events and psychological symptoms. *Journal of Abnormal Child Psychology* 18:591–605.

Baruch, G. K. 1984. The psychological well-being of women in the middle years.

In *Women in midlife*, ed. G. K. Baruch and J. Brooks-Gunn, 161–80. New York: Plenum Press.

Blatter, C. W., and J. J. Jacobsen. 1993. Older women coping with divorce: Peer support groups. *Women and Therapy* 14:141–55.

Bolger, N., A. DeLongis, R. C. Kessler, and E. A. Schilling. 1989. Effects of daily stress on negative mood. *Journal of Personality and Social Psychology* 57:808–18.

Bond, K. 1992. Osteoporosis. *NAACOG'S Clinical Issues in Perinatal and Women's Health Nursing* 3:497–508.

Brim, O. G., and C. D. Ryff. 1980. On the properties of life events. In *Life-span development and behavior,* ed. P. B. Baltes and O. G. Brim, Jr., 3:363–87. New York: Academic Press.

Brown, G. W., and T. O. Harris. 1978. *Social origins of depression: A study of psychiatric disorder in women.* London: Tavistock.

Chiriboga, D. A. 1997. Crisis, challenge, and stability in the middle years. In *Multiple paths of midlife development,* ed. M. E. Lachman and J. B. James, 293–322. Chicago: University of Chicago Press.

Cohen, F. 1980. Coping with surgery: Information, psychological preparation, and recovery. In *Aging in the 1980's: Psychological issues,* ed. L. W. Poon. Washington, D.C.: American Psychological Association.

Costa, P. T., R. R. McCrae, A. B. Zobderman, H. E. Barbano, B. Lebowitz, and D. M. Larson. 1986. Cross-sectional studies of personality in a national sample. 2. Stability in neuroticism, extraversion, and openness. *Psychology and Aging* 1:144–49.

Datan, N., and L. H. Ginsberg, eds. 1975. *Life-span developmental psychology: Normative life crises.* New York: Academic Press.

Dohrenwend, B. S., and B. P. Dohrenwend. 1974. *Stressful life events: Their nature and effects.* New York: John Wiley.

Eckenrode, J., and N. Bolger. 1995. Daily and within-day event measurement. In *Measuring stress: A guide for health and social scientists,* ed. S. Cohen, R. C. Kessler, and L. U. Gordon, 80–101. New York: Oxford University Press.

Etaugh, C. 1993. Women in the middle and later years. In *Psychology of women: A handbook of issues and theories,* ed. F. L. Denmark and M. A. Paludi, 213–46. Westport, Conn.: Greenwood Publishing.

Evans, M. S., and M. A. Nies. 1997. Effects of daily hassles on exercise participation in perimenopausal women. *Public Health Nursing* 14:129–33.

Fogel, C. I., and N. F. Woods. 1995. Midlife women's health. In *Women's health care: A comprehensive handbook,* ed. C. I. Fogel and N. F. Woods, 79–96. Thousand Oaks, Calif.: Sage Publications.

Gallant, S. J., and P. S. Derry. 1995. Menarche, menstruation, and menopause: Psychosocial research and future directions. In *The psychology of women's health: Progress and challenges in research and application,* ed. A. L. Stanton, and S. J. Gallant, 199–260. Washington, D.C.: American Psychological Association.

Gilligan, C. 1982. *In a different voice: Psychological theory and women's development.* Cambridge: Harvard University Press.

Gove, W. R. 1972. The relationship between sex roles, marital status, and metal illness. *Social Forces* 52:992–1003.

Gove, W. R., and J. F. Tudor. 1973. Adult sex roles and mental illness. *American Journal of Sociology* 98:812–35.

Gruber-Baldini, A. L., and L. M. Verbrugge. 1993. Differences in activity pat-
terns due to chronic conditions in the Baltimore Longitudinal Study of Aging.
Paper presented at the meetings of the Gerontological Society of America, New
Orleans.

Grzywacz, J. G., D. M. Almeida, S. D. Neupert, and S. L. Ettner. In press. Stress and
socioeconomic differentials in physical and mental health: A daily diary approach.
Journal of Health and Social Behavior.

Henderson, S., D. G. Byrne, and P. Duncan-Jones. 1981. *Neurosis and the social environment.* New York: Academic Press.

Holmes, T. H., and R. H. Rahe. 1967. The social readjustment rating scale. *Journal of
Psychosomatic Research* 11:213–18.

Horn, M. C., and D. M. Almeida. 2000. Women's daily health during middle adulthood. In *Psychology and Health,* forthcoming.

Horowitz, M. J., and N. Wilner. 1980. Life events, stress, and coping. In *Aging in the
1980's: Psychological issues,* ed. L. W. Poon, 363–74. Washington, D.C.: American
Psychological Association.

Hultsch, D. F., and J. K. Plemons. 1979. Life events and life-span development. In
Life-span development and behavior, ed. P. B. Baltes and O. G. Brim, Jr., 3:1–31.
New York: Academic Press.

Kanner, A. D., J. C. Coyne, C. Schaefer, and R. S. Lazarus. 1981. Comparison of two
models of stress measurement: Daily hassles and uplifts versus major life events.
Journal of Behavioral Medicine 4:1–39.

Kessler, R. C., J. D. McLeod, and E. Wethington. 1985. The costs of caring: A perspective
on sex differences in psychological distress. In *Social support: Theory, research,
and applications,* ed. I. G. Sarason and B. R. Sarason, 491–507. Dordrecht, The
Netherlands: Martinus Nijhoff.

Lachman, M. E., and J. B. James, eds. 1997. *Multiple paths of midlife development.*
Chicago: University of Chicago Press.

Lachman, M. E., C. Lewkowicz, A. Marcus, and Y. Peng. 1994. Images of midlife
development among young, middle-aged, and older adults. *Journal of Adult
Development* 1:201–11.

Larsen, R. J., and M. Kasimatis. 1991. Day-to-day physical symptoms: Individual
differences in the occurrence, duration, and emotional concomitants of minor
daily illnesses. *Journal of Personality* 59:388–423.

Lazarus, R. S., and A. DeLongis. 1983. Psychological stress and coping in aging.
American Psychologist 38:245–54.

Lazarus, R. S., and S. Folkman. 1984. *Stress, appraisal, and coping.* New York: Springer-
Verlag.

Levinson, D. J. 1978. *Season's of a man's life.* New York: Knopf.

Lowenthal, M. F., and D. A. Chiriboga. 1972. Transition to the empty nest: Crisis,
change, or relief? *Archives of General Psychiatry* 26:8–14.

Lowenthal, M. F., M. Thurner, and D. A. Chiriboga. 1975. *Four stages of life: A comparative study of men and women facing transitions.* San Francisco: Jossey-Bass.

Mitchell, V., and R. Helson. 1990. Women's prime of life: Is it in the 50's? *Psychology
of Women Quarterly* 14:451–70.

Neugarten, B. L. 1968. The awareness of middle age. In *Middle age and aging,* ed.
B. L. Neugarten, 93–98. Chicago: University of Chicago Press.

Older Women's League. 1988. The picture of health for midlife and older women in America. *Women and Health* 14:53–91.

Pearlin, L. I. 1983. Role strains and personal stress. In *Psychological stress: Trends in theory and research,* ed. H. B. Kaplan, 3–32. New York: Academic Press.

Pearlin, L. I., E. G. Menaghan, M. A. Lieberman, and J. P. Mullan. 1981. The stress process. *Journal of Health and Social Behavior* 22:337–56.

Pearlin, L. I., and C. Schooler. 1978. The structure of coping. *Journal of Health and Social Behavior* 19:2–21.

Rollins, B. C. 1989. Marital quality at midlife. In *Midlife myths: Issues, findings, and practice implications,* ed. S. Hunter and M. Sundel, 184–94. Newbury Park, Calif.: Sage.

Rossi, A. S. 1980. Life-span theories and women's lives. *Signs* 6:4–32.

Ryff, C. D. 1989. In the eye of the beholder: Views of psychological well-being among middle-aged and older adults. *Psychology and Aging* 4:195–210.

Sales, E. 1978. Women's adult development. In *Women and sex roles: A social psychological perspective,* ed. I. H. Frieze, J. E. Parsons, P. B. Johnson, D. N. Ruble, and G. L. Zellman, 157–90. New York: W. W. Norton.

Serido, J., D. M. Almeida, and E. Wethington. In press. Conceptual and empirical distinctions between chronic stressors and daily hassles. *Journal of Health and Social Behavior.*

Stone, A. A. 1992. Selected methodological concepts: Mediation and moderation, individual differences, aggregation strategies, and variability of replicates. In *Stress and disease process,* ed. P. McCabe, N. Schneiderman, and A. Baum, 55–71. Hillsdale, N.J.: Lawrence Erlbaum Associates.

Stone, A. A., R. C. Kessler, and J. A. Haythornthwaite. 1991. Measuring daily events and experiences: Decisions for the researcher. *Journal of Personality* 59:575–607.

Vaillant, G. E. 1977. *Adaptation to life.* Boston: Little, Brown.

Wethington, E., D. Almeida, G. W. Brown, E. Frank, and R. C. Kessler. 2002. The assessment of stress exposure. In *Assessment in behavioral medicine,* ed. A. K. Vingerhoets, 113–34. New York: Taylor and Francis.

Zautra, A. J., J. F. Finch, J. W. Reich, and C. A. Guarnaccia. 1991. Predicting the everyday life events of older adults. *Journal of Personality* 59:507–38.

CHAPTER SIXTEEN

Psychological Well-Being across Three Cohorts: A Response to Shifting Work–Family Opportunities and Expectations?

Deborah Carr

The life course of women—and men, to a lesser degree—has undergone considerable transformation in the past four decades. The occupational and educational opportunities available to women and men have expanded drastically, with each cohort of young adults completing more years of school than their parents did (Bell 1973; Bianchi and Spain 1996; Meyer et al. 1977). At the same time, norms and expectations guiding appropriate gender-role behavior in the home and work place have undergone a "subtle revolution" (Gerson 1985, 1993). Men and women raised in the 1940s and 1950s could look forward to holding clearly demarcated gender roles in adulthood; married men would serve as the primary breadwinner and leave childrearing responsibilities to their wives, who would typically exit the labor force all together when their children were young (Baruch, Barnett, and Rivers 1983; Bernard 1981; Coontz 1992). In contrast, women and men who came of age in the late 1960s and beyond faced an entirely new set of expectations for appropriate work and family roles. Although men of the baby boom and baby bust cohorts are still expected to fulfill the traditional role of breadwinner, they are also expected to be involved fathers who play a larger role in childrearing and housekeeping tasks than their own fathers did (Gerson 1993; Hochschild 1989; Kaufman and Uhlenberg 2000; Wilkie 1993). Women, too, are now expected to maintain a household and care for their children as their mothers did but also to fulfill their career potential by working for pay outside the home.

These recent changes in structural opportunities and normative expectations raise an interesting puzzle for research on psychological well-being in different birth cohorts. On one hand, expanded opportunities for higher education and autonomous, white-collar work over the past four decades may have created a context in which younger cohorts have better psychological health than their parents did, given the widely documented linkages between socioeconomic status, broadly defined, and psychological well-being (e.g., Rosenberg and Pearlin 1978; Kessler and

Cleary 1980; Ross and Mirowsky 2002). Yet cultural changes that promote "having it all" among younger cohorts, that is, achieving a balance between fulfilling professional lives and involved family lives, may lead to decrements in psychological well-being across recent cohorts, as men and women strive to fulfill this lofty and potentially elusive expectation.

Using data from MIDUS, I answer three questions in this chapter: (1) Do the baby bust, baby boom, and silent generation cohorts differ in terms of their psychological well-being? (2) To what extent do these cohort differences reflect historical shifts in access to important structural opportunities, such as higher education and rewarding employment? and (3) Do work and family roles affect psychological well-being differently for the three cohorts, reflecting cultural shifts in the meaning, desirability, and importance of these roles? The cohorts considered are the silent generation, born between 1931 and 1943 (ages 52–64); the baby boom cohort, born between 1944 and 1959 (ages 37–52); and the baby bust cohort, born between 1960 and 1970 (ages 25–36). These research questions have important implications for understanding psychological well-being during a period of marked social change, when opportunities and expectations for fulfilling one's work and family roles may be in flux.

Cohort Influences on Personal Experiences

A birth cohort is a group of individuals born at the same point in history and who "experience the same event within the same time interval" (Ryder 1965, 845). Given their shared age at a given point in history, members of a birth cohort also may face similar opportunities and constraints as they pass through the life course. For example, levels of educational attainment have risen steadily across recent birth cohorts, the result of expanding educational opportunities throughout the twentieth century (Meyer et al. 1977). Cohort shifts in educational opportunities are particularly pronounced for women. Although women earned approximately one-third of all college degrees in the early 1950s, they earned more than half (55 percent) by the 1990s (U.S. National Center for Educational Statistics 1995).

The transformation of the U.S. economy from a manufacturing to a postindustrial or service-based economy over the past fifty years also has presented the baby bust, baby boom, and pre–World War II cohorts with very different occupational opportunities and trajectories (Bell 1973). Men born in the 1930s and early 1940s entered the labor force during the postwar years, when the U.S. economy was prospering. Even men with relatively limited education were able to secure stable and reasonably well-paying jobs in the manufacturing sector. In contrast, members of the large baby boom cohort, born between 1944 and 1959, faced intense competition for well-paying jobs when they entered the labor market during the recession years of the early 1970s (Easterlin 1980; Levy 1998). Spells of recession and widespread unemployment again in the late 1970s and early 1980s, declining employment in the manufacturing sector, job growth in the service sector, a tripling in the number of corporate mergers and acquisitions between 1976 and 1986 (*Mergers and acquisitions* 1987, 216), and the glut of workers created by the baby boom (Easterlin 1980) have created a context in which the men of the baby bust cohort may have had less stable occupational prospects than did earlier cohorts (Dunn 1993; Levy 1998; Schrammel 1998).

The labor market prospects and experiences of women also have changed dramatically over the past fifty years. The proportion of women who work for pay has increased steadily, and this increase has been sharpest among mothers of young children. The proportion of mothers of preschool children working for pay increased from just 19 percent in 1960 to approximately 64 percent in 1995 (U.S. Bureau of the Census 1996, 399). Thus, having young children does not constrain paid employment for young women today, as it did for their mothers in the 1950s and 1960s. Additionally, the gender gap in earnings has declined for recent cohorts. In 1994, women ages 20–24 earned approximately 95 cents for each dollar earned by men, whereas that proportion drops to approximately 80 cents for women ages 25–34, 73 cents for women ages 35–44, and 66 cents among women ages 55–64 (U.S. Bureau of Labor Statistics 1995).[1] Thus, for current cohorts of young women, paid employment is both a more common and more financially rewarding role than it was for earlier cohorts.

Changes in women's labor force participation are due, in part, to a rising demand for workers in the service sector. Women's employment patterns also reflect historical changes in family structure (Bianchi and Spain 1996; Goldin 1990). Fertility rates have dropped steadily in the United States since the mid-1960s, largely a result of increased availability of effective birth control, changing gender roles in the home and workplace, and the changing economic and social costs of children (Butz and Ward 1979; Easterlin 1980; Cherlin and Walters 1981). These new family formation patterns, in turn, have created a context in which current cohorts of young women spend fewer years bearing and rearing children than their mothers did; consequently, they may have greater access to continuous employment and rewarding occupational opportunities (Watkins, Menken, and Bongaarts 1987).

Implications of Macrosocial Change for Psychological Well-Being

Macrolevel changes in family structure, educational attainment, and industrial shifts may have important implications for understanding cohort differences in two important dimensions of psychological well-being: environmental mastery and self-acceptance. Environmental mastery refers to the process of shaping one's social environment to reflect one's needs and personality, as well as to the ability to manage one's environment and daily affairs (Ryff 1989). A large body of research demonstrates that levels of perceived mastery and personal control are highest for persons with advanced education, higher incomes, and more intellectually challenging occupations. Education promotes the development of proactive problem-solving strategies, which in turn increases one's perceived mastery over the environment. Moreover, those with higher-status, well-paying occupations have greater economic resources for molding their environments to their tastes, and may face fewer unanticipated and uncontrollable life events that may threaten their sense of control (e.g., Kessler and Cleary 1980). Occupations that allow for self-directed, autonomous work (i.e., typically white-collar and managerial jobs) tend to promote autonomous and self-directed behavior in other life domains (Andrisani 1978; Bird and Ross 1993; Kohn 1969; Kohn and Schooler 1973; Mirowsky and Ross 1998; Pearlin et al. 1981; Ross and Mirowsky 2002; Wheaton 1980).

Self-acceptance is also positively related to one's social and economic resources. Self-acceptance is conceptually similar to self-esteem—one of the most widely examined aspects of psychological well-being (e.g., Rosenberg and Pearlin 1978). It refers to having positive attitudes toward oneself, acknowledging and accepting multiple aspects of one's self, and feeling positive about one's past accomplishments (Ryff 1989). Socioeconomic status is an important predictor of adult self-esteem for at least three reasons. Social class is a salient or identity-relevant trait for most adults; social class is typically achieved rather than ascribed (or inherited) among adults and is thus perceived as an indicator of one's ability and self-worth; and persons of lower social classes who compare themselves unfavorably to more successful peers may develop negative self-attitudes (Rosenberg and Pearlin 1978).

At first inspection, the changing life-course patterns of women and men over the past forty years would suggest that each successive cohort should have higher levels of self-acceptance and mastery than did the previous cohort. Given the increases in educational attainment among recent cohorts (Meyer et al. 1977), and shifts in the economy whereby younger cohorts are more likely than prior cohorts to hold white-collar or professional occupations that offer opportunities for autonomous and self-directed work (Bell 1973; Levy 1998), one may conclude that baby bust men and women should have higher levels of mastery and self-esteem than baby boom men and women, who in turn would have higher levels of well-being than men and women born before World War II. Moreover, because historical changes in work and educational opportunities have been more drastic among women than men, the psychological benefits enjoyed by younger cohorts may be pronounced among women.

The psychological consequences of a role or status, such as education, one's job, or parental status, may not be so clear-cut, however, and may be contingent upon the meaning or importance the role holds for members of a birth cohort. Members of a birth cohort not only face similar structural opportunities and obstacles; they also may share a unique culture, or a "set of cognitive and evaluative beliefs about what is or what ought to be" (House 1981, 543). A cohort is most likely to develop a set of beliefs that are distinct from those of preceding cohorts during periods marked by rapid social changes, such as stark changes in gender roles in the home and workplace over the past forty years (Mannheim 1952, 291).

The baby bust, baby boom, and pre–World War II birth cohorts may hold very different standards for evaluating their successes, and thus their work and educational accomplishments may have very different consequences for their psychological well-being. For example, Inglehart (1977, 1985) proposed that in advanced industrial societies, cohorts born before World War II often grew up under conditions of poverty or scarcity, and consequently developed "materialist" concerns about economic and physical security. The baby boom and baby bust cohorts, born after World War II, grew up in conditions of relative affluence and found their material needs satisfied, and thus are believed to seek rewards such as self-expression rather than high pay, status, or job security in their work lives (Inglehart 1985). Consequently, the linkage between extrinsic work rewards, such as occupational status, may be more strongly linked to the psychological well-being of the older cohorts, for whom economic concerns were particularly salient.

Cohorts may also differ in their beliefs and expectations about appropriate gender roles in the home and workplace. Married women and men raised in the mid-1960s and earlier were socialized to exchange services according to the traditional marriage contract, that is, women maintain the household and raise children, and men support the family financially (Bernard 1972, 1981). Women were socialized to believe that that their families should take priority over their own careers and that they would exit the labor force completely when their children were young (Bernard 1972; Hartmann 1981; Hochschild 1989; Levant, Slattery, and Loiselle 1987; Shelton and John 1993). In contrast, men and women of the baby boom and baby bust cohorts generally expect that both partners will participate in homemaking responsibilities and work for pay, even when their children are young (Bohannon and Blanton 1999; Moen, Erickson, and Dempster-McClain 1997; Morgan, Hayes, and Affleck 1989; Thornton 1989).

These generational differences in expectations about the way that work and family roles should mesh may have important implications for the psychological well-being of members of the silent generation, baby boom, and baby bust cohorts. The psychological consequences of having made a work–family trade-off (and of possible outcomes of those trade-offs, such as holding a lower-status occupation) may be heightened for baby bust and baby boom women. The baby boom cohort's formative years were punctuated by the women's rights movement; the passage of Title VII of the Civil Rights Act of 1964, which promised to remove official barriers to hiring and promotion of women and minorities; and the passage of the Equal Pay Act of 1963, which prohibited employers from paying women less than men for equivalent work (Reskin and Padavic 1994). These social movements and policies may have encouraged the baby boom and bust cohorts (especially their women members) to form idealized, although more difficult to attain, expectations about how their work and family lives should unfold. Interviews with young women growing up in the 1970s and 1980s revealed that their expectations for occupational opportunities were identical to those of their male peers, and that they believed parenthood and household tasks should impinge equally on husbands and wives (Hesse-Biber and Carter 2000, xiii–xv; Sidel 1990). Consequently, despite the higher absolute levels of educational attainment and the higher-status occupations generally enjoyed by the younger cohorts of women, they may suffer poorer psychological well-being than older women if their work and family lives do not match the expectations formed earlier in life.

For men, as well, the implications for psychological well-being of blending work and family roles (and the socioeconomic consequences thereof) may vary across the birth cohorts. As noted earlier, men who were raised in the 1930s and 1940s, and who entered the labor market and formed families in the 1950s, were expected to provide economically for their families; any activity that reduced a man's earnings potential—for example, cutting back on his work hours to care for children—may have chipped away at an important source of his self-worth (Baruch, Barnett, and Rivers 1983). For younger generations of men, however, successfully combining the roles of involved parent and breadwinner may bolster psychological well-being. Because baby bust and baby boom men are more likely than their fathers to have wives who work for pay, the pressure of fulfilling the breadwinner role is less acute than it was for earlier generations of men (Bianchi and Spain 1996). Moreover, because of changing expectations regarding male gender roles, men who limit their labor force participation in order to play a greater role in family responsibilities may actually view themselves more favorably for complying with prevailing norms (Gerson 1993; Kimmel 1996; Levant and Kopecky 1995; Pleck 1974).

Do Psychological Consequences of Social Roles Differ by Age?

Thus far, the MIDUS participants have been characterized as members of three distinctive birth cohorts, each of which faced unique historical, economic, and normative contexts as they came of age, entered the labor force, and developed strategies for balancing their work and family responsibilities. Yet these three cohorts also represent three distinct stages in the life course; members of a birth cohort are at the same maturational stage or chronological age at a given point in time. The age at which an individual experiences a given event or holds a certain role also may condition its psychological consequences.

Age stratification theory (Riley 1996) suggests that age is an important basis for ascribing status or social roles. For example, work lives are loosely structured by age. In the first stage, young adults explore different employment opportunities. The second stage, occurring at young adulthood through midlife, involves the selection of an occupation and the establishment of a stable career. An assumption is that individuals should have more challenging work, higher status, and more income as they progress through the life course, with this upward trajectory leveling off at about age 50 for white-collar workers and slightly younger for blue-collar workers (Featherman and Hauser 1978; Spilerman 1977). Although younger workers typically anticipate upward occupational mobility in the future, midlife individuals may come to terms with their past work accomplishments and in some cases may abandon hopes of further promotions. Older adults begin a deceleration or "disengagement" that prepares them for retirement (Super 1957).

The extent to which one's occupational pursuits are constrained by family roles also varies over the life course (although these constraints are more pronounced for women than men at every point in the life course). Young adults generally enter into a permanent union, bear children, and care for young children; thus family responsibilities tend to place the greatest constraints on their work life at this stage in the life course. The time and labor intensiveness of family demands generally diminish over the life course, yet challenges exist even for midlife and later-life adults. Midlife adults are believed to be caught between the competing demands imposed by young adult children and aging parents. Older adults often must tend to sick or aging spouses, parents, siblings, and peers (Cowan 1991; Rexroat and Shehan 1987). Thus, both work–family strategies and work rewards, such as occupational status, may have different effects on psychological well-being at different stages of the life course.

Age group/cohort differences in psychological well-being may reflect developmental, role-related, or historical differences in the experience of individuals. Because the MIDUS is a cross-sectional data set, it is not possible to ascertain whether the patterns evidenced in the data are attributable to age or cohort effects. However, in the findings and discussion sections, both sets of explanations are considered.

Strengths of the MIDUS

Despite the limitation of being a cross-sectional survey, the MIDUS data are ideally suited for examining cohort differences in psychological well-being. The MIDUS includes data on a full age range—men and women ages 25–74 in 1995—so it is possible to investigate differences between three cohorts exposed to very different opportunities, obstacles, and normative contexts over the life course. Few data sets obtain information on both the baby bust cohort and those men and women born before World War II. The baby bust cohort is the first to come of age in an era in which women and men have educational equity, and this cohort is more likely than other generations to have had two working parents. Their experiences may provide an important comparison when examining the effects of macrosocial conditions on three generations of adults.

The MIDUS is also particularly well suited to exploring work–family strategies and their implications for psychological well-being. The data set is unique in that it measures whether one has *ever* adjusted one's work life to accommodate family responsibilities. If only current work–family strategies were evaluated, we would not have a complete picture of the work and family lives of the older adults who have completed their childrearing years. Moreover, information on work–family trade-off histories allows for a new perspective on an old sociological question: How do competing work and family roles affect psychological well-being? Most research on the work–family interface is guided by the assumption that combinations of work and family duties impact mental health in one of two ways. Role strain theory holds that multiple roles are stressful in the short term and may impair psychological well-being because competing work and family demands outstrip an individual's abilities and resources for juggling these demands (Verbrugge 1986). The alternate hypothesis, the role enhancement hypothesis, suggests that multiple roles contribute to greater psychological well-being because shortcomings in one domain are offset by benefits achieved in other life domains. Multiple roles also provide multiple sources of meaning and access to more sources of social support (Sieber 1974; Thoits 1983).

Neither of these perspectives considers the longer-term view—that the strategies one takes to manage competing roles in the short term may have important longer-term consequences for psychological well-being. Men and women who adjust their work lives to accommodate childrearing demands end up diminishing their earnings and prospects for occupational mobility (Mincer and Polachek 1974; Goldin 1990). Given the widely documented linkages between socioeconomic status and psychological well-being, it is possible that work–family trade-offs are a critical explanatory pathway that has previously been overlooked.

Data and Methods

Analyses are based on the 2445 adults (1308 men and 1137 women), aged 25–64, who completed both the telephone survey and the self-administered questionnaire of MIDUS, and who are currently employed.

Dependent Variables

Two dependent variables are considered: self-acceptance and environmental mastery. These two dimensions of well-being are among the six subscales of the Ryff (1989) psychological well-being scale, which also encompasses autonomy, positive relations with others, purpose in life, and personal growth (Ryff and Keyes 1995). Respondents indicate their level of agreement or disagreement with three self-descriptive statements for each subscale. Response categories are based on a seven-point

Likert scale, ranging from "strongly disagree" to "strongly agree." Sub-scale scores range from 1 to 7, on the basis of one's average response across the three items. Self-acceptance and environmental mastery were selected as outcomes because of their widely documented linkages to social structural characteristics, including occupational status, educational attainment, family roles, and gender (e.g., Rosenberg and Pearlin 1978; Ross and Mirowsky 2002).

Self-acceptance ($\alpha = .62$) is assessed with three items: (1) I like most parts of my personality; (2) When I look at the story of my life, I am pleased with how things have turned out so far; and (3) In many ways I feel disappointed about my achievements in life (reverse-coded). *Environmental mastery* ($\alpha = .58$) is measured by participants' response to three statements: (1) The demands of everyday life often get me down (reverse-coded); (2) In general, I feel I am in charge of the situation in which I live; and (3) I am good at managing the responsibilities of daily life.

Independent Variables

The main objective of this research is to explore cohort differences in psychological well-being. Three cohorts are considered: *older adults,* born between 1931 and 1943 (ages 52–64); *baby boom cohort/midlife adults,* born between 1944 and 1959 (ages 37–51); and *baby bust cohort/young adults,* born between 1960 and 1970 (ages 36 and younger). Although these categories differ slightly from those typically used in demographic research (persons born between 1960 and 1964 are often referred to as "late baby boomers" rather than as members of the baby bust cohort), each of these three cohorts faced distinct opportunities in terms of work, education, and gender-role expectations as they matured (Baruch, Barnett, and Rivers 1983; Coontz 1992).[2] Each category also represents a distinct stage in an individual's work and family life course (Hagestad 1990; Settersten and Hagestad 1996).

OCCUPATION. Occupational status is assessed with the Stevens–Featherman (1981) TSEI scale, a widely used indicator of occupational ranking, based on occupation-specific education and income data from male and female job holders in the 1980 U.S. Census. This scale is an updated version of the Duncan socioeconomic index. Lower scores represent lower-status occupations such as domestic servant, and the highest scores represent prestigious and well-paying occupations such as physician and lawyer.

HUMAN CAPITAL CHARACTERISTICS. Access to rewarding work opportunities is affected by human capital characteristics, including *educational attainment, total years of work experience,* and the number of hours worked per week, that is, *full- or part-time status. Educational attainment* is coded into four categories: less than 12 years, 12 years (reference group), 13–15 years, and 16 or more years of schooling. *Total years of work experience* is the total number of years a respondent has worked for pay, including both part- and full-time work. *Full/part-time status* is a dummy variable set equal to 1 if an individual works at least thirty-five hours per week, in the average week, on his/her main job. (The reference group is those working fewer than thirty-five hours per week.)

CURRENT FAMILY CHARACTERISTICS. Current family characteristics include *marital status* and *number of children.* Marital status is captured with two dummy variables: *currently married* and *formerly married* (i.e., widowed, divorced, or separated). The reference group is *never married.* In preliminary analyses, I considered using two separate indicators for married persons, to denote those persons married to employed spouses and those married to non-employed spouses. The two coefficients did not differ significantly from one another, and thus the single indicator is used. Number of children (including biological, adopted, and step-children) is indicated with two dummy variables: one signifies persons with *no children;* the other signifies persons with *three or more children.* The reference group refers to those with one or two children only.

WORK–FAMILY TRADE-OFFS. The extent to which family and childrearing demands impinge on men's and women's work lives is captured with the following questions: "We are interested in how having children may have changed your work situation. Which of the following changes did you make because you were living with children? Did you: (1) stop working at a job to stay home and care for the children; (2) cut back on the number of hours worked at a job to care for the children; (3) switch to a different job that was less demanding or more flexible to be available to the children?" A dummy variable is set equal to 1 if a respondent reports *any* of the three behaviors.[3]

CONTROL VARIABLES. Race and adolescent health status are controlled in all analyses.[4] Early physical and mental health are controlled in order to address the possibility that one's educational and occupational prospects may have been impeded by early life health problems—which may also affect adult psychological well-being (see Dohrenwend, Levav, and Shrout 1992 for a review). Respondents were asked: "Think about when you were 16 years old. Was your [physical] and [mental] health at that time poor, fair, good, very good, or excellent?" For each question, responses of fair or poor are coded as 1; the reference group includes responses of good, very good, or excellent. *Race* is a dummy variable equal to 1 for those who indicate that they are not white (i.e., African American, Asian, or Native American).[5] Racial minorities account for a larger proportion of the baby bust cohort than older cohorts (U.S. Bureau of the Census 1996) and also tend to be disadvantaged in terms of occupational and educational attainment (see Hacker 1992). Descriptive statistics for all variables, by age/cohort and sex, are presented in table 1.

MISSING DATA. The sample mean value is imputed to item-specific missing data on continuous variables, and the median value is imputed for dichotomous variables. Dummy variables are constructed to indicate item-specific missing data and are included in all models.

Methodology

Ordinary least squares (OLS) regression models are used. Preliminary analyses using gender-interaction terms indicate the independent variables that have significantly different effects ($p \leq .05$) on men's and women's psychological well-being. Sex-specific models are presented in tables 2–4, and significant gender differences in coefficients are noted with superscripts.

FINDINGS
Bivariate Analyses

Table 1 presents descriptive statistics by birth cohort and gender. Two-tailed *t*-tests were conducted to evaluate significant differences in means (1) by cohort, for men and women, and (2) by sex, within each cohort. The older adults (b. 1931–43) comprise the reference group for the cohort comparisons. The bivariate analyses reveal significant differences in psychological well-being and educational, work, and family experiences across the cohorts, especially for women.

No single birth cohort has a clear advantage in terms of psychological well-being. Rather, the oldest adults fare best in terms of environmental mastery, while the baby bust cohort reports the highest levels of self-acceptance. Among both women and men, self-acceptance levels are significantly higher for each successive generation. In contrast, the oldest cohort fares significantly better than the younger two cohorts in terms of environmental mastery; the scores of the older women and men are approximately .2 higher than the scores of the baby bust

463

TABLE 1 Descriptive Statistics, by Gender and Age

	Men ($N = 1308$)		
Variables	Age 52–64 (b. 1931–43)	Age 37–51 (b. 1944–59)	Age 25–36 (b. 1960–70)
Dependent variables	5.41	5.64*	5.69**
Self-acceptance	(1.36)	(1.16)	(1.14)
Environmental	5.57	5.41+	5.42+
mastery	(1.17)	(1.17)	(1.08)
Independent variables			
Occupational status,	40.97	43.04*	41.92
current/last job	(13.64)	(14.01)	(14.93)
Human capital	0.095	.043***	.057+
<12 years	(.293)	(.203)	(.232)
13–15 years	0.233	.297*	.302*
	(.423)	(.457)	(.460)
16 years +	0.167	.216+	.277***
	(.374)	(.412)	(.448)
Total years work	39.67	26.39***	14.27***
experience	(10.41)	(9.69)	(10.85)
Full-time worker,	0.826	.919***	.923***
current/last job	(.380)	(.273)	(.266)
Current family characteristics			
Currently married	0.796	.741+	.602***
	(.403)	(.438)	(.490)
Formerly married	0.178	0.167	.111*
	(.383)	(.373)	(.315)
Has no children	0.073	.149***	.473***
	(.260)	(.357)	(.500)
Has 3 or more	0.571	.381***	.134***
children	(.496)	(.486)	(.341)
Has made at	0.087	.162***	.139***
least one	(.283)	(.369)	(.346)
work–family			
trade-off			
N	275	629	404

Notes: Two-tailed *t*-tests were conducted to assess within-gender cohort differences (significant differences denoted with superscripts) and within-cohort gender differences (significant differences denoted by asterisks). The 1931–43 cohort is the reference group, where $^+ p \leq .10$; $^* p \leq .05$; $^{**} p \leq .01$; $^{***} p \leq .001$. For the within-cohort gender difference analysis, [a] denotes a gender difference among older adults, [b] denotes a gender difference among baby boomers, [c] denotes a gender difference among baby bust cohort. Only gender differences significant at $p \leq .05$ are noted.

and baby boom cohorts. Interestingly, the gender gap in environmental mastery appears to converge with age. Baby boom and baby bust men have significantly higher scores than their female peers, yet the oldest men and women do not differ significantly from one another. This gender convergence may reflect the fact that the demands of balancing work ȝroup/Cohort, of Men and Women of the MIDUS

Women ($N = 1137$)		
Age 52–64 (b. 1931–43)	Age 37–51 (b. 1944–59)	Age 25–36 (b. 1960–70)
5.46	5.58	$5.72^{**a,c}$
(1.14)	(1.26)	(1.34)
5.44	5.24^*	$5.21^{*b,c}$
(1.17)	(1.15)	(1.22)
38.00	40.06^*	$39.82^{a,b,c}$
(14.49)	(13.94)	(14.12)
0.081	0.052	$.032^{***}$
(.273)	(.222)	(.176)
0.311	0.321	0.356^a
(.464)	(.467)	(.479)
0.099	$.189^{***}$	$.257^{***a}$
(.299)	(.392)	(.438)
30.95	21.88^{***}	$12.81^{***a,b,c}$
(15.53)	(10.83)	(8.33)
0.733	0.724	$0.723^{a,b,c}$
(.443)	(.447)	(.448)
0.546	0.556	$0.549^{a,b}$
(.498)	(.499)	(.499)
0.392	0.363	$.156^{***a,b}$
(.489)	(.481)	(.363)
0.062	$.126^{***}$	$.425^{***}$
(.242)	(.332)	(.495)
0.568	$.386^{***}$	$.121^{***}$
(.496)	(.481)	(.327)
0.637	$.569^+$	$.390^{***a,b,c}$
(.482)	(.496)	(.488)
273	518	346

and family attenuate with age, and thus an important threat to women's sense of mastery weakens with age when their stressful roles disappear. These cohort differences in mastery and self-acceptance underscore the importance of examining separately the subscales of the Ryff well-being scale; if cohort differences in the *aggregate* (i.e., the six subscales) well-being scale had been examined, the opposite patterns documented among the subscales may have cancelled out one another.

Both occupational status and educational attainment differ significantly across the cohorts/age groups. Occupational status scores are highest among the midlife group for both men and women, likely reflecting the widely documented pattern whereby career trajectories peak and then plateau at midlife (Spilerman 1977). Younger workers are beginning their careers and can expect to experience some career advancement in the coming years. Older workers, in contrast, often enter "bridge jobs" before retirement; these are relatively low-status and low-paying jobs clustered in a small set of industries and occupations (Barth, McNaught, and Rizzi 1995; Couch 1998). Moreover, older workers may be disproportionately represented in lower-status blue-collar jobs and farming jobs, given secular shifts in educational attainment and historical shifts in occupational availability over the past half-century (Bell 1973).

Educational opportunities have improved considerably for recent cohorts, especially for women members. Each successive cohort has a higher proportion of college graduates than the last. Women's educational attainment has converged with men's for the most recent two cohorts; although silent generation women are significantly less likely than their male peers to have graduated college, the proportions of baby bust and boom men and women who have graduated college are very similar. Despite the educational strides made by women in recent years, women are still concentrated in less financially rewarding jobs than men are. Women's occupational status scores lag behind their male peers' by approximately three points, for each of the birth cohorts. This may be partly because women (regardless of birth cohort) are far more likely than men to have cut back on their paid work in order to accommodate their family responsibilities, and thus they receive fewer extrinsic work rewards.

Less than 10 percent of the oldest group of men have made a work–family trade-off, whereas 64 percent of the oldest women have made such a sacrifice, reflecting traditional gender-based allocation of work and family roles among those who made the transition to adulthood in the 1950s and early 1960s (Baruch, Barnett, and Rivers 1983). The gender gap is smaller, yet still pronounced, for the younger two cohorts. Among women, generational changes are also pronounced. Baby bust women are significantly less likely than the older two cohorts of women to have made a work–family trade-off. On the one hand, this may reflect a more egalitarian division of labor in the home currently enjoyed by cohorts of young adults. Baby bust women are significantly more likely than the baby boom and older women to report that their *spouses* have at some point adjusted their work schedules to accommodate family demands: 13 percent versus 7 percent and 2 percent, respectively. (The percentages are not shown in the table.) On the other hand, this pattern may reflect life-course stage; women under age 36 may not yet have made the transition to parenthood or marriage. Because the MIDUS data are cross-sectional, however, it is not possible to ascertain whether this pattern reflects cohort differences in fertility behavior, or the fact that the youngest cohort has not yet completed its childbearing.

Multivariate Analyses

The first two questions addressed by the multivariate analyses are (1) Do the three birth cohorts differ in their levels of self-acceptance and environmental mastery? and (2) To what extent can these differences be explained by the different structural opportunities and constraints—such as education, work, and family experiences—facing the three co-horts? Results from OLS regression models are presented in tables 2 (self-acceptance) and 3 (environmental mastery). The baseline model displays the effect of cohort/age group only, model 2 incorporates occupational status, model 3 includes human capital characteristics, model 4 includes family status variables, and model 5 adjusts for whether one has made a work–family trade-off. By adding variables in a stepwise fashion, it is possible to identify the mediators, or pathways, linking cohort status to psychological well-being.[6]

Cohort Differences in Self-Acceptance

The bivariate analyses revealed that each birth cohort has significantly higher levels of self-acceptance than the preceding cohort does. The mul-tivariate analyses show that the baby bust women's self-esteem advantage is mediated largely by their occupational status, educational attainment, and family roles. Although the baby bust women have self-acceptance levels .30 points higher than older women do in the baseline model, their advantage drops to .23 after occupational status, educational attainment, and work characteristics are controlled (model 3). Thus, the richer edu-cational and occupational opportunities afforded to the youngest cohort of women accounts for approximately 25 percent of their advantage in self-acceptance scores. This young cohort of women is further advan-taged in the labor market—relative to their mothers and grandmothers—because marriage and childbearing are less constraining to their work options. After family characteristics are controlled (see model 4), the baby bust women's advantage further declines ($\beta = .187$, $p \leq .05$), and it is only marginally significant when work–family trade-offs are ad-justed ($\beta = .187$, $p \leq .10$). Thus, if the baby bust, baby boom, and silent

TABLE 2 OLS Regression Predicting Self-Acceptance

Independent Variables	Women ($N = 1137$)				
	Model 1	Model 2	Model 3	Model 4	Model
Age/cohort					
Baby boom cohort	0.134	0.099	0.079	0.062	0.062
	(.089)	(.087)	(.091)	(.117)	(.092)
Baby bust cohort	.304***	.267***	.229*	0.187*	0.187+
	(.096)	(.087)	(.109)	(.091)	(.117)
Occupational status					
Stevens-Featherman TSEI score, current occupation		.017***	.008**	.007*	0.007*
		(.002)	(.003)	(.003)	(.031)
Human capital					
Total years work experience			0.001	0.001	0.001
			(.003)	(.003)	(.003)
Full-time worker, current/last job			0.015	0.061	0.061
			(.078)	(.079)	(.080)
<12 years			−.374*	−.344*	−.344*
			(.162)	(.162)	(.162)
13–15 years			0.139	.162+	.163+
			(.089)	(.089)	(.089)
16 years +			.452***	.466***	.466**
			(.106)	(.109)	(.109)
Current family characteristics					
Currently married				.273*	.273*
				(.130)	(.130)
Formerly married				−.008	−.008
				(.138)	(.138)
Has no children				0.029	0.027
				(.119)	(.132)
Has 3 or more children				−.067	−.066
				(.080)	(.080)
Made work–family trade-off					−.004
					(.083)
Constant	5.49	4.83	5.02	4.85	4.86
	(.072)	(.002)	(.158)	(.208)	(.218)
Adjusted R^2	0.012	0.052	0.071	0.081	0.08

Notes: Unstandardized regression coefficients and standard errors are shown. Models were also estimated for a pooled sample of men and women, and all gender interaction terms were tested. No gender interaction terms were statically significant. Physical and mental health at age 16 and race are controlled in all models.

$^+ p \le .10.\ ^* p \le .05.\ ^{**} p \le .01.\ ^{***} p \le .001.$

Women and Men of MIDUS ($N = 2445$)

	Men ($N = 1308$)			
Model 1	Model 2	Model 3	Model 4	Model 5
.235**	.285**	.347**	.355**	.372**
(.086)	(.092)	(.122)	(.125)	(.126)
.301***	.202*	.221**	.218*	.229*
(.093)	(.085)	(.095)	(.095)	(.095)
	.016***	.010***	.010***	.010***
	(.002)	(.003)	(.003)	(.003)
		0.003	0.003	0.003
		(.003)	(.003)	(.003)
		0.058	0.016	0.013
		(.109)	(.109)	(.109)
		−.448**	−.453**	−.463**
		(.149)	(.148)	(.148)
		−.009	−.003	−.003
		(.090)	(.089)	(.089)
		.247*	.254**	.254**
		(.097)	(.098)	(.098)
			.311*	.311*
			(.124)	(.124)
			−.062	−.051
			(.140)	(.140)
			0.009	−.014
			(.108)	(.109)
			−.071	−.068
			(.076)	(.076)
				−.121
				(.096)
5.42	4.77	4.78	4.64	4.65
(.073)	(.118)	(.205)	(.239)	(.239)
0.015	0.049	0.063	0.076	0.077

generation women had equal levels of educational attainment and occupational status, and had similar marriage and childbearing patterns, their levels of self-acceptance would not differ significantly ($p \leq .05$) from one another.

For men, a different scenario is evidenced. Even when work, human capital, and family characteristics are controlled, men of the baby bust and baby boom cohorts have significantly higher levels of self-acceptance than the older men do. The baby bust men's advantage is mediated

TABLE 3 OLS Regression Predicting Environmental Mastery,

Independent	Women ($N = 1137$)				
Variables	Model 1	Model 2	Model 3	Model 4	Model 5
Age/cohort					
Baby boom cohort	−.176*	−.192*	−.161[+]	−.194*	−.201*
	(.088)	(.088)	(.092)	(.093)	(.093)
Baby bust cohort	−.179[+]	−.197*	−.135	−.236*	−.242*
	(.096)	(.096)	(.111)	(.119)	(.119)
Occupational status					
Stevens-Featherman		.008***	0.005	0.004	0.004
TSEI score, current occupation		(.002)	(.003)	(.003)	(.003)
Human capital			0.005	0.004	0.004
Total years work experience			(.003)	(.003)	(.003)
Full-time worker, current/ last job			0.048	0.042	0.021
			(.079)	(.081)	(.082)
Less than 12 years			−.116	−.098	−.110
			(.165)	(.165)	(.165)
13–15 years			0.079	0.06	0.067
			(.091)	(.092)	(.092)
16 years +			.204*	0.161	0.168
			(.107)	(.111)	(.111)
Current family characteristics					
Currently married				0.101	0.101
				(.133)	(.133)
Formerly married				0.043	0.046
				(.141)	(.141)
Has no children				0.132	0.028
				(.122)	(.134)
Has 3 or more children				−.147[+c]	−.145[+•]
				(.082)	(.082)
Made work–family trade-off					−.156*
					(0.82)
Constant	5.47	5.16	5.08	5.11	5.23
	(.072)	(.118)	(.161)	(.213)	(.222)
Adjusted R^2	0.013	0.021	0.023	0.025	0.027

Notes: Unstandardized regression coefficients and standard errors are shown. Models were also estimated for a pooled sample of men and women, and all gender interaction terms were tested. Significant gender differences are noted by superscripts: [a]($p \leq .10$); [b]($p \leq .05$); and [c]($p \leq .01$).
[+] $p \leq .10$. * $p \leq .05$. ** $p \leq .01$. *** $p \leq .001$.

somewhat through occupational status; their self-esteem advantage declines by approximately 33 percent when occupational status is controlled. In contrast, educational attainment and family-role variables do little to mediate the effect of baby bust status on self-acceptance levels; the coefficient changes only vary slightly when these variables are controlled.

Vomen and Men of MIDUS ($N = 2445$)

| | Men ($N = 1308$) | | | |
Model 1	Model 2	Model 3	Model 4	Model 5
-.156*	−.165*	−.122	−.111	−.098
(.081)	(.082)	(.092)	(.093)	(.093)
-.145+	−.149+	−.058	−.018	0.003
(.089)	(.089)	(.118)	(.123)	(.123)
	.004*	0.004	0.004	0.004
	(.002)	(.003)	(.003)	(.003)
		0.004	0.004	0.003
		(.003)	(.003)	(.003)
		0.124	0.097	0.094
		(.107)	(.106)	(.106)
		−.055	−.055	−.067
		(.145)	(.145)	(.145)
		−.072	−.060	−.060
		(.087)	(.088)	(.088)
		0.023	0.039	0.039
		(.095)	(.095)	(.095)
			.269*	.269*
			(.122)	(.121)
			0.161	0.174
			(.137)	(.138)
			0.049	0.021
			(.105)	(.107)
			0.025[c]	0.029[e]
			(.074)	(.074)
				−.146
				(.093)
5.54	5.36	5.15	4.92	4.94
(.069)	(.114)	(.199)	(.233)	(.233)
0.015	0.017	0.017	0.019	0.02

For baby boom men, in contrast, their self-esteem advantage cannot be explained by increased access to education and high-status occupations among recent cohorts. To the contrary, the advantage of the baby boom cohort ($\beta = .235$) shown in the baseline model *increases* by a full 50 percent (from .24 to .35) when occupational status is controlled. The addition of human capital and family variables does little to further alter relationship. The self-esteem advantage of the baby boom men is actually suppressed—rather than mediated—by work, and educational and family characteristics.

Other significant predictors of men's and women's self-acceptance are consistent with past research on the social correlates of self-esteem. Not one of the gender interaction terms (evaluated in preliminary models) was statistically significant, suggesting that the correlates of self-acceptance are generally similar for women and men. Those with richer social and economic resources—college graduates, married persons, and those with higher-status occupations—have significantly higher levels of self-acceptance. Childbearing status, however, is not significantly linked to self-acceptance. As later analyses will reveal, however, *adjustments* to childrearing—or work–family strategies—have distinct effects for each of the three cohorts.

Cohort Differences in Environmental Mastery

The bivariate analyses revealed that older adults have a significant advantage in terms of environmental mastery. The multivariate analyses show that although the cohort gap in environmental mastery levels is mediated fully by work experiences for men, the advantage of the older women persists even when mediating pathways are considered.

Results in table 3 show that baby boom and baby bust men have environmental mastery scores approximately .15 points lower than those of the older men, and this effect persists even after occupational status is controlled. However, when educational attainment is adjusted, the effect of cohort on environmental mastery is no longer statistically significant. In contrast, the lower environmental mastery scores reported by the baby bust and baby boom women persist even when their work and family roles are controlled. Models 1 and 2 show that the baby boom and bust women have mastery scores nearly .2 lower than those of older women. Interestingly, when family characteristics and work–family trade-offs are controlled, the disadvantage of the baby bust and boom cohorts *increases* (see models 4 and 5). This finding suggests that if the younger two cohorts had the same childbearing histories and work–family strategies as the oldest cohort of women (i.e., higher fertility and a higher proportion of members making career sacrifices to raise their children), they would have even lower levels of mastery.

Few other characteristics are significantly linked to environmental mastery for either men or women. Marital status is a large positive predictor of men's but not women's mastery. Moreover, having three or more children negatively affects women's mastery ($\beta = -.15$, $p \leq .10$), and this effect is significantly larger for women than men. Given that women typically bear the brunt of childrearing responsibilities, it is not surprising that having a large family takes a larger toll on women's sense of control.

Changing Meaning of Work–Family Strategies across Three Cohorts

The third objective of the multivariate analysis is to explore whether work and family characteristics have different psychological consequences for members of the three birth cohorts. If an independent variable has significantly different effects for each of the three birth cohorts, this pattern could reflect changing cultural views, evaluations, or expectations across the three cohorts. To address this objective, cohort interaction terms were added individually to model 5 (of tables 2 and 3). Surprisingly few interaction terms were statistically significant. Of the 44 possible interactions (birth cohort by each of the 11 independent variables, for each of the two dependent variables), only a handful were significant. Only occupational status and work–family strategies have different psychological consequences for members of the three birth cohorts.

Occupational status has significantly different effects on the self-acceptance levels of the three cohorts of women and men (models not presented). For women, the relationship between occupational status and self-acceptance is significantly stronger for midlife/baby boom women than for the older or younger age groups. Each one-point increase in occupational status increases baby boom women's well-being by .013 points, yet only .004 points for baby bust and .002 points for older women. This pattern may reflect either the elevated importance that work pursuits have for women at midlife or the importance of one's own accomplishments for women of the baby boom cohort. In contrast, occupational status has a significantly larger effect on the self-acceptance levels of the older men than either the baby boom or baby bust men. Each one-point increase in occupational status increased older men's self-acceptance levels by .021, compared with just .005 points for baby bust men and .008 points for the baby boom men. Men who came of age in the 1940s and 1950s were expected to be good economic providers and to support their families (Easterlin 1980). Pre–World War II cohorts are also believed to have "materialist" concerns, and thus they may place greater importance on economic well-being than do younger generations (Inglehart 1985). Consequently, their self-evaluations may be particularly closely tied to their occupational and financial success.

The work–family trade-off variable also has significantly different consequences for psychological well-being across the three cohorts. The cohort by work–family trade-off interaction term is statistically significant

473

for women in models predicting both self-acceptance and environmental mastery, and for men in models of self-acceptance only. Regression models are presented in table 4, and interaction terms are plotted in figures 1 (self-acceptance) and 2 (environmental mastery).

Older men who have ever altered their labor force participation in order to fulfill family duties had self-acceptance levels .55 points (i.e., one-half standard deviation) lower than their peers who did not make such a trade-off (see table 4, col. 3). Older men who altered their work behavior to meet family demands not only have significantly lower levels of self-acceptance than that of their peers who did not make such adjustments, but they also have significantly lower levels of self-acceptance than do the men of the younger two cohorts who made similar adjustments. In contrast, baby bust men who altered their work lives to meet family demands have self-acceptance levels that are .285 points higher than that of their peers whose work schedules were untouched by family demands. Among the baby boom men, having made a work–family trade-off did not significantly affect a man's self-evaluation. These findings suggest that social norms and expectations guiding gender-appropriate behavior and, consequently, the benchmarks used for evaluating one's self-worth may have shifted in recent decades. As noted earlier, men who came of age in the 1940s and 1950s were expected to work continuously to support their families, abiding by the "good provider" norm (Bernard 1972, 1981). The baby bust men, in contrast, are expected both to provide financially for their families and to be active involved parents (Gerson 1993). Current cohorts of young men who both work for pay and who modify their work schedules to accommodate family responsibilities may be fulfilling the new expectations of the "good father" role, and may derive positive self-evaluations from the recognition that they are living up to this cultural ideal.

Among women, work–family strategies affect psychological well-being differently for the three cohorts. Among the oldest cohort of women, those who either quit work, reduced their hours, or changed jobs while raising children have self-acceptance levels .37 points *higher* than that of their peers who did not alter their work lives in response to family demands ($p \leq .05$). Older women who made such a trade-off presumably complied with the social expectations imposed on young mothers in the 1950s and 1960s, whereby for women, paid employment would be second in importance to family responsibilities (Coontz 1992). Moreover, they have higher levels of self-acceptance than those of the baby bust and boom women who adopted a similar work–family

TABLE 4 OLS Regression Predicting the Effect of Cohort by Work–Family Trade-offs on Environmental Mastery and Self-Acceptance, Women and Men of MIDUS ($N = 2445$)

Independent Variables	Women ($N = 1137$)		Men ($N = 1308$)
	Environmental Mastery	Self-Acceptance	Self-Acceptance
Age/cohort			
Baby boom cohort	0.066	.414**	.203*
	(.171)	(.144)	(.099)
Baby bust cohort	0.056	.466**	.259*
	(.147)	(.168)	(.131)
Occupational status			
Stevens-Featherman	0.004	.007*	.009***
TSEI score, current	(.003)	(.003)	(.003)
occupation			
Human capital			
Total years work	0.005	0.002	0.002
experience	(.003)	(.003)	(.003)
Full-time worker,	−.015	0.025	0.026
current/last job	(.083)	(.081)	(.109)
<12 years	−.091	−.323*	−.465**
	(.165)	(.162)	(.148)
13–15 years	0.063	.162+	0.001
	(.091)	(.090)	(.089)
16 years +	0.161	.470***	.263**
	(.111)	(.108)	(.097)
Current family characteristics			
Currently married	0.083	.254*	.302*
	(.133)	(.130)	(.124)
Formerly married	0.034	−.023	−.050
	(.140)	(.138)	(.140)
Has no children	−.044	−.015	0.019
	(.139)	(.136)	(.109)
Has 3 or more children	−.153+c	−.073	−.053
	(.081)	(.080)	(.076)
Made work–family	0.154	.372*c	−.551*c
trade-off	(.150)	(.147)	(.248)
Trade-off * baby	−.396*	−.562**c	0.323c
boom cohort	(.181)	(.178)	(.277)
Trade-off * baby bust	−.509*	−.432*c	.836**c
cohort	(.209)	(.204)	(.300)
Constant	5.07	4.66	4.69
	(.116)	(.116)	(.239)
Adjusted R^2	0.031	0.086	0.082

Notes: Unstandardized regression coefficients and standard errors are shown. Models were also estimated for a pooled sample of men and women, and all gender interaction terms were evaluated. Significant gender differences are noted by superscripts: [a]($p \leq .10$); [b]($p \leq .05$); and [c]($p \leq .01$). Physical and mental health at age 16 and race are controlled in all models.
[+]$p \leq .10$. [*]$p \leq .05$. [**]$p \leq .01$. [***]$p \leq .001$.

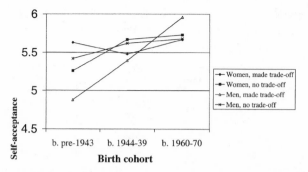

FIGURE 1. Self-acceptance, by gender, cohort, and work–family strategy.

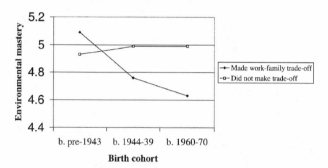

FIGURE 2. Environmental mastery by cohort and work–family strategy among women.

strategy. Among the baby boom and bust women, in contrast, having made a workplace sacrifice for their children is linked to significantly *lower* levels of self-acceptance. Women who do not make work–family trade-offs have work lives that are similar to most men's; their continuous employment generally brings with it the benefits of more rapid occupational mobility, higher earnings, and greater responsibilities on the job (Goldin 1990). For the younger two cohorts who came of age during and after the women's rights movement of the 1960s, the financial rewards and personal fulfillment associated with paid work may be much more closely tied to a woman's sense of self-worth than they are for the older women.

A different set of patterns emerges for environmental mastery. Among those women who did not make work–family trade-offs (i.e., women who worked continuously despite having children), the three birth cohorts are nearly identical in their levels of environmental mastery. In contrast, among those women who did make a trade-off, each successive cohort of women has significantly lower levels of environmental mastery (see fig. 2). Among the oldest women, the effect of having made a work–family trade-off is not statistically significant ($\beta = .154$, $\text{SD} = .150$). However, among the baby bust and baby boom cohorts, having made a trade-off is linked to significantly lower levels of environmental mastery. These findings likely reflect age differences rather than cohort differences in the psychological meaning and relevance of work–family strategies. The baby bust women are at the stage in the life course when they are currently rearing young children, thus their lower levels of mastery may reflect the contemporaneous pressures of managing work and family. For the older women, work–family trade-offs were likely made in the distant past and may no longer pose a threat to the women's sense of mastery and control.

Discussion

This chapter explored three questions: Do the baby bust, baby boom, and silent generation cohorts differ in terms of their psychological well-being? Can these cohort differences be explained by historical shifts in access to opportunities and resources that may enhance psychological well-being? Finally, do work and family roles have different psychological consequences for members of the three birth cohorts, reflecting cultural shifts in the meaning and desirability of these roles? The empirical analyses revealed five important findings. First, the elevated levels of self-acceptance enjoyed by baby bust women can be explained fully by the young women's greater access to self-esteem-enhancing resources, such as higher education, higher status occupations, and fewer family-related obstacles to their work lives. Second, baby bust and baby boom women have significantly lower levels of environmental mastery than do older women, likely reflecting the intense pressures of balancing work and family which threaten young adult and midlife women's sense of mastery. Third, the three cohorts of men do not differ in terms of environmental mastery, once occupational status and education are controlled. Fourth, baby bust and baby boom men have significantly higher levels of self-acceptance than the silent generation men do. Fifth, cohort differences in psychological well-being are conditioned by one's work–family strategies. These specific findings also have broader implications for understanding historical shifts in structural opportunities and normative expectations, and the implications of these macrosocial patterns for individual-level psychological well-being.

Historical Change in Access to Resources May Promote Well-Being

Macrosocial changes over the past four decades have created a context in which the baby bust, baby boom, and silent generation cohorts faced very different opportunities and obstacles to occupational success, particularly during their young adult years. On average, members of each cohort have more education than their parents. Economic restructuring has created a context in which younger cohorts are more likely to hold white-collar or professional occupations and less likely to hold manufacturing or farming jobs. Reduced fertility means that childbearing and rearing tasks are less of a constraint to young women's work lives today than they were for earlier generations (e.g., Bell 1973; Bianchi and Spain 1996; Easterlin 1980; Meyer et al. 1977). The linkages between social and economic resources (such as higher education, income, and occupational status) and psychological well-being have been widely documented (Andrisani 1978; Bird and Ross 1993; Kohn 1969; Kohn and Schooler 1973; Mirowsky and Ross 1998; Pearlin et al. 1981; Rosenberg and Pearlin 1978; Ross and Mirowsky 2002; Wheaton 1980). However, few studies have explored explicitly the possibility that cohort differences in access to such resources may, in part, explain cohort differences in psychological well-being.

The research presented here suggests that historical transitions in the availability of important resources do, in part, explain cohort differences in well-being. For instance, although the baby bust women appear to have significantly higher levels of self-acceptance than those of earlier cohorts of women, this advantage is explained mainly by their higher levels of educational attainment, higher-status occupations, and lower levels of childbearing. Thus, if the educational and occupational opportunities and constraints imposed by family demands were identical for the three cohorts of women, they would enjoy equivalent levels of self-acceptance.

Historical Change in Norms and Values May Condition Psychological Effects

This research has also shown that a role or status, in and of itself, may not be sufficient for explaining subgroups' differences in psychological well-being. Rather, cohort-related cultural changes—such as the shifting normative context surrounding one's behaviors or the evaluative criteria used for determining success—must also be considered. The analyses have shown that the psychological ramifications of one particular behavior—cutting back on (or quitting) work in order to fulfill parenting demands—have very different consequences for the psychological well-being of the baby bust, baby boom, and silent generation men and women. Cutting back on one's work to tend to childrearing responsibilities enhanced the self-acceptance levels of silent generation women and baby bust men. In contrast, the same behavior is associated with significantly lower self-acceptance scores for silent generation men and both baby bust and boom women.

These patterns suggest that historical changes in the meaning and perceived appropriateness of a behavior may condition the behavior's effect on well-being. Engaging in a behavior that conforms to prevailing norms and expectations may enhance one's self-evaluations (see Jackson 1966, 25). For instance, older women who earlier cut back on work to raise their children abided by the prevailing expectation of the 1950s and 1960s—that mothers should give higher priority to their family responsibilities than to their occupational pursuits (Baruch, Barnett, and Rivers 1983). Similarly, for young men who entered adulthood in the 1970s and beyond, fulfilling the "good father" role means both supporting the family financially and playing an active role in childrearing (Gerson 1993; Kaufman and Uhlenberg 2000). Consequently, adjusting one's work life to accommodate family responsibilities is an appropriate and positively evaluated activity for older women and baby bust men.

In contrast, for silent generation men and the baby bust and baby boom women, making a work–family trade-off may indirectly chip away at one's self-evaluations. For the oldest men, altering one's work behavior (and presumably, forsaking earnings and mobility prospects in the process) may violate the norms that prevailed during their young adult years—that men should be primary breadwinners (Bernard 1981). Likewise, the baby bust and baby boom women may be less willing than their mothers to accept the career hindrances that inevitably accompany making work–family trade-offs (Budig and England 2001). Women who expect to achieve equity in the workplace may be particularly disappointed and self-critical upon finding their career trajectories curtailed. In sum, these findings suggest that behaving in a way that either violates one's personal goals and preferences or violates society's expectations for appropriate behavior may take a psychological toll.

Considering Age- and Cohort-Based Explanations for Social Phenomena

These analyses also have underscored the importance of considering both age- and cohort-related explanations when exploring subgroup differences in well-being, where appropriate. For instance, the strong relationship between occupational status and self-acceptance among the midlife/baby boom might reflect either cohort- or age-related factors. Jung (1933) and Giele (1993) have argued that at middle age, a role "crossover" occurs in which women experience a heightened interest in activities earlier associated with typically "male" domains, such as employment and the pursuit of personal accomplishment. At midlife, women are also at the stage in the life course when their childrearing responsibilities diminish, and they are free to pursue their own goals and interests. Consequently, work accomplishments may be a particularly meaningful source of self-esteem. The strong relationship between occupational status and self-acceptance might also reflect a cohort phenomenon. Women who came of age during the women's rights movement of the late 1960s and 1970s are characterized as a generation who placed great emphasis on personal fulfillment and career pursuits; thus their occupational status may be a particularly powerful influence on their self-esteem (Fodor and Franks 1990). Although women of the baby bust cohort also were raised to place great importance on occupational attainment, they are still young enough that they will likely anticipate job promotions in the future, and thus their current occupational status is not necessarily a strong correlate of their self-acceptance levels.

In conclusion, this chapter has investigated the processes through which macrosocial patterns have implications for microlevel outcomes: the self-acceptance and environmental mastery scores of three cohorts of adults. Although historical changes in educational and employment opportunities and family structure explain, in part, why older adults enjoy higher levels of mastery and younger adults report higher levels of self-acceptance, structural factors alone are not sufficient for understanding cohort differences in well-being. Rather, the values, attitudes, and normative expectations facing each of the three cohorts must be considered when exploring the psychological consequences of their life-course experiences. In doing so, scholars may obtain a richer understanding of how both structural and cultural aspects of social change affect the inner lives of American men and women.

NOTES

1. These statistics may also reflect women's declining earnings capacity over the life course. Young women who work full time have earnings higher than those of women in their thirties and forties who are working part time while raising children.

2. I present analyses here that define the baby bust cohort as those born between

1960 and 1970. I also conducted preliminary analyses in which this group was subdivided into "late boom cohort" (b. 1960–64) and "baby bust cohort" (b. 1965–70), in order to ascertain whether the two cohorts differed significantly in their psychological well-being. The coefficients for the two groups were nearly identical (i.e., < .05 of a standard deviation difference), and the regression models with two cohort indicators did not fit the data significantly better than did models with only one indicator. Thus, the final analyses use the single indicator only to capture the baby bust cohort.

    3. A continuous variable ranging from 0 to 3 trade-offs was also considered. The dichotomous and continuous variables behaved in generally similar ways in the multivariate analyses. The dummy variable is used here because a small proportion of men (12 percent) made any form of work–family adjustment.

    4. Social background characteristics *(parental education, urban/rural status, number of siblings, maternal employment,* and *family structure at age 16)* were controlled in earlier analyses because such characteristics are significant correlates of occupational achievements in adulthood (see Sewell and Hauser 1975 for a review), as well as values, gender-role attitudes, and one's criteria for evaluating adequate standards of living (Baumrind 1971; Brown and Harris 1978; Easterlin 1980; Kohn 1969). The social background indicators were not significant predictors of psychological well-being net of education and occupational status, nor did they mediate the effect of birth cohort, and thus they are omitted from the analysis.

    5. Racial minorities are coded simply as white or nonwhite, because more fine-grained subgroup analyses are beyond the scope of the chapter.

    6. Physical and mental health at age 16, and race are controlled in all models.

References

Andrisani, P. J. 1978. Internal–external attitudes, personal initiative, and labor market experience. In *Work attitudes and labor market experience: Evidence from the National Longitudinal Surveys,* ed. P. J. Andrisani, 101–33. New York: Praeger.

Barth, M., W. McNaught, and P. Rizzi. 1995. Older Americans as workers. In *Older and active: How Americans over 55 are contributing to society,* ed. S. A. Bass. New Haven: Yale University Press.

Baruch, G. K., R. Barnett, and C. Rivers. 1983. *Lifeprints: New patterns of love and work for today's women.* New York: New American Library.

Baumrind, D. 1971. Current patterns of parental authority. *Developmental Psychology* 41:1–103.

Bell, D. 1973. *The coming of post-industrial society: A venture in social forecasting.* New York: Basic Books.

Bernard, J. 1972. *The future of marriage.* New York: Bantam.

———. 1981. The good provider role: Its rise and fall. *American Psychologist* 36:1–12.

Bianchi, S., and D. Spain. 1996. Women, work, and family in America. *Population Bulletin* 513:1–47.

Bird, C. E., and C. E. Ross. 1993. Houseworkers and paid workers: Qualities of the work and effects on personal control. *Journal of Marriage and the Family* 55:913–25.

Bohannon, J. R., and P. W. Blanton. 1999. Gender role attitudes of American mothers and daughters over time. *Journal of Social Psychology* 1392:173–79.

Brown, G. W., and T. Harris. 1978. *Social origins of depression: A study of psychiatric disorder in women.* New York: Free Press.

Budig, M. J., and P. England. 2001. The wage penalty for motherhood. *American Sociological Review* 66:204–25.

Butz, W. P., and M. P. Ward. 1979. The emergence of countercyclical U.S. fertility. *American Economic Review* 69June:318–28.

Cherlin, A., and P. Barnhouse Walters. 1981. Trends in U.S. men's and women's sex role attitudes: 1972 to 1978. *American Sociological Review* 46:453–60.

Coontz, S. 1992. *The way we never were: American families and the nostalgia trap.* New York: Basic Books.

Couch, K. 1998. Later life job displacement. *Gerontologist* 38:7–17.

Cowan, P. A. 1991. Individual and family life transitions: A proposal for a new definition. In *Family transitions,* ed. D. A. Cowan and M. Hetherington, 3–30. Hillsdale, N.J.: Lawrence Erlbaum Associates.

Dohrenwend, B. P., I. Levav, and P. E. Shrout. 1992. Socioeconomic status and psychiatric disorders: The causation-selection issue. *Science* 255:946–51.

Dunn, W. 1993. *The baby bust: A generation comes of age.* Ithaca, N.Y.: American Demographics Books.

Easterlin, R. 1980. *Birth and fortune: The impact of numbers on personal welfare.* New York: Basic Books.

Featherman, D., and R. M. Hauser. 1978. *Opportunity and change.* New York: Academic Press.

Fodor, I. G., and V. Franks. 1990. Women in midlife and beyond: The new prime of life. *Psychology of Women Quarterly* 14:445–49.

Gerson, K. 1985. *Hard choices: How women decide about work, career and motherhood.* Berkeley: University of California Press.

———. 1993. *No man's land: Men's changing commitments to family and work.* New York: Basic Books.

Giele, J. 1993. Women in adulthood: Unanswered questions. In *Women in the middle years,* ed. J. Z. Giele, 1–35. New York: Free Press.

Goldin, C. 1990. *Understanding the gender gap: An economic history of American women.* New York: Oxford University Press.

Hacker, A. 1992. *Two nations: Black and white, separate, hostile, unequal.* New York: Ballantine.

Hagestad, G. 1990. Social perspectives on the life course. In *Handbook of aging and the social sciences,* ed. R. Binstock and L. George, 151–86. San Diego, Calif.: Academic Press.

Hartmann, H. I. 1981. The family as the locus of gender, class, and political struggle: The example of housework. *Signs* 366–94.

Hesse-Biber, S., and G. Carter. 2000. *Working women in America: Split dreams.* New York: Oxford University Press.

Hochschild, A. 1989. *The second shift.* New York: Avon.

House, J. S. 1981. Social structure and personality. In *Social psychology: Sociological perspectives,* ed. M. Rosenberg and R. H. Turner, 525–61. New York: Basic Books.

Inglehart, R. 1977. *The silent revolution.* Princeton, N.J.: Princeton University Press.

————. 1985. Aggregate stability and individual-level flux in mass belief systems: The level of analysis paradox. *American Political Science Review* 79:97–116.

Jackson, J. 1966. Structural characteristics of norms. In *Role theory: Concepts and research*, ed. B. J. Biddle. New York: John Wiley.

Jung, C. G. 1933. *Modern man in search of a soul*. New York: Harcourt, Brace, and World.

Kaufman, G., and P. Uhlenberg. 2000. The influence of parenthood on the work effort of married men and women. *Social Forces* 78:931–41.

Kessler, R. C., and P. Cleary. 1980. Social class and psychological distress. *American Sociology Review* 45:463–78.

Kimmel, M. 1996. *Manhood in America: A cultural history*. New York: Free Press.

Kohn, M. L. 1969. *Class and conformity: A study in values*. Homewood, Ill.: Dorsey Press

Kohn, M. L., and C. Schooler. 1973. Occupational experience and psychological functioning: An assessment of reciprocal effects. *American Sociological Review* 38:97–118.

Levant, R. F., and G. Kopecky. 1995. *Masculinity reconstructed: Changing the rules of manhood at work, in relationships and in family life*. New York: Dutton.

Levant, R. F., S. C. Slattery, and J. E. Loiselle. 1987. Father's involvement in housework and child care with school-aged daughters. *Family Relations* 36:152–57.

Levy, F. 1998. *The new dollars and dreams: American incomes and economic change.* New York: Russell Sage Foundation.

Mannheim, K. 1952. The problem of generations. In *Essays in the sociology of knowledge*, ed. and trans. P. Kecskmeti, 276–322. London: Routledge and Kegan Paul.

Mergers and acquisitions. 1987. Almanac and index. Philadelphia: Thomson Media.

Meyer, J. W., F. O. Ramirez, R. Rubinson, and J. Boli-Bennett. 1977. The world educational revolution, 1950–70. *Sociology of Education* 50:242–58.

Mincer, J., and S. Polachek. 1974. Family investments in human capital and earnings of women. *Journal of Political Economy* 82:76–97.

Mirowsky, J., and C. E. Ross. 1998. Education, personal control, life style and health: A human capital hypothesis. *Research on Aging* 20:415–49.

Moen, P., M. A. Erickson, and D. Dempster-McClain. 1997. Their mother's daughters? The intergenerational transmission of gender attitudes in a world of changing roles. *Journal of Marriage and the Family* 59:281–93.

Morgan, C. S., M. P. Hayes, and M. Affleck. 1989. The influence of gender role attitudes on life expectations of college students. *Youth and Society* 20:307–19.

Pearlin, L. I., E. G. Menaghan, M. A. Lieberman, and J. T. Mullan. 1981. The stress process. *Journal of Health and Social Behavior* 22:337–56.

Pleck, J. 1974. *Men and masculinity*. Englewood Cliffs, N.J.: Prentice-Hall.

Reskin, B., and I. Padavic. 1994. *Women and men at work*. Thousand Oaks, Calif.: Pine Forge Press.

Rexroat, C., and C. Shehan. 1987. The family life cycle and spouses' time in housework. *Journal of Marriage and the Family* 49:737–50.

Riley, M. 1996. Age stratification. *Encyclopedia of Gerontology* 1:81–92.

Rosenberg, M., and L. I. Pearlin. 1978. Social class and self-esteem among children and adults. *American Journal of Sociology* 841:53–77.

Ross, C., and J. Mirowsky. 2002. Age and the gender gap in the sense of personal control. *Social Psychology Quarterly* 65:125–45.

Ryder, N. 1965. The cohort as a concept in the study of social change. *American Sociological Review* 30:843–61.

Ryff, C. D. 1989. Happiness is everything, or is it? Explorations on the meaning of psychological well-being. *Journal of Personality and Social Psychology* 57:1069–81.

Ryff, C. D., and C. L. Keyes. 1995. The structure of psychological well-being revisited. *Journal of Personality and Social Psychology* 694:719–27.

Schrammel, K. 1998. Comparing the labor market success of young adults from two generations. *Monthly Labor Review*, February, 3–9.

Settersten, R., and G. Hagestad. 1996. What's the latest? Cultural age deadlines for family transitions. *Gerontologist* 36:178–88.

Sewell, W. H., and R. M. Hauser. 1975. *Education, occupation and earnings: Achievement in the early career.* New York: Academic Press.

Shelton, B. A., and D. John. 1993. Does marital status make a difference? Housework among married and cohabiting men and women. *Journal of Family Issues* 14:401–20.

Sidel, R. 1990. *On her own: Growing up in the shadow of the American dream.* New York: Penguin.

Sieber, S. D. 1974. Toward a theory of role accumulation. *American Sociological Review* 39:567–78.

Spilerman, S. 1977. Careers, labor market structure, and socioeconomic achievement. *American Journal of Sociology* 833:551–93.

Stevens, G., and D. L. Featherman. 1981. A revised socioeconomic index of occupational status. *Social Science Research* 104:364–95.

Super, D. E. 1957. *The psychology of careers.* New York: Harper and Row.

Thoits, P. 1983. Multiple identities and psychological well-being: A reformulation and test of the social isolation hypothesis. *American Sociological Review* 48:174–87.

Thornton, A. 1989. Changing attitudes toward family issues in the United States. *Journal of Marriage and the Family* 51:873–93.

U.S. Bureau of Labor Statistics. 1995. *Employment and earnings.* Washington, D.C.: U.S. Government Printing Office.

U.S. Bureau of the Census. 1996. *Statistical abstract of the United States.* Washington, D.C.: U.S. Government Printing Office.

U.S. National Center for Educational Statistics. 1995. *Digest of education statistics.* Washington, D.C.: U.S. Government Printing Office.

Verbrugge, L. 1986. Role burdens and physical health of men and women. *Women and Health* 11:47–77.

Watkins, S. C., J. Menken, and J. Bongaarts. 1987. Demographic foundations of family change. *American Sociological Review* 52:346–58.

Wheaton, B. 1980. The sociogenesis of psychological disorder: An attributional theory. *Journal of Health and Social Behavior* 21:100–124.

Wilkie, J. R. 1993. Changes in U.S. men's attitudes toward the family provider role, 1972–1989. *Gender and Society* 7:261–79.

Williams, J. 2000. *Unbending gender: Why work and family conflict and what to do about it.* New York: Oxford University Press.

CHAPTER SEVENTEEN

Work, Family, and Social Class

Alison Earle and S. Jody Heymann

Parents Living in Poverty

In August of 1996, the United States Congress passed the most sweeping changes in poverty policy in sixty years. The Personal Responsibility and Work Opportunity Reconciliation Act ended the guarantee of income support for single parents and their children living in poverty and replaced it with block grants to the states, time limits, and work requirements for both food stamps and income support (U.S. Congress 1996). Under the new law, the majority of welfare recipients are required to find work within two years, and no individual is allowed to receive even intermittent support for more than a total of five years during his or her lifetime. Poverty policy may now be more aptly considered a component of family labor policy. Whether and how poor working parents manage the challenges of balancing work and family under these conditions have important consequences for poor children.

Poor working parents and those who have successfully left welfare for work typically hold low-paying jobs. With low wages and few assets, these families have far less financial resources than middle-class families to pay for routine and emergency child care that would enable them to keep a job and meet the demands of parenting. Because of their financial constraints, low-income parents often rely on unpaid substitute care when they have no paid leave. In the past, many parents who received welfare provided unpaid support to friends, relatives, and neighbors who were working (Edin and Lein 1996). However, as a result of welfare reform, poor working parents may now have fewer people in their communities to rely on for unpaid or minimally paid help.

Not only do parents living in poverty have fewer financial resources, but children growing up in poverty are at higher risk of having developmental and educational problems (Duncan et al. 1998; Reynolds and Ross 1998; Hill and Sandfort 1995; McLeod and Shanahan 1996; Haveman, Wolfe, and Spaulding 1991; Duncan 1988). Numerous studies have shown that childhood poverty, particularly persistent poverty, has significant negative effects on children's outcomes, including lowering adult earnings, high school completion rates, and adult employment rates (Duncan et al. 1998; Haveman, Wolfe, and Spaulding 1991; Caspi et al. 1998). In addition, living in poverty or in a low-income family has been shown to compromise children's physical growth, cognitive development, and social and emotional functioning (Hill and Sandfort 1995; Reynolds and Ross 1998; McLeod and Shanahan 1996).

Parental Work Across Social Class

Although understanding how parents manage work and family is critical to improving the well-being of poor working parents, many of the issues they face are common to parents of all social classes. How parents combine work and family has important effects on the children of all employed parents. It has been shown that parental time plays a central role in children's cognitive, educational, and social development, and conversely that parental absence and loss of contact are detrimental (Benson, Medrich, and Buckley 1980; Biller 1993; Coleman 1998; Long and Long 1984; Parcel and Menaghan 1990, 1994; Radin and Russell 1983; Rossi 1984). Among adolescents who have already developed behavioral problems, parental involvement has been shown to be critical in reducing socially destructive behaviors and improving social competence (Waugh and Kjos 1992).

Parental availability is also critical for children's physical health (Woods 1972; LaRosa-Nash and Murphy 1997; George and Hancock 1993). Studies have shown that sick children have shorter recovery periods, better vital signs, and fewer symptoms when their parents participate in their care (Bowlby 1953; Robertson 1958; Van der Schyff 1979; Muhaffy 1965; Palmer 1993). For example, the presence of parents has been shown to reduce hospital stays by 31 percent (Taylor and O'Connor 1989). When parents are involved in children's care, children recover more rapidly from outpatient procedures as well (Kristensson-Hallstron, Elander, and Malmfors 1997). Research has shown that parents play important roles in the care of children with chronic as well as acute conditions (Wolman et al. 1994; Hanson et al. 1992). The importance of parental involvement has been demonstrated for children with epilepsy (Carlton-Ford et al. 1995), asthma, and diabetes (Hamlett, Pellegrini, and Katz 1992; LaGreca et al. 1995; Anderson et al. 1981).

Receiving care from their parents is important for children's mental as well as physical health (Waugh and Kjos 1992; Sainsbury et al. 1986). The detrimental effects of separating young children from their parents when they are sick have been repeatedly demonstrated (McGraw 1994; Robertson 1958; Bowlby 1953). When parental involvement in the care of sick children is increased, children's anxiety decreases (Cleary et al. 1986; Sainsbury et al. 1986; Gauderer, Lorig, and Eastwood 1989; Hannallah and Rosales 1983).

Understanding how working parents balance the needs of their children and their work is particularly important for families that contain children with chronic or serious health conditions. Nationwide, approximately one out of five children, or a total of more than twelve million children, have chronic conditions or special health care needs requiring ongoing care (Aron, Loprest, and Steuerle 1996; Johnson 1994; Newacheck et al. 1998). Parental involvement is often crucial to meeting the daily medical needs of children with chronic conditions, such as monitoring diet and blood glucose levels, and administering medications (LaGreca et al. 1995). The emotional support parents provide can be equally important (Hauser et al. 1990; Johnson 1994; Holden et al. 1997). If parents are available, they can play an important role in easing the child's psychological adjustment to having a serious disease (Wolman et al. 1994; Hamlett, Pellegrini, and Katz 1992).

Work and Family across Social Class

Recent changes in social policy were based on the assumption that poor and nonpoor working parents face similar conditions in trying to balance work and family. Regardless of income and social class, all parents were assumed to have similar caretaking responsibilities as well as the same opportunities and resources available to care for their family's physical, emotional, and educational well-being.[1] In the debate of how best to ensure that poor parents work to support themselves, there has been surprisingly little large-scale research in the United States regarding the caretaking responsibilities that poor parents will be managing while they try to meet the demands of a job, or the resources they will have to meet their dual demands.

Past research has examined the relationship between individuals' income and their sick days (D'Arcy 1998; Dewa and Lin 2000; Andresen and Brownson 2000; Rutledge, Eve, and Doering 1988). However, to our knowledge, there has been no research that examines the relationship between income and the caretaking burden resulting from family illness. There is some evidence from outside the United States that caretaking responsibilities, including those related to family illness, are distributed differently across socioeconomic status when measured as occupation, education, ethnicity, or race. One recent study of 6500 Canadians found that men with the lowest levels of education (defined as less than a high school diploma) were more likely to provide personal care to an elderly person (Matthews and Campbell 1995). Using a 1986 survey of more than 18,000 adults in Great Britain, researchers found that working-class women and men are more likely than their middle-class counterparts to provide care for an elderly, handicapped, or disabled individual (Arber and Ginn 1992).

Caretaking responsibilities are one of many factors determining whether employed adults can balance work and family demands. Employed parents' availability to care for their family is often determined by job benefits, working conditions, and the availability of social supports. All parents need time off from work to meet their family's health, emotional, and educational needs. Among other things, they may need to take their children to sick- and well-child doctor visits and to attend meetings with a child's teacher. The need for time off is even more critical and frequent for parents of children with special needs. These parents may need to meet with specialists during regular work hours to discuss, monitor, and plan treatment for their children's problems, and these meetings may need to take place on a frequent basis. These families also face a myriad of unpredictable child-care needs such as visits to the emergency room when an asthma exacerbation occurs.

Employed caregivers are likely to need more than one of these forms of support. Because many of the responsibilities for children, the elderly, or the disabled are unpredictable—such as the occurrence of a medical emergency—vacation leave, which generally must be scheduled ahead of time, may not be adequate. Having flexibility in the scheduling of one's work hours can enable a parent to take a few hours off during the work day to ensure that young children are not left alone, to address problems that arise in child care, and to meet with teachers when children are having problems at school or elsewhere. However, family responsibilities such as caring for children when school or child-care centers are closed can require time off for at least one full day of work.

Although working caregivers who have at least one form of paid leave or flexibility may still face difficulties meeting their family's needs, those families whose members lack all sources of support are in greatest danger. Working caregivers who cannot take days off often cannot care for their children when they are sick. Employed parents who have no flexibility in when they start and end their workday may have to leave a young child home alone before or after school. The families of caregivers who lack any paid time off—sick, vacation, or personal leave—will find it doubly difficult to meet family members' needs. We examined how many working caregivers find themselves in this double jeopardy. We also examined how many working caregivers lack flexibility in their schedules as well as paid leave and thus are placed in multiple jeopardy.

Although the risks of working caregivers who are in double and multiple jeopardy ought to be of special concern, we know little about the prevalence of this problem from past research. National data exist on the availability of paid sick or vacation leave (U.S. Department of Labor 1997, table 1, Percent of full-time employees participating in selected employee benefit programs). These data do not, however, look at the risk at the family level. The national estimates do not document the availability of benefits for working caregivers. Furthermore, these estimates are not broken down by income or social class. Finally, the national estimates do not include data on the fraction of families whose working caregivers are at double jeopardy—lacking both paid sick and vacation leave—nor those at multiple jeopardy, who lack both paid time off and schedule flexibility.

There is a larger literature on the availability of supports outside the workplace; however, studies in this area have not been focused on how they influence working adults and their particular challenges. Although some have looked at low-income populations, most focus on the middle class. Few directly examine differences across social class (see, e.g., Wijnberg and Weinger 1998; Lindblad-Goldbert and Dukes 1985; Belle 1982; Andress, Lipsmeier, and Salentin 1995).

In sum, what has been missing from the literature on caretaking responsibilities and resources is the ability to look in detail at the conditions faced by low-income parents and how their experience compares with that of middle- and upper-income parents. This study fills this important gap.

Organization

In this chapter, we examine whether there are differences across social class in the degree and amount of caretaking burden adults face during midlife, and in the availability of social and working conditions that would enable employed adults to meet their caretaking burdens. This chapter builds on our previous work about the conditions faced by low-income working parents (Heymann and Earle 1997, 1998, 1999, 2000; Heymann, Toomey, and Furstenberg 1999; Heymann, Earle, and Egleston 1996). It summarizes the findings from our previous studies in this area and presents new findings.

The chapter is organized as follows. The data section describes our three sources of data. The results section reviews our findings. First, we describe our analysis of whether caretaking burdens vary by social class. Because concrete working conditions such as paid leave and formalized flexible scheduling can make an obvious difference in enabling parents and caretakers to meet their family's needs, we next review our findings on the prevalence of these types of benefits across social class. When no formalized policies for time off from work are in place, job flexibility is an important predictor of whether caregivers can meet work demands while caring for their children. Because of this, our next section reviews our analyses of the degree of decision-making latitude that working parents have experienced at their jobs. Although quantifiable measures of support are important to employed caregivers, it is clear that the attitudes of co-workers and supervisors often determine whether employees can actually take advantage of the benefits offered within a workplace or job. The next section reviews our findings on the degree of informal support that is available from supervisors and co-workers and how it varies by social class. Last, we examine social supports and networks that working parents in midlife might use when the workplace leaves a gap in the support they need because paid time off and schedule flexibility are not available or cannot be used.

DATA

Our analyses use three data sets to examine aspects of both family caretaking burdens and working conditions of poor and nonpoor working parents. These data sets are the Survey of Midlife in the United States (MIDUS), the National Longitudinal Survey of Youth (NLSY), and the National Medical Expenditure Survey (NMES). Each contributes unique information regarding the health and developmental needs of families and the characteristics of jobs held by employed midlife parents.

Survey of Midlife in the United States

The Survey of Midlife in the United States (MIDUS) has been previously described in chapter 1 of this volume. To understand the experiences of the working poor, it is critical to understand the social supports available to them, the nature of that support, and the flexibility available in the workplace. The MIDUS survey is an excellent source for examining these issues, and it allows us to explore them as they are experienced by adults from all ages in midlife, from 25 to 74. MIDUS explored the degree of job autonomy of its respondents by asking how often they have a choice in deciding how they do their tasks at work, deciding what tasks they do, planning their work environment, and making decisions about work in general. These are aspects of a person's work environment that are generally not measured well or at all in other surveys. MIDUS also collected data on the number of days that respondents changed their work schedule to meet family responsibilities, including staying home or making arrangements for their child when their child was ill, their usual caregiver was not available, or a day care center or school was closed.

The MIDUS subsample used for analysis in this study was comprised of 908 working parents who had children under 18 years of age. A respondent was considered to be low income if the total family income was equal to or below 150 percent of the Federal Poverty Threshold for the respondent's family size. MIDUS surveyed 146 low-income working parents and 743 middle- or upper-income working parents. Nineteen parents did not report income.

National Longitudinal Survey of Youth

In order to study the working poor who have been on welfare, we sought a longitudinal data set with a substantial sample of low-income respondents. The National Longitudinal Survey of Youth (NLSY) met both criteria. The initial sampling design included an oversampling of poor and minority populations. In addition, the NLSY provides monthly indicators of welfare use over time, allowing us to determine a more complete and accurate picture of an individual's welfare history.[2] The NLSY also has current and historical data on employment and concrete working conditions, including how much paid leave and scheduling flexibility parents receive in jobs held over a period of time.

The NLSY has current and historical data on the specific medical conditions and illnesses of children as well as behavioral and school outcomes. Because the NLSY provides detailed longitudinal data on children's health outcomes, the survey was also used to estimate the fraction of parents caring for a child with a chronic health condition such as asthma.

The NLSY consists of a nationally representative probability sample of 11,406 civilian men and women aged 14–21 in 1979 when they were first surveyed (Center for Human Resources Research 1995). Respondents are currently aged 38–45. Multistage, stratified area sampling was used to select the civilian respondents. Female respondents were interviewed annually and had been observed biannually with their children since 1986.

Our NLSY sample consists of 2261 full-time employed mothers with children under age 18 in the household. A full-time employed mother was defined as one who reported working twenty hours per week or more and was not self-employed. We think it is equally important to examine fathers' working conditions; however, the NLSY does not provide data on fathers that can be linked to their children. Therefore, analyses using the NLSY examined only mothers working twenty hours per week or more. Because many employees who work less than half time are ineligible for many employer-provided benefits, our estimates of the proportion of employed parents who lack benefits are likely to be conservative.

National Medical Expenditure Survey

We estimate health-related family caretaking responsibilities using our third data set, the National Medical Expenditure Survey (NMES). The NMES provides data on whether and how often, over a one-year period, individual family members missed school or work or otherwise limited daily activities because of illness. NMES surveyed civilian, noninstitutionalized families living in the United States and interviewed a national sample of all adults 18 and older at the time of the 1987 survey. Households were selected through an area sampling technique. Interviews of each family were held at four points in time during a sixteen-month period. Certain population groups, including African Americans, Hispanics, families near or below the poverty line, the elderly, and the functionally impaired were oversampled. Our NMES sample consists of 3213 employed parents and their children under the age of 18 living in the respondent's household. A total of 514 of these 3213 were living in poverty at the time of the survey.

Results
Family Caretaking Responsibilities

We examined the caretaking responsibilities that working parents face across social class, including days needed to care for an ill family member, to care for children with special needs, and to meet all of children's needs.

Family Illness Burden

We used the NMES to examine health-related family caretaking responsibilities: the number of days a family member is ill and requires care. In NMES, data were collected on the number of days a person's activity is limited, the number of days spent in bed, the number of school loss days—that is, days when a 5- to 17-year-old cannot attend school because of illness—and the number of days an adult misses work. The family illness burden for poor families in which the parents are employed was compared with that of nonpoor families, where poor is defined as having an income at or below 150 percent of the poverty threshold.

We found that more than one in three families face a family illness burden of two weeks or more each year. Approximately one in four families faces a family illness burden of three weeks or more each year. Poor working parents are more likely to have over three weeks a year of illness burden to manage than nonpoor families ($p < .001$). A total of 27 percent of working poor parents faced a family illness burden of more than three weeks compared with 23 percent of nonpoor parents.

Caring for a Child with Special Needs

Using a sample of employed mothers from the NLSY, we examined how frequently parents were needed to care for children with special needs. We first examined how frequently parents were called on to care for children with asthma, and second, how frequently parents needed to attend to children with any special needs whose care was likely to place greater demands on the parents. The frequency of parents needing to care for a child with asthma was assessed both because asthma is the most common chronic childhood condition and because children who suffer from it need frequent health care. In assessing all special needs, we considered a child to have special needs if the parent described the child as having a physical, emotional, or mental condition that required frequent attention or treatment from a doctor, the regular use of medicine, or the use of special physical equipment, or if the child had a condition that limited his or her ability to attend school regularly, to complete regular school work, or to participate in typical children's activities (Center for Human Resources Research 1990).

We found that mothers who have been on AFDC are significantly more likely than mothers who have never been on AFDC to have at least one child with asthma ($p < .001$) and at least one child who has a chronic condition ($p < .001$) for whom they need time to care. Fourteen percent of working mothers who have been on AFDC for more than two years in the past and 11 percent of working mothers who have been on AFDC for two years or less have a child with asthma compared with 7 percent of mothers who have never been on AFDC ($p < .001$) (see fig. 1). Forty-one percent of mothers who have been on AFDC for more than two years in the past and 32 percent of mothers who have been on AFDC for two years or less have at least one child with a chronic condition whose health and developmental needs they must address compared with 21 percent of mothers who have never been on AFDC ($p < .001$). Those mothers

493

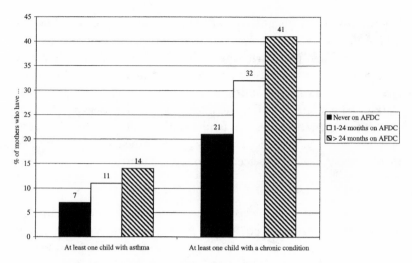

FIGURE 1. Family caretaking burden. This figure is based on analyses the authors conducted using data from the NLSY.

who have been on AFDC the longest are the most likely to have a child with a chronic condition ($p < .001$).

Work Cutbacks to Meet Family Needs

Although the needs of sick children require most parents to take time off from work, children have other types of needs that require parental attention. We used MIDUS to examine the extent of these broader types of family responsibilities and their effect on work, and then compared and contrasted the experiences of families living above and below 150 percent of the poverty threshold.

In the MIDUS survey, we asked respondents the number of days in the past three months that they or their spouses had changed or dropped their normal schedule to care for children, including days when parents stayed home or made arrangements for child care when a child was ill, when the usual caregiver was not available, or when a day care center or school was closed.

We found that, on average, parents needed to take 1.84 days of work cutbacks in a three-month period to care for their children. However, single and low-income parents who face additional challenges in meeting the needs of their children reported having even greater needs (see fig. 2). Low-income single parents reported needing to take 3.4 days of cutbacks in a three-month period for their children. However, single parents who

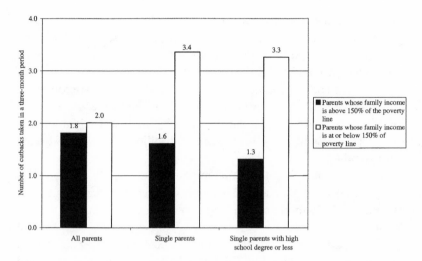

FIGURE 2. Comparison of days taken to meet children's needs. This figure is based on analyses the authors conducted using data from the MIDUS.

were living above 150 percent of the poverty line reported needing to take only 1.6 days. Single parents with a high school education or less (who were more likely to have a low-wage job) who were also living in poverty reported that cutbacks for their children affected nearly three and a half days of work over a three-month period. This is almost three times greater than single parents with a high school degree or less who were not low income.

Concrete Working Conditions

Using the NLSY, we examined the availability of paid sick leave, paid vacation leave, and flexible work schedules to help working parents meet children's needs. Because those parents with no paid leave or flexibility are likely to be the least able to take time off to care for their children, we examined the extent to which parents leaving welfare for work had at least one benefit or working condition that would facilitate their meeting their children's health care and developmental needs. Because parents need to have time off from work not just at one point in time but consistently over their working lives, the availability of paid leave and flexibility over five years was examined.

Analyses using the NLSY compared the working conditions for employed women who had at some point received welfare with those who had never been on welfare. Because the overwhelming majority of working parents who had received welfare were women, and because women may receive different benefits than men, working women who had never received AFDC were used as the comparison group for working women who had received AFDC. In addition, we calculated total years of welfare receipt between January 1978 and December 1993. We compared the benefits and flexibility available to mothers who had received welfare for a lifetime total of more than two years before their current job and two years or less with the benefits and flexibility available to working mothers who had never received welfare.

Of our sample of 2261 working mothers in the NLSY, 736 had been on welfare at some point and 1525 had never been on welfare. Our analyses included 410 mothers who used welfare for more than twenty-four months.

Last, we examined the working conditions faced by those parents with the greatest caretaking responsibilities—those with children with special needs. Having good working conditions is particularly important for parents whose children have chronic physical or mental health conditions that require ongoing and frequent care. We examined the 2261 working mothers in the NLSY, which included 308 who had children with a chronic physical, emotional, or mental condition. The experience of mothers who had children with these special needs was compared and contrasted with the experience of mothers who did not have children with special needs.

Consistent Availability of Paid Leave from Work

Mothers who had received welfare in the past were significantly less likely to have paid sick leave than were other mothers (see table 1). Only

TABLE 1 Working Conditions of Parents Leaving Welfare for Work

Working Conditions	Never on AFDC	1–24 months on AFDC	>24 Months on AFDC	p Value
Had sick leave the entire time they worked	51.3	27.9	21.4	<.001
Had vacation leave the entire time they worked	61.3	44.0	38.2	<.001
Had flexible schedules the entire time they worked	30.1	16.3	18.6	<.001
Had sick leave and vacation leave the entire time they worked	45.9	24.2	19.0	<.001
Had sick leave, vacation leave, and flexibility the entire time they worked	15.1	6.2	5.2	<.001

Note: This table is based on analyses the authors conducted with data from the NLSY.

21 percent of mothers who had received welfare for more than two years had paid sick leave the entire time they worked between 1990 and 1994, compared with 51 percent of mothers who had never received AFDC ($p < .001$). Fifty-eight percent of mothers who had received welfare in the past received paid sick leave less than half of the time they worked, compared with 34 percent of working mothers who never received AFDC ($p < .001$).

Mothers leaving welfare for work received fewer days of paid sick leave when they did receive paid sick leave. Less than 14 percent of mothers who had received welfare in the past received more than 10 days of paid sick leave, compared with 27 percent of mothers who had never received AFDC ($p < .001$).

Mothers leaving welfare for work were also significantly less likely than mothers who had never received AFDC to have paid vacation leave when they worked ($p < .001$). Only 38 percent of mothers who had been on welfare more than two years and 44 percent of those who had been on it for less than two years received paid vacation leave the entire time they worked. In contrast, 61 percent of working mothers who had never received AFDC had paid vacation consistently available to them. Twenty percent of mothers returning to work from welfare received paid vacation leave none of the time they worked, compared with 14 percent of working mothers who had never received AFDC ($p < .001$).

When they did receive paid vacation leave, mothers with a history of welfare receipt were given significantly fewer days of paid vacation than mothers who had never received welfare. Although more than one in three mothers who had never received AFDC in the past received more than two weeks of paid vacation leave, less than one in six mothers who had received AFDC for more than two years received that much paid vacation leave ($p < .001$).

Mothers leaving welfare for work were significantly less likely to have a flexible schedule ($p < .001$). Only 18 percent of mothers who had received welfare in the past consistently found jobs that provided them with flexible schedules, compared with 30 percent of mothers who had never received AFDC. Fifty-seven percent of past welfare recipients found jobs that provided flexible schedules less than half of the time they worked ($p < .001$).

During the five-year period from 1990 to 1994, parents of children with chronic conditions were significantly less likely to have paid leave or flexibility when compared with parents who had no children with chronic physical or mental health conditions ($p < .001$). Parents who

TABLE 2 Working Conditions of Employed Parents of Children
with Chronic Conditions

Working Conditions	No Children with a Chronic Condition	One Child with a Chronic Condition	More than One Child with a Chronic Condition	p Value
Had sick leave the they entire time worked	45.7	40.4	30.1	0.002
Had vacation leave the entire time they worked	57.8	50.3	43.4	0.021
Had flexible schedules the entire time they worked	26.9	31.5	40.7	0.058
Had sick leave and vacation leave the entire time they worked	40.7	35.5	30.1	0.006
Had sick leave, vacation leave, and flexibility the entire time they worked	6.4	15.5	12.6	0.141

Note: This table is based on analyses the authors conducted with data from the NLSY.

had more than one child with a chronic condition were in the most difficult position (see table 2). Thirty percent of parents with multiple children with chronic conditions had sick leave the entire time they worked. In contrast, 46 percent of parents with no children with chronic conditions had sick leave all their working years. Compared with parents with no children with chronic conditions, parents who had more than one child with a chronic condition were significantly less likely to have both sick and vacation leave while they worked ($p = .006$).

The families with the fewest resources to manage a child's special health needs—low-income parents—were significantly less likely than middle- and higher-income parents to have sick leave and vacation leave the entire time they worked. Eighteen percent of parents of children with chronic conditions who live below the poverty line had sick leave the entire time they worked, compared with 44 percent of parents with incomes greater than 100 percent of the poverty threshold ($p = .007$). Thirty-three percent of parents of children with chronic conditions living below the poverty line had vacation leave the entire time they worked, compared with 54 percent of those with incomes greater than 100 percent of the poverty threshold ($p = .014$).

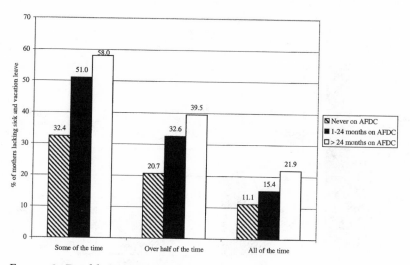

FIGURE 3. Double jeopardy: lacking sick and vacation leave. This figure is based on analyses the authors conducted using data from the NLSY.

Working Parents Facing Double or Multiple Jeopardy over Time

We found that one-quarter of all working mothers lacked both sick and vacation leave over half of their working years between 1990 and 1994. More than one in eight lacked sick and vacation leave the entire time they worked. More than one in five working mothers lacked any paid leave or schedule flexibility some of their working years. One in ten working mothers faced these same working conditions more than half of the time they worked between 1990 and 1994.

Mothers leaving welfare for work were significantly more likely to lack both paid sick leave and vacation leave than were mothers who had never received AFDC (see fig. 3). Nearly 60 percent of mothers who had received welfare for more than two years lacked any type of paid leave for some of their working years. Among mothers who had never received welfare, only 32 percent, or half as many mothers as those on welfare for more than two years, lacked paid leave for some of their working years. One in five mothers who had received AFDC for more than two years lacked any type of paid leave the entire time they worked between 1990 and 1994. In contrast, only one in ten mothers who never received AFDC in the past lacked paid sick and vacation leave the entire time they worked between 1990 and 1994 ($p < .001$).

Those mothers who lack scheduling flexibility in addition to paid sick and vacation leave face the most problematic working conditions when

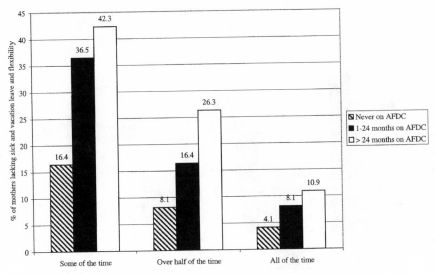

FIGURE 4. Multiple jeopardy: lacking sick and vacation leave and flexibility. This figure is based on analyses the authors conducted using data from the NLSY.

it comes to meeting their children's needs. Although more than one in four mothers who had received AFDC for over two years in the past and one in six mothers who had received AFDC for two years or less lacked flexible schedules and paid leave the majority of the time they worked, less than one in ten mothers who never received AFDC lacked all three benefits for the majority of the time they worked ($p < .001$) (see fig. 4.).

Parents who had at least one child with a chronic condition were significantly more likely to find themselves in double jeopardy, that is, lacking both sick and vacation leave, than parents who had no children with chronic conditions (see fig. 5). Families who were caring for more than one child with a chronic condition were more likely to find themselves in double jeopardy than families who had only one child with a chronic condition. Twenty-eight percent of families who had more than one child with a chronic condition lacked sick leave and vacation leave all of the time they worked, compared with 17 percent of families who had one child with a chronic condition and 12 percent of families who had no children with chronic conditions ($p = .003$).

Parents who had multiple children with chronic conditions were the most likely to find themselves in multiple jeopardy, that is,

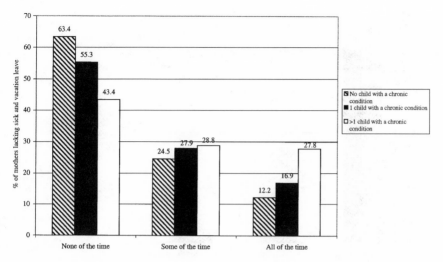

FIGURE 5. Double jeopardy: lacking sick and vacation leave. This figure is based on analyses the authors conducted using data from the NLSY.

lacking sick and vacation leave as well as flexibility in work hours (see fig. 6).

Decision Latitude

Because parents with more say in decisions about their work have greater flexibility in meeting work demands while caring for their children, the degree of decision-making latitude that working parents had at their jobs was also examined.

The MIDUS survey contains questions regarding four aspects of job autonomy. Respondents were asked how often they have a choice in deciding how they do their tasks at work, how often they have a choice in deciding what tasks they do, how often they have a say in planning their work environment, and how often they have a say in decisions about work in general. We examined whether low-income parents have the same degree of decision-making latitude that higher-income working parents had at their jobs, where low income was defined as having an income at or below 150 percent of the 1995 poverty threshold.

Table 3 compares working conditions broken down by income level and shows that low-income working parents were significantly less likely than middle- and upper-income parents to be able to decide how their job was done ($p = .024$) and what jobs were done ($p = .014$), to have a say in planning their work environment ($p < .001$), and to have a say in

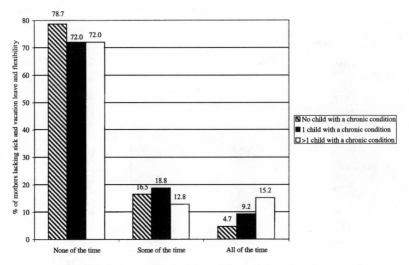

FIGURE 6. Multiple jeopardy: lacking sick and vacation leave and flexibility. This figure is based on analyses the authors conducted using data from the NLSY.

TABLE 3 Decision Latitude at Work: Does It Differ
for Low-Income Parents?

Measure of Decision Latitude	Above 150% of the Poverty Line	At or Below 150% of the Poverty Line	*p* Value
Rarely or never decide how job is done	6.4	11.0	0.024
Rarely or never decide what jobs are done	17.4	25.9	0.014
Rarely or never have a say in planning your work environment	17.9	30.4	<0.001
Rarely or never have a say in decisions about your work	13.0	23.2	0.004

Note: This table is based on analyses the authors conducted with data from the MIDUS.

decisions about their work in general ($p = .004$). One in four working parents whose family income was at or below 150 percent of the poverty threshold did not have a say in general decisions about his or her work or in decisions about what jobs are done. Nearly one in eight did not decide how his or her job is done. Almost one in three did not have a say in planning his or her work environment.

TABLE 4 Working Conditions and Workplace Supports:
Do They Differ for Low-Income Parents?

	Above 150% of the Poverty Line	At or Below 150% of the Poverty Line	*p* Value
Support at the workplace			
Do not receive help and support from co-workers	9.3	13.0	0.008
Do not receive help and support from supervisor	16.6	17.9	0.738
Double jeopardy			
Poor working conditions and no workplace support[a]	4.8	8.9	0.067

Notes: This table is based on analyses the authors conducted with data from the MIDUS.
[a]This category indicates that a person was in the bottom quartile of respondents in terms of decision latitude as well as never or rarely receiving support at the workplace.

Informal Support at the Workplace

Informal support within the workplace assists parents in meeting dual demands of family and employment. Two questions asked in the MIDUS survey are relevant to this issue: "How often do you get help and support from your co-workers?" and similarly, from "your immediate supervisor."

We find that one in six employed parents felt they do not receive support from their immediate supervisor. One in ten report that they do not receive help or support from co-workers. Table 4 summarizes differences in the availability of workplace support across income groups. Employed parents with incomes at or below 150 percent of the poverty level were significantly less likely to get help and support from co-workers ($p = .008$). Almost twice as many low-income working parents as higher-income parents found themselves in the lowest quartile of respondents in terms of both work place support and decision latitude.

Social Supports

Social support from family, friends, and neighbors can serve as a partial substitute for job autonomy and flexibility when parents are seeking to meet work demands at the same time as caring for their children. MIDUS examined the extent to which working parents could rely on family, friends, and neighbors for help. Respondents were first asked to describe the frequency of contact with any member of their family. They were then asked "How much can you rely on them for help if you have a serious problem?" The same series of questions was asked regarding friends and then neighbors.

TABLE 5 Working Conditions and Social Supports:
Do They Differ for Low-Income Parents?

	Above 150% of the Poverty Line	At or Below 150% of the Poverty Line	p Value
Social support outside of work			
Do not feel you can rely on family for help	10.9	19.8	0.005
Do not feel you can rely on a friend for help	19.5	23.6	0.054
Do not feel you can rely on a neighbor for help	13.1	28.9	<0.001
Double jeopardy			
Poor working conditions and no outside support[a]	2.3	7.9	<0.001

Note: This table is based on analyses the authors conducted with data from the MIDUS.
[a]This category indicates that a person was in the bottom quartile of respondents in terms of decision latitude and could not rely on social support as indicated above.

One in five parents did not feel they could rely on friends to help them when a serious problem occurs. One in eight employed parents did not feel they could call on family members in a crisis.

There were no significant differences in the amount of contact that low-income and higher-income working parents had with their neighbors, family members, and friends. However, low-income working parents were significantly more likely to state that they could not rely on a neighbor ($p < .001$) or on family ($p < .001$) for help (see table 5). Twice as many low-income as higher-income working parents stated that they could not rely on family or neighbors for help, perhaps because the friends, family, and neighbors of low-income parents are likely equally overburdened trying to balance working and caring for their families with limited resources. Low-income working parents were also significantly more likely than higher-income parents to lack both decision latitude in the workplace and social supports ($p < .001$). More than three times as many low-income working parents found themselves in the lowest quartile of respondents, in terms of both decision latitude and outside support, as did higher-income parents.

SUMMARY AND POLICY IMPLICATIONS

In this chapter we have explored and documented the work and caretaking challenges facing employed adults at midlife. Using three complementary data sets, we were able to examine the scope and types of responsibilities workers face outside their jobs as well as the full range of supports that would help them manage their dual roles. Concrete benefits such as paid sick and vacation leave that are measured in NLSY can make an obvious and important difference in whether employed caregivers can meet the needs of their families. Equally important are job flexibility and the informal supports in the workplace from co-workers and supervisors, which are asked about in the MIDUS survey. The MIDUS questions on decision latitude and social supports provide us with a measure of the availability of employed adults to care for their families that is not often included or gathered with much depth or accuracy in other surveys.

Analyzing three data sources provided other advantages. The NLSY and NMES surveys are excellent resources because of their large sample size and their oversampling of minority and low-income populations. MIDUS is unique in that it gathered detailed information on autonomy and decision-making in the workplace as well as on social supports from adults across a wide age spectrum, between the ages of 25 and 74.

Prior to this study, there had been little investigation of the caretaking burden of the working poor. The analyses in this chapter show that low-income working parents and those leaving welfare for work have more illness days to cover and are more likely to have a child with a chronic condition than are other working parents. Our analyses also show that poor working parents have greater caretaking responsibilities. These findings are consistent with the small but growing body of research on caretaking that uses samples from outside the United States (Arber and Ginn 1992; Matthews and Campbell 1995; Schofield et al. 1997).

Despite the substantial literature on social supports, there is strikingly little research that focuses on employed caregivers or that examines differences across social class. Research on the availability of workplace benefits is also lacking in these two respects. In this chapter, we examined the availability of supports for employed parents both within and outside the workplace, including paid leave benefits provided by employers, job flexibility, and social support networks. In each area, low-income working parents have fewer resources available to them.

Our analyses show that nearly one-quarter of all employed parents lack paid vacation and paid sick leave the majority of the time they work. Of those who do have leave, many do not have adequate time off. Nearly one-quarter of mothers with paid leave have less than two weeks of paid sick and vacation leave. Low-income working parents and those leaving welfare for work are less likely to have paid leave at their jobs than are other working parents. Seventy-six percent of mothers who returned to work from AFDC lacked sick leave some of the time they worked, and 58 percent lacked sick leave more than half of the time they worked.

The evidence is strong that the universal availability of paid leave makes a difference in addressing children's and family needs. Parents who have paid leave are five times more likely to stay home and care for their sick children (Heymann, Toomey, and Furstenberg 1999). A detailed evaluation of the national Family and Medical Leave Act showed that 64 percent of those who needed leave but did not take it said it was because they could not afford to give up the income (Commission on Family and Medical Leave 1996). Furthermore, women working in Rhode Island—some of whom are eligible for paid leave through a state Temporary Disability Insurance (TDI) program that offers maternity leave with partial wage replacement—are more likely to take leave and take more of it than are women in neighboring states without TDI (Wever 1996).

There is evidence that recent economic restructuring means that good jobs with fringe benefits and promotion opportunities are vanishing from the low-skill job market (Blank 1995, 1996). One approach to increasing the availability of paid leave among low-income parents would be to help the working poor and welfare mothers obtain the education and job skills they need to compete successfully for jobs that offer better benefits. Under the previous set of rules governing the receipt of welfare benefits, individuals could receive benefits while obtaining education and training in the form of basic and secondary education, classes in English as a second language, job skills training, and job readiness training. States could, and some did, count postsecondary education as an acceptable "work activity."

Under the new law, the Personal Responsibility and Work Opportunity Reconciliation Act of 1996, the activities allowed to be counted toward the work requirements generally do not include education and training but only paid work, subsidized work, and unpaid community service. Individuals may participate in education directly related to employment or a GED program only after they are already working twenty hours per week. Given their family responsibilities and the cost of child care, parents living in poverty are likely to find it extremely difficult to increase their educational credentials to a level that would enable them to enhance their employment prospects.

Policy changes not specifically targeted to the poor would also be effective at improving the working conditions of employed parents living in poverty, just as Medicare was effective at ensuring that elderly

Americans have health insurance. One universal approach to parental leave is to expand on the Family and Medical Leave Act (FMLA), the federal policy that addresses the needs of working parents to have time off from work to care for family members. Passed by the U.S. Congress in 1993, the FMLA requires employers to provide up to twelve weeks of unpaid leave to those who have a major illness or whose immediate family members have major illnesses, as well as providing for unpaid leave around the time of the birth or adoption of a child.

As it currently stands, the FMLA leaves many working families unable to meet their children's needs. The stipulations of the FMLA result in only half of all parents being covered. The other half work for firms that do not meet the size requirement, or they have worked too few hours or for too few months. Even among employees who are covered by FMLA, many cannot take advantage of it because it is unpaid and therefore unaffordable. In addition, the FMLA does not address the majority of children's sick care needs—frequent common illnesses and injuries that require care—because it limits medical leave to the care of major illnesses. Altering FMLA so that it covers a larger percentage of workers, provides paid leave or partial wage replacement, and allows coverage of short-term illnesses would assist all families but especially low-income families.

A number of other options exist that might increase the availability of paid leave for parents. State or federal government could provide paid leave through family leave insurance, using a system that parallels disability or unemployment insurance. Tax incentives could be used to encourage employers to provide paid leave for employees who need time to care for their children, in the same way that companies have long been provided with tax incentives for conserving energy. Certainly protecting children's health is as important a public good as protecting our energy reserves.

Our results suggest that changes in the availability of flexibility in the workplace are also needed. A small fraction of public and private employers offer flextime, which allows employees more choice about which hours they work during the day. Although some companies have raised concerns that flextime would disrupt operations, make supervision of employees more difficult, or cause the firm to fail to meet clients' needs, other companies have found that it has led to increased productivity, increased employee satisfaction in the long run, and reduced tardiness and absences (Nollen 1979; Bohen and Viveros-Long 1981; Christensen 1989). Many more companies could offer flexible schedules while still meeting their goals.

These employer-based solutions would go a long way toward improving parents' ability to balance work and family. However, implementation of family-friendly policies is not sufficient if the structures and norms in the workplace and community do not also change. Many community resources and services for working families could be expanded. For example, providing care for children before and after school, and during summer and school vacations, would help parents use less of their time off for predictable demands of children and save it for the unpredictable but inevitable needs such as illness. Meeting the educational needs of children can also be difficult when parent–teacher meetings and conferences are held during the school day. A willingness on the part of teachers and administrators to meet with parents before or after the workday would also assist working parents and their children. Similarly, physicians' offices and clinics might offer evening hours for both sick and well visits so that parents who work during the day do not need to take time off from work to adequately meet their children's health needs.

These community supports are important for all families, but they are critical for the working poor, who are less likely to have the financial resources necessary to arrange and pay for substitute care. Furthermore, their children are in even greater need of the health and educational services that a community can provide because they are at a higher risk for significant health problems as well as for failure to grow and develop at the same rate as their peers who are not living in poverty (Montgomery, Kiely, and Pappas 1996; Bradley et al. 1994; Issler et al. 1996; McGaughey et al. 1991; McLoyd 1990; Starfield 1992; Watson et al. 1996; Wise and Meyers 1988).

Until new employer- and community-based policies are developed to improve parents' ability to balance work and family, parents may be forced to choose to meet the needs of one at the expense of the other. Parents who work at jobs that provide no paid leave or flexibility but who take time off to meet a child's health, developmental, or educational needs at best lose wages and at worst lose their jobs. For families whose income is barely above the poverty level, taking unpaid leave to meet children's health, developmental, or child-care needs and losing wages for multiple weeks during the course of the year can bring them below the poverty line. When parents who lack leave or flexibility choose not to be with their children in order to preserve their job, children's health and developmental needs often go unmet. At present, too many parents are forced to make untenable choices between caring for their children's health and well-being and working to keep a job on which they and their family rely.

ACKNOWLEDGMENTS

This work was made possible by additional funding from the National Institutes of Child Health and Development, the William T. Grant Foundation, and the Canadian Institute for Advanced Research. This work was greatly enriched by the thoughtful comments of members of the MacArthur Foundation Research Network on Successful Midlife Development. We are indebted to Sara Toomey for her assistance with statistical programming and to Lisa Berk, Christine Kerr, and Cara Bergstrom for their invaluable staff assistance.

NOTES

1. While the term *caretaking* sometimes refers to the direct care of impaired adults, in this chapter this term is defined in the broader sense as the provision of direct care of another person. Although this chapter focuses on the care of children by their parents, *caretaking* was used instead of the term *parenting* to highlight that providing direct care for a child is one specific aspect of the general notion of parental responsibilities.

2. In this chapter, the term *welfare* is used to refer to the federal program that provided income support to families living in poverty. Before 1996, this program was called Aid to Families with Dependent Children (AFDC). Currently, this program is called Temporary Assistance to Needy Families.

REFERENCES

Anderson, B. J., J. P. Miller, W. F. Auslander, and J. V. Santiago. 1981. Family characteristics of diabetic adolescents: Relationship to metabolic control. *Diabetes Care* 4 (6):586–94.

Andresen, E. M., and R. C. Brownson. 2000. Disability and health status: Ethnic differences among women in the United States. *Journal of Epidemiology and Community Health* 543:200–206.

Andress, H., G. Lipsmeier, and K. Salentin. 1995. Social isolation and lack of social support in the lower classes? Comparative analyses of survey data. *Zeitschrift fur Soziologie* 244:300–315.

Arber, S., and J. Ginn. 1992. Class and caring: A forgotten dimension. *Sociology* 264:619–34.

Aron, L. Y., P. J. Loprest, and C. E. Steuerle. 1996. *Serving children with disabilities: A systematic look at the programs.* Washington, D.C.: Urban Institute Press.

Belle, D. 1982. The impact of poverty on social networks and supports. *Marriage and Family Review* 54:89–103.

Benson, C. S., E. A. Medrich, and S. Buckley. 1980. A new view of school efficiency: Household time contributions to school achievement. In *School finance policies and practices: The 1980's, a decade of conflict,* ed. J. Guthrie. Cambridge, Mass.: Ballinger Publishers.

Biller, H. B. 1993. *Fathers and families: Paternal factors in child development.* Westport, Conn.: Auburn House.

Blank, R. 1995. Outlook for the U.S. labor market and prospects for low-wage entry jobs. In *The work alternative: Welfare reform and the realities in the job market*, ed. D. Nightingale and R. Haveman. Washington, D.C.: Urban Institute Press.

———. 1996. *It takes a nation: A new agenda for fighting poverty*. Princeton, N.J.: Russell Sage Foundation.

Bohen, H., and A. Viveros-Long. 1981. *Balancing jobs and family life: Do flexible schedules help?* Philadelphia: Temple University Press.

Bowlby, J. 1953. *Child care and the growth of love*. Baltimore: Penguin Books.

Bradley, R. H., L. Whiteside, D. J. Mundfrom, P. H. Casey, K. J. Kelleher, and S. Pope. 1994. Early indications of resilience and their relations to experiences in the home environments of low birthweight, premature children living in poverty. *Child Development* 652:346–60.

Carlton-Ford, S., R. Miller, M. Brown, N. Nealeigh, and P. Jennings. 1995. Epilepsy and children's social and psychological adjustment. *Journal of Health and Social Behavior* 363:285–301.

Caspi, A., T. Moffit, B. Wright, and P. Silva. 1998. Early failure in the labor market: Childhood and adolescent predictors of unemployment in the transition to adulthood. *American Sociological Review* 633:424–51.

Center for Human Resource Research. 1990. *National Longitudinal Survey of Labor Force Behavior: Child Supplement 1986–1990*. Columbus: Ohio State University.

———. 1995. *National Longitudinal Survey of Labor Force Behavior. 1995 users' guide*. Columbus: Ohio State University.

Christensen, K. 1989. *Flexible scheduling and staffing*. Conference board research bulletin 240. New York: Conference Board.

Cleary, J., O. P. Gray, D. J. Hall, P. H. Rowlandson, C. P. Sainsbury, and M. M. Davies. 1986. Parental involvement in the lives of children in hospital. *Archives of Disease in Childhood* 618:779–87.

Coleman, J. S. 1998. Social capital in the creation of human capital. *American Journal of Sociology* 94:S95–S120.

Commission on Family and Medical Leave. 1996. *A workable balance: Report to congress on family and medical leave policies*. Washington, D.C.: Department of Labor.

D'Arcy, C. 1998. Social distribution of health among Canadians. In *Health and Canadian society: Sociological perspectives*, 3d ed., ed. D. Coburn, C. D'Arcy, and G. M. Torrance. Ontario: University of Toronto Press.

Dewa, C. S., and E. Lin. 2000. Chronic physical illness, psychiatric disorder and disability in the workplace. *Social Science and Medicine* 511:41–50.

Duncan, G. J. 1988. The volatility of family income over the life-course. In *Life-span development and behavior*, vol. 9, ed. P. Baltes, D. Featherman, and R. M. Lerner. Hillsdale, N.J.: Lawrence Erlbaum Associates.

Duncan, G. J., J. Brooks-Gunn, W. J. Yeung, and J. Smith. 1998. How much does childhood poverty affect the life chances of children? *American Sociological Review* 633:406–23.

Edin, K., and L. Lein. 1996. *Making ends meet: How single mothers survive welfare and low-wage work*. New York: Russell Sage Foundation Press.

Gauderer, M. W., J. L. Lorig, and D. W. Eastwood. 1989. Is there a place for parents in the operating room? *Journal of Pediatric Surgery* 247:705–6.

George, A., and J. Hancock. 1993. Reducing pediatric burn pain with parent participation. *Journal of Burn Care and Rehabilitation* 141:104–7.

Hamlett, K. W., D. S. Pellegrini, and K. S. Katz. 1992. Childhood chronic illness as a family stressor. *Journal of Pediatric Psychology* 171:33–47.

Hannallah, R. S., and J. K. Rosales. 1983. Experience with parents' presence during anesthesia induction in children. *Canadian Anaesthetists Society Journal* 303, pt. 1:286–89.

Hanson, C. L., M. J. DeGuire, A. M. Schinkel, S. W. Henggeler, and G. A. Burghen. 1992. Comparing social learning and family systems correlates of adaptation in youths with IDDM. *Journal of Pediatric Psychology* 175:555–72.

Hauser, S. T., A. M. Jacobson, P. Lavori, J. I. Wolfsdorf, R. D. Herskowitz, J. E. Milley, R. Bliss, D. Wertlieb, and J. Stein. 1990. Adherence among children and adolescents with insulin-dependent diabetes mellitus over a four-year longitudinal follow-up. 2. Immediate and long-term linkages with the family milieu. *Journal of Pediatric Psychology* 154:527–42.

Haveman, R., B. Wolfe, and J. Spaulding. 1991. Childhood events and circumstances influencing high school completion. *Demography* 281:133–57.

Heymann, S. J. 2000. *The widening gap: Why America's working families are in jeopardy and what can be done about it.* New York: Basic Books.

Heymann, S. J., and A. Earle. 1997. Working conditions faced by poor families and the care of children. *Focus* 191:56–58.

———. 1998. The work family balance: What hurdles are parents leaving welfare likely to confront? *Journal of Policy Analysis and Management* 172:312–21.

———. 1999. The impact of welfare reform on parents' ability to care for their children's health. *American Journal of Public Health* 894:502–5.

———. 2000. Low-income parents: How do working conditions affect their opportunity to help school-age children at risk? *American Educational Research Journal* 374:833–48.

Heymann, S. J., A. Earle, and B. Egleston. 1996. Parental availability for the care of sick children. *Pediatrics* 982:226–30.

Heymann, S. J., S. Toomey, and F. Furstenberg. 1999. Working parents: What factors are involved in their ability to take time off from work when their children are sick? *Archives of Pediatrics and Adolescent Medicine* 1538:870–74.

Hill, M., and J. Sandfort. 1995. Effects of childhood poverty on productivity later in life: Implications for public policy. *Children and Youth Services Review* 171–72:91–126.

Holden, E. W., D. Chimielewski, C. C. Nelson, V. A. Kager, and L. Foltz. 1997. Controlling for general and disease-specific effects in child and family adjustment to chronic childhood illness. *Journal of Pediatric Psychology* 221:15–27.

Issler, R. M. S., E. R. R. J. Giugliani, G. T. Kreutz, C. F. Meneses, E. B. Justo, V. M. Kreutz, and M. Pires. 1996. Poverty levels and children's health status: Study of risk factors in an urban population of low socioeconomic level. *Revista Saude Publica* 306:506–11.

Johnson, K. 1994. Children with special health needs: Ensuring appropriate coverage and care under health care reform. *Health Policy and Child Health* 13:1–5.

Kristensson-Hallstron, I., G. Elander, and G. Malmfors. 1997. Increased parental participation on a pediatric surgical daycare unit. *Journal of Clinical Nursing* 64:297–302.

LaGreca, A. M., W. F. Auslander, P. Greco, D. Spetter, E. B. Fisher, and J. V. Santiago. 1995. I get by with a little help from my family and friends: Adolescents' support for diabetes care. *Journal of Pediatric Psychology* 204:449–76.

LaRosa-Nash, P. A., and J. M. Murphy. 1997. An approach to pediatric perioperative care: Parent-present induction. *Nursing Clinics of North America* 321:183–99.

Lindblad-Goldberg, M., and J. Dukes. 1985. Social support in black, low-income, single-parent families: Normative and dysfunctional patterns. *American Journal of Orthopsychology* 551:42–58.

Long, T. J., and L. Long. 1984. Latchkey children. In *Current topics in early education,* vol. 5, ed. L. G. Katz. Norwood, N.J.: Ablex Publishing.

McGaughey, P., B. Starfield, C. Alexander, and M. Ensminger. 1991. The social environment and vulnerability of low birth weight children: A social-epidemiological perspective. *Pediatrics* 885:943–53.

McGraw, T. 1994. Preparing children for the operating room: Psychological issues. *Canadian Journal of Anaesthesia* 4111:1094–1103.

McLeod, J., and M. Shanahan. 1996. Trajectories of poverty and children's mental health. *Journal of Health and Social Behavior* 373:207–20.

McLoyd, V. 1990. The impact of economic hardship on black families and children: Psychological distress, parenting and socioemotional development. *Child Development* 612:311–46.

Matthews, A. M., and L. D. Campbell. 1995. Gender roles, employment, and informal care. In *Connecting gender and ageing: A sociological approach,* ed. S. Arber and J. Ginn. Buckingham, U.K.: Open University Press.

Montgomery, L. E., J. L. Kiely, and G. Pappas. 1996. The effects of poverty, race and family structure on U.S. children's health: Data from the NHIS 1978–1980 and 1989–1991. *American Journal of Public Health* 8610:1401–5.

Muhaffy, P. 1965. The effects of hospitalization on children admitted for tonsillectomy and adenoidectomy. *Nursing Research* 141:12–19.

Newacheck, P. W., B. Strickland, J. P. Shonkoff, J. M. Perrin, M. McPherson, M. McManus, C. Lauver, H. Fox, and P. Arango. 1998. An epidemiologic profile of children with special health care needs. *Pediatrics* 1021:117–23.

Nollen, S. D. 1979. Does flextime improve productivity? *Harvard Business Review* 57 (September–October): 12–22.

Palmer, S. J. 1993. Care of sick children by parents: A meaningful role. *Journal of Advanced Nursing* 182:185–91.

Parcel, T. L., and E. G. Menaghan. 1990. Maternal working conditions and children's verbal facility: Studying the intergenerational transmission of inequality from mothers to young children. *Social Psychology Quarterly* 532:132–47.

———. 1994. *Parents' jobs and children's lives.* New York: Aldine de Gruyter.

Radin, N., and G. Russell. 1983. Increased father participation and child development outcomes. In *Fatherhood and family policy,* ed. M. Lamb and A. Saji. Hillsdale, N.J.: Lawrence Erlbaum Associates.

Reynolds, J. R., and C. E. Ross. 1998. Social stratification and health: Education's benefit beyond economic status and social origins. *Social Problems* 452:221–47.

Robertson, J. 1958. *Young children in hospital.* New York: Basic Books.

Rossi, A. S. 1984. Gender and parenthood. *American Sociological Review* 491:1–19.

Rutledge, E. M., S. B. Eve, and T. A. Doering. 1988. Use of health care services by older blacks and whites: Implications for health care policy. Association paper. Society for the Study of Social Problems, University of Tennessee, Knoxville.

Sainsbury, C. P. Q., O. P. Gray, J. Cleary, M. M. Davies, and P. H. Rowlandson. 1986. Care by parents of their children in hospital. *Archives of Disease in Childhood* 616:612–15.

Schofield, H. L., H. E. Herrman, S. Bloch, A. Howe, and B. Singh. 1997. A profile of Australian family caregivers: Diversity of roles and circumstances. *Australian and New Zealand Journal of Public Health* 211:59–66.

Starfield, B. 1992. Effects of poverty on health status. *Bulletin of the New York Academy of Medicine* 681:17–24.

Taylor, M. R. H., and P. O'Connor. 1989. Resident parents and shorter hospital stay. *Archives of Disease in Childhood* 642:274–76.

U.S. Congress. 1996. Personal Responsibility and Work Opportunity Reconciliation Act. 104th Congr., 2d sess. Public Law No. 104–193.

U.S. Department of Labor, Bureau of Labor Statistics. 1997. *Employee benefits in medium and large private establishments 1997.* Retrieved on November 17, 2000, from http://stats.bls.gov:80/news.release/ebs3.t01.htm].

Van der Schyff, G. 1979. The role of parents during their child's hospitalization. *Australian Nursing Journal* 811:57–61.

Watson, J. E., R. S. Kirby, K. J. Kelleher, and R. H. Bradley. 1996. Effects of poverty on home environment: An analysis of three-year outcome data for low-birth weight premature infants. *Journal of Pediatric Psychology* 213:419–31.

Waugh, T. A., and D. L. Kjos. 1992. Parental involvement and the effectiveness of an adolescent day treatment program. *Journal of Youth and Adolescence* 214:487–97.

Wever, K. S. 1996. *The Family and Medical Leave Act.* Changing Work in America series. Radcliffe Public Policy Institute, Radcliffe College, Cambridge.

Wijnberg, M. H., and S. Weinger. 1998. When dreams wither and resources fail: The social-support systems of poor single mothers. *Families in Society* 79 (2): 212–19.

Wise, P. H., and A. Meyers. 1988. Poverty and child health. *Pediatric Clinics of North America* 35 (6): 1169–86.

Wolman, C., M. D. Resnick, L. J. Harris, and R. W. Blum. 1994. Emotional well-being among adolescents with and without chronic conditions. *Adolescent Medicine* 15 (3): 199–204.

Woods, M. B. 1972. The unsupervised child of the working mother. *Developmental Psychology* 6:4–25.

CHAPTER EIGHTEEN

Family Roles and Well-Being during the Middle Life Course

Nadine F. Marks, Larry L. Bumpass, and Heyjung Jun

As we embark on the early years of a new millennium, considerable consternation and debate about what is happening to the family as a social institution in the United States and elsewhere continue (Waite 2000). During the twentieth century, family demography charted historic changes in rates of mortality, marriage, fertility, divorce, remarriage, and household composition (Bumpass 1990). Today both men and women live significantly longer than they did in 1900, a smaller proportion of the adult life course is spent married, a higher proportion of adults cohabit before marriage or in lieu of marriage, a higher proportion of marriages end in divorce, fewer remarriages follow a divorce, fewer children are born to each woman, a higher proportion of the population lives in single-person households, and a higher proportion of adults have parents who live beyond the age of 65 (and thus are at risk of dependency on their adult children because of their own frailty and/or chronic illness) (Bumpass 1990; Bumpass and Sweet 1989a, 1989b; Bumpass, Sweet, and Castro-Martin 1989; Castro-Martin and Bumpass 1989; Cherlin 1992; Glick 1988; Schoen et al. 1985; Schoen and Weinick 1993; Watkins, Menken, and Bongaarts 1987). All of these changes have led some scholars to proclaim the decline if not the demise of the traditional family (Popenoe 1988, 1993; Skolnick 1991). Others have suggested that although, indeed, the American family is changing, this dynamism is nothing new; rather, it is a continuation of long-term trends and patterns (Bane 1976). Families in twenty-first-century America are increasingly diverse in structure and process, yet they still constitute a resilient social institution that continues to provide an important emotional and economic foundation for the life course of adults as well as children (Stacey 1990, 1993; Waite 2000).

Life experience within family roles, including the partner role, the parent role, and the adult child role vis-à-vis aging parents, has been previously documented to be a significant determinant of the well-being of men and women (Ross, Mirowsky, and Goldsteen 1990). Yet the dynamism of family change currently in process has considerably altered expectations for these family roles and family-role enactments. A life-course structural symbolic interactionist theoretical perspective (Stryker and Statham 1985; Wells and Stryker 1988) would predict that such changes in role meaning and role expectations could lead to changing consequences of occupying these roles for adult well-being. For example, marital partners are now struggling with changed and sometimes conflicting expectations about women's and men's responsibilities for marital emotional and instrumental support (Goldscheider and Waite 1991). Divorce is a more normative potential outcome for contemporary marriage cohorts if marital expectations are not met. Many marriages are remarriages, where one or both partners come to the institution with a history of disenchantment or, at least, disappointment (Cherlin 1992). Cohabitation has grown from a rare and deviant behavior to the majority experience among cohorts of marriageable age (Bumpass and Lu 2000; Bumpass and Sweet 1989b).

Parenthood is no longer necessarily a role shared with a single partner across the life course (Bumpass and Sweet 1989a; Cherlin 1992). Research on intergenerational relations has documented the continuing emotional and instrumental ties that characterize parenting for children aged 19 and older, as well as for children aged 18 and younger (Hogan, Eggebeen, and Clogg 1993; Rossi and Rossi 1990; Marks 1995). Parenthood responsibilities are more often shared by fathers and mothers, and caring for children is more often juggled with work and other caregiving responsibilities by contemporary women and men (Marks 1996c).

Experience in the adult child role vis-à-vis aging parents has been less well studied—possibly a holdover from the extended period in family studies when structural functionalism was the dominant theoretical paradigm, emphasizing the relative isolation of the elderly from their grown children (Parsons 1942). One exception is the growing literature on caregiving to aging parents (e.g., Brody 1990; Stone, Cafferata, and Sangl 1987; Marks 1996a, 1998). However, again, as families become more vertical (i.e., more typically comprised of persons from three or more generations) and less horizontal (i.e., more typically comprised of fewer persons from the same generation, such as siblings and cousins) in structure, continuing relations and interdependency across generations become even more common (Rossi and Rossi 1990; Hogan, Eggebeen, and Clogg 1993; Cooney and Uhlenberg 1992). Across the middle adult years, men and women are more and more likely to have living parents who may provide them with varying degrees of emotional, instrumental, and financial support and/or whom they watch gradually, or sometimes suddenly, decline in health and possibly become more dependent on them (Rossi and Rossi 1990; Watkins, Mencken, and Bongaarts 1987).

In this chapter we use data from the primary respondent sample ($N = 3032$; 1318 men, 1714 women) of the 1995 National Survey of Midlife in the United States (MIDUS) (see chap. 1 of this volume for more design details) to describe how the distribution of the adult population occupying marital/partner, parenthood, and adult child (in relationship to older parents' health and mortality) roles varies across ages 25–74 for contemporary men and women in the United States. Additionally, we examine how marital status, parental status, and adult child status are currently associated with physical, mental, and social well-being, and whether these associations differ across gender and age groups (young adults, ages 25–39, representing birth cohorts from 1956 to 1970; midlife adults, ages 40–59, representing birth cohorts from 1936 to 1955; and older adults, ages 60–74, representing birth cohorts from 1920 to 1935). The MIDUS data offer a particularly rich resource for the investigation of these issues because the survey's development by an interdisciplinary team resulted in the inclusion of expansive and innovative measurements of health, psychological, and social constructs for a large representative sample of American adults across a wide adult age span. Sampling weights that correct for selection probabilities and nonresponse allow this sample to match the composition of the U.S. population on age, sex, race, and education.

Marital/Partnership Status during the Middle Life Course

Although in general there has been a major upheaval in the stability of marriage, most Americans continue to develop partnerships during the middle adult years. Marriage now, compared with that of fifty years ago, is occurring at older ages for both women and men (Schoen et al. 1985; Schoen and Weinick 1993). Ever more typically, contemporary marriages occur after a period of cohabitation (Bumpass and Sweet 1989b; Bumpass and Lu 2000). Although a high proportion of marriages occurred before age 25 for older cohorts, younger cohorts are increasingly waiting until after age 25 to marry. Additionally, across the middle life course, many adults are married more than once (Schoen et al. 1985; Schoen and Weinick 1993).

Table 1 describes the distribution of number of marriages reported across the sample of MIDUS respondents aged 25–74 in 1995 (weighted distribution estimates here and in other descriptive tables are provided to estimate U.S. population distributions). Overall, only about one in ten women and one in eight men reported having never been married when

TABLE 1 Weighted Percentage Distribution (unweighted *n*) of the Number of
Times Married, U.S. Adults Aged 25–74

Number of Marriages	Total Sample		Women		Men	
	Unweighted N	Weighted %	Unweighted N	Weighted %	Unweighted N	Weighted %
0	351	11.5	163	10.9	188	12.4
1	1980	65.8	1030	66.1	950	65.4
2	557	18.3	292	18.8	265	17.8
3	117	3.7	63	3.7	54	3.7
4	23	.6	11	.5	12	.7
5	3	.1	2	.1	1	.1
TOTAL	3031	100.0	1561	100.0	1470	100.0

Source: National Survey of Midlife Development in the United States (MIDUS).
Note: Percentage columns do not always total 100.0 due to rounding error.

we considered the entire population at these ages. About two-thirds of
the population in this age range have been married only once. A little
over one in five adults these ages report two or more marriages.

A further examination of current marital status by age provided in table 2 indicates that although a little more than one in five women at young
adult ages 25–39 have never been married (5.8 percent cohabiting and
14.7 percent noncohabiting) and just under one in four young adult men
has never been married (7.1 percent cohabiting and 15.7 percent noncohabiting), by midlife ages 40–59, only about one in twenty American
women and men have not tried marriage at least once. For all the rhetoric
about a "retreat from marriage," Americans remain a "marrying people,"
much more so than some Western Europeans (Popenoe 1988).

Considered in cross-sectional, one-point-in-time perspective, we find
that about half of young and midlife adult men and women are in first
marriages. At young adult ages, another one in ten men and women
are in second or higher-order marriages. By the midlife years, for those
members of birth cohorts who have moved through young adulthood
during a period of relatively high divorce rates, a full one in five women
and one in four men are remarried. By contrast, for members of the
older adult age group, representing somewhat older birth cohorts that
historically experienced lower divorce rates during the young adult ages
when divorce is most likely, only about one in eight women and one in
five men are remarried.

Cohabitation has become a much more common type of union in the
last few decades (Bumpass and Sweet 1989b). About one in ten young

TABLE 2 Weighted Percentage Distribution

| | Young Adults Aged 25–39 | | | |
| | Women | | Men | |
Marital Status	Unwgtd *n*	Wgtd %	Unwgtd *n*	Wgtd %
First marriage	244	50.6	258	55.1
Remarried	52	11.2	45	10.7
Sep/div–cohabiting	22	5.6	9	2.3
Widow–cohabiting	0	.0	0	.0
Never married–cohabiting	24	5.8	34	7.1
Sep/div–not cohabiting	76	11.7	49	8.9
Widow–not cohabiting	2	.3	1	.3
Never married–not cohabiting	89	14.7	94	15.7
TOTAL	509	100.0	490	100.0

Source: MIDUS.
Note: Percentage columns do not always total 100.0 due to rounding error.

adult MIDUS respondents reported living in a cohabiting, marriage-like union. By midlife these rates had reduced by half to about one in twenty for both men and women. Cohabitation was seldom reported by older adults.

At young adult ages, 17.3 percent of women (5.6 percent cohabiting, 11.7 percent noncohabiting) reported being separated or divorced. At midlife for these birth cohorts, separated and divorced rates had risen to include almost one in four women (3 percent cohabiting, 20.2 percent noncohabiting). By older ages for these birth cohorts, about one in ten women reported being separated or divorced (almost exclusively noncohabiting).

Men's rates of reporting separated or divorced status are somewhat lower than women's rates due mainly to their propensity to remarry more quickly if divorced (Schoen and Weinick 1993). For example, in the MIDUS sample, about 11.2 percent of young adult men report being separated or divorced (2.3 percent cohabiting, 8.9 percent noncohabiting). At midlife ages about 15.5 percent of men were separated or divorced (3.6 percent cohabiting, 11.9 percent noncohabiting). At older ages about 7.6 percent of older men reported being separated or divorced (almost exclusively noncohabiting).

The prevalence of widowhood at young adult ages is extremely low.[1] At midlife the rates begin to increase for women (4.4 percent) but not for of Marital Status, by Age and Gender

Midlife Adults Aged 40–59				Older Adults Aged 60–74			
Women		Men		Women		Men	
Unwgtd n	Wgtd %	Unwgtd n	Wgtd %	Unwgtd n	Wgtd %	Unwgtd n	Wgtd %
301	47.1	354	53.5	135	48.9	171	62.4
118	20.0	153	24.6	36	12.9	56	19.1
17	3.0	20	3.6	2	.5	1	.7
0	.0	3	.4	1	.1	1	.3
2	.4	7	1.0	1	.7	0	.0
187	20.2	100	11.9	45	10.0	25	6.9
38	4.4	7	.6	104	25.4	20	5.3
37	5.0	38	4.5	10	1.5	14	5.3
700	100.0	682	100.0	334	100.0	288	100.0

men; at older adult ages about one in four women is a widow and about one in twenty men is a widower.

MARITAL/PARTNERSHIP STATUS AND WELL-BEING

Marital status and its association with well-being have been an important topic of study in the family studies literature. Historically, being married has been associated with better mental health than being unmarried (e.g., Booth and Amato 1991; Glenn 1975; Gove, Hughes, and Style 1983; Gove, Style, and Hughes 1990; Menaghan and Lieberman 1986; Pearlin and Johnson 1977). However, as marriage has become more delayed, cohabitation more common, divorce more common, and a period of single living more typical and acceptable for young adults, there has been some speculation and even some evidence that marriage per se may have become less important for adult happiness (e.g., Glenn and Weaver 1988; Lee, Seccombe, and Shehan 1991). Overall, however, population research continues to suggest that marriage is associated with less psychological distress for both men and women (e.g., Marks 1996b; Marks and Lambert 1998).

Previous research on marriage and well-being often has been limited, however, in that (1) it has seldom included important contemporary categories reflecting the full range of marital/partnership status, such as remarried and cohabitor, to contrast with first-marriage status (Ross 1995); (2) it has seldom examined age differences in the importance of marriage

519

for well-being (e.g., young adult versus midlife adult versus older adult differences in the influence of marriage on well-being); and (3) it has often been limited to studying only depression and/or life satisfaction, and sometimes health, as outcomes.

To address these gaps, we used the MIDUS data to examine how marital/partner status might be related to four dimensions of well-being: negative affect (dysphoria), positive psychological wellness, global self-assessed health, and generativity. Examining this range of psychological, physical, and social well-being is congruent with the multidimensional approach to considering positive human health that was first suggested by the World Health Organization in 1946 (i.e., health defined as not just the "absence of disease" but as "a state of complete physical, mental, and social-well-being"). A similar expansive conceptualization of health was further developed by the MIDMAC Network, which chose to focus on physical health, mental health, and social responsibility as three key criteria for defining successful midlife development. Examining dysphoria allows us to examine an indicator of negative affect or psychological dysfunction—the most typically studied aspect of mental health, thereby building on and replicating previous work. Negative affect, or dysphoria, was operationalized with a six-item, highly reliable scale ($\alpha = .87$) developed for MIDUS (see Mroczek and Kolarz 1998 for additional details on reliability and validity). Respondents were queried: "During the past 30 days, how much of the time did you feel (1) so sad nothing could cheer you up? (2) nervous? (3) restless or fidgety? (4) hopeless? (5) that everything was an effort? (6) worthless?" Response categories ranged from 1, "none of the time," to 5, "all of the time." (See the appendix for descriptives for all variables used in the analyses.)

Positive psychological wellness is much less typically studied, yet it represents an important related, but distinct, domain of mental health (Ryff 1989; Ryff and Keyes 1995). Much previous work studying more positive psychological well-being has focused singularly on either happiness or life satisfaction. However, attention to these outcomes has arisen from a largely atheoretical basis. Addressing this gap in studying psychological wellness among adults, Ryff and her colleagues have used adult development theories to guide the development and validation of six new psychological wellness scales. Three-item versions of these scales were included in the MIDUS. For this investigation we created a psychological wellness index ($\alpha = .81$) by summing across the eighteen Ryff items that assessed autonomy (e.g., "I have confidence in my own opinions, even if they are different from the way most other people think"), environmental mastery (e.g., "I am good at managing the responsibilities of daily life"), positive relations with others (e.g., "People would describe me as a giving person, willing to share my time with others"), self-acceptance (e.g., "When I look at the story of my life, I am pleased with how things have turned out so far"), purpose in life (e.g., "Some people wander aimlessly through life, but I am not one of them"), and personal growth (e.g., "For me, life has been a continuous process of learning, changing, and growth") (for more details on reliability and validity, see Ryff 1989; Ryff and Keyes 1995).

Global physical health was measured using a standard one-item self-report: "In general, would you say your physical health is poor (1), fair (2), good (3), very good (4), or excellent (5)?" This one item has been shown to have high predictive validity for future mortality and morbidity in a wide range of studies (Idler and Benyamini 1997).

The most atypical well-being outcome we considered is a measure of social well-being: generativity. Erikson's (1950) developmental theory suggests that during middle adulthood, the most important developmental task is to engage in activity that extends benefit beyond the self and supports the growth and development of others. This often includes support offered to one's own children, but it is conceptually and operationally by no means limited to this. In the context of family roles, we might expect that individuals have a rich opportunity to realize gains in this area of personal development; however, generativity has seldom been previously examined in research on family roles and well-being (McAdams and de St. Aubin 1992, 1998).

The measure of generativity we used from the MIDUS was adapted from the McAdams generativity scale (McAdams and de St. Aubin 1992) by Alice Rossi (see also Rossi, chap. 19, in this volume). This summed index, which includes six items, asks respondents, "To what extent does each of the following statements describe you? (1) Others would say that you have made unique contributions to society. (2) You have important skills you can pass along to others. (3) Many people come to you for advice. (4) You feel that other people need you. (5) You have had a good influence on the lives of many people. (6) You like to teach things to people." Response categories, ranging 1–4, were defined as "not at all," "a little," "some," and "a lot" ($\alpha = .84$).

Because our aim was to examine gender differences as well as age differences in the influence of marital status on well-being, we undertook our analyses in two steps: the first step included an evaluation of gender differences, and the second step examined age differences. Specifically, in the first step for the marital-status analyses, to investigate gender differences we estimated models for men and women together, regressing each of the four outcome variables on variables for the following: gender (female = 1); age (coded categorically: age1 = 25–39 years, age3 = 60–74 years, contrasted with age2 = 40–59 years); marital status (coded categorically: remarried, cohabiting [any type], formerly married [separated, divorced, widowed, but not cohabiting], never married [not cohabiting], contrasted with first marriage); gender × marital-status interaction variables; and demographic control variables for race/ethnicity (dichotomous, black = 1); employment status (dichotomous, employed = 1); education (coded categorically and then used as a continuous measure: 1 = less than high school, 2 = high school graduate or GED, 3 = some college, and 4 = college graduate or more); household income (summed across respondent and spouse and coded continuously in thousands of dollars); parental status (dichotomous, 1 = has child); and adult child status (dichotomous, 1 = both parents alive and healthy).

Although it might have been preferable to examine the marital role, parental role, and adult child role concurrently, we were not able to do this, due to cell-size limitations, and still allow for the degree of differentiation in categories for each of these roles that we wished to investigate. Therefore, we undertook a separate analysis for each of these roles, and in each analysis, we controlled for the other two family roles in a simplified way. Specifically, in the marital-role analysis, we controlled for parental status and adult child status with dichotomous variables as just noted. For the parental-role analysis, we controlled for marital status with a dichotomous variable (first married = 1) and adult child status with a dichotomous variable. Likewise, in the adult-child-role analysis, we controlled for marital status and parental status with dichotomous variables.

In a second step of our marital-status analytic sequence, to further examine age differences, we created as many viable contrasts (i.e., age × marital-status interaction variables) as we could based on the population distribution of marital status (see table 2) and examined these contrasts in separate models for men and women. Specifically, we were able to create categories to contrast remarried young adults and remarried older adults with remarried midlife adults, and formerly married young adults and formerly married older adults with formerly married midlife adults. However, because so very few cohabitors exist at older ages, we created only a contrast of young cohabitors with predominantly midlife (plus a few older) cohabitors; and because so few never-married adults exist at older ages, we created only a contrast of young never-married adults with predominantly midlife (plus a few older) never-married adults.

All models were estimated both with and without population weighting. The overall patterns of results for both weighted and un-weighted models were similar; therefore, unweighted results are reported (Winship and Radbill 1994).

Table 3 provides the results of our analyses of the effects of marital status on well-being. (Fig. 1 graphically illustrates predicted well-being scores for population subgroups based on the estimates from models reported in table 3.)

Gender Differences

In our preliminary models (first step of analyses) examining men and women together (results not shown in full but denoted on table 3 with superscripts), we found trend-level evidence of two gender differences. In the models estimated for both psychological wellness and generativity, it appeared that never-married men were reporting less positive psychological wellness and generativity than never-married women, when they were both compared with their first-married peers.

Age Differences

To better view these potential gender differences and also to more easily consider age-group differences, we proceeded to estimate a second model for men and women separately by adding the age interaction variables. The resulting estimates from these models displayed in table 3 suggest that noncohabiting formerly married (separated, divorced, or widowed) women and men clearly reported more negative affect than did those in a first marriage (the omitted contrast category). There was also suggestive evidence (trend-level effect) that remarried men might experience more negative affect than first-married men (the omitted contrast category).

One robust age-group difference was also in evidence for both women and men but working in opposite directions: younger never-married women reported significantly more dysphoria than did midlife never-married women (the omitted contrast category); however, younger never-married women reported less dysphoria than did midlife never-married men.

When we considered positive psychological wellness, our results from the analyses of women and men separately suggested that age has an

TABLE 3 Unstandardized Regression Coefficients for

	Dysphoria		Psychological Wellness (Ryff)	
Predictors	Women	Men	Women	Men
First marriage (omitted)	—	—	—	—
Remarried	.56	.63[+]	1.97	−1.06
Cohabiting	.36	.61	2.53	−2.54
Formerly married	.75*	1.05**	−.36	−2.91*
Never married	−.91	1.87**	−2.47[a]	−7.14***[a]
Age1 (25–39 yrs)	−.14	.98**	1.99[+]	.45
Age2 (40–59 yrs) (omitted)	—	—	—	—
Age3 (60–74 yrs)	−1.25**	−1.32***	.91	3.65***
Age1 × remarried	.60	−.30	−5.35**	.51
Age3 × remarried	−1.02	.35	−2.42	−2.43
Age1 × cohabiting	−.02	−.08	−5.99*	2.38
Age1 × formerly married	.98	−.93	−5.61**	.03
Age3 × formerly married	−.41	.28	1.28	−1.30
Age1 × never married	1.84*	−2.01**	−1.95	4.66*
Constant	12.17***	9.93***	54.14***	57.84***
R^2	.06	.07	.09	.08

Source: MIDUS.

Note: All models also included controls for race/ethnicity, employment status, education, household income, parental status, and adult child status. Analyses used unweighted data.

[a]Model estimated with men and women together revealed a trend-level gender difference ($p \leq .10$).

[+]$p \leq .10$. *$p \leq .05$. **$p \leq .01$. ***$p \leq .001$ (two-tailed test).

important moderating effect on the influence of marriage on women's wellness. Younger remarried women, younger cohabiting women, and younger formerly married women all reported significantly less psychological wellness than did their marital-status counterparts at midlife ages. Among men, in a pattern similar to that found for dysphoria, we found formerly married and never-married men doing more poorly than first-married men, although the negative effect for younger never-married men was significantly less than for midlife never-married men.

We found only limited evidence that marital-status differences were associated with physical health differences in this sample. In our model estimated for men, we found remarried men overall reported poorer health than first-married men (although fig. 1 indicates this global effect is mainly driven by the relatively poorer health of midlife remarried men). There were no significant marital-status differences in health for women, and no significant age-group differences for either men or women.

In terms of generativity, in the separate analyses for women and men, an interesting age pattern for remarried women came into evidence. A trend-level age interaction effect suggested that remarried midlife women the Effects of Marital Status on Well-Being, by Gender

Self-Assessed Global Health		Generativity	
Women	Men	Women	Men
—	—		
.03	−.21*	1.11**	.07
−.03	.07	.21	.98
−.07	−.16	.66+	.33
.03	−.05	.38[a]	−1.24[+a]
.16+	.05	.05	−.82*
—	—	—	—
−.01	.04	.29	.07
−.16	.27	−1.35+	.46
−.04	.15	−1.46	−.12
−.31	−.13	−.56	.23
−.19	.16	−.27	−.80
.16	.21	−.72	.88
−.19	.09	−.24	1.75*
2.50***	2.47***	13.59***	14.75***
.13	.14	.09	.06

may experience more generativity than remarried young adult women. There was also trend-level evidence that formerly married midlife women were reporting somewhat more feelings of generativity than first-married midlife women. Among men, again, never-married status (in contrast to first-married status) at midlife ages was associated with a trend toward reporting less generativity, but the young adult never-married men reported significantly more generativity than the midlife never-married men did.

Conclusions

Overall, these results suggest several broad conclusions. First, being in a first marriage is associated with less negative affect than being formerly married at all adult ages. This replicates a relatively consistent finding in the marital-status and mental health literature.

Second, there are few robust gender differences in the association between marital status and well-being. The issue of whether and how gender may moderate the association between marriage and well-being has been hotly contested over the years—beginning with Bernard's (1972) thesis that marriage benefits men more than women. However, more recently evidence from population studies has been shifting to suggest that the benefits of marriage may be more even across women and men than was previously thought (Marks and Lambert 1998; Waite 2000).

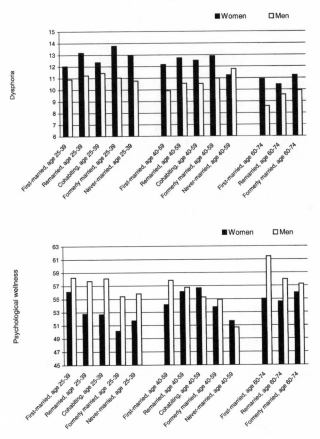

FIGURE 1. Predicted well-being scores by marital status, age, and gender.

Our results here are generally congruent with the hypothesis of relatively similar well-being benefits of marriage for women and men.

Third, never-married status contributes to more negative effects for midlife men than it does for younger men. This finding supports other work that suggests that never-married young men are happier now than in the past (Glenn and Weaver 1988), possibly because a new life-course period of semiautonomous young adult single living is increasingly more normative and less stigmatized (Goldscheider and Waite 1991). Yet the fact that midlife never-married men are disadvantaged in psychological wellness (a measure that includes many adult development subscales) and possibly generativity in comparison to men in a first marriage suggests that marriage may be particularly important for psychological and social development for men as they age into middle adulthood.

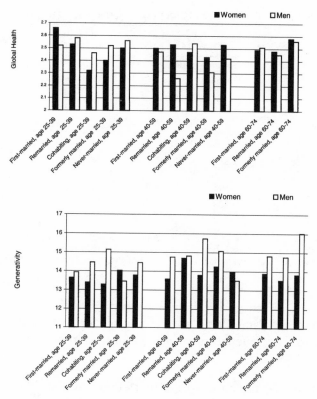

FIGURE 1. *(continued)*

Fourth, younger remarried, cohabiting, and formerly married women experience less psychological wellness than do midlife women in these statuses. Additionally, midlife women who experience nontraditional marital careers that include remarriage or formerly married status may experience some benefits in terms of generativity not experienced by their first-married counterparts. These results highlight the importance of considering age effects in family roles and are suggestive that some of the growing life expertise and life management skills that may go along with the midlife years (cf. Brim 1992) are an asset for women in nontraditional marital statuses (see also a similar pattern of results reported in Marks and Lambert 1998).

Finally, differences in physical health for married persons in contrast to single persons are not obvious when viewed cross-sectionally and with many demographic factors controlled. We found only one difference among the married: remarried men reported poorer health than

TABLE 4 Weighted Percentage Distribution (unweighted n

| | Young Adults Aged 25–39 | | | |
| | Women | | Men | |
Marital Status	Unwgtd n	Wgtd %	Unwgtd n	Wgt« %
Age of youngest child: 5 yrs or less	174	37.4	153	33.!
Age of youngest child: 6 yrs to 18 yrs	178	37.8	121	28.1
Age of youngest child: 19 yrs or older	4	.8	1	.:
No child	144	24.0	201	38.1
TOTAL	500	100.0	476	100.«

Source: MIDUS.
Note: Definition of parent here includes all biological or adoptive parents together with stepparents and others who indicated they played a significant role in rearing a child in their household for five or more years. Percentage columns do not always total 100.0 due to rounding error.

first-married men. Marriage has been consistently associated with longevity (Lillard and Panis 1996), but the findings for health status have been less robust; we found no evidence of a self-assessed health disadvantage of single status.

PARENTAL STATUS ACROSS THE MIDDLE LIFE COURSE

Although great advances in birth control across the last several decades have increasingly made it possible to separate sex from child-bearing, parenthood remains a normative role during the American adult life course (Marks 1996c). The middle adult years tend to be a time when adults are participating in the development of their children: beginning with infancy and preschool years, moving on to school-age years, and finally, to the "launching" phase of young adulthood and older ages.

Table 4 describes the population distribution of parental status for men and women across young, middle, and older ages. For these analyses we defined parents of a child as (1) anyone who reported that they had a biological child, and/or (2) anyone who reported that they had any "other children . . . including step children, adopted children, and any others you helped to raise for at least five years."[2] Using this operational definition, we found that among young adults about three in four women and more than three in five men reported being parents of a child. The age of the youngest child (usually an indicator of the heaviest level of child of Parental Status by Age and Gender, U.S. Adults Aged 25–74

	Midlife Adults Aged 40–59				Older Adults Aged 60–74			
	Women		Men		Women		Men	
	Unwgtd *n*	Wgtd %	Unwgtd *n*	Wgtd %	Unwgtd *n*	Wgtd %	Unwgtd *n*	Wgtd %
	16	3.1	38	7.2	0	0.0	0	0.0
	213	35.7	267	45.4	1	.3	9	2.9
	380	53.8	261	37.7	296	92.5	237	87.1
	58	7.4	77	9.6	24	7.2	23	10.0
	667	100.0	643	100.0	321	100.0	269	100.0

dependency) was about evenly split, at these young adult ages, between having a youngest child under age 5 and having a youngest child traversing middle childhood or adolescence. It was rare to report a youngest child age 19 or older at young adult ages.

By examining evidence from adults at midlife, we can determine relatively good estimates of lifetime incidence of childbearing/childrearing. At ages 40–59, only about 7.4 percent of women and 9.6 percent of men from these birth cohorts report not having any children. These rates are also quite similar for the older birth cohorts of women and men. Overall, therefore, even with greater control over childbearing, and greater public attitudinal acceptance of childfree adults (Thornton 1989), the vast majority of adults from these birth cohorts continue to experience a parenting role during their adult life course.

By midlife, a much smaller proportion of women and men has a preschool child, and about half of women and over a third of men report that their youngest child is an adult (age 19 or older). By older ages, almost all children are adult children.

Parental Status and Well-Being

Overall, the evidence has suggested that parenthood is associated with a greater degree of psychological distress than is being childfree (McLanahan and Adams 1987). However, research on the association between parenthood and well-being is typically missing an important examination of moderating factors, such as age of children and also age of parents, which might influence the pattern of associations (Seltzer and Ryff 1994; Umberson 1989; Umberson and Gove 1989). Additionally,

TABLE 5 Unstandardized Regression Coefficients for

Predictors	Dysphoria		Psychological Wellness (Ryff	
	Women	Men	Women	Men
No children (omitted)	—	—	—	—
Age of youngest 5 yrs or less	2.87*	−.84	−9.62***[a]	.59[a]
Age of youngest 6 yrs to 18 yrs	.66	−.26	−3.22+[b]	2.02[b]
Age of youngest 19 yrs or older	.47	−1.05*	−.87[c]	2.88*[c]
Age1 (25–39 yrs)	1.33*	.14	−.24	3.11*
Age2 (40–59 yrs) (omitted)	—	—	—	—
Age3 (60–74 yrs)	−.10	−1.44+	−5.40+	3.26
Age1 × age of youngest 5 yrs or less	−3.39**	1.05	6.72+	−.61
Age1 × age of youngest 6 yrs to 18 yrs	−1.58*	−.14	1.39	−2.53
Age3 × age of youngest 19 yrs or older	−1.41	.23	6.09*	−.77
Constant	12.38***	11.44***	55.51***	53.28***
R^2	.06	.07	.09	.07

Source: MIDUS. Analyses used unweighted data.

Note: All models also included controls for race/ethnicity, employment status, education, household income, marital status, and adult child status.

[a]Model estimated with men and women together revealed a significant gender difference ($p \leq .01$).

[b]Model estimated with men and women together revealed a significant gender difference ($p \leq .05$).

[c]Model estimated with men and women together revealed a trend level gender difference ($p \leq .10$).

+$p \leq .10$. *$p \leq .05$. **$p \leq .01$. ***$p \leq .001$ (two-tailed test).

examinations of parenthood and well-being have typically focused on psychological distress or life satisfaction as outcomes. An examination of only these outcomes does not provide evidence about whether parenthood might actually have positive effects on other domains of well-being, such as psychological wellness (including here dimensions of adult development such as purpose in life, self-acceptance, positive relations with others, and personal growth) and generativity, which might be posited to be enhanced by the experiences, and even challenges, of parenthood.

In our analyses we aimed to better examine child age differences, parent age differences, and differences that might occur in reports of psychological wellness, generativity, and physical health, as well as psychological dysphoria, in the effects of parenthood among contemporary American parents. Therefore we constructed an analysis similar to the one previously described for marital-status contrasts, this time including greater differentiation for parental status. For age contrasts in these analyses, we the Effects of Parental Status on Well-Being, by Gender

Self-Assessed Global Health		Generativity	
Women	Men	Women	Men
—	—	—	—
−.50+	−.08	−2.10[+c]	1.45[+c]
−.25+	−.09	.42	1.14*
−.34**	−.11	.31[b]	1.51**[b]
−.27+	.03	−.16	.57
—	—	—	—
−.24	−.09	−.33	.12
.62*	.09	1.97+	−1.40
.29	.10	−.12	−1.70**
.35	.22	.13	−.16
2.72***	2.45***	13.86***	13.78***
.14	.13	.09	.05

were again limited by population age composition considerations to the following contrasts: (1) because so few older adults have a youngest child under age 5, only young adults with children under age 5 (age1 × age of youngest under 5) could be contrasted with midlife adults with children under age 5; (2) because so few older adults have a youngest child aged 6–18 years, only young adults with children aged 6–18 (age1 × age of youngest 6–18) could be contrasted with midlife adults (and a few older adults) with a youngest child aged 6–18; and (3) because so few young adults have a youngest child age 19 and older, only older adults with a youngest child 19 or older (age3 × age of youngest 19 or older) could be contrasted with midlife adults (and a few younger adults) with a youngest child 19 or older.

Table 5 describes the associations between having children of varying ages with well-being, also by gender and age group. (Fig. 2 graphically illustrates predicted well-being scores for population subgroups on the basis of the estimates from models reported in table 5.)

Gender and Age Differences

Among women, two significant age-group differences were in evidence. Although it appears that among midlife women, having a youngest aged 5 years or less is associated with more dysphoria than having no children (the omitted parental-status contrast category), this effect was significantly reduced for women aged 25–39. Similarly, the association

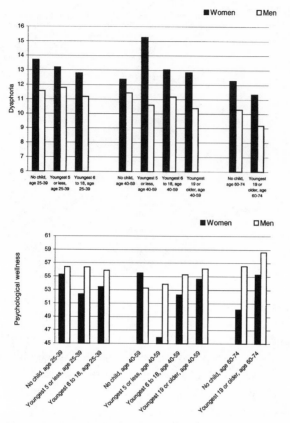

FIGURE 2. Predicted well-being scores by parental status, age, and gender.

between having school-aged youngest children and having more dyspho-ria was significantly less among young adult women than midlife women (the omitted age-contrast category).

Among men there were no significant age-group differences. Overall, evidence indicated well-being benefits of parenthood for men, in contrast to being childfree. Having only adult children was associated with less dysphoria than having no children.

In terms of psychological wellness, there were clear gender differences in evidence regarding the impact of parenthood on well-being. In our preliminary model, estimated across men and women together, we found that for all categories of parenting (in contrast to being childfree), women reported less psychological wellness than did men in the comparable

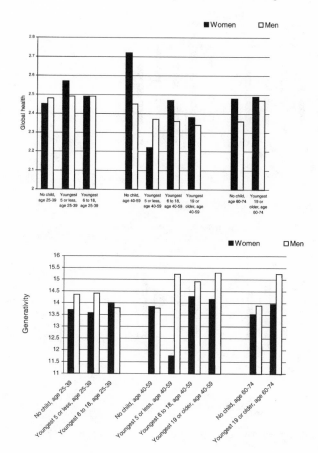

FIGURE 2. (*continued*)

parenting category. In the separate analyses by gender that added age-group contrasts, we found that women with a youngest child under age 6 reported significantly less psychological wellness than did women with no children (although a trend-level effect suggested that this negative effect might be attenuated for younger women in contrast to midlife women). Additionally, a trend-level effect suggested that having school-aged children was associated with less wellness for women than having no children. However, the age contrasts allowed us to also observe that for women at older ages, having adult children was associated with significantly greater wellness than it was at midlife ages (perhaps because children are likely to be even more mature and independent when mothers are at these ages). Figure 3 graphically illustrates how at older ages, mothers of adult

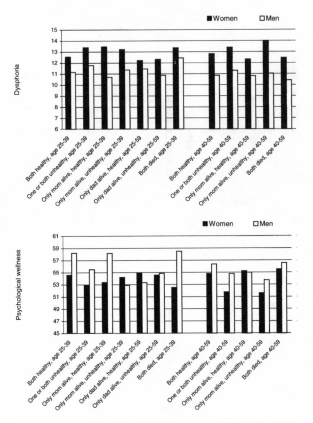

FIGURE 3. Predicted well-being scores by adult child status, age, and gender.

children are actually at a psychological wellness advantage in comparison to women without children.

The models estimated separately for men and women, and including an analysis of age-group differences, revealed that parental status had more implications for women's than men's reports of physical health. Younger women reporting a youngest child aged 5 or under reported significantly better physical health than did midlife women reporting a youngest aged 5 or under. Across this sample of women, women reporting a youngest 19 or older reported poorer health than women without children. No significant differences in health by parental status were observed among men when they were examined in a separate model with age interaction variables added.

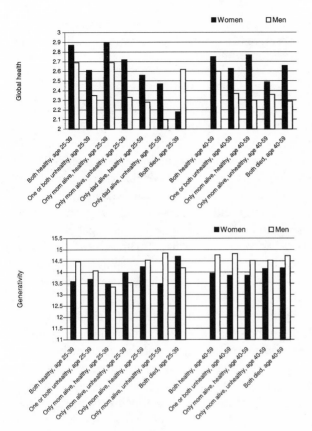

FIGURE 3. (*continued*)

The combined analysis of men and women also revealed two gender differences in the influence of parenthood on generativity. Men with adult children report significantly more generativity than do women with adult children, and men with preschool children show evidence of possibly reporting more generativity than do women with preschool children.

The separate analysis of women that added age contrasts suggested that midlife women with a preschool-aged youngest child may experience less generativity than midlife women with no children. However, this negative effect appeared to be attenuated for younger women with a preschool-aged youngest child.

Men, by contrast, clearly benefited in terms of their experience of generativity when they had children in contrast to not having children.

The only age-group exception was young men whose youngest child was school-aged, and whose predicted generativity scores were lower than those for young men without children (see figure 2).

Conclusions

Overall, our results suggest several conclusions in terms of the parent role and well-being. First, parenting children is more challenging to the well-being of women than men. This is likely a result of the greater emotional and instrumental responsibility for children that women internalize and enact (Rossi and Rossi 1990). Second, the challenge of parenting a preschool-aged child is associated with more negative mental health consequences but better physical health and generativity reports for women at midlife ages than at young adult ages. These findings highlight the importance of considering age differences. They also illustrate how a family role can have costs and benefits at the same time, such that in examining only one dimension of well-being (e.g., dysphoria), we would miss the complexity of the story.

Third, having only adult children in contrast to no children is associated with increased psychological wellness for men and older women. Additionally, parenthood is particularly important in contributing to men's experience of generativity. These findings again illustrate the importance of considering different age periods of childrearing when considering the association of parenthood with well-being (Seltzer and Ryff 1994; Umberson 1989). They also demonstrate the significant benefits for development that parenting has for men. The finding regarding parenthood and generativity among men provides convergent support from population data for a finding that has previously been suggested in earlier psychological research with more limited samples (McAdams and de St. Aubin 1992, 1998). These results overall also suggest that a monolithic examination of parenthood and its association with only one dimension of well-being—psychological distress—is likely to miss the benefits as well as costs of parenthood for men as well as women.

Adults and Their Aging Parents across the Middle Life Course

An important part of adult life is spent now in relationship to parents who are still alive or who over time become ill and die. More men and women reach adulthood with both parents alive than was true early in the twentieth century, and men and women from contemporary adult birth cohorts are likely to spend more years with one or more parents aged 65 and older than they are with children under age 18 (Watkins, Menken, and Bongaarts 1987). Despite these demographic trends, relatively little social demography and family research to date have focused on midlife adults in their adult child role vis-à-vis their aging parents, and how this adult child role might be related to the well-being of midlife adults.

Table 6 describes the population distribution of men and women who have parents alive and who have parents in good or poor health. For these analyses, MIDUS respondents' reports of whether father and mother were alive were combined with respondents' reports about the relative health of their parents ("How would you rate your biological mother's/father's current physical health? Excellent, very good, good, fair, poor?") to create seven mutually exclusive and exhaustive categories of respondents. The first category included respondents who reported both parents were alive and both were "healthy" (i.e., rated global health for each as good, very good, or excellent, in contrast to fair or poor). The second category included respondents who reported both parents alive, but one or both were "unhealthy" (i.e., rated global health for at least one living parent as fair or poor). The third category included respondents who reported that only their mother was alive but that she was healthy. The fourth category included respondents who reported that only their mother was alive but that she was unhealthy. The fifth category included respondents with only a father alive who was healthy. The sixth, only a father alive who was unhealthy. And the final category included respondents who reported both parents had died prior to their adult children's interview in 1995.

The population estimates provided in table 6 show the dramatic changes in adult child role status vis-à-vis aging parents that occur across the middle life course. At young adult ages, a little more than one-third of the sample reported that both parents were alive and healthy. About half the young adult population reported only healthy living parent(s) (i.e., either both alive and healthy or only mom or dad alive and healthy). Reflecting gender differences in mortality rates, our findings indicated that young adults were about three times more likely to have a sole-surviving mother than a sole-surviving father. Less than one in twenty young adults had lost both parents to death.

By midlife ages 40–59, only about one in nine adults overall (10.5 percent of women and 12.8 percent of men) reported having both parents alive and both parents healthy. Another approximately one in three reported at least one unhealthy parent. About one in five midlife adults reported having a sole-surviving parent in poor health, most typically

TABLE 6 Weighted Percentage Distribution of

	Young Aged 25–39			
	Women		Men	
Adult Child Status	Unwgtd n	Wgted %	Unwgtd n	Wgted %
Both parents alive, both healthy	164	35.0	161	36.0
Both parents alive, 1 or both unhealthy	174	37.7	161	35.3
Only mom alive, healthy	57	11.2	60	12.5
Only mom alive, unhealthy	35	7.6	26	6.1
Only dad alive, healthy	16	3.8	17	4.0
Only dad alive, unhealthy	7	1.4	10	1.9
Both parents dead	15	3.3	22	4.2
TOTAL	468	100.0	457	100.0

Source: MIDUS.

Note: Percentage columns do not always total 100.0 due to rounding error.

a mother. Already by midlife ages, less than one in ten adults reported having a father alive, healthy or not, and more than one-quarter reported the loss of both parents.

By older ages, it is quite uncommon to have both parents still alive. The vast majority of adults (80.5 percent of women and 90.3 percent of men) have experienced the death of both parents by these ages. The relatively small proportion of adults who do have living parents is comprised mainly of persons whose mothers are still alive.

ADULTS, AGING PARENTS, AND WELL-BEING

Overall, there is little literature examining how the health and mortality of parents affects the well-being of adult children. The literature that does exist in this area tends to emphasize filial caregiving and typically focuses on the stressful well-being consequences of becoming a caregiver for an aging parent (e.g., Brody 1990; Horowitz 1985; Marks 1998; Marks, Lambert, and Choi 2002; Montgomery 1992).

In this study, we wished to make a further contribution to the literature that considers the continuing potential influence of aging parents and their health status on the well-being of adult children. Because the population estimates provided in table 6 suggest that most of the variance in the adult child role differentiated by the relative health and mortality

Adult Child Status, by Age and Gender

Midlife Adults Aged 40–59				Older Adults Aged 60–74			
Women		Men		Women		Men	
Unwgtd *n*	Wgted %	Unwgtd *n*	Wgted %	Unwgtd *n*	Wgted %	Unwgtd *n*	Wgted %
70	10.5	85	12.8	1	.2	2	.3
105	18.3	105	16.5	7	2.9	3	.7
123	18.1	117	18.5	26	6.1	12	3.8
110	17.6	94	14.8	28	8.7	15	3.7
28	3.9	36	5.8	2	.8	3	.6
20	3.0	22	3.8	2	.8	2	.5
189	28.6	185	27.9	250	80.5	227	90.3
645	100.0	644	100.0	316	100.0	264	100.0

of their parents is confined to the young adult and midlife adult years as we have defined them here, for our adult child role analyses, we limited our analytic sample only to respondents aged 25–59. Again we began by estimating a preliminary model, including both men and women together, which included gender interaction variables to explore potential gender differences. We subsequently estimated models for women and men separately, adding age by adult child role interaction variables where cell sizes for both young adults made such a comparison possible (specifically, for contrasts of both parents alive, one or both unhealthy; only mom alive and healthy; only mom alive and unhealthy; and for both parents dead).

The results of these analyses are provided in table 7. (Fig. 3 graphically illustrates predicted well-being scores for population subgroups on the basis of the estimates from models reported in table 7.)

Gender and Age Differences

The preliminary models that included men and women together suggested one robust gender difference: having a mother alive and unhealthy was associated with significantly higher levels of dysphoria for women than for men. The models for women and men separately further demonstrated this gender difference. Specifically, among women, those who had a sole-surviving, unhealthy mother reported significantly higher rates of

TABLE 7 Unstandardized Regression Coefficients for the Effects of Adult

	Dysphoria		Psychological Wellness (Ryff	
Predictors	Women	Men	Women	Men
Both parents alive, both healthy (omitted)	—	—	—	—
Both parents alive, 1 or both unhealthy	.58	.45	-3.01^+	-1.58
Only mom alive, healthy	$-.49$	$-.04$	.46	-1.39
Only mom alive, unhealthy	1.20^{*a}	$.19^a$	-3.18^+	-2.62^+
Only dad alive, healthy	$-.61$	.58	.14	-3.07^+
Only dad alive, unhealthy	$-.50$	.01	$-.25$	-1.54
Both parents died	$-.35$	$-.41$	.76	.22
Age1 (29–39 yrs)	$-.27$	.30	$-.23$	1.83
Age2 (40–59 yrs) (omitted)	—	—	—	—
Age1 × both parents alive, 1 or both unhealthy	.25	.15	1.34	-1.13
Age1 × only mom alive, healthy	1.39	$-.43$	-1.67	1.35
Age1 × only mom alive, unhealthy	$-.54$	.01	2.80	-2.72
Age1 × both parents dead	1.16	1.70^+	-2.80	.07
Constant	12.82^{***}	10.85^{***}	54.79^{***}	56.38^{***}
R^2	.07	.06	.09	.08

Source: MIDUS.
Note: All models also included controls for race/ethnicity, employment status, education, household income, marital status, and parental status. Analyses used unweighted data.
^{a}Model estimated with men and women together revealed a significant gender difference ($p \le .05$).
$^+p \le .10$. $^*p \le .05$. $^{**}p \le .01$. $^{***}p \le .001$ (two-tailed test).

dysphoria than their women peers who continued to have two healthy parents. Among men, differences in the health and mortality of parents did not appear to have robust effects on dysphoria, although a trend-effect age interaction suggested that having both parents dead by young adult ages was associated with higher levels of dysphoria among men than having both parents dead by midlife ages.

For women, trend effects suggested that having both parents alive but one or both unhealthy, or having only a mother alive but unhealthy, was associated with lower psychological wellness for women than having both parents alive and healthy. Among men, trend effects suggested that having a mother alive but unhealthy, or having a father alive and healthy, might be associated with less wellness. No age-group differences were in evidence for men or women.

Again for global health, having a sole-surviving unhealthy mother appeared possibly to compromise women's self-rated health (trend effect).

Child Status on Well-Being by Gender, U.S. Adults Aged 25–59

Global Health		Generativity	
Women	Men	Women	Men
—	—	—	—
−.12	−.23+	−.10	.06
.02	−.30*	−.10	−.25
−.26+	−.24+	.20	−.24
−.19	−.32*	.29	−.23
−.28	−.50**	−.47	.08
−.09	−.31**	.23	−.03
.12	.09	−.37	−.30
—	—	—	—
−.14	−.11	.20	−.47
.01	.30+	−.00	−.87
.11	−.12	.19	−.69
−.60*	.24	.89	−.24
2.75***	2.60***	13.96***	14.77***
.11	.14	.09	.05

Additionally, a significant age interaction effect indicated that having both parents dead at young adult ages was associated with reporting significantly poorer health among women than having both parents dead at midlife adult ages.

All the adult child contrasts other than having both parents alive and healthy were associated with reporting poorer physical health among men, although trend-level age interaction effects suggested that the negative effect of this status may be more problematic for midlife men than young adult men. Differences in adult child status were not associated with differences in reports of generativity among men or women.

Conclusions

Overall, our results from this analysis of the adult child role in relation to aging parents suggest the following: First, having unhealthy parents, particularly an unhealthy sole-surviving mother, can undermine the mental health and self-assessed physical health of young and midlife adults. We speculate (but cannot empirically verify with these data) that an unhealthy sole-surviving father is more likely to be remarried and therefore less worrisome because of care provided by the new spouse. Second, the negative effects of having a sole-surviving unhealthy mother are greater for women than for men. This is congruent with what we know about the gendered nature of the schemas for family roles (Rossi and Rossi 1990), which have traditionally led women to assume greater emotional and instrumental caregiving responsibilities for family members (often leading to added stress) than men assume.

Third, the early death (i.e., by young adulthood) of both parents (in contrast to having both parents remain alive and healthy) may be associated with greater dysphoria among men and poorer assessments of physical health among women. It is difficult to reliably interpret these findings because we do not know exactly when parental deaths occurred (e.g., in childhood or young adulthood) or to what degree genetic selection is at work here. However, these suggestive findings lead us to recommend that scholars studying midlife further explore the possible importance of ongoing relationships with parents in adulthood for mental and physical well-being.

Summary and Conclusions

In this chapter we have taken advantage of the unique strengths of the MIDUS population data to examine gender and age variation in marital, parenting, and adult child vis-à-vis aging parent roles, and to investigate how these family-role differences are associated with differences in physical, mental, and social well-being. We have used the opportunity provided by these rich data to highlight the increased contemporary diversity within marital, parental, and adult child roles across the middle life course—by considering, for example, cohabiting and re-married partner statuses, parenting experiences across different ages of children, and variation in types of adult child role diversity based on differences in the health and mortality status of parents. Considering age-group differences in population distributions across these roles also helped us draw attention to the implicit life-course trajectories that take place in marital, parenting, and adult child roles. In other words, these roles each involve an age-related "career" that is likely to have different opportunities, challenges, constraints, and consequences for well-being. Early adulthood first marriage may be followed by divorce and possibly midlife remarriage or continued formerly married status. Parenting young children is followed by parenting adolescents, "launching" children, and finally, continued parental involvement with adult children. Young adult children may begin by having both parents still alive and providing them with support, but over time experience the loss of health of one or both parents, and the death of one or both parents.

We also use the MIDUS physical, mental, and social health measurements to highlight here the value of considering a wider range of different well-being outcomes in relation to these family roles than is typically employed in the literature, as well as gender and age differences in the impact of these role differences. The inclusion of a measure of social well-being—that is, generativity—proved to be particularly illuminating. Examining multiple well-being outcomes, we were better able to demonstrate the combination of both gains and strains that can be associated with family roles. For example, we found evidence that although being a parent can be associated with more psychological distress than being childfree, being a parent can also result in reports of greater psychological wellness and generativity.

Examining gender differences, we found fewer marital-status effect differences than some of the literature may have led us to expect. However, we found important gender differences in the effects of a parenting role; men clearly evidenced greater psychological wellness benefits and generativity benefits from parenting than women did. Women in an adult child role having only an unhealthy mother alive also reported more dysphoria than did their male peers. However, young adult and midlife men without two healthy parents all reported some degree of poorer physical health; this pattern was not replicated among women.

In the literature on family roles, potential age differences in the consequences of roles for well-being are typically ignored. However, we found age moderation results to be some of the most interesting findings of our study—highlighting the importance of considering substantive differences in the experience of adulthood in young adult versus midlife adult versus older adult years and demonstrating that, indeed, midlife is to some extent distinct. For example, in our marital-status analyses we found never-married midlife men reporting more dysphoria and less generativity than never-married young adult men. We also found midlife women in nontraditional marital statuses (cohabiting, remarried, and formerly married) to be reporting more psychological wellness than younger women in these statuses. Midlife women parenting children under 19 reported more dysphoria than younger women parenting children these ages. Older women with young adult children (aged 19 or older) reported more psychological wellness than midlife women with young adult children. Women with both parents dead at young adult ages reported significantly poorer overall health than women reporting both parents dead at midlife ages.

In sum, we believe there is sufficient evidence here to recommend that future research on family roles and well-being continue to investigate diverse dimensions of well-being to better gauge the costs and benefits of family roles. We also believe it is important to continue to consider both gender and age moderation of effects.

However, we also acknowledge the many limitations of this broad-brush study. Although we have made efforts to take a more differentiated approach to examining family roles and well-being, we have still not taken into full account additional important axes of variance. For example, we have not fully addressed the considerable differences in prevalence of family-role categories by race/ethnicity and socioeconomic status (Marks 1996c), and the potential these differences might have on moderating family-role effects on well-being. For parsimony's sake, we have also ignored here important differences in role quality and role history (Wheaton 1990) that we expect would also have a significant impact on how differences in family-role incumbency influence multiple dimensions of well-being. We have not carefully examined different combinations of roles and evaluated how this might influence the impact of role experience. We used cross-sectional data here, so our inferences of causality occurring from family roles to well-being are not definitive. Nor can we necessarily infer that differences across the range of our different birth cohorts are telling us a story of developmental change. We are certain that important period and cohort effects are embedded in this analysis, given the considerable family and social changes we outlined at the outset; therefore we urge reader caution in making developmental inferences.

Future research is needed to address these many limitations and to keep apace of tracking the continuing evolution in family-role variance in the years to come. Nonetheless, we believe the results of our work here confirm the continued significance of family roles, responsibilities, opportunities, and constraints for the ongoing development and well-being of adults across the middle life course at the beginning of the twenty-first century. We see no evidence to suggest that the family is an obsolete institution that will not remain a significant context and constituting factor for adult well-being in the century ahead.

Descriptive Statistics for Analysis Variables

	Total Sample Mean (SD) ($n = 3032$)	Women Mean (SD) ($n = 1714$)	Men Mean (SD) ($n = 1318$)
Outcome variables			
Dysphoria	9.50 (3.89)	9.88 (4.14)	9.01 (3.49)
Psychological wellness (Ryff)	63.26 (10.89)	62.67 (10.99)	64.02 (10.71)
Self-assessed global health	3.41 (1.00)	3.37 (1.02)	3.46 (.97)
Generativity	16.94 (3.74)	17.02 (3.77)	16.83 (3.71)
Demographic characteristics			
Female	.57		
Age	45.30 (13.78)	45.49 (13.69)	45.05 (13.20)
Age1 (25–39 yrs)	.41	.41	.40
Age2 (40–59 yrs)	.40	.39	.42
Age3 (60–74 yrs)	.19	.20	.18
Marital status			
First marriage	.52	.49	.56
Remarried	.16	.15	.18
Cohabiting	.06	.06	.06
Formerly married	.17	.22	.11
Never married	.09	.08	.09
Parental status			
Age of youngest child: <5 yrs	.17	.17	.17
Age of youngest child: 6 to 18 yrs	.30	.29	.31
Age of youngest child: 19 or older	.36	.39	.31
No child	.17	.14	.21
Adult child status			
Both alive, both healthy	.19	.18	.20
Both alive, 1 or both unhealthy	.22	.23	.21
Only mom alive, healthy	.13	.13	.14
Only mom alive, unhealthy	.11	.12	.09
Only dad alive, healthy	.04	.03	.04
Only dad alive, unhealthy	.02	.02	.02
Both parents died	.29	.29	.29
Black	.11	.13	.10
Employed	.73	.66	.81
Level of education[a]	2.58 (.98)	2.52 (.96)	2.67 (1.01)
Household income (in thousands)	50.75 (43.88)	45.47 (39.71)	57.61 (47.93)

Source: MIDUS.

Note: Descriptive statistics were calculated using weighted data. Dichotomous variable means are proportions.

[a] Range for level of education: 1, less than high school graduation; 2, high school graduation; 3, some college; 4, college graduation or more.

Notes

1. Because this is a cross-sectional profile, remarried widows are included in the remarried category.

2. Only about 3.3 percent of parents, so defined, were exclusively stepparents; in total, only 3.5 percent of parents, so defined, were exclusively nonbiological parents.

References

Bane, M. J. 1976. *Here to stay: American families in the twentieth century.* New York: Bantam.

Bernard, J. 1972. *The future of marriage.* New York: Bantam.

Booth, A., and P. Amato. 1991. Divorce and psychological stress. *Journal of Health and Social Behavior* 32:396–407.

Brim, O. B. 1992. *Ambition.* New York: Basic Books.

Brody, E. M. 1990. *Women in the middle:* Their parent care years. New York: Springer-Verlag.

Bumpass, L. 1990. What's happening to the family: Interactions between demographic and institutional change. *Demography* 27:483–98.

Bumpass, L., and H.-H. Lu. 2000. Trends in cohabitation and implications for children's family contexts in the U.S. *Population Studies* 541:29–41.

Bumpass, L., and J. A. Sweet. 1989a. Children's experience in single-parent families: Implications of cohabitation and marital transitions. *Family Planning Perspectives* 216:256–60.

———. 1989b. National estimates of cohabitation: Cohort levels and union stability. *Demography* 26:615–25.

Bumpass, L. L., J. A. Sweet, and T. Castro-Martin. 1989. Changing patterns of remarriage. *Journal of Marriage and the Family* 52:747–56.

Castro-Martin, T., and L. L. Bumpass. 1989. Recent trends and differentials in marital disruption. *Demography* 26:37–51.

Cherlin, A. 1992. *Marriage, divorce, remarriage.* Rev. ed. Cambridge: Harvard University Press.

Cooney, T. M., and P. Uhlenberg. 1992. Support from parents over the life course: The adult child's perspective. *Social Forces* 71:63–84.

Erikson, E. 1950. *Childhood and society.* New York: W. W. Norton.

Glenn, N. D. 1975. Psychological well-being in the postparental stage: Some evidence from national surveys. *Journal of Marriage and the Family* 37:105–10.

Glenn, N. D., and C. N. Weaver. 1988. The changing relationship of marital status to reported happiness. *Journal of Marriage and the Family* 50:317–24.

Glick, P. 1988. Fifty years of family demography: A record of social change. *Journal of Marriage and the Family* 50:861–74.

Goldscheider, F. K., and L. J. Waite. 1991. *New families, no families?* Berkeley: University of California Press.

Gove, W. R., M. Hughes, and C. B. Style. 1983. Does marriage have positive effects on the psychological well-being of the individual? *Journal of Health and Social Behavior* 24:122–31.

Gove, W. R., C. B. Style, and M. Hughes. 1990. The effect of marriage on the well-being of adults. *Journal of Family Issues* 11:4–35.

Hogan, D. P., D. J. Eggebeen, and C. C. Clogg. 1993. The structure of intergenerational exchanges in American families. *American Journal of Sociology* 98:1428–58.

Horowitz, A. 1985. Sons and daughters as caregivers to older parents: Differences in role performance and consequences. *Gerontologist* 25:612–17.

Idler, E. L., and Y. Benyamini. 1997. Self-rated health and mortality: A review of twenty-seven community studies. *Journal of Health and Social Behavior* 38:21–37.

Lee, G., K. Seccombe, and C. Shehan. 1991. Marital status and personal happiness: An analysis of trend data. *Journal of Marriage and the Family* 53:839–44.

Lillard, L. A., and C. W. A. Panis. 1996. Marital status and mortality: The role of health. *Demography* 33:313–27.

Marks, N. F. 1995. Midlife marital status differences in social support relationships with adult children and psychological well-being. *Journal of Family Issues* 16:5–28.

———. 1996a. Caregiving across the lifespan: National prevalence and predictors. *Family Relations* 45:27–36.

———. 1996b. Flying solo at midlife: Gender, marital status, and psychological well-being. *Journal of Marriage and the Family* 58:917–32.

———. 1996c. Social demographic diversity among American midlife parents. In *When children grow up: Development and diversity in midlife parenting*, ed. C. D. Ryff and M. M. Seltzer, 29–75. Chicago: University of Chicago Press.

———. 1998 Does it hurt to care? Caregiving, work-family conflict, and midlife well-being. *Journal of Marriage and the Family* 60:951–66.

Marks, N. F., and J. D. Lambert. 1998. Marital status continuity and change among young and midlife adults: Longitudinal effects on psychological well-being. *Journal of Family Issues* 19:652–86.

Marks, N. F., J. D. Lambert, and H. Choi. 2002. Transitions to caregiving, gender, and psychological well-being: Prospective evidence from a U.S. national study. *Journal of Marriage and Family* 64:657–67.

McAdams, D. P., and E. de St. Aubin. 1992. A theory of generativity and its assessment through self-report, behavioral acts, and narrative themes in autobiography. *Journal of Personality and Social Psychology* 62:1003–15.

———, eds. 1998. *Generativity and adult development: Psychosocial perspectives on caring for and contributing to the next generation.* Washington, D.C.: American Psychological Association.

McLanahan, S. S., and J. Adams. 1987. Parenthood and psychological well-being. *Annual Review of Sociology* 5:237–58.

Menaghan, E. G., and M. A. Lieberman. 1986. Changes in depression following divorce: A panel study. *Journal of Marriage and the Family* 48:319–28.

Montgomery, R. J. V. 1992. Gender differences in patterns of child–parent caregiving relationships. In *Gender, families, and elder care*, ed. J. W. Dwyer and R. T. Coward, 65–83. Newbury Park, Calif.: Sage.

Mroczek, D. K., and C. M. Kolarz. 1998. The effect of age on positive and negative affect: A developmental perspective on happiness. *Journal of Personality and Social Psychology* 75:1333–49.

Parsons, T. 1942. Age and sex in the social structure of the United States. *American Anthropologist* 45:22–38.

Pearlin, L. I., and J. S. Johnson. 1977. Marital status, life-strains and depression. *American Sociological Review* 42:704–15.

Popenoe, D. 1988. *Disturbing the nest: Family change and decline in modern society.* New York: Aldine de Gruyter.

———. 1993. American family decline, 1960–1990: A review and appraisal. *Journal of Marriage and the Family* 55:527–55.

Ross, C. E. 1995. Reconceptualizing marital status as a continuum of social attachment. *Journal of Marriage and the Family* 57:129–40.

Ross, C. E., J. Mirowsky, and K. Goldsteen. 1990. The impact of the family on health: The decade in review. *Journal of Marriage and the Family* 52:1059–78.

Rossi, A. S., and P. H. Rossi. 1990. *Of human bonding: Parent–child relations across the life course.* New York: Aldine de Gruyter.

Ryff, C. 1989. Happiness is everything, or is it? *Journal of Personality and Social Psychology* 6:1069–81.

Ryff, C. D., and C. L. M. Keyes. 1995. The structure of psychological well-being revisited. *Journal of Personality and Social Psychology* 69:719–27.

Schoen, R., W. L. Urton, K. Woodrow, and J. Baj. 1985. Marriage and divorce in 20th century American cohorts. *Demography* 22:101–14.

Schoen, R., and R. M. Weinick. 1993. The slowing metabolism of marriage: Figures from 1988 U.S. marital status life tables. *Demography* 30:737–46.

Seltzer, M. M., and C. D. Ryff. 1994. Parenting across the lifespan: The normative and nonnormative cases. In *Life-span development and behavior,* ed. D. L. Featherman, R. M. Lerner, and M. Perlmutter, 12:1–40. Hillsdale, N.J.: Lawrence Erlbaum Associates.

Skolnick, A. 1991. *Embattled paradise: The American family in an age of uncertainty.* New York: Basic Books.

Stacey, J. 1990. *Brave new families: Stories of domestic upheaval in late 20th century America.* New York: Basic Books.

———. 1993. Good riddance to "the family": A response to David Popenoe. *Journal of Marriage and the Family* 55:545–47.

Stone, R., G. L. Cafferata, and J. Sangl. 1987. Caregivers of the frail elderly: A national profile. *Gerontologist* 27:616–26.

Stryker, S., and A. Statham. 1985. Symbolic interaction and role theory. In *The handbook of social psychology,* vol. 1. *Theory and method,* 3d ed., ed. G. Lindzey and E. Aronson, 311–78. New York: Random House.

Thornton, A. 1989. Changing attitudes toward family issues in the United States. *Journal of Marriage and the Family* 51:873–93.

Umberson, D. 1989. Parenting and well-being: The importance of context. *Journal of Family Issues* 10:427–43.

Umberson, D., and W. Gove. 1989. Parenthood and psychological well-being: Theory, measurement, and stage in the family life course. *Journal of Family Issues* 10:440–62.

Waite, L. J., ed. 2000. *The ties that bind: Perspectives on marriage and cohabitation.* Hawthorne, N.Y.: Aldine de Gruyter.

Watkins, S. C., J. A. Mencken, and J. Bongaarts. 1987. Demographic foundations of family change. *American Sociological Review* 50:689–98.

Wells, L. E., and S. Stryker. 1988. Stability and change in self over the life course. In *Life-span development and behavior,* ed. P. B. Baltes, D. L. Featherman, and R. M. Lerner, 8:191–229. Hillsdale, N.J.: Lawrence Erlbaum Associates.

Wheaton, B. 1990. Life transitions, role histories, and mental health. *American Sociological Review* 55:209–23.

Winship, C., and L. Radbill. 1994. Sampling weights and regression analysis. *Sociological Methods and Research* 23:230–63.

CHAPTER NINETEEN

Social Responsibility to Family and Community

Alice S. Rossi

For more than a decade now, there have been pronouncements to the effect that American society is undergoing a fundamental process of social breakdown and alienation. Such alarms have been prevalent in academe, politics, and the media. Within academe, scholars across a wide spectrum of disciplines—sociology, political science, and moral philosophy, in particular—have written much about the presumed breakdown of the family, the alienation of the public from the political process, the decline of civic participation in voluntary associations, the loss of civility in public encounters with each other.[1]

A major example of such a critique is Robert Putnam's research on the decline of civic virtue and participation, which first came to public attention in journal articles (Putnam 1995a, 1995b), especially "Bowling Alone," and subsequently greatly expanded in a book, *Bowling Alone: The Collapse and Renewal of American Community* (Putnam 2000). The title of this volume is misleading because for all but a few pages in the last chapter, the book focuses on the collapse, not the renewal, of American community. At the heart of Putnam's book is an empirical reanalysis of three national surveys repeated over the years from the 1970s to the mid-1990s. These data permitted Putnam to demonstrate cohort change in support of his thesis of long-term decline in social trust and social-political values during the last quarter of the twentieth century. For example, compared with young adults surveyed in the 1970s, young adults in the 1990s are less trustful of major social institutions or individuals encountered during their daily rounds, less engaged in civic affairs, and more highly focused on their own private pursuits in life rather than on the common good. The chief culprit, according to Putnam's analysis of these trends, is a turning away from social engagement into excessive amounts of time devoted to television and Internet scanning. The effects of such "thin" social networks and withdrawal into solitary pursuits are illustrated, he claims, by the rising rates of suicide and depression among young people today compared with young adults of twenty-five years ago.

Indeed, exposure to these alarmist articles and books gives the impression that there are hardly any social indicators suggesting that life is good in America or that Americans are good people. If we were to take personally all the bad news and faults one hears and reads about, we should all be in a state of deep depression. Americans are berated in almost every aspect of their lives: for being too individualistic and neglectful of their civic and family responsibilities; for spending too much and saving too little; for either neglecting or overindulging their children; for not taking their marriage vows seriously enough or bypassing marriage all together in preference for cohabiting; for eating too much of the wrong foods and being overweight if not obese.

A wide array of reasons for the presumed social and moral breakdown has been argued: excessive individualism with its attendant overemphasis on individual rights and downplaying of social responsibility; the residue of counterculture lifestyles from the 1960s; the loss of religious faith (or attraction to deviant religious cults); overdependence on a bloated federal bureaucracy; excessive stridency of the feminist movement; the pervasive focus on sex and violence on television; the fragility of families as a consequence of premarital cohabitation, births outside marriage, and the high divorce rate; the breakdown of social networks and stable communities; and as illustrated by Putnam's work discussed above, the withdrawal from social interaction in favor of countless hours of TV viewing and Web surfing.

There is evidence to support some but not all of these explanations. From opinion polls conducted over the past twenty-five years, it is indeed the case that increasing numbers of Americans have little confidence and trust in major institutions in society, in particular the legislative and executive branches of government and the press, a trend consistent with Putnam's cohort analysis (Rossi 2001). Americans vote in elections at much lower rates than do citizens of any western European nation. It is also true that the American diet has deteriorated as a consequence of the vast increase in the consumption of sugar, salt, and fat combined with the sedentary lifestyle that goes with sitting before a TV screen or computer for so many hours every week, with the result that very large numbers of Americans are overweight from puberty through late midlife.[2]

On the other hand, there are important points that are missed or given insufficient attention in these alarmist criticisms and explanations. An important but neglected fact is that there have been numerous times in our history when contemporary critics claimed the social fabric was being frayed irrevocably, that people were losing trust in social institutions, that alienation was on the increase, crime rampant, behavior in public crude. In the 1934 final report of the President's Research Committee on Social Trends in the United States, editor William Ogburn and his contributing authors took note of trends during the period 1900–1930, trends that would be familiar to us today: declining parental supervision of children; increasing sexual freedom; declining membership in churches; and a sharply declining percentage of eligible voters who actually voted in presidential elections (Ogburn 1934). There were similar cycles of change during the nineteenth century in American history, as illustrated by the steady rise in the serious crime rate from the beginning of the 1800s, peaking in the 1840s, and gradually declining by the end of the nineteenth century. Drunkenness was far more prevalent in the nineteenth century than it is today, and time spent in saloons or taverns exceeded time spent at church services, at least among men if not women (Fukuyama 1999).

The more recent past is often viewed through a rosy lens. Today's social critics who look back with nostalgia to the 1950s forget many things that marked that decade: the pervasive fear that the United States would become involved in a nuclear war or would plunge back into another depression like that of the 1930s; the world population explosion, and the early warnings of dire consequences for quality of life that attend the doubling of huge human populations every thirty years (air and water pollution and acute competition for dwindling natural resources); the "problem that has no name" among suburban women, as Betty Friedan described the 1950s scene in the early 1960s (Friedan 1963); and the still unresolved issues of civil rights for minorities. As Alan Ehrenhalt (1995, 259) reminds us, "there is a pendulum at work in the manners and values of a society, and . . . it can swing when no one expects it to." Such a pendulum is likely to swing again in the decades ahead, much as it did throughout our history.

Two important factors are commonly neglected when this diverse array of contemporary alarmist criticisms is touted. One factor, perhaps the most important and conspicuous by its absence, is any criticism of Americans as workers and rarely any reference to the changes taking place in the American economy and the effect those changes have on other aspects of employed adults' lives. Any assessment of the cohesiveness of a society must surely take into account how well or poorly people are performing in their work roles. On this score, Americans show a high and positive profile: they are hard-working, committed workers, rarely absent from their jobs, and for the most part, loyal to the firms, farms, or bureaus they work for. In light of the pressures and requirements of the jobs Americans hold, this is a very significant point. Americans work longer hours with less vacation time than workers in any other Western nation, and at a pace that has sharply increased over the past several decades as a result of the demands for ever-greater productivity per worker (Robinson and Godbey 1997; Schor 1992). Just as the transition from an agricultural to an industrial economy involved as much hardship as potential gains, the transition in our time to an information and service economy affects workers at all levels of society, and such transitions involve human tolls not just gains. At the bottom of the occupational hierarchy, workers are being displaced from good-paying manufacturing jobs to lower pay, nonunion jobs in the service sector; at the top rungs of the occupational hierarchy, trained workers in the high-tech computer and telecommunications industries hold down jobs that absorb great amounts of time and energy against ever-shorter deadlines, leaving little time for other domains of life.

A second neglected factor in the contemporary debate about American civic and social responsibility is the consequences that flow from the rapid increase in labor force participation of women over the past several decades. Women rarely move in and out of the workplace today, as they did in the past while rearing young children: with only one or two children and short maternity leaves after each birth, most women today have work histories increasingly more like those of men. Co-breadwinning is the most prevalent pattern in American families. Further, more women work full time just as their husbands do, and increasing numbers work in occupations with high demands on time and energy. Time is one of the most precious commodities in the lives of both women and men. Is it any wonder that priorities center on work and family obligations, or surprising that after exhausting days there is little energy or motivation left for attending community meetings or formal get-togethers with friends and neighbors? As seen in the analysis in this chapter, what is surprising in our findings is how deeply involved most adults are in both family and community, despite the severe constraints imposed by long hours of work and commuting.

Design Considerations in the Development of the MIDUS National Survey
Earlier Work on Community Participation

Earlier studies of community involvement and participation that have been published and widely discussed in recent years have been excellent sources for tracing aggregate-level changes in voting, volunteer service, political values, and judgments of confidence in major social institutions, particularly when repeat surveys using the same questions appear in a sequence of years. A good example is provided by the Independent Sector on the extent of volunteer work reported by adults 18 years or older. From such reports we learn that in 1995, 93 million adults served as volunteers, a number that represents 49 percent of the adult population; that they served an average of 4.2 hours a week; that the total amount of adult volunteer time in 1995 totaled 20.3 billion hours, with a dollar value of $202 billion (Hodgkinson and Weitzman 1996). The Gallup Organization surveys over the years since 1977 show a steady increase in the proportion of adults who say they have been involved in some "charity or social service activities," from 26 percent in 1977, to 39 percent in 1987, to a high of 46 percent in 1991 (Wuthnow 1998).[3] This trend alone puts in question Putnam's thesis of widespread withdrawal from public life and neglect of communal responsibility.

Unique Advantages of the MIDUS Research Design

Such aggregate-level trend data do not inform us about who does volunteer service and who does not, or whether volunteer service varies by any individual characteristics such as sex, age, income level, or educational attainment, much less more interesting factors that compete for the time adults can contribute to volunteer service. The MacArthur Research Network on Midlife had as its major interest an understanding of individual lives, and to study, within the same individuals, such major characteristics as their health, well-being, and the social roles that define the contours of those lives on a daily basis. This required crossing the barriers among the medical, psychological, and social sciences, which led to a study design centered on three major outcome criteria: physical and mental health, psychological well-being, and social responsibility. This chapter represents a sampler of the work we have done on social responsibility. The larger work is available in the book I was privileged to edit, *Caring and Doing for Others: Social Responsibility in the Domains of Work, Family, and Community* (Rossi 2001).

A second major concern in all the research we have conducted as life-course analysts with a special concern for midlife was to collect a representative sample that permitted us to place midlife in this larger life-course context. Any analysis worth its salt is premised on a comparative method: what is unique to women cannot be established without a comparison with men. So too, this criterion required being able to compare midlife adults with adults both younger and older, and guided by the question of what, if anything, is unique to midlife, and what is similar in earlier and later phases of the life course. Hence the MIDUS survey included adults 25–74 years of age, providing us with young adults old enough to be fairly well settled into major adult roles and old adults still young enough to be healthy and active.

Many of the major social-demographic variables are interrelated, and only with a large representative sample and multivariate analysis can we assess the net effect of one variable, controlling for all others. An interesting example of this is our finding that it is not employment per se that affects the amount of time that women spend performing volunteer service but how satisfied they are with their jobs. It may come as a surprise to learn that it is women with low ratings of job satisfaction who are most likely to engage in volunteer work. A moment's reflection suggests a likely explanation for this finding: with volunteers in high demand and tasks of a very varied nature to choose among, combined with the fact that most women work in routinized clerical, retail, and factory occupations, many women seek in volunteer work the gratifications they do not experience in the work they do to support themselves and their families (reported in Rossi 2001, chap. 11). An example from my own work and volunteer experience is the contrast between a very dull routinized job I held as an adolescent in a bookbinding firm repairing thousands of school textbooks by erasing or scotch-taping page after damaged page, compared with the intense gratification I experienced serving as a volunteer in a community library reading stories to young children.

Another advantage of the multidimensional content of the MIDUS survey is the delightful surprise of serendipitous discoveries, which is more likely to occur in studies designed by researchers from diverse fields. A good example of this was the inclusion in MIDUS by my medical colleagues of a scale on sensitivity to internal body sensations (known as somatic amplification), familiar to medical and psychiatric researchers concerned with chronic diseases but a construct I was not familiar with. Yet the scale turned out to be a major predictor of elevated menopausal symptoms, a variable not previously considered in research on menstrual and menopausal discomfort and pain. It was also of interest to learn that women show higher scores on this scale than men do, which no doubt reflects women's many years of experiencing cyclic changes of body sensation and mood associated with the female menstrual cycle. Another example of serendipity stemmed from having comparable measures of normative obligations to family and community: midlife has long been associated with a peaking of multiple role responsibilities, but in a broader life-course framework we found that during midlife, as family responsibilities decline, civic obligations and participation increase, suggesting that midlife is a watershed period of significant change from being turned inward to private family affairs to turning outward to more public involvement. This is strikingly the case for better-educated midlife adults but less so for the less well educated, who tend to remain within the confines of family and parish or congregation throughout their lives.

The Life Domains Covered in the Module on Social Responsibility

A major decision guiding the design of the module on social responsibility in the 1995 national survey flowed from our conviction that little was to be gained by following in the footsteps of earlier work in sociology and political science that focused narrowly on research on voluntary associations and political participation, the two dimensions on which the contemporary dialogue about the decline of social and community cohesion has concentrated. The level of felt obligation and actual behavior as responsible adults cannot be judged merely in terms of voting behavior or community participation. The most vital roles adults fulfill are those involving the two primary functions of providing goods and services for self and others, and bearing and rearing the young. From this perspective, work and family roles are of equal if not greater significance than any roles adults play in the larger community because they assure the maintenance and continuity of society and of the human species itself.

A very special focus in approaching the design of modules on family roles is of particular importance. Almost all the criticism about family "breakdown" is premised on a narrow conception of family; marriage and divorce rates, cohabitation, and out-of-wedlock birth rates all refer only to adults as married or cohabiting partners, and as mothers or fathers. This neglects the fact that throughout the human life span we live a "three-generational life." That is, the emotional and social life for most people is lived out within such three-generation units, which change in composition as each generation moves from one stage of life to the next, from the youngest of three generations in childhood, to the middle or "sandwich" generation in midlife, to the elderly stratum in old age, when grown children and grandchildren round out the three-generational kindred (Riley, Abeles, and Teitelbaum 1982; Riley and Riley 1993, 1994). Hence, in the design of the survey instruments, our concern was not merely with the marital and parental roles of our subjects but also with their obligations, interaction, and support to adult children and siblings, parents, in-laws, grandchildren, and other kin.

If one thinks of the age pyramid used by demographers to describe the age and sex distribution of the U.S. population, today's distribution is not that of a pyramid but of a slim tall beanpole, as compared with the squat, wide-bottomed triangle of the age pyramid earlier in the last century, in which there were many more young children at the base than elderly adults at the top. In human contact terms, this means that as family size has declined from four or more children to one or two in each generation, with each generation living longer, adults may have fewer siblings, cousins, aunts and uncles compared with adults in the past, but they have a much enlarged kindred composed of as many as four or five generations of older or younger kinfolk, depending on their generational position. Let a crisis strike in the life of a young or old member of such kindreds and a wide array of concerned relatives are available to provide social and emotional support. Studies repeatedly show that family members provide 70 percent to 80 percent of long-term care to the elderly (Stone, Cafferata, and Sangl 1987). As hospital stays have been severely curtailed and outpatient care more common, much caregiving of convalescent young and middle-aged individuals is also provided by family members—spouses, adult children, and parents (Fisher and Tronto 1990). For young people, the presence of relatives two or three generations older is an important new source for acquiring a deeper understanding of what lies ahead in their own lives: all the trials and joys confronted by a grandparent or great grandparent become known within intimate relationships that reach the heart in a way not matched by any amount of reading about the "problems of the elderly" or political debates about prescription drugs and Social Security policies.

The Dimensions Measured in the Domains of Family, Work, and Community

After we decided to give major attention to the three domains of work, family, and community, our next question was what about each of these domains shall we investigate, and to what extent can we develop measures that are appropriate to and preferably equivalent on all three of these domains? The very differences among the three domains impose limitations on the development of equivalent measures, because these domains vary in the degree to which there are restraints on individual choice and preference. What one does on a job is in large measure determined not by employees but by employers: tasks, hours, and one's co-workers tend to be givens, not subject to choice by workers beyond the selection of one job over another. The higher the qualifications of a job applicant, the greater the latitude of job choice; an adult with limited training or skills has very little choice, often no greater than choosing between working for MacDonald's or Taco Bell.

By contrast, in the domain of community participation, volunteers find great leeway in choice: we can join and participate in clubs, organizations, and political parties congenial to our own preferences, interests, and skills. No one is forced to work as a volunteer, and one can choose the kind of setting of interest to us, whether a hospital, church, cub scouts, parent-teacher organization, or political party.

When contributing to individuals and groups, people find that the domain of family falls between work and community in the latitude of choice. Feelings of indebtedness and obligation are internalized, while we are growing up, toward parents, siblings, and close kin. As we know, the occasions of family gatherings may not be all fun and games; many of us bring ambivalent feelings to such occasions. But let a serious crisis develop or a special celebratory event be announced, and family members rally around. By contrast, the frequency with which we phone or e-mail family members and the extent to which we provide them with social and emotional support have a higher quotient of preference over obligation. I attended the weddings of both my siblings, but I had very frequent contact with my brother and very little contact with my sister.[4]

Our decision in the design of the social responsibility module in MIDUS was to measure the degree of obligation adults feel in all three domains. Social norms where work and family are concerned are assumed to be laid down during youth, in part from parental modeling of a work ethic and childrearing values, to say nothing of the numerous occasions during which children observe their parents interacting with relatives. Children pick up subtle cues from their parents to differences in feelings toward kin of various degrees of relatedness; to a surprising extent, those differences are retained in adulthood when respondents rank the degree of obligation they feel toward different kin as a function of degree of relatedness (Rossi and Rossi 1990). School and church contribute further to the laying down of primary social norms. For those exposed to religious beliefs at home or through religious affiliations, there are opportunities during childhood to develop deeply felt obligations toward not only family and friends but extended to the wider community and the common good. The significance of early family and religious beliefs for adult social responsibility is illustrated in this chapter, but fuller detail on how characteristics of respondents' families of origin relate to their adult norms and behavior is covered in our book on social responsibility (Rossi 2001).

Pilot surveys helped in the selection of items that yielded meaningful scales on normative obligations.[5] Norms can be measured on a very general level, independent of whether or not an individual has actually confronted the situations posed in an item. The question series was therefore prefaced with the statement "If the situation does not apply to you, please think about how much obligation you would feel if you *were* in this situation." This enabled respondents who were not in the work force to rate an item asking how much obligation they *would* feel "to work hard even if you didn't like or respect your employer or supervisor?" or for adults with only preschool children to say how much obligation they *would* feel "to call, write, or visit your adult children on a regular basis."

Whether social norms are invoked and relied on in actual behavior is subject to numerous existential circumstances not only in the lives of respondents but in those of kin and friends as well. You can feel high levels of obligation to elderly parents, but whether you see them once a week or only a few times a year depends on the geographic distance between your home and theirs, and the array of other obligations both generations carry that may preclude frequent visits. As I report later in the chapter, poorly educated adults tend to give of their time and social support to family members more than well-educated adults do, who rely to a greater extent on financial assistance in helping other family members. This contrast by education or social class is to a large extent a reflection of the greater geographic scope of the labor market for the highly educated.

Implicit in these illustrations is the fact that we focused on two types of behavioral measures in designing the dimensions of family and community domains that we would cover; one measure was of time, the other of financial contributions. Hence, we asked about the amount of time given to family, close friends, and kin, as measured by how many hours per month a respondent provided hands-on assistance (e.g., help around the house, transportation, or child are) and how many hours per month he or she spent giving informal emotional support (e.g., comforting, listening to problems, or giving advice) to spouse, parents, in-laws, children or grandchildren, or any other family members or close friends. Summary scores on time given over to caregiving and emotional support are the two behavioral measures in the family domain used in the empirical analysis reported in this chapter.

The analogue in the community domain are two measures of time contributions: the hours per month devoted to doing formal volunteer work (summed across specified types of volunteer work: health-related, school or youth-related, political organizations or causes, and any other), and the times per month respondents attended a variety of meetings (religious groups, unions or professional groups, sports or social groups, or any other group, excluding those required by their jobs).

The second major type of behavioral measure in MIDUS consists of estimates of the amount of money that respondents contributed to the same array of specified family members in the family domain, and in the community domain, the estimated amount of money that respondents contributed to religious groups, political organizations or causes, or any other organizations, causes, or charities (including donations made through monthly payroll deductions).

In the work domain, clearly we only get *from*, we do not give money *to* our employers, and our time is largely determined by job requirements, not our own preferences. For the dimensions analyzed in the work domain, therefore, we rely on normative obligations to work, the reported amount of personal earnings, hours spent at work plus commuting between home and workplace, and what hours of the day and/or night respondents typically spent on the job. A variety of additional measures were included in the instrument, such as the degree of stress at work and at home, and the extent of positive and negative spillover between work and family, but these variables are not included in the analysis reported in this overview chapter on the social-demographic patterning of social responsibility; they are dealt with in detail in the volume on social responsibility (Rossi 2001).

In this chapter I show age trends in normative obligations to family and community, and use characteristics of the jobs that respondents held as control variables, constraining the time available for either help to family members or participation in the larger community.

DESCRIPTIVE OVERVIEW OF SOCIAL RESPONSIBILITY MEASURES

Table 1 provides specific descriptions of the measures of responsibility discussed in the previous section. These scores, scales, and ratings are itemized in the table by domain, dimension, and name of the actual measures, with illustrative items on each. As noted in the column titled "Descriptive Detail," all three normative obligation scales (family obligation, civic obligation, and altruism) have good reliability (alphas from .78 to .82) and considerable variation in scale range. The family obligation scale refers to degree of obligation to family members and close friends; the civic obligation scale refers to civic and political obligations.

TABLE 1 Domains and Dimensions Tapped by Major Social
Responsibility Measures

Domain	Dimension	Measures	Descriptive Detail
Family	Time	Hands-on care	Summated score of hours per month providing unpaid assistance (help around the house, transportation, child care) to four types of recipients: parents, in-laws, children/grandchildren, other family or close friends.
		Emotional/social support	Summated score of hours per month providing emotional support (comforting, listening to, advising) to five types of recipients: spouse, parents, in-laws, children/grandchildren, other family or close friends.
	Money	Family financial help	Summated score of dollars per month that respondents, or family living with them, contribute (including dollar value of food, clothing, or other goods) to four types of recipients: parents, in-laws, grandchildren, other family members or close friends.
	Norms	Family obligations	Eight-item scale of 11-point ratings of degree of obligation felt toward children, parents, spouse, friends, from $0 =$ No obligation to $10 =$ Very great obligation, (0–80 scale range, alpha $= .82$, mean $= 60$, $\text{SD} = 13.2$).
Community	Time	Volunteer work	Summated score of hours per month doing volunteer work to four types of organizations/causes: hospital/health related, school/youth related, political organization/causes, other organizations/causes/charities.
		Meeting attendance	Summated score of number of meetings attended involving four groups: religious groups, unions or other professional groups, sports or social groups, any other groups (not required by job).
	Money	Amount of public contribution	Summated score of dollars per month contributed to three types: religious groups, political organizations/causes, other organizations/causes or charity.
	Norms	Civic obligation	Four-item scale of 11-point ratings of degree of obligation felt toward civic participation, e.g., "to serve on a jury if called" or "to vote in local and national elections" (0–40 scale range, alpha $= .78$, mean $= 30.7$, $\text{SD} = 7.8$).
		Altruism	Four-item scale of 11-point ratings of degree of obligation felt in situations involving helping others at expense to self, e.g., "to pay more for your health care so that everyone had access to health care" (0–40 scale range, alpha $= .80$, mean $= 23.4$, $\text{SD} = 8.9$).
Overall Self-rating		Contributions to others	Single-item rating of contribution to welfare and well-being of other people, 11-point rating from 0 (worst) to 10 (best).

The altruism scale differs from the civic scale by referring to obligations to be helpful to others but at some expense to oneself.[6] The last measure in table 1 is an overall self-rating of the extent to which respondents felt they contributed to the welfare and well-being of "others" (who are not specified in terms of life domain).

Table 2 shows the matrix of correlation coefficients between all pairs of these ten measures of social responsibility, organized to distinguish between the four family variables (shown in the upper left triangle) and the five community variables (shown in the lower right triangle). Of the 36 coefficients in this matrix, 5 do not reach statistical significance, and 15 show significant but low correlations ($<.10$); only 5 coefficients are $>.20$, with 5 of them $>.30$. Closer inspection suggests several points of substantive interest:

1. The highest correlation in the matrix (.48) is between hands-on caregiving and emotional support given in the family domain—hardly surprising in light of the fact that any caregiving activity almost invariably entails listening to and comforting the recipient of care, although it is not necessarily the case that those to whom we provide emotional support require hands-on care as well.

2. The three measures with the highest intercorrelations are the three measures of normative obligations (.36, .46, and .45), tapping a general predisposition toward helpfulness to others, with no necessary implication that such values are carried into actual behavior. Note, too, that the three highest correlations with the overall self-rating of contributions to others are precisely the three normative obligation scales (.28, .24, and .33), along with the behavioral measure of civic obligation—volunteer work (.22). In a regression analysis of the overall self-rating on contribution to others, eight of the nine normative and behavioral predictor variables make independent contributions to these self-ratings (data not shown). Interestingly, the single exception is frequency of meeting attendance, perhaps because the motivation for such participation may be grounded as much in self-interest and promotion as in concern for the welfare of others, for example, local businessmen and lawyers who find organizational meetings a good opportunity to cultivate contact with potential customers and clients.

3. Normative obligations and social behavior are only modestly correlated, and only within domains, with correlations only ranging from .08 to .14 in the family domain, and slightly higher in the community domain (.09 to .19). Norms indicate predispositions to help or participate: in family interaction, existential circumstances of donor and recipient

TABLE 2 Correlation Coefficients between Social Responsibility Measures

Measures	Family				Community					
	1	2	3	4	5	6	7	8	9	10
Family										
1. Hands-on care	—									
2. Emotional support	.48	—								
3. Financial help	.13	.13	—							
4. Family obligations	.18	.14	.08	—						
Community										
5. Volunteer work	.02	.07	.08	.08	—					
6. Meeting attendance	.02	.04	.08	.05	.35	—				
7. Financial contribution	−.03	−.02	.18	.05	.24	.21	—			
8. Civic obligations	−.02	−.02	.05	.36	.13	.11	14	—		
9. Altruism	.04	.04	.07	.46	.19	.12	.09	.45	—	
Overall Self-rating										
10. Contribution to others	.09	.10	.11	.28	.22	.11	.14	.24	.33	—

Note: Underlined coefficients are not statistically significant; all others are significant at $p < .05$ to $p < .001$.

dictate whether such norms are acted upon or not; in the community domain, as-yet-unspecified characteristics of respondents' life circumstances are critical factors in giving time or money, independent of normative predispositions to do so. In research on volunteerism, the major reasons given for not doing volunteer work was "lack of time" and "no one asked me to help" (Verba, Schlozman, and Brady 1995; Wilson and Musick 1999).

4. Among the behavioral measures themselves (highlighted by enclosure in the rectangle to the bottom left of table 2), only one of the nine coefficients is above .10: those who contribute financial aid to family members are also somewhat predisposed to contribute money to community organizations and charities ($r = .18$). As we see in the section to follow, money contributions are far more dependent on educational attainment and financial resources than are caregiving or providing informal emotional support.

The overall profile projected by the correlation matrix implies that our major construct—social responsibility—is highly differentiated by both domain of life and dimension of expression. I assume that general normative obligations are rooted in early socialization, whereas behavioral manifestations of social responsibility are more affected by the circumstances in the individual lives of our respondents, their immediate families, relatives, and friends, and the time and resource constraints imposed by job requirements.

TABLE 3 Regressions of Behavioral Measures of Social Responsibility or

Predictor Variables	Family Domain		
	Hands-on Care	Emotional Support/ Advice	Financia Contributi
Age	−.777***	−.250***	.064**
Sex[a]	.058**	.149***	−.017
Resources			
Education	−.086***	−.090***	.042*
Household income	−.012	−.024	.211***
Constraints			
Hours worked per week	−.027	−.004	.038
Family status			
Marital status[b]	.008	.168***	−.063***
Number of children	.111***	.114**	.116***
R^2	.032***	.113***	.068***
N	(2845)	(2845)	(2845)

[a]Men = 1, women = 2.
[b]Married = 1, not married = 0.
*$p < .05$. **$p < .01$. ***$p < .001$.

SOCIAL DEMOGRAPHY OF SOCIAL RESPONSIBILITY

I begin the analysis of what predicts level of social responsibility with attention to those characteristics that have the greatest relevance to an individual's predisposition and ability to be of help to others in the family network and to be involved in the larger community. In keeping with the priority given to age and sex in all our research network analysis, these two social-demographic characteristics top the array of major predictors. From earlier research on help exchange among family members, we expect women to play a greater role in caregiving and emotional support, and men in providing financial assistance to family members, but it is not known if this same distinction holds for women's and men's involvement with the community. Marriage and parenthood enlarge the kinship network and intensify both personal desire for and social pressure toward greater involvement with both kin and local organizations in the community (O'Donnell 1983; Rossi and Rossi 1990).

In addition, status position is an expected determinant of the amount of time and financial contributions an individual makes to kin and community. Educational attainment itself is a gateway to higher social status in a community, leading to higher earnings and both a predisposition and ocial-Demographic Characteristics (standardized beta coefficients)

	Community Domain	
1eetings ttended	Volunteer Time	Financial Contribution
020	−.008	.092***
018	.047*	−.020
,159***	.158***	.162***
021	.014	.210***
010	−.070**	−.035
011	.051**	.068***
018	.073***	.037***
,030***	.036***	.117***
(2866)	(2866)	(2866)

general social expectation that an individual will contribute to charitable causes and community organizations. Adults today also vary greatly in their time commitments to their jobs. Few professionals and executives work a thirty-five- or forty-hour week; more typical for top professionals is a workweek that approximates the sixty-hour workweek of nineteenth-century factory workers. The variables entered into the regression equations in table 3 therefore include family status (married or not, and number of children), resources (education, household income), constraints (hours worked per week), and our major variables of age and sex.

Table 3 shows several significant differences in the pattern of predictors by both domain and dimension of social responsibility, as follows.

1. *Age.* Age is a significant predictor of socially responsible behavior. The largest single standardized beta coefficient shown in table 3 is the negative relationship between age and giving care and emotional support to family members and friends ($-.777$ and $-.250$, significant at $p < .001$): young adults are very much more active in this regard than older adults. This is less surprising than it might seem at first sight, because young adults not only give more caregiving and emotional support than older adults do but they also get more such help from family and friends. In identical equations that predict receiving emotional support, the standardized beta coefficient of age is also negative ($-.172$) (data not shown).

Thus in personal support involving time contributions in the family domain, reciprocity rules: those who give help to others also get help from others. This is not the case when comparing giving with receiving financial help. Whereas table 3 shows that older adults give more money than younger adults do (.064, significant at $p < .001$), analysis of the amount of money received from others shows a negative sign on age ($-.172$): older adults give financial support; young adults get financial help from family members.

2. *Time versus money contributions.* This difference is most sharply shown in the family domain: those who are most likely to provide hands-on care and emotional support to others are less well-educated, married, young, and women, whereas those contributing financial aid to family members are better-educated, high-income, older, unmarried adults.

Major predictors of time and money contributions are less sharply differentiated in the community domain: the major predictors of *both* time and money are high education, marriage, and having a number of children. Predictors of volunteer service are somewhat different: women, those who are either not employed or put in fewer hours on the job, are more likely to contribute more time to volunteer service.

From the larger perspective of social structure, note how different the interpretation of social responsibility would be if we were analyzing only community-level participation as the exclusive domain of social responsibility, which would suggest that well-educated, high-income married adults are the most socially responsible members of the community. Such an interpretation is clearly qualified by the very different profile shown for socially responsible behavior in the family domain, in which it is the less well-educated, low-income, young adults who report higher levels of personal caregiving and emotional support than do well-educated, high-income adults. This pattern was a long-familiar one to me; for many years my high-school-graduate brother and his wife were the major caregivers to our mother in her declining years, while I, many hundreds of miles away, consoled myself with a weekly note and an occasional check.

Normative Precursors of Socially Responsible Behavior in Adulthood

The social-demographic variables in the analysis to this point provide only a bare-bones profile of what prompts socially responsible behavior, focusing largely on current family and status characteristics. Human motivation draws on many longstanding values and personality

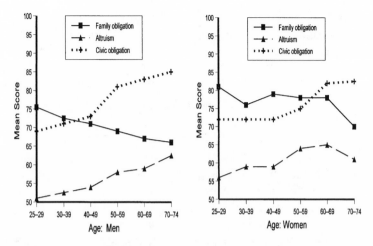

FIGURE 1. Normative obligations by domain, age, and sex (means are converted to a 0–100 range). All age trends are significant at a $p < .01$ or $p < .001$ level. Women scored significantly higher than men on family obligation and altruism, but sex differences on civic obligation scale are not significant.

predispositions not captured by demographic variables. My next step in this analysis is to introduce the normative obligation scales discussed in the previous section and described in table 1. A detailed analysis of a developmental trajectory model, explored in depth in chapter 7 of the comprehensive volume on social responsibility (Rossi 2001), found these normative obligations to be strongly influenced by early family life, in particular the affection and discipline that respondents' parents demonstrated in their childrearing values, the stability of the family of origin, the degree to which religion was important in family life, and the extent to which the parents were models of helpfulness toward people outside the family (a measure of parental models of generativity).

Figure 1 shows the life-course trajectory of our major normative obligation scales, separately for men and women. A major pattern shown in the graphs, which holds for both men and women, is a decline in the mean ratings of obligation toward family and close friends with increasing age (the family obligation scale), and a highly significant increase in the average scores on the civic obligation and altruism scales, a pattern already noted in the relationship of age to the major behavioral measures of current time contributions to family and community in table 3. The implication is that as childrearing is completed in midlife, and fewer adults have living parents, family obligations subside whereas commitments deepen and expand to the larger world of community and to the welfare of others in need.

Interpreting Age Differences: Maturation versus Cohort

The interpretation of age differences in cross-sectional data must be approached with caution because it is difficult to disentangle cohort from maturational factors. Were we to find that scores on all three normative obligation scales increased with age, we might be tempted to explain the results as a cohort change reflecting the alienation of the young from major social institutions, consistent with the charge of social critics discussed in the introduction. But the fact that young adults espouse higher levels of obligation in the family domain puts a cohort interpretation in question, because it is precisely the family domain that has shown significant demographic change in recent decades as indexed by lower marriage and fertility rates, more cohabitation and births outside marriage, and a higher divorce rate (Bumpass 1990, 1994; Rossi 1993). Indeed, our younger MIDUS respondents themselves report much higher endorsement than older respondents of the view that neither marriage nor having children is important to living a full happy life. But note that here again the family reference is only to marriage and parenting, and that the general attitudinal perspective espoused is for most of us a world apart from the lives we prefer for ourselves; this pattern is analogous to that shown in the political domain, in the frequency with which citizens who hold very low expectations and distrust toward congressional politicians in general have high regard for their own representatives.

Our developmental analysis also showed significant influences of two characteristics of the family of origin that are relevant to further analysis of social responsibility. We asked respondents to rate the extent to which each of their parents showed generosity, helpfulness, and sociability in their relations with people outside their family. This was our effort to measure parents as generativity models, on the hypothesis that such parental modeling would be a significant precursor of the respondent's own development of generativity. Our generativity scale is a modified version of the Loyola generativity scale (McAdams and de St. Aubin 1992) and measures the extent to which adults report that they are sought out for advice, that other people need them, that they have made unique contributions to society, and that they have had a good influence on the lives of many people.

The second important early family characteristic is the extent to which religion was salient in the family in which respondents grew up.[7] Figure 2 shows graphically, the relationship of both measures—religiosity and generativity—to age, separately by sex. For both men and women, religiosity shows a highly significant linear increase over the life course. By contrast, the age profile on generativity shows a peaking in the middle years. The generativity pattern is consistent with Erikson's life-stage developmental task theory, that is, generativity develops with maturity: as skills are acquired, self-confidence builds, particularly but not necessarily through childrearing, and through many occupations such as teaching, counseling, or social work, or through volunteer work to improve the quality of life for future generations (de St. Aubin and McAdams 1995; Erikson 1963, 1964; Ryff and Heincke 1983; Vaillant 1993). It is not clear why generativity declines in old age. One possibility is that in Western societies, the elderly experience either a loss of respected status or their skills are no longer relevant to the young. By contrast, in non-Western societies, the elderly have historically not lost but gained status as major sources of wisdom worthy of high respect, with the result that generativity in such societies may show the same positive linear increase with age that religiosity has. My colleague Carol Ryff suggests that, as Erikson might argue, the later age decline in generativity reflects moving to other developmental tasks, in particular ego integrity. This interpretation is clearly in keeping with a maturational interpretation of the age pattern shown on generativity.

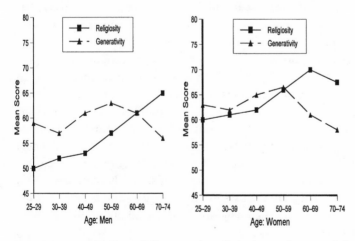

FIGURE 2. Age and sex differences in religiosity and generativity (means converted to a 0–100 range).

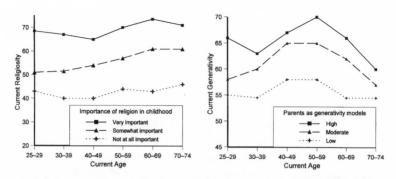

FIGURE 3. Age differences in current religiosity and generativity, by comparable characteristics of parents and family of origin (means converted to a 0–100 range).

But what of the pattern shown for religiosity? Many scholars claim that the lower level of religiosity of young adults compared with that of older adults reflects historic change away from religious values (a cohort interpretation) rather than maturational change, that is, older adults become more religious as they age. Andrew Greeley (1995) has provided evidence in favor of a maturational interpretation, showing that when cohorts are followed through the life cycle and measured for church attendance and prayer frequency, such indicators of religiosity did not vary once age was taken into account. Whether surveyed in the 1980s or the 1930s, older adults were more apt to attend church and to pray more frequently than young adults. In fact, frequency of prayer has actually increased, according to a comparison of surveys that had been conducted in the 1980s and the 1930s.[8]

Additional support for a maturational interpretation of the age profile shown in figure 2 can be seen by relating the early family markers of generativity and religiosity to the current ratings of MIDUS respondents, also by age and sex. Figure 3 shows the age profile of current values by three levels of early family religious importance and by three comparable levels of parental generativity. Note, first of all, the high degree to which there is cross-generational continuity on both measures: at any age, respondents from highly religious backgrounds, or whose parents rated high on generativity, are themselves more religious and generative than those from families in which religion was not at all important or whose parents were low in generativity.

Second, the same age profile is found within each of the three levels of early family religiosity or parental generativity: religiosity increases

significantly with age, whereas generativity peaks in midlife.[9] A maturational interpretation of age differences in religiosity is further supported
by our finding that women are currently much more religious than men,
although the sexes do not differ in the importance of religion in their families of origin, suggesting a greater upturn in religiosity among women
during their lifetime than among men. It is also of interest that early family religiosity has no significant correlation with generativity for adults
under 40 years of age but that it turns increasingly significant from early
midlife on. This pattern implies a sleeper effect of early exposure to
religious values and beliefs, re-activated during the middle years by increased concern for the welfare of others, a midlife transition consistent
with the shift from higher emphasis on family rather than civic obligations in early adulthood to higher emphasis on civic rather than family
obligations during mid and late adulthood, as shown earlier in figure 1.

Cross-sectional data do not allow a definitive interpretation, but from
what special analyses we have performed, and in light of the fact that
comparable age differences were found in a study of intergenerational
relations in data gathered a decade before the MIDUS survey, in the
mid-1980s (Rossi and Rossi 1990), we conclude that the age differences
reported in this chapter are essentially maturational in nature.

The Relationship of Generativity and Religiosity to Major Social Responsibility Measures

To round out this discussion of generativity and religiosity and pave the
way for the next step in the multivariate analysis of social responsibility,
table 4 shows the correlation coefficients of religiosity and generativity to
each of the ten major measures of social responsibility. Included as well is
a measure of frequency of religious service attendance. The reason for the
inclusion of the latter is that earlier analysis showed actual participation
in religious services was more important than religiosity in an analysis of
community participation. One can hold strong religious beliefs without
involvement in congregations or parishes; actual attendance provides
occasions for interaction with others who share one's faith—neighbors,
friends, acquaintances. Beliefs can be held close to the heart; church
attendance provides access to extended networks of others.

All but seven of the thirty coefficients in the matrix shown in table 4
are statistically significant. Substantively, however, most of the correlations are modest. Fifteen fall within the range of .09 and .20; six between
.21 and .30; only two above .30. Generativity shows the highest correlation with the self-rating of overall contribution to others (.43), hardly

TABLE 4 Correlation Coefficients between Social Responsibility Measures and Generativity, Religiosity and Religious Attendance

Domain	Dimension	Generativity	Religiosity	Religious Attendance
Family				
	Hands-on care	.05	<u>.04</u>	−<u>.00</u>
	Emotional/social support	.09	<u>.01</u>	−<u>.01</u>
	Financial assistance	.11	<u>.02</u>	<u>.01</u>
	Family obligation	.22	.12	.10
Community				
	Volunteer work	.21	.13	.20
	Meeting attendance	.19	.15	.25
	Financial contribution	.14	.27	.35
	Civic obligation	.22	.16	.16
	Altruism	.23	.18	.13
Overall self-rating on helping others		.43	.14	.13

Note: All correlations are significant except those underlined.

surprising because both measures share some common features. That the correlation is not higher is, we believe, due to the fact that the overall self-rating is an assessment based on what respondents are currently doing for others, as measured by all the more specific ratings in the battery of responsibility measures, whereas generativity is more likely to be a predisposition rooted in early family life and reinforced by the gradual development of confidence and experience between early and mid life.

The major contrast between religiosity and religious attendance is shown by the higher correlations between attendance and giving time and money in the community domain than is shown for religiosity, illustrating the point suggested earlier in the section, that actual church attendance opens opportunities, and perhaps introduces some social pressure, to participate in church and community-related projects quite apart from religious services themselves. As Olasky (1996) and Wuthnow (1991, 1994) have noted, many churches today are settings for all manner of activities and projects only peripherally related to the specific theology of a church, with child care and homeless centers, food distribution projects, and mentoring of youngsters high among them.

AN EXPANDED MULTIVARIATE ANALYSIS OF SOCIAL RESPONSIBILITY

We are now in a position to greatly expand the multivariate analysis of what determines the level of responsible behavior in the domains of

TABLE 5 Regressions of Time and Money Contributions
in the Family Domain (standardized beta coefficients)

Predictor Variables	Time Contributions (hours per month of emotional/social support)	Money Contributions ($ amount per month)
Age	−.231***	.091***
Sex	.124***	−.052**
Resources		
Education	−.094***	.038*
Total household income	−.030	.209***
Constraints		
Hours per week on job	−.015	.028
Physical health rating[a]	−.016	−.011
Normative predispositions		
Family obligations	.061***	.089***
Generativity	.088***	.067***
Social embeddedness		
Marital status	.174***	−.059***
Number of children	.093***	.091***
Frequency contact with kin	.086***	.125***
Positive regard of ego by kin	.032	−.074***
Frequency religious attendance	−.041*	−.023
R^2	.133***	.099***
N	(2845)	(2845)

[a]Single-item rating of health: poor = 1 to excellent = 5.
*$p < .05$. **$p < .01$. ***$p < .001$.

family and community, from the narrowly social-demographic analysis reported in table 2 to an enlarged set of variables, including normative obligations, generativity, and religious attendance. In addition, I round out the family measures with the frequency of contact with relatives and the extent to which relatives react to respondents in a positive or critical way. (In regressions in the community domain, I include frequency of contact with friends rather than relatives as the more appropriate network measure.) Also included are self-ratings of physical health to test whether poor health constitutes a restraint on helpful behavior. To simplify this expanded analysis, we confine attention to one measure each of time and money contributions in the two domains: emotional support and financial assistance in the family domain, volunteer work and financial contributions in the community domain. Tables 5 and 6 report the results in detail. Table 7 summarizes the significant results from both previous

TABLE 6 Regressions of Time and Money Contributions in the
Community Domain (standardized coefficients)

Predictor Variables	Time Contribution (hours per month of volunteer work)	Money Contribution ($ amount per month to organizations/charities)
Age	−.038	.047*
Sex	.002	−.062***
Resources		
Education	.113***	.114***
Total household income	.014	.226***
Constraints		
Hours per week on job	−.081***	−.032
Hours of hands-on caregiving	.008	−.003
Physical health rating	−.010	−.001
Normative predispositions		
Civic obligation	.001	.020
Altruism	.126***	.026
Generativity	.124***	.040*
Social embeddedness		
Marital status	.054**	.040*
Number of children	.058**	.020
Frequency contact with friends	.094***	.049***
Frequency religious attendance	.140***	.323***
R^2	.118***	.235***
N	(2866)	(2866)

$*p < .05.$ $**p < .01.$ $***p < .001.$

TABLE 7 Significant Predictors of Social Responsibility by Domain
and Dimension (as reported in tables 5 and 6)

DOMAIN OF CONTRIBUTION	DIMENSION OF CONTRIBUTION		
	Only Time	Both Time and Money	Only Money
Only family	Low-educated Women Low religious attendance	High family obligation Large no. of children High contact with kin	High-educated Not married Kin critical of ego
Both family and community	Married Large no. children	HIGH GENERATIVITY	Old High income Men
Only community	High altruism Low hours work	Married High contact with friends High religious attendance High-educated	

tables, viewed together to pinpoint the variables that significantly predict one or both domains of social responsibility (family and community) and one or both dimensions of social responsibility (time and money).

With the additional predictor variables added to the array of social-demographic variables, the amount of explained variance is increased (as indexed by the larger R^2's in all four equations in tables 5 and 6, compared with those shown previously, in table 3). There is no significant change in the direction of effect or statistical significance of the social-demographic predictors; hence we restrict discussion of these tables to the effect of the new variables, as follows:

1. The most striking finding is that the generativity scale is a significant predictor of all four dependent variables: the higher the score on generativity, the greater the likelihood that adults provide time and money to both the family and the community. As highlighted in table 7, generativity stands alone in this regard.

2. Normative obligation scales are tailored to one or the other of the two domains. Table 5 shows that the family obligation scale predicts time and money contributions to family members. Table 6 shows that high scores on the altruism scale are stimulants for volunteer work, although not significantly so for financial contributions to organizations and charities. By contrast, the civic obligation scale contributes nothing independent of the more general altruism measure, perhaps because the items in the civic obligation scale refer to such things as voting and jury service rather than volunteer work in youth or health-related organizations, the major types of service in the four-item score on volunteer work.

3. Physical health has no significant effect as a constraint against time or money contributions in either domain, although the sign is negative in all four equations. To some extent this reflects the overall skewness of the health self-rating: very few MIDUS respondents report being in poor health; most report good to excellent health. Very seriously ill adults, especially ones in a hospital or convalescent facility, or at home but too ill to participate, would not be in the pool of likely respondents to a survey. The negative sign on the health measure in the regression equations does not mean sick people are high volunteers. There is hardly any difference in volunteer rate between those rating their health as good, very good, or excellent: some 46 percent of all those in the three top categories of health report doing some volunteer work (compared with only 23 percent among those with "poor" health ratings).

What does stand out is the finding that the amount of time devoted to volunteer work is highest among those reporting only "fair" health.

Why should this be? One possibility is that those in very good or excellent health may prefer to spend their leisure hours in more active pursuits, such as jogging, tennis, or golf, rather than in the more sedentary activities of most volunteer work in hospitals, schools, or political groups. Consistent with this interpretation is that we find a linear increase in the amount of vigorous exercise that respondents engage in: a gradual increment in average exercise score from 11 (on a scale range of 4–24) among those in poor health to a high of 20 among those in very good or excellent health.[10] In light of the time bind so many adults experience today, it may well be that an increasing proportion of adults give priority to their own participation in exercise and athletic regimens over time devoted to volunteer service. It remains for future research to establish whether this is an instance of the midlife watershed transition discussed above, involving some shifting from vigorous activity in leisure time to more sedentary service in community organizations and projects.

4. Religious attendance shows a strong effect, but only in the community domain: the more frequent such attendance, the greater the extent of volunteer service, and even more so, the greater the financial contributions to organizations and charities. Indeed, religious attendance has the largest net effect on financial contributions (beta coefficient of .323, significant at the $p < .001$ level) of all the predictors in this regard. As noted earlier, our six-item scale on religiosity contributed only modestly to community service, suggesting that it is actual social participation at services and social interaction with parishioners that stimulate adults to contribute time and money to organizations and charities, rather than religiosity per se. There are echoes in these results of a finding by Wilson and Musick (1999) on persistence in volunteer service over a three-year time span; they found that it was church attendance and not religiosity that predicted such volunteer persistence from first to second contact with survey respondents.

The finding that low religious attendance is associated with providing more emotional support to family members is at first sight surprising, and we can offer only a possible explanation for this finding; it is not something we can pursue with other variables in our MIDUS data set. Our untested hypothesis is that adults who are deeply religious and involved in church affairs can draw on their faith to help them through life's crises, whereas those without such anchoring in faith are more likely to come from families like their own, and therefore both seek solace from and provide solace to close family members of similar low levels of faith. This is premised on the view that religious faith provides the confidence and lack of fear of death that makes it easier to survive health crises, as recent research has shown in positive surgical outcomes and survival rates when highly religious people are compared with those of little faith (Ellison and Levin 1998; Koenig et al. 1998; Ryff and Singer 2000).

5. Frequency of contact with friends may operate in much the way religious attendance does: the greater the frequency of such contact, the greater are both volunteer service and dollar contributions. It seems likely that friendships are formed in the course of volunteer work in the community, and friendship networks themselves may provide access to and motivation for volunteer service in sports or social clubs, parish, school, or health-related organizations.

6. Worth special note because it was *not* expected is the finding that respondents who report that family members have a high regard for them (that is, who care for and understand them; and with whom they can open up with personal problems) contribute not more but less money to family members. On a parallel scale measuring negative feelings toward ego (that is, kin making too many demands, getting on their nerves, or criticizing them), a comparable pattern is found: respondents reporting high criticism by members of their family give more money than those with low scores on the negative kin affect scale. This pattern may reflect reliance on money to sooth troubled kin relations, or it may involve kin with troubled personalities with whom it is difficult to get along but who nonetheless are in need of financial assistance. Examples would include a depressed hypochondriacal elderly parent or a grown child who cannot hold down a steady job or sustain an intimate peer relationship.

Table 7 helps to distill the findings from tables 5 and 6, allowing us to identify simultaneously the cluster of characteristics associated with one or both domains with the cluster of characteristics associated with one or both time and money dimensions of contributions to others. For example, the upper left of the first row of table 7 contains adults who contribute only time and only in the family domain; they tend to be low-educated, young females who rarely if ever attend religious services. By contrast, the middle cell of the last row of the table contains adults who contribute both time and money but only in the community domain, not the family; they tend to be high-educated, married adults who have frequent contact with friends and high religious attendance.

Close inspection of these profiles of net predictors of adult responsibility suggests a differentiation by both social structure and phase of the life course. Adults of low social status (indexed here by education and income) are heavy providers of emotional support to family members, as they are of hands-on caregiving as well (data not shown). If they are also married women with a number of children, they contribute time to both family and community. Their social world is densely peopled by family and kin, with infrequent excursions into the larger social world of community organizations. By contrast, it is high-income, well-educated adults who are more apt to limit their contribution in the family domain to financial assistance but provide both time and money in the community domain. Their social world extends away from the family domain to more involvement with friends, parish, and community organizations. These findings intersect nicely with the findings from qualitative analyses by Hazel Markus, Carol Ryff, Katherine Curhan, and Karen Palmersheim (chap. 10, this volume) to the effect that low-education adults define their well-being very much in terms of close proximal relationships, whereas high-education individuals define well-being in much more self-oriented terms involving personal striving and pursuit of goals as well as more concerns about society and larger world issues. This set of findings illustrates important points of convergence in analyses targeted on two of our main outcomes: social responsibility and psychological well-being.[11]

Phase of the life course is a second axis of social differentiation: the family preoccupies young people, whereas older adults show greater involvement in community affairs, a pattern shown both in the multivariate analysis reported in tables 5 and 6, and in the age trajectory of normative obligations shown earlier in figure 1. For both men and women, obligations felt toward family and close friends show a significant decline with age, whereas mean scores on both the civic obligation scale and the altruism scale show significant increases with age.

CONCLUSION

In concluding this chapter, I summarize the major findings on the social, normative, and resource pressures that predict levels of adult social responsibility in the domains of family and community, and then discuss these findings with special attention to the question of what, if anything, is unique to midlife.

Major Findings

1. Social responsibility is a multidimensional construct and social phenomenon, highly differentiated by life domain—family, work, and community—and by its major dimensions—normative obligations, time, and financial contributions. This alerts us to the caution necessary in

interpreting whether the social fabric is fragmenting or not, and whether individuals within a society are socially responsible or not, because such an assessment depends on whether we rely on a wide or a narrow range of empirical indicators of social responsibility. With a narrow range, one researcher may characterize a nonvoter as low in social responsibility, yet such a person may be a heavy provider of care to an elderly parent who restricts hours of employment in order to do so. Those who devote a great deal of time to local politics may be viewed as highly responsible by one analyst but be found wanting if such politically active adults hardly ever extend a helping hand or sympathetic ear to friends or kin. *A pluralist society seems best served by a great diversity of arenas in which adults show social responsibility tailored to their preferences and abilities.* It is because we defined social responsibility within a broad and multidimensional framework that the results of our analyses project a far more optimistic image of Americans at turn of the twenty-first century than the alarmist voices so critical of their fellow citizens that have dominated public discussion.

2. Empirical measures on each of the three domains and their major dimensions contribute independently to an adult's self-perception as someone who contributes a great deal or very little to the welfare of others. The high endorsement of normative obligations to family, work, and community that our respondents show provides a foundation for actual behavior that contributes to the well-being of others. Such norms are in part grounded in religious beliefs and in early family life, when basic personality and values are laid down. Whether adults act in conformity to their sense of obligation depends on a variety of factors: the press of job and family responsibilities, which limits the time and energy available to do well by others outside the immediate family; the needs of potential recipients for support and caregiving by others; their place on life's trajectory from early adulthood to old age; and their sex. There are also many adults in our society whom I call "frustrated altruists," people willing to give more than anyone or any organization wishes to get from them. In this connection, I think of parents more than willing to lend a hand (or send a check) to grown children unwilling to accept help as they struggle to make it on their own; or colleagues more than willing to serve as dean or department chair but who are not acceptable to others; or a neighbor frustrated because we declined his help in struggling to start a gas tiller in the garden.

3. The extent of social responsibility is strongly influenced by social structure and phase of the life course: members of the lower social strata of

society (as indexed by education and income) have higher commitments to hands-on caregiving and social support to primary-group family members and their close friends, whereas members of the higher social strata predominate in the contribution of both time and money to the larger community through a heightened sense of civic obligations, more volunteer work, and financial contributions to organizations and charities. Young adults report higher obligations to family, older adults to broader civic participation. Note, too, that well-educated members of society are more likely to be approached by representatives of community organizations to serve in some capacity in community affairs, whether personally inclined to do so or not. A poorly educated plumber, though a master of his craft, is far less likely to be recruited to serve in a community organization, chair a fund drive, or become a lay deacon of a mainstream church than a successful businessman or professional woman is. Hence social class plays an important role in who is recruited to contribute both time as a volunteer and money.

4. Sex differences remain pervasive and significant in the patterning of social responsibility. Women exceed men in caregiving and social-emotional support to family and friends, and in much of the volunteer work in youth and health-related community groups and institutions. Men exceed women in financial contributions to both family and community. There are echoes here of the distinctions drawn by Joan Tronto between caregiving as "fate" versus caregiving as "opportunity": women's roles as wives, mothers, and daughters predispose them to hands-on caregiving not merely out of personal desire but out of social expectations held by others (Tronto 1993). Men drawn to caregiving may find opportunities for social recognition in the public domain by "taking care of" others' needs in indirect ways, a role differentiation seen, for example in doctors "taking care of" patients while nurses "give care." In this view, fated direct caregiving links women to other lower-status direct providers of care—janitors, servants, slaves. Or as the saying goes, men tend to the important matters like tax policy or foreign affairs, while women attend to the needs of others in direct personal relationships. But women's acts of kindness and sacrifice are at the heart of what provides the lifeblood of continuity to any society.

What Is Unique to Midlife?

A backward look over the terrain covered in this chapter, and drawing on research reported elsewhere, suggests an interesting cluster of findings concerning several important characteristics unique to the middle years.

1. In the family domain, with childrearing largely completed during the middle years, parents undergo a significant transition in their relations with grown children, renegotiating the relationship toward a more peer-like quality that is facilitated by the child's own experience of childbearing and a new appreciation for what trials their own parents underwent in rearing them (Nydegger and Mitteness 1996). Particularly striking is the high degree of reciprocity between the generations, as indexed by the strong relationship between giving and getting social support from family members, undoubtedly facilitated by the high frequency of social contact between members of the kindred. Actual face-to-face visits may be less frequent due to the pressure of work commitments, but the phone lines buzz with frequent conversations between relatives, and as more older adults adapt to the computer and rely on e-mail, these exchanges between the generations become even more frequent and spontaneous. Whatever romantic hopes parents held for their children's future are clearly tempered by reality as adult children's abilities are tested in the job and marriage markets. But most parents are no less concerned for their children when they are grown and living independently than when they were young and members of the household. In an analysis of the problems confronting MIDUS respondents that worry them, we found a steady rise in problems that worry parents about their children the older the respondent, and hence the older the child (Rossi 2001).

2. Other analyses of MIDUS data suggest that the experience of midlife is strongly influenced by the experience of aging: the menopausal transition for women, and the onset of serious illnesses for men and their male friends, involves coming to grips with mortality and the meaning of life, which may be related to the increase in religiosity among those in the middle years. In the chapter on menopause and aging (chap. 6, this volume), I report that midlife adults are very aware of the physical changes they are undergoing in fitness, weight, physique, and energy level: many more adults report that they are "worse off" now than five years ago on these aspects of aging than report "no change" or, much less, "better now."

We can only know for sure what troubles and pleasures we experienced in the past, not whether there are calm waters or a sea of troubles ahead. For most of us, at least some portion of the middle years may be the "prime of life"; for a fortunate few, old age may yield even richer rewards. Few adults wish to be older than they are, but at the same time few wish to be adolescents again. From many points of view, midlife permits many of us to feel on top of the world, in control of our lives, and well enough pleased with what we have accomplished to seek new outlets of both self-expression and giving back to society some of what we have earned—and learned.

NOTES

1. A highly selective number of such critiques includes the following: Ehrenhalt 1995; Fukuyama 1999; Glendon and Blankenhorn 1995; Olasky 1996; Poponoe, Elshtain, and Blankenhorn 1996; Putnam 2000; Seligman 1992; Verba, Schlozman, and Brady 1995; Wilson 1993; Wolfe 1998; Wright 1994; and Wuthnow 1991, 1994. A review of this work on civil society and social responsibility can be found in chapter 1 of the author's edited volume, *Caring and Doing for Others: Social Responsibility in the Domains of Family, Work, and Community* (Rossi 2001).

2. An interested reader will find evidence of weight characteristics of respondents to the MIDUS survey in chap. 6 on menopause and aging, in this volume.

3. These levels of volunteer work are of roughly the same magnitude in the 1995 MIDUS survey, despite slight differences in the questions used and the restriction of the MIDUS sample to adults 25–74 years of age, thus excluding young adults 18–24, or older adults over 74 who were included in the Gallup surveys.

4. It is more typical to find greater intimacy, social interaction, and help exchanged between women (mother–daughter, sister–sister pairs in particular) than between men (e.g., father–son, brother–brother) or cross-sex pairs (e.g., brother–sister) (Rossi and Rossi 1990).

5. Six pilot surveys of approximately one thousand respondents were conducted in advance of launching the MIDUS survey. Data from these telephone interviews consisted largely of new measures for constructs of importance to the larger research endeavor. A major goal of these pilot surveys was to develop as small a number of items for scales of major constructs as possible, a necessity in a study covering so many domains of life. An example is provided by the pilot survey on social responsibility, in which we included thirteen items as candidates for a revised measure of generativity. Data analysis resulted in a six-item scale that explained more than 90 percent of the variance on the full thirteen-item scale. Similar procedures were followed to produce short but reliable measures of psychological well-being, mastery and control, personality, depression, and anxiety and panic attacks, among others.

6. The altruism items were expected to load on the same construct as the civic obligation items, but factor analysis identified them as a related but separate dimension.

7. Regrettably, this is a single-item rating. We did not foresee how important religiosity and religious attendance would be in our overall analysis of adult social responsibility, much less the extent to which there is a high degree of cross-generational transmission of religious values, a not uncommon oversight on the part of social science research generally. It seems likely that this neglect will be short-lived, as research increasingly shows the importance of faith not only for adult responsibility and social support networks but in contributing to health and longevity (Ellison and Levin 1998; Koenig et al. 1998; Ryff and Singer 2000).

8. Greeley (1995) reports that in the European Study of Values, "belief in life after death" increased from the 1930s to the 1990s; it is most frequently espoused by Americans (78 percent) but much less so by people of other countries, for example, the British (56 percent) and the Germans (54 percent).

9. An interesting example of the emergence of generativity in midlife was offered by Nancy Moses, who explained her career shift from managing partner of a marketing communications firm to director of a Philadelphia museum: "When I was hit by a *midlife urge to give something back to the community*, I sold my interest in the firm and dusted off my master's degree in historic museum management" (Moses 1997, A18, emphasis added).

10. Unfortunately the MIDUS survey did not contain measures on leisure-time activities or preferences apart from the exercise scales to test whether such activities compete or not with volunteer service in the community.

11. The volume on social responsibility reports some similar results in chapters by Diane Hughes and Katherine Newman, who conducted research with largely low-status black, Puerto Rican, and Dominican minority residents in New York City. A dominant finding in their research is that the entire concept of social responsibility is defined narrowly in these communities, centering on a conviction that they make their major contribution to society by doing a reasonably good job in rearing their children.

References

Bumpass, L. L. 1990. What is happening to the family? Interaction between demographic and institutional change. *Demography* 27:483–98.

———. 1994. The declining significance of marriage: Changing family life in the United States. NSFH Working Paper No. 66. Madison, Wisc.: Center for Demography and Ecology.

de St. Aubin, E., and D. P. McAdams. 1995. The relation of generative concern and generative action to personality traits, satisfaction/happiness with life, and ego development. *Journal of Adult Development* 2:99–112.

Ehrenhalt, A. 1995. *The lost city: The forgotten virtue of community in America.* New York: Basic Books.

Ellison, C. G., and J. S. Levin. 1998. The religion–health connection: Evidence, theory, and future directions. *Health Education and Behavior* 25:700–720.

Erikson, E. H. 1963. *Childhood and society.* 2d ed. New York: W. W. Norton.

———. 1964. *Insight and responsibility.* New York: W. W. Norton.

Fisher, B., and J. Tronto. 1990. Toward a feminine theory of caring. In *Circles of care: Work and identity in women's lives,* ed. E. K. Abel and M. K. Nelson, 35–62. Albany: State University of New York Press.

Friedan, B. 1963. *The feminine mystique.* New York: W. W. Norton.

Fukuyama, F. 1999. *The great disruption: Human nature and the reconstitution of social order.* New York: Free Press.

Glendon, M. A., and D. Blankenhorn, eds. 1995. *Seedbeds of virtue: Sources of competence, character, and citizenship in American society.* Landam, Md.: Madison Books.

Greeley, A. 1995. *Religion and poetry.* New Brunswick, N.J.: Transaction Publishers.

Hodgkinson, V. A., and M. S. Weitzman. 1996. *Giving and volunteering in the United States*. Washington, D.C.: The Independent Sector.

Koenig, H. G., L. K. Georg, H. J. Cohen, J. C. Hays, D. B. Larson, and D. G. Blazer. 1998. The relationship between religious activities and cigarette smoking in older adults. *Journal of Gerontology* 53A:M416–24.

McAdams, D. P., and E. de St. Aubin. 1992. A theory of generativity and its assessment through self-report, behavioral acts, and narrative themes in autobiography. *Journal of Personality and Social Psychology* 62:1003–15.

Moses, N. 1997. The nonprofit motive. *Wall Street Journal,* March 17, A18.

Nydegger, C. N., and L. S. Mitteness. 1996. Midlife: The prime of fathers. In *The parental experience in midlife*, ed. C. D. Ryff and M. Seltzer, 533–59. Chicago: University of Chicago Press.

O'Donnell, L. 1983. The social world of parents.*Marriage and Family Review* 5:9–36.

Ogburn, C. M., ed. 1934. *Recent social trends*. New York: Whittlesey House.

Olasky, M. 1996. *Renewing American compassion*. New York: Free Press.

Poponoe, D., J. B. Elshtain, and D. Blankenhorn, eds. 1996. *Promises to keep: Decline and renewal of marriage in America*. Lanham, Md.: Rowman and Littlefield.

Putnam, R. D. 1995a. Bowling alone: America's declining social capital. *Journal of Democracy* 6:65–78.

———. 1995b. Tuning in, tuning out: The strange disappearance of social capital in America. *PS: Political Science and Politics* 28:664–83.

———. 2000. *Bowling alone: The collapse and renewal of American community*. New York: Simon and Schuster.

Riley, M. W., R. P. Abeles, and M. S. Teitelbaum, eds. 1982. *Aging from birth to death: Sociotemporal perspectives*. AAAS Symposium, no. 79. Boulder, Colo.: Westview Press.

Riley, M. W., and J. W. Riley, Jr. 1993. Connections: Kin and cohort. In *The changing contract across generations*, ed. B. L. Bengtson and A. Achenbaum, 169–82. New York: Aldine.

———. 1994. Structural lag: Past and future. In *Age and structural lag*, ed. M. W. Riley, R. L. Kahn, and A. Foner, 15–36. New York: John Wiley.

Robinson, J. P., and G. Godbey. 1997. *Time for life: The surprising ways Americans use their time*. University Park: Pennsylvania State University Press.

Rossi, A. S. 1993. The future in the making: Recent trends in the work–family interface. *American Journal of Orthopsychiatry* 63:166–76.

———, ed. 2001.*Caring and doing for others: Social responsibility in the domains of family, work, and community*. Chicago: University of Chicago Press.

Rossi, A. S., and P. H. Rossi. 1990. *Of human bonding: Parent–child relations across the life course*. New York: Aldine de Gruyter.

Ryff, C. D., and S. G. Heincke. 1983. The subjective organization of personality in adulthood and old age. *Journal of Personality and Social Psychology* 44:807–16.

Ryff, C. D., and B. H. Singer. 2000. Biopsychosocial challenges of the new millennium. *Psychotherapy and Psychosomatics* 69:170–77.

Schor, J. B. 1992. *The overworked American: The unexpected decline in leisure*. New York: Basic Books.

Seligman, A. B. 1992. *The idea of civil society*. Princeton, N.J.: Princeton University Press.

Stone, R., G. L. Cafferata, and J. Sangl. 1987. Caregivers of the frail elderly: A national profile. *Gerontologist* 27:616–26.

Tronto, J. C. 1993. *Moral boundaries: A political argument for an ethic of care.* New York: Routledge.

Vaillant, G. E. 1993. *The wisdom of the ego.* Cambridge: Harvard University Press.

Verba, S., K. L. Schlozman, and H. E. Brady. 1995. *Voices and equality: Civic voluntarism in American politics.* Cambridge: Harvard University Press.

Wilson, J., and M. S. Musick. 1999. Attachment to volunteering. *Sociological Forum* 14:243–72.

Wilson, J. Q. 1993. *The moral sense.* New York: Free Press.

Wolfe, A. 1998. *One nation, after all.* New York: Viking.

Wright, R. 1994. *The moral animal: Why we are the way we are: The new science of evolutionary psychology.* New York: Pantheon Books.

Wuthnow, R. 1991. *Acts of compassion: Caring for others and helping ourselves.* Princeton, N.J.: Princeton University Press.

———. 1994. *Sharing the journey: Support groups and America's new quest for community.* New York: Free Press.

———. 1998. *Loose connections: Joining together in America's fragmented communities.* Cambridge: Harvard University Press.

CHAPTER TWENTY

Turning Points in Adulthood

Elaine Wethington, Ronald C. Kessler, and Joy E. Pixley

One important task of the MIDUS study was to chart the psychological landscape of adulthood, including the meaning that Americans in midlife typically assign to their everyday tasks and social roles. What can Americans expect to encounter as they enter and progress through midlife? How do middle-aged Americans knit the experiences of daily life into a coherent sense of meaning and purpose? How do middle-aged people differ from younger and older people in how they interpret their current and accumulated accomplishment in life as successes or failures?

The midlife crisis holds a remarkably dominant place in the experiences Americans expect to encounter as they age (Menon 2001). It predominates over the alternate perspective that positive development and experiences accumulate in midlife, typified by the hopeful phrase "life begins at 40" (e.g., Chiriboga 1997; Pitkin 1932). As Menon (2001) suggests, Americans dread aging and decline because of the consequent threat to their independence and control over life. The recent assertion that early adulthood is a more trying time for the average person, the so-called quarter life crisis (e.g., Robbins and Wilner 2001), has not (yet) had the same impact on the American imagination. The quarter life crisis, brought about by an overabundance of opportunities, decisions, and fateful choices, may not seem as threatening as the midlife crisis to most Americans, most particularly to the numerous and culturally dominant baby boomers.

Yet there is relatively little evidence to support the idea that most Americans experience a midlife crisis or, more generally, a universal course of life with expectable periods of crisis and stability. Brim's (1992) review of studies on midlife changes found that about 10 percent of adult males experience the period of emotional and personal turmoil called the midlife crisis, suggesting that serious emotional disturbance at midlife is not the modal experience for men (or women). Studies on self-perceived life turning points (e.g., Clausen 1995, 1998; Thurnher 1983) and general adaptation in adulthood (Vaillant 1977) also have not found self-reported psychological change and turmoil to be more common in midlife than in other periods of adulthood. Analyzing the Institute for Human Development (IHD) studies in Berkeley and Oakland, California, Clausen (1995) found that the majority of self-perceived "most important" turning points in life were reported as occurring in early adulthood, some even in adolescence and childhood. Midlife turning points were rare. In another longitudinal study of life transitions and turning points, Thurnher (1983) reported a general decline in the number of turning points reported by successively older age groups, from youth to retirement age. Thus in at least two important longitudinal samples of Americans, participants were more likely to report that emotionally significant changes took place early in life, when the groundwork was being laid for the career and relationship trajectories of adult life. Big changes of life trajectories were relatively rare in midlife.

In a previous paper (Wethington 2000), data from the MIDUS survey and one of its follow-up studies, the Psychological Turning Points (PTP) study, showed that for many Americans the term *midlife crisis* names a widely held belief about experiences thought to be prevalent in midlife. The term connotes personal turmoil and sudden changes in personal goals and lifestyle, brought about by the realization of aging. Intensive studies of self-perceived personality change in adult life (e.g., Rosenberg, Rosenberg, and Farrell 1999) suggest that the term *midlife crisis* is used by many American men as a metaphor for changes in personality and attitudes they perceive that they have undergone in their forties.

Why then do Americans focus on midlife as a time of crisis? In common lore, midlife (age 40) is a time for taking stock (Brandes 1985). Taking stock is an evaluation of how well one has met goals set earlier in life, in other words, an assessment of whether life has been a success or a failure up to this point. More recently, McAdams and colleagues (1996, 2001), in a series of research studies of how people narrate their lives, have argued that people tell stories that are representative of the meaning they give to the trajectories of their lives, and these stories, or plots, are related to culturally held ideas about expectable changes in life (as well as to events that shaped the experience of a birth cohort). The narratives tend to focus on themes of aging and development and its relationship to cultural stories, or themes. These themes represent a culturally shared meaning of life—what makes it good, and what constitutes evidence of success or failure.

Social scientists, particularly sociologists, have studied the themes of the "plots" people use to describe the meaning of their lives. Three major themes emerged from this work on the contemporary American or "Western" character. The first of those themes is work, career, and measures of economic success (Bellah et al. 1985; Keegan 1994; Swidler 1986). The second theme is the role of love and other intense emotional bonds in the calculus of maturity and a life well lived (Bellah et al. 1985; Bourdieu 1977; Swidler 1986). The third theme, which crosscuts the themes of love and work, relates to the characteristics assigned to the successful "mature" adult personality, or "character."

The themes of character that typically emerge among Americans are a sense of control over the environment, confidence to undertake new actions, independence in judgment, and self-reliance (Baumeister 1986; Bellah et al. 1985; Giddens 1991). Aging and its threat to physical control symbolically, if not in fact, pose a threat at all levels—to work and career, the maintenance of love relationships, and self-reliance (see Menon 2001). To return to Brandes (1985), his work posits that attaining the age of 40 is to reach a midpoint or peak in the power to apply new resources toward a personal goal or the attainment of maturity, with subsequent life viewed as a shortened future.

In this chapter we describe research on psychological experiences in adulthood, specifically contrasting the clinical and popular image of the midlife crisis (Rosenberg, Rosenberg, and Farrell 1999) with the concept of the turning point, defined as a significant change in the trajectory of a person's life (Clausen 1995, 1998). The chapter presents data from two national studies, collected in response to questions about both the midlife crisis and self-perceived turning points.

We address three major themes. First, we report the types of life situations that Americans describe as significant changes in the trajectories of their lives, or turning points. Second, we examine how these experiences vary across gender, age, and the life course. Third, we analyze these themes and their variations for insights into the views that American hold of what constitutes success and failure and the expectations for judging optimal performance and attaining "the good life."

Previous Studies of Life Turning Points

Clausen's study of turning points (1995) constitutes an anchor by which one can compare the experiences of succeeding generations of Americans in reflecting on the important and significant events of their lives. Clausen (1990, 2) interviewed 244 men and women aged 50–62 in

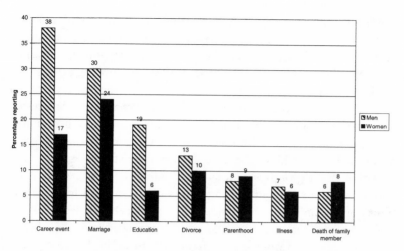

FIGURE 1. Types of life turning points ever experienced, by gender.
Source: Clausen 1990 (124 men and 144 women, aged 50–62 in 1982).

1982, asking them to "pick out any point or points along your life course that you would call 'turning points'—where your life took a different direction." Figure 1 briefly summarizes Clausen's findings. Participants were encouraged to report all of the important turning points they had experienced across their lives.

Gender differences were evident in reports of significant life experiences. Men reported turning points about career most frequently (38 percent), followed by marriage (30 percent), and education (19 percent). Women most frequently reported marriage as a turning point (24 percent), followed by career (17 percent). Most notably, nearly everyone, when reviewing life experiences from the perspective of later middle age, could report a turning point of some kind over the course of their lives, but unexpectedly most of the turning points involved events and transitions in early stages of life, not in midlife. Clausen interpreted these findings as indicating that in retrospect, participants saw decisions in early adulthood as critical for setting the subsequent course of life, and also as more significant than transitions in midlife, which participants interpreted as mostly dependent on previous decisions they had made.

Another major study of turning points, using a question very like Clausen's, reported similar gender differences in reported important turning points. The study, led by Thurnher (1983), reported data on turning points from a longitudinal study of 180 adults who had been selected to represent four major transitions in adulthood. Those four major transitions were the transition from high school to adulthood, recent marriage, departure of children from the household, and retirement. Each of the four groups contained between 43 and 48 people, with equal numbers of men and women. Eight years after first enrolling in the study, participants were asked about life situations that they now perceived as constituting important turning points. Participants had progressed through the major transitions defining adulthood and adult responsibilities, establishing a career, maintaining a stable marital relationship, having and raising children, or bringing career to a close.

Although the groups were small, the findings were suggestive. Work dominated as a source of turning points for men, in all four age–life transition groups (Thurnher 1983, table 1, p. 54). Overall, work was the most frequently nominated source of life turning points. The recently graduated group of women most frequently mentioned marriage as a life turning point, whereas the recently married group of women most frequently mentioned parenthood. For older women, work became the predominant source of life turning points. Unlike Clausen's (1990) study, Thurnher's found that parenthood was overall the second most nominated turning point (the finding was probably a result of the design of Thurnher's study, which was intended to capture the transition to parenthood). The third most nominated type of turning point involved the purchase of a home, an event not often mentioned in Clausen's study (1990) but which, on reflection, seems a major indicator of success in attaining the American dream of material comfort.

The MIDUS Studies

Following Clausen (1995, 1998), our study defines a turning point as a period or point in time in which a person has undergone a major transformation in views about the self, commitments to important relationships, or involvement in significant life roles (e.g., career, marriage, parenthood). A turning point involves a fundamental shift in the meaning, purpose, or direction of a person's life and must include a self-reflective awareness of, or insight into, the significance of the change. Major life events, life difficulties, normatively expected life transitions, and internal, subjective changes such as self-realizations or reinterpretations of past experiences may bring on a turning point. Such "triggers," as well as the turning points, may be either positive or negative in character, or both. According to Clausen's study (1998), many of the reported turning points were entirely psychological in nature, involving not so much objective change in life circumstances as a resolution or commitment to make a change. Some of these situations were relatively minor but had gained significance over time.

To explore the meanings that Americans assign to different stages of life and age, we report from two studies conducted to explore self-reported psychological change about how beliefs and self-reports about psychological change are distributed by age and gender. In the first study, data on self-perceived turning points were collected in the MIDUS national telephone sample (weighted $n = 3032$). In the second, 724 respondents were randomly selected from the same national telephone sample and interviewed more intensively about turning points. (They were also asked a series of questions about the midlife crisis.) The primary methods employed are conceptual coding and analysis of brief narratives supplied by participants in the second study, and statistical comparison of those who volunteered these narratives versus those who did not. The major questions addressed are as follows:

1. How are self-perceived psychological changes, or turning points, distributed across the life span and by gender?

2. What types of events and situations are reported as important turning points?

3. How are self-reported turning points and midlife crises related to other life events and transitions?

4. How do turning points relate to the meanings Americans derive from their lives?

Turning Points and Beliefs about the Midlife Crisis

In the MIDUS survey, respondents were asked seven questions about the occurrence of turning points in the last twelve months. The seven questions, including follow-up probes, are reported in table 1. The first six questions, modified for telephone administration, were repeated in the PTP study (see table 1). The questions about turning points were developed in three successive pilot studies (Wethington, Cooper, and Holmes 1997). Following Clausen's recommendation (1990), the aim of these questions was to study turning points in the contexts of specific life roles rather than as a general evaluation of life. (Clausen [1995] also noted that recalling turning points over the entire life course was a very difficult task for many of his respondents.) Because the course of life is influenced by the expectations of work and family roles, focusing on role-related turning points would enable us to detect shifts in the way success and failure are gauged across the life course, as was done in the Thurnher (1983) study of turning points.

TABLE 1 Turning Point Questions Used in the MIDUS and PTP Studies

Questions Used in Both Studies	Questions Used in MIDUS Only	Questions Used in PTP Only
	Introduction	
The following questions are about what we call psychological turning points. Psychological turning points are major changes in the ways people feel about an important part of their lives, such as work, family, and beliefs about themselves and the world. Turning points involve people changing their feelings about how important or meaningful some aspect of life is or how much commitment they give it.		
	Work Turning Point	
With this definition in mind, in the past 12 months (MIDUS)/last 5 years (PTP), did you have a psychological turning point that involved your job or career?	This could be an experience like increasing the amount of effort you put into your job or career, cutting back on your job to spend more time with your family, deciding to change careers, now or in the future, or leaving your job to do something different. Probe: Briefly, what happened? What impact has this had on you?	Probe: In what year did that happen? In what month? Briefly, what happened? What impact did this have on you?
	Learning Upsetting Thing about Other	
Another kind of psychological turning point involves learning something new and very important about a person close to you.	This would be things like someone close to you making a major change for the better, finding out that he or she is doing	Probes: In what year did that happen? In what month? Briefly, what happened? What impact did this have on you?

TABLE 1 *continued*

Questions Used in Both Studies	Questions Used in MIDUS Only	Questions Used in PTP Only
What these turning points have in common is the realization that this person is not the person you thought they were, either for the better or for the worse. First, in the past 12 months (MIDUS)/last 5 years (PTP), have you had a psychological turning point like this where you learned something very upsetting about a close friend or relative?	something you disapprove of strongly, or learning that he or she is a stronger person than you thought. Probes: Briefly, what happened? What impact has this had on you?	

Learning Good Thing about Other

What about the opposite situation: in the past 12 months (MIDUS)/last 5 years (PTP), did you discover that a close friend or relative was a much better person than you thought they were?	Probes: Briefly, what happened? What impact has this had on you?	Probes: In what year did that happen? In what month? Briefly, what happened? What impact did this have on you?

Learning Upsetting Thing about Oneself

Sometimes things happen that force people to learn upsetting things about themselves. This can lead to a big change in your feelings about who you are, what you stand for, and what your life is all about. Did you have a major psychological turning point like this in the past 12 months (MIDUS)/last 5 years (PTP)?	Probes: Briefly, what did you learn? What impact has learning this had on you?	Probes: In what year did that happen? In what month? Briefly, what happened? What impact did this have on you?

(continued)

593

TABLE 1 *continued*

Questions Used in Both Studies	Questions Used in MIDUS Only	Questions Used in PTP Only
Learning Good Thing about Oneself		
What about the opposite situation, discovering important good things about yourself that changed your view of who you are, what you stand for, or how you should lead your life? Did you have a major psychological turning point like this in the past 12 months (MIDUS)/last 5 years (PTP)?	Probes: Briefly, what did you learn? What impact has learning this had on you?	Probes: In what year did that happen? In what month? Briefly, what happened? What impact did this have on you?
Fulfilling a Dream		
Most people have dreams for their future. Sometimes they're realistic, sometimes not, but often they are important. During the past 12 months (MIDUS)/last 5 years (PTP), were you able to fulfill a special dream?	Probe: Briefly, what was that about?	Probes: In what year did that happen? In what month? Briefly, what was this about? What impact has this had on you?
Giving Up a Dream		
	During the past 12 months, did you give up for good on fulfilling one of your dreams? Probe: Briefly, what was that about?	

Note: Questions in the MIDUS survey asked about the past twelve months; questions in the PTP survey asked about the past five years.

The concept of *turning point* was defined in the first question. In the MIDUS survey, if a respondent checked "yes" to having one of the turning points in the past twelve months, he or she then was asked to describe what had happened and what impact it had had on him or her. Questions about turning points were asked of everyone in the sample. There were some major disadvantages to the strategy used in the MIDUS study. First, the questions were located in the self-administered portion of the study and required respondents to write descriptions of the turning point; many of the respondents' descriptions were fairly cryptic, or missing altogether. (There were particular problems with the seventh question in the series, "giving up a dream.") Second, the recall period of twelve months (rather than a lifetime) led to respondents reporting what Clausen referred to as "little" turning points, memorable events to be sure, but not likely to lead to big changes in the direction of one's life. Third, the twelve-month recall period might have been too short to allow for adequate time to have elapsed for a person to know whether an event was a turning point or not. Fourth, the questions themselves were in some cases too leading. The question about work turning points (see table 1) included examples of what were meant by turning points, and some of these examples (e.g., "leaving your job to do something different") are not necessarily major or life changing. The examples were useful for helping define what a turning point might be, but they may have in fact affected responses.

In the follow-up PTP study, we used a very different assessment strategy. To address concerns that the twelve-month recall period had been inappropriate, respondents were asked to report turning points "over the last five years." The follow-up survey was by telephone, and responses could be consistently probed by interviewers. This resulted in more detailed responses. The examples were dropped from the work turning point and other turning points questions to reduce their influence on people's responses. Finally, because of its relatively infrequent endorsement and missing data in the MIDUS study, the turning point question about "giving up a dream" (Levinson et al. 1978) was not repeated in the PTP survey. The decision was made reluctantly, but there was considerable evidence that the question did not fulfill its purpose.[1]

In the PTP survey, detailed information was coded regarding the content of self-reported turning points. (The MIDUS responses, embedded in a self-administered survey, did not yield the same quality of data as the personal interviews in the PTP survey, and thus they were not coded in the same manner.) The codes are based on a classification scheme proposed by Clausen (1995). First, this information includes the self-reported "trigger" of the experience. A trigger can be an objective event, an anticipated event, or various types of self-reflection. Up to two causes were coded as triggers. The specific coding system for triggers is based on that developed by Wethington, Brown, and Kessler for the Structured Life Event Interview (1995).

TABLE 2 Question Texts for Midlife Crisis Questions (PTP only)

1. People often use the term *midlife crisis* to describe important experiences during their middle years. What does that term mean to you?
2. At what age do you believe someone might have a midlife crisis?
3. Have you ever experienced something you would consider a midlife crisis?
4. How old were you when this happened?
5. Briefly, what was that about?

Second, the codes include perceived impacts or consequences of the experience. These are events that came about as a result of the triggering events, objective changes in roles or behavior that the respondent undertook as a consequence of the triggering events, or psychological changes.

All entries were double-coded. Discrepancies were resolved by the first author. The coding scheme required several iterations before coders could distinguish triggers and impacts reliably. After the final iteration, coders agreed on average 85 percent of the time in their coding of the experiences.

In the PTP survey, respondents were asked five questions about the midlife crisis. The questions were placed after the turning point questions and before a series of questions about life events. The five questions about the midlife crisis, including probes for positive responses, are reported in table 2.

The midlife crisis questions were coded for content. First, we coded them for beliefs about what constitutes a midlife crisis. Second, for people who reported they had had midlife crises, we coded what these crises were about. All entries were coded independently by two trained coders, and discrepancies were resolved by the first author. Interrater agreement between the coders was .81.

PSYCHOLOGICAL EXPERIENCES IN ADULTHOOD
Definitions of the Midlife Crisis

Despite findings in the research literature that the midlife crisis is not particularly common (Chiriboga 1997; McCrae and Costa 1990), the idea remains very popular. The term *crisis* itself implies that midlife is a time of stress and difficulties brought about by aging, and by turning age 40 in particular. Using the PTP study, Wethington (2000) examined the disjunction between popular and researcher views of midlife and its "crisis."

The PTP study confirms that the term is very recognizable to the majority of Americans. Over 90 percent of the PTP participants provided a definition of the midlife crisis, and these definitions coincided very well with the definitions used in psychological and psychoanalytic theories of the midlife crisis. Consistent with the popular portrayal, the midlife crisis was described by most people in negative terms. Twenty-six percent of the PTP participants over age 40 reported that they had had a midlife crisis sometime in the past. This is higher than the proportion reported from other studies (e.g., McCrae and Costa 1990) in which an investigator definition was applied rather than relying on self-report. Subsequent qualitative analyses of the data applying various types of investigator definitions showed that the PTP participants used a much wider definition of what constitutes a midlife crisis than that used by researchers estimating the prevalence of the crisis.

Multiple points of discrepancy involved who typically has these crises, when they occur, and what causes them. Perhaps the most notable discrepancy was that despite the identification of the term *midlife crisis* with male personality development, women were as likely as men to report having had one. Another source of discrepancy was the range of ages reported for midlife crises. More than half of the reported crises occurred before age 40 and after age 50. The average age reported for a midlife crisis shifted up with the age of respondents who believed they had had one, with respondents over age 60 reporting midlife crises in their fifties and even in their sixties. Although the reports of "off-time" midlife crises were in most cases serious events or crises, from a theoretical standpoint they did not meet one typical criterion of what constitutes a midlife crisis (e.g., Chiriboga 1997), which is a crisis at or around ages 40–50.

Another discrepancy was the reported cause of midlife crises. Most participants did not attribute their self-reported midlife crises to aging itself but rather to major life events that posed a severe threat and challenge during a very broadly defined period of midlife. These were major negative life events that caused a searching reassessment of life. A number were linked to episodes of serious depression (Wethington 2000). Moreover, those who believed they had not experienced a midlife crisis defined the midlife crisis as a time of reassessment, brought about by serious events in one's life.

To summarize the major findings, we found that women were as likely as men to report a midlife crisis. Most self-reported midlife crises occurred before age 40 or after age 50; relatively few people report having a midlife crisis in their forties. Finally, Americans tended to report serious crises that occur in a very broad period of "midlife" as midlife crises, rather than as crises brought on solely by turning 40 (or any other age).

597

Midlife Crises, Turning Points, and Life Events

The preceding findings suggest, consistent with previous research, that the experience of the midlife crisis is not a universal factor of adult life, for either men or women. Why do so many Americans believe that they have experienced a midlife crisis? And are these crises "real"?

Almost certainly some of these reports came about because the boundary of what constitutes midlife has now stretched to include the years leading up to retirement (Moen and Wethington 1999). Another reason respondents reported midlife crises that occurred outside the 40–50 age range is that self-perceived psychological changes are prevalent across the life course, as Clausen (1995) and Thurnher (1983) demonstrated. Although researchers make fine distinctions between different types of psychological experiences, those who are less familiar with the theories justifying the concepts are more inclusive about "what counts." A midlife crisis is a crisis in "midlife," a period with ever-widening boundaries. Another possibility is that crises occurring in early adulthood and in old age pose greater emotional and practical difficulties than crises in midlife (cf. Clausen 1993; Erikson 1963). The earlier crises threaten the subsequent course of life ("forks in the road"), whereas the later crises threaten the most precious of resources for maintaining control over life, physical health.

Another possible explanation for why the midlife crisis persists as the major descriptor for adulthood is that there is no other widely available alternate term applied to expected, normal development in this period of life. Coupled with the observation that most Americans view aging in negative terms (e.g., Menon 2001), the term *midlife crisis* becomes a way to make meaning of negative events that occur during a period that is also expected to be a time when people are at the peak of their achievements. Thus a belief that the midlife crisis is common and expected provides a kind of comfort to those who experience the types of very serious events described by the PTP respondents who believed they had had midlife crises.

Some might note another explanation for why most reports of having a midlife crisis did not fit the traditional definition of the term. Our questions were not directed specifically at the age 40 transition itself. (If we had asked separate questions about crises associated with turning 30, 40, 50, and 60, we might have had different findings.) Another possibility is that many people, particularly men, may deny having had a crisis around age 40 (Rosenberg, Rosenberg, and Farrell 1999). The state of crisis in the prime of life implies that one may be mentally ill or unable to cope effectively with normal challenges.

The PTP data, although very rich, do not provide all of the measures necessary to come to a firm conclusion about why Americans did not frequently report crises around the age of 40. But they do provide one way (albeit imperfect) to examine how self-perceived psychological changes of other types are distributed across the life course, and whether their distribution implies that midlife is a period of particular crisis in ways that the midlife crisis questions did not capture. Four of the turning point questions refer explicitly to psychological changes believed to "peak" in midlife, from the midlife crisis perspective: experiencing turning points in job or career, learning upsetting things about oneself, learning good things about oneself, and fulfilling dreams (Gould 1978; Levinson et al. 1978; Vaillant 1977). Data are available from both the MIDUS and PTP surveys to examine the distribution of such turning points by age and to explore their meaning.

The Distribution of Turning Points across the Life Course

MIDUS survey data on the gender and age distribution of turning points are reported in figure 2. These data document self-reported turning points over the last year before the interview. People could report up to seven types of turning points, although doing so was rare (52 percent

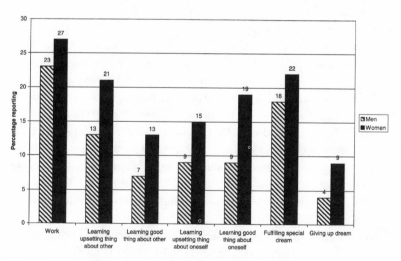

FIGURE 2. Turning points in the past twelve months, by type and gender. *Source:* MIDUS ($n = 3032$).

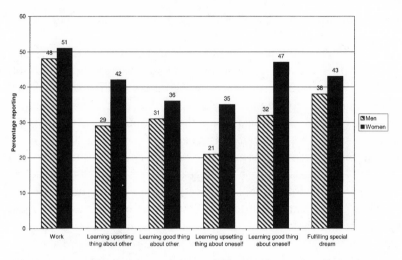

FIGURE 3. Turning points in the past five years, by type and gender. *Source:* PTP ($n = 724$).

report no turning point, and the mean number of turning points is 1.08 (SD $= 1.46$)). Overall, women report significantly more turning points than men.

Work turning points are the most frequently endorsed, which is consistent with Clausen's (1990) data reported in figure 1 (23 percent of men and 27 percent of women report them). The second most frequently endorsed in the MIDUS survey is fulfilling a dream, by 18 percent of men and 22 percent of women. (The third most endorsed was learning something upsetting about someone else.) The least endorsed is giving up a dream; only 4 percent of men and 9 percent of women report this.

Figure 3 summarizes reports on turning points, as described in the PTP survey, over a five-year retrospective period. Recall that in the PTP survey, both the method of collecting data and the recall period were different from those of the MIDUS survey. As a consequence of both of these changes, endorsement rates are higher. (The endorsement rate for the last twelve months is very similar to that of the MIDUS survey, however. Endorsement rates "fall off," with most turning points reported as taking place in the two years before the interview.) Only 16 percent do not report a turning point over the five-year recall period, and the mean number of turning points reported (out of six) is 2.23 (SD $= 1.66$). The high rate of reporting turning points is consistent with Thurnher's (1983) study.

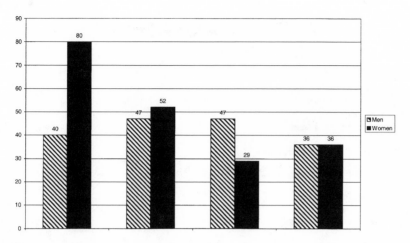

FIGURE 4. Percentage reporting work turning points in the past five years, by age and gender. *Source:* PTP.

Both men and women are most likely to report a turning point involving work (48 percent and 51 percent, respectively). For men, the second most common turning point reported is fulfilling a dream, and the third most common is learning something good about oneself. For women, the second most common is learning something good about oneself, and the third is fulfilling a dream.

We now examine how the content of frequently reported turning points differs by age, gender, and life circumstances.

Turning Points at Work

Figure 4 examines the age distribution of work turning points by gender. The age distribution varies by gender, although the difference is not statistically significant. Men's reports of work turning points peak in early and later midlife, and decline at retirement. Women's reports peak in early adulthood and decline until retirement age, where there is a small increase in reports. The age trends by gender may reflect the different average course of women's lives in contrast to men's. In early adulthood, many women must adjust their work lives to accommodate marriage and the demands of childrearing, even if they remain committed to careers (Wethington 2002). The middle of most men's lives remains dominated by work and career responsibilities. Although the peak of work turning points comes at midlife for men, there is little evidence from detailed qualitative analyses that these events are connected to classic midlife crises

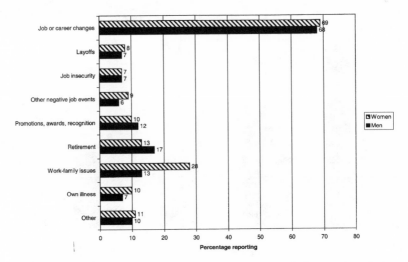

FIGURE 5. Reported causes of turning points at work, by gender. *Source:* PTP.

(Wethington 2000). For the same respondents in the PTP study, reports of turning points at work are distinct from reports of midlife crises.

Wethington (2002) analyzed the causes to which people attribute turning points involving work or career. Findings from these analyses, using the PTP data, are summarized in figure 5. The predominant cause reported was a job or career change. Overall, 68 percent of men and 69 percent of women reported that their turning point at work was triggered by the process or the fact of a job or career change. A small proportion (7 percent) named job insecurity as a trigger for a work or career turning point. Five to 7 percent attributed their work turning points to actual layoffs.

Those who reported work or career turning points attributed them to positive as well as negative events and situations. For example, retirements were reported sometimes as positive events leading to turning points, and sometimes as negative events leading to turning points. Many of the job and career changes reported were also reported as positive events, because they were voluntary or self-directed to improve a career (Wethington 2002).

What meaning do people attach to work turning points? McAdams, Josselon, and Lieblich (2001) reported that the narratives Americans produce to explain changes in their lives emphasize psychological growth in response to stress and adversity. Because work is a major source of meaning and purpose in life, it is likely that many of those who reported work turning points spontaneously reported personal growth as an outcome of the experience.

In the PTP study, consistent with McAdams's research, most men (61 percent) and women (62 percent) reported that the work or career turning point had a positive impact on them. This was the case even when the event or situation that triggered the turning point had been a negative event. The positive impacts reported include successful mastery or resolution of the situation that caused the turning point, such as a career change that turned out well, or an impending layoff that was resolved by starting a successful business of one's own. Intrinsic rewards (e.g., a sense of growth and confidence) outnumber extrinsic rewards (a higher salary) among the positive impacts reported.

For example, the most frequently reported positive impact (11 percent) of participants was a positive shift of energy away from career to personal life. These are instances not only of scaling back at work to spend more time with family (Becker and Moen 1999) but also of scaling back to pursue volunteering, community action, and other, more rewarding interests such as hobbies. Many participants reported gaining more self-confidence, enjoying new challenges and achievements, and finding relief from stress. The most frequently mentioned negative impacts of work turning points reflect a lack of perceived mastery over work and life in general. Whether or not a turning point is perceived as having a positive or negative impact is also related to whether the job or career change was brought about by personal choice (deciding to pursue a new career) or external events (a layoff).

Changes in the Self: Lessons Learned from Events

Another type of turning point that could be related to popular ideas about midlife change and turmoil is self-perceived changes in oneself, or character. Wethington (2000) found that learning something upsetting about oneself was significantly correlated with reporting a midlife crisis, although only for men.

It was the women, however, who reported significantly more turning points involving changes in how they viewed themselves over the past twelve months (MIDUS survey) and in the last five years (PTP survey) (see figs. 6 and 7). Women were significantly more likely to report discovering something upsetting about themselves, as well as more likely to report discovering something good about themselves. Among the men and women who specifically reported learning something upsetting about

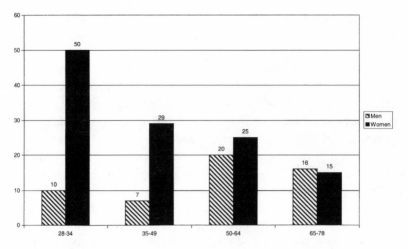

FIGURE 6. Percentage reporting learning something upsetting about themselves in the past five years, by age and gender. *Source:* PTP.

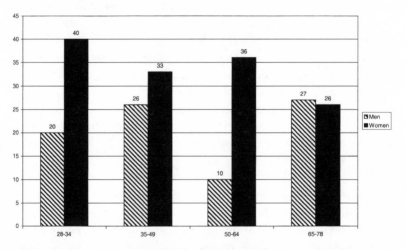

FIGURE 7. Percentage reporting learning something good about themselves in the past five years, by age and gender. *Source:* PTP.

themselves in the PTP survey, 49 percent also reported learning something good about themselves.

Younger women were most likely to report learning something upsetting about themselves, whereas young men were relatively less likely than older men to do so. The proportion of men and women who reported

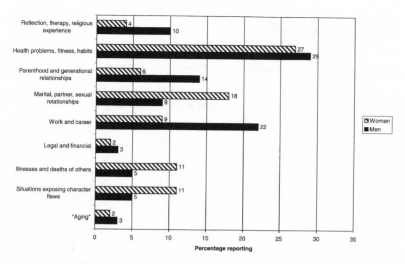

FIGURE 8. Self-reported causes of learning something upsetting oneself. *Source:* PTP.

learning something upsetting about themselves was nearly equal in the oldest age group (fig. 6). Younger women were also the most likely to learn something good about themselves, although the age trend was not significant.

Wethington (2003) examined the PTP survey responses more closely to characterize the reasons people give for learning something upsetting or good about themselves. These analyses give some insight into the age and gender distributions of this type of turning point. The causes are summarized in figures 8 and 9.

Respondents attributed changes in the way they viewed themselves to a variety of situations. The majority who reported these turning points attributed them to objective changes in the environment, either major negative events or long-lasting difficulties. Less then one in ten reported that they found out something upsetting about themselves through reflection, therapy, or religious contemplation. What these triggering situations had in common were the challenge they posed or the way they revealed one's character or personality.

Health problems were the most commonly reported cause of learning something upsetting about oneself (fig. 8). (Health problems accounted for the increase in reports of learning something upsetting among older men.) Work was the second most commonly reported cause of learning something upsetting about oneself. Work was also the most commonly

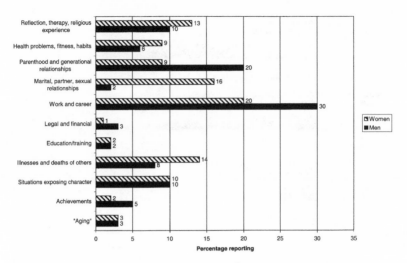

FIGURE 9. Self-reported causes of learning something good about oneself. *Source:* PTP.

self-reported cause of learning something good about oneself (fig. 9), followed by parenthood.

At first glance, health problems might seem to be an incorrect answer to the question about learning something upsetting about oneself, because health does not obviously pertain to character. Did people misunderstand this question? An examination of the PTP responses shows, however, that people understood the question. Health problems led to revelations about the need to change health-related behavior. They also led to the realization that the cause of the health problem may have been in previous behavior. Many of the respondents who reported health problems described blaming themselves for their health problems and the steps they were taking to increase their expected span of life.

As expected from past research on Americans' definitions of success, many respondents attributed learning something upsetting about themselves to problems and failures at work and in their families. No respondents attributed learning something upsetting to educational or other personal achievements, although some reported that achievements led them to learn good things about themselves.

Reports of learning something upsetting about oneself were often related to learning something good about oneself. In the PTP study, 45 percent who reported learning something upsetting about themselves also reported that the same situation led them to learn something good about themselves. In other words, a substantial number of people used the question about finding out something good about themselves to elaborate or balance their description of the upsetting thing they had learned about themselves. Most people whose responses followed this pattern were describing their adjustment to stressful events and difficulties.

Those participants who reported learning only something good about themselves were more likely to attribute its cause to a positive event. The situations reported frequently involved positive events and transitions that symbolize maturity. These included getting married, finishing school, having a child, adopting a child, and starting a new business. Other respondents reported learning something good about themselves from experiencing approbation and affirmation from important others, at work, from their families, or from social groups. Another type of situation reported was success in challenging situations, such as managing the care of a disabled child or accomplishing difficult tasks at work. Other respondents reported learning good things about themselves from mastering new tasks and difficult hobbies.

Wethington (2003) also examined what sorts of personality and situational factors (from the MIDUS survey) predicted the reporting of turning points of this type in the PTP survey. A consistent finding was that reporting stressful difficulties or recent life events in important life roles related significantly to reporting learning both upsetting and good things about oneself. This finding holds when we control for demographic factors (age in years, female gender, and completion of college) and respondent personality. Conventional theory and research on life events and psychological distress successfully explain why negative events would be correlated to the reporting of learning upsetting things about oneself. It is not so obvious, however, why negative events and difficulties are related to reporting good things about oneself. Analyses of the qualitative data in PTP revealed that respondents reported not only negative impacts on views of themselves but also positive impacts.

As noted earlier, many of those who described negative impacts on self-views also went on to describe how the same challenging situations had had positive impacts on self-views. In the PTP responses, these reported changes are best described as lessons learned rather than positive reappraisals of the situations that caused the turning points (e.g., Aldwin, Sutton, and Lachman 1996). The majority of narratives about positive impact were extended reports of coping with the situation that caused the turning point, or plans for avoiding such problems in the future.

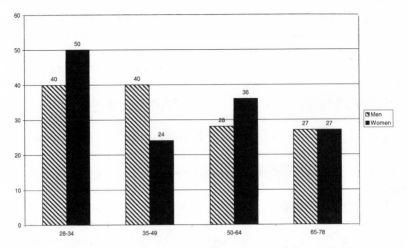

FIGURE 10. Percentage reporting fulfilling a special dream in the past five years, by age and gender. *Source:* PTP.

Dreams Fulfilled

Figure 10 reports the age and gender distribution of persons who reported fulfilling dreams. Fulfilling dreams peaks for women in early adulthood (as did work turning points and learning something upsetting or good about themselves). For men, fulfilled dreams peak in early to middle adulthood, that is, about the time the midlife crisis is believed (at least popularly) to occur.

The most common dream fulfilled involves personal finances or property acquisition (see fig. 11). Reminiscent of Thurnher's findings (1983), buying a new home, extensively remodeling an older home, or acquiring a second home was perceived as a significant transition in life. Others nominated the achievement of financial freedom or security, or the acquisition of boats and cars as significant milestones. Surely this is a reflection of the American dream; material possessions symbolize how well we have managed all of our other responsibilities and provided for others. (As one participant said, "look at what I had left over to give myself.") They also may reflect the increasing prosperity of the years over which the PTP study asked respondents to reflect, from 1993 to 1998.

For men, work was the second most common type of dream fulfilled. For women, parenthood and accomplishments outside of work and education were the second most common types of dream fulfilled, reflective of a continuing division by gender in American society as a whole.

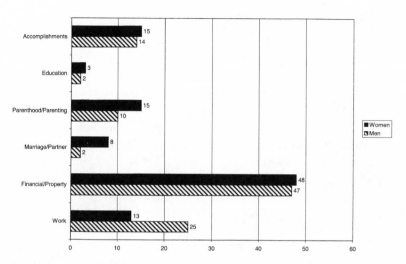

FIGURE 11. Types of dreams fulfilled in the past five years, by gender. *Source:* PTP.

DISCUSSION

This study of turning points has found support for some of its guiding ideas. First, not surprisingly, events and situations symbolizing appropriate enactment of adult social roles are associated with self-perceived psychological change in adulthood. The more detailed analyses demonstrate that reports of the four types of turning points we examined are associated with characteristics of marriage, work, parenting, and family relationships. People frequently report that major changes or disturbances in these important social roles are triggers of turning points that have a negative impact on them, at least initially. Moreover, successes and recognition in these roles are frequently nominated as causes of turning points that turned out well.

Specifically, this study examined self-reports of personal growth and change that related to work and career, and reported by respondents as "turning points at work." Research and theory in adult development and the life course suggest that work turning points would be associated with characteristics of work life that define success, such as promotions. Work turning points are related to adapting to negative work events, particularly situations that were resolved successfully. Turning points at work are also related to achieving success at work. Analyses of the intensive data suggest that promotions and getting better jobs are perceived as contributing to perceived positive growth and change for many who experience them.

It is important that many of the improvements in career are described as self-directed. In fact, perceptions of experiencing growth and change are more frequently mentioned as impacts than are increased extrinsic rewards from a better job, such as more pay.

The study also found that challenge and stress at work produce adaptation and change that is in retrospect construed positively (Vaillant 1977). Reports of turning points were strongly related to involuntary job loss (and other situations indicating job insecurity). However, it is notable that not all of the reported long-term impacts of work turning points involving job loss are negative. The qualitative data suggest that people believe they derive positive feelings of growth and change from stressful situations that they were able to resolve well (Pearlin and Schooler 1978; Thoits 1994).

Third, the data show that turning points involving perceived changes in oneself, both positive and negative, are associated by Americans with stressors and challenges. Chronic stressors in marriage, at work, and in parenting are consistently related to reporting a turning point involving one's character. The qualitative data confirm this interpretation.

The analyses of the qualitative data on turning points involving learning something good or upsetting about oneself raise several additional important points. When people reported the negative psychological impacts of learning upsetting things about themselves, they described depression, devaluation of previous beliefs or views, or devaluation of the self. When they described positive impacts of learning upsetting things about themselves, they reported how they coped with the consequences of the events or the difficulties that caused the turning point. People report experiencing positive psychological growth because they believe they coped well (see also Schaefer and Moos 1992). They attribute success to taking action and solving the problem, to taking steps to avoid similar problems in the future, to minimizing the impact of chronic stress on other aspects of their lives, to acquiring new knowledge and self-knowledge, and to renewing their faith and hope in the future.

Another important finding is that self-reported turning points are more prevalent in early adulthood than in midlife. Clausen (1993) found no evidence of prevalent midlife crises in his in-depth studies of life history. Both the MIDUS and the PTP studies confirm Clausen's general finding. In general, turning points were most likely to be reported in young adulthood, with some important exceptions. Except for one instance—learning an upsetting thing about oneself—reporting a turning point was not significantly correlated with reporting a midlife crisis (Wethington 2000), and then only for men.

What we have called turning points often occur earlier in the life span than what was defined as the age of midlife crisis. In fact, we found considerable evidence that the "age 30 transition" described by Levinson et al. (1978) or the decade of life before age 30 is more psychologically disruptive to more people than is the age 40 transition. This is consistent with previous research (Clausen 1995, 1998) on psychological turning points: people in the Clausen study nominated early adulthood (and even adolescence) as the time period of "most important" turning points. It is also consistent with Levinson's writings about the age 30 transition (see Levinson et al. 1978), an aspect of his work that has been less integrated into popular beliefs about adulthood.

Nevertheless, the term *midlife crisis* remains a powerful metaphor in the stories told about adulthood. Its ubiquity in descriptions of middle-aged men and women in contemporary literary novels (e.g., Oates 2001) speaks to its standing as a phenomenon of popular culture and its power as a belief. We suggest that the notion's persistence is indicative of its symbolism to Americans of the hidden potential of their aging to threaten control over their lives, rather than its presence in everyday life. In everyday life, the decade of the forties is likely to be experienced as a time when material and emotional dreams are fulfilled.

NOTE

1. About 20 percent of the MIDUS survey respondents skipped the question, and another 3 percent answered the question incorrectly. This may have been the result of an inadvertently confusing questionnaire page, which implied that the question could be skipped. In telephone pilots for the PTP study, moreover, respondents often protested the question angrily, saying that people should "never give up dreams."

REFERENCES

Aldwin, C. M., K. J. Sutton, and M. Lachman. 1996. The development of coping resources in adulthood. *Journal of Personality* 64:837–71.

Baumeister, R. F. 1986. *Identity.* New York: Oxford University Press.

Baumeister, R. F., and B. Wilson. 1996. Life stories and the four needs for meaning. *Psychological Inquiry* 4:322–25.

Becker, P., and P. Moen. 1999. Scaling back: Dual-career couples' work–family strategies. *Journal of Marriage and the Family* 61:995–1007.

Bellah, R. N., R. Madsen, W. H. Sullivan, A. Swidler, and S. M. Tipton. 1985. *Habits of the heart: Individualism and commitment in American life.* Berkeley: University of California Press.

Bourdieu, P. 1977. *Outline of a theory of practice.* Cambridge: Cambridge University Press.

Brandes, S. H. 1985. *Forty: The age and the symbol.* Knoxville: University of Tennessee Press.

Brim, O. G. 1976. Theories of the male midlife crisis. *Counseling Psychologist* 6:2–9.

———. 1992. *Ambition: How we manage stress and failure in our lives.* New York: Basic Books.

Brown, G. W., and T. O. Harris. 1978. *Social origins of depression: A study of psychiatric disorder in women.* New York: Free Press.

Chiriboga, D. A. 1997. Crisis, challenge, and stability in the middle years. In *Multiple paths of midlife development,* ed. M. E. Lachman and J. B. James, 293–322. Chicago: University of Chicago Press.

Clausen, J. 1990. *Turning point as a life course concept.* Paper presented at the Annual Meeting of the American Sociological Association, Washington, D.C.

———. 1993. *American lives: Looking back at the children of the Great Depression.* New York: Free Press.

———. 1995. Gender, contexts, and turning points in adults' lives. In *Examining lives in context: Perspectives on the ecology of human development,* ed. P. Moen, G. Elder, and K. Lüscher, 365–89. Washington, D.C.: American Psychological Association.

———. 1998. Life reviews and life stories. In *Methods of life course research: Qualitative and quantitative approaches,* ed. J. Z. Giele and G. H. Elder, 189–212. Thousand Oaks, Calif.: Sage.

Erikson, E. H. 1963. *Childhood and society.* New York: W. W. Norton.

Giddens, A. 1991. *Modernity and self-identity.* Stanford, Calif.: Stanford University Press.

Gould, R. 1978. *Transformations: Growth and change in adult life.* New York: Simon and Schuster.

Heckhausen, J. 2001. Adaptation and resilience in midlife. In *Handbook of midlife development,* ed. M. E. Lachman, 345–94. New York: John Wiley.

Keegan, R. 1994. *In over our heads: The mental demands of modern life.* Cambridge: Harvard University Press.

Levinson, D., C. N. Darrow, E. B. Klein, M. H. Levinson, and B. McKee. 1978. *The seasons of a man's life.* New York: Knopf.

Lowenthal, M. J., M. J. Thurnher, and D. A. Chiriboga. 1975. *Four stages of life.* San Francisco: Jossey-Bass.

McAdams, D. P. 1996. Personality, modernity, and the storied self: A contemporary framework for studying personality. *Psychological Inquiry* 4:295–321.

McAdams, D. P., R. Josselon, and A. Lieblich. 2001. *Turns in the road: Narrative studies of life in transition.* Washington, D.C.: American Psychological Association.

McCrae, R., and P. Costa. 1990. *Personality in adulthood.* New York: Guilford.

McFarland, C., M. Ross, and M. Giltrow. 1992. Biased recollections in older adults: The role of implicit theories of aging. *Journal of Personality and Social Psychology* 57:1069–81.

Menon, U. 2001. Middle adulthood in cultural perspective: The imagined and the experienced in three cultures. In *Handbook of midlife development,* ed. M. E Lachman, 40–74. New York: John Wiley.

Moen, P., and E. Wethington. 1999. Midlife development in a life course context. In *Life in the middle,* ed. S. L. Willis and J. D. Reid, 3–23. San Diego: Academic Press.

Mroczek, D. K., and C. Kolarz. 1998. The effect of age on positive and negative affect: A developmental perspective on happiness. *Journal of Personality and Social Psychology* 75:1333–49.

Oates, J. C. 2001. *Middle age: A romance.* New York: Ecco Press.

Pearlin, L., and C. Schooler. 1978. The structure of coping. *Journal of Health and Social Behavior* 19:2–21.

Pitkin, W. B. 1932. *Life begins at forty.* New York: Whittlesey House, McGraw-Hill.

Robbins, A., and A. Wilner. 2001. *The quarterlife crisis: The unique challenges of life in your twenties.* New York: Tarcher/Putnam.

Rosenberg, S. D., H. J. Rosenberg, and M. P. Farrell. 1999. The midlife crisis revisited. In *Life in the middle,* ed. S. L Willis and J. D. Reid, 47–73. San Diego: Academic Press.

Schaefer, J., and R. Moos. 1982. Life crises and personal growth. In *Personal coping: Theory, research, and application,* ed. B. N. Carpenter, 149–70. Westport, Conn.: Praeger.

Swidler, A. 1986. Culture in action: Symbols and strategies. *American Sociological Review* 51:273–86.

Thoits, P. 1994. Stressors and problem-solving: The individual as psychological activist. *Journal of Health and Social Behavior* 35:143–60.

Thurnher, M. 1983. Turning points and developmental change: Subjective and "objective" assessments. *American Journal of Orthopsychiatry* 53:52–60.

Vaillant, G. E. 1997. *Adaptation to life.* Boston: Little, Brown.

———. 2000. Adaptive mental mechanisms: Their role in a positive psychology. *American Psychologist* 55:89–98.

Wethington, E. 2000. Expecting stress: Americans and the "midlife crisis." *Motivation and Emotion* 24:85–102.

———. 2002. The relationship of work turning points to perceptions of psychological growth and change. In *Advances in life course research: New frontiers in socialization,* ed. R. Settersten and T. Owens, 111–31. Stamford, Conn.: JAI Press.

———. 2003. Turning points as opportunities for psychological growth. In *Flourishing: The positive person and the life well-lived,* ed. C. L. Keyes and J. Haidt, 37–53. Washington, D.C.: American Psychological Association.

Wethington, E., G. W. Brown, and R. C. Kessler. 1995. Interview measurement of stressful life events. In *Measuring stress: A guide for health and social scientists,* ed. S. Cohen, R. C. Kessler, and L. U. Gordon, 59–79. New York: Oxford University Press.

Wethington, E., H. Cooper, and C. S. Holmes. 1997. Turning points in midlife. In *Stress and adversity across the life course: Trajectories and turning points,* ed. I. H. Gotlib and B. Wheaton, 215–31. New York: Cambridge University Press.

CHAPTER TWENTY ONE

Well-Being in America: Core Features and Regional Patterns

Hazel Rose Markus, Victoria C. Plaut, and Margie E. Lachman

> True happiness comes from just having to adjust to what you
> have, not from choosing. Like ice fishing in Minnesota, you have
> cold weather, so you make the best of it. Choice can make you
> miserable.
>
> > Garrison Keillor, *A Prairie Home Companion* (1997)

> People accustomed to mountains and tree cover go crazy out here
> [Texas]. But I just hate trees and mountains. I went to Virginia
> once. I felt so fenced in by the landscape that I could scream.
> When I was in Chicago, the skyscrapers made me feel the same
> way. I can't imagine spending your life in a place where you can't
> see for miles in all directions.
>
> > R. D. Kaplan, *An Empire Wilderness* (1998)

When it comes to what gives rise to the good life or a global sense of well-being, place matters. As the epigraphs to this chapter suggest, moving from one region to another can give rise to an unsettling feeling that something is not quite right. The North and the South, and the East and the West, diverge from one another, just as the city does from the country, and the mountains from the coasts. These places differ not only in their geography, or physical space, but also in their ideological landscape, or collective meaning space. And it is the lay of the land with respect to well-being that concerns us here.

Even though there is some consensus across people, places, and time about what counts for well-being, it is increasingly evident that well-being can also take a variety of forms (King and Napa 1998; Markus, Ryff, Curhan, and Palmersheim, chap. 10, this volume; Ryff and Singer 1998). We propose here that both the consensus and the diversity in well-being can be systematically linked to the ideas and practices that are common in particular sociocultural contexts.

We first use the MIDUS data to determine some of the core features of well-being in the United States, and then we examine some points of regional variation. We suggest that American well-being at midlife is importantly constituted both by widely distributed American ideas and practices and by regionally specific ones.

THE SOCIOCULTURAL MATRIX OF WELL-BEING

In exploring regional variation in well-being, we use the framework of mutual constitution—the notion that psyche and culture, or person and community, "make each other up" (Berry, Poortinga, and Pandey 1997; Cole 1996; Fiske et al. 1998; Shweder 1990, 24; Triandis 1995). According to this perspective, psychological tendencies require and are shaped by engagement with the culture-specific meanings, practices, artifacts, and institutions of particular cultural contexts, and these psychological tendencies serve to perpetuate these particular cultural contexts. Research in cultural psychology and cultural anthropology reveals that even such presumably basic processes as cognition, motivation, and emotion are culturally patterned (Fiske et al. 1998; Markus and Kitayama 1991; Shweder 1990). For example, recent studies suggest that in the United States, where independence and autonomy of the self are emphasized, well-being is associated with the pursuit of individual success and control (Lachman and Weaver 1998), whereas in Japan, where interdependence or relationality are more focal, well-being is linked to fitting in and maintaining sympathy (Diener and Suh 2000; Kitayama and Markus 2000).

"Being well" is a collective and context-specific project, and to be well depends on the incorporation of particular understandings and practices of wellness and being. Different sociocultural and sociostructural environments (e.g., different regions of the world, or of the United States, that differ in ecology, history, sociopolitical circumstances, economic position, and ethnic background of inhabitants) are associated with somewhat different distributions of ideas and practices about well-being. It is not difficult, therefore, to imagine that people in diverse regional contexts have understandings and representations of what is good, right, and moral that diverge from one another, and that these differences are manifest in the nature of well-being.

The sociocultural analysis we are pursuing here does not, of course, imply that two people in a given cultural context—for example, a 30-year-old male banker and 45-year-old female administrative assistant both living in New York—will have exactly the same understandings of well-being. People engage with context-specific practices and meanings in ways that are selective and creative, including resisting and contesting them. Moreover, each person is influenced by the practices and meanings associated with other cultural contexts, such as those of gender, age, and occupation. Yet, we hypothesize that their psychological responses will show some patterns that can be linked to regionally prevalent ideas and practices, just as the banker will also show some similarities to other bankers or 30-year-olds and the administrative assistant may show some similarities to other administrative assistants or to other women. These similarities are not essential or inherent but attributable to the specific meanings and practices that are necessarily engaged in the course of being an appropriate person in the various contexts.

This analysis systematically links the ideological landscape, or prevalent ideas and practices, in the United States as a whole and in various geographic regions to patterns of well-being. We first describe the well-being indicators, or features of well-being, used in our analysis. We then turn our attention to consensual features of well-being. We delineate ideas and practices that are prevalent across American cultural contexts and form hypotheses based on these ideas and practices about what features of well-being are likely to be consensual, or commonly endorsed by Americans. Finally, we ask if well-being is valued and represented differently across regions in the United States. On the basis of the perspective of mutual constitution and some limited empirical research on regional variation, we propose that how people see their roles in a community and in society, how much control they feel over their lives, and even their physical and mental health—all of these—can be regionally patterned. These regional ways of being, in turn, serve to maintain and perpetuate the reality of regional differences. In examining regional differences in patterns of well-being, we first depict the ideas and practices that are prevalent in a given region as well as demographic indicators from our sample and from U.S. Census data. On the basis of these qualitative and quantitative accounts, we then develop hypotheses about what features of well-being are likely to be endorsed more commonly in one region than in others. The goal of our analysis, however, is not just to determine if well-being varies by region; our larger aim is to examine the ways in which culturally prevalent ideas and practices can shape individual well-being.

Well-Being Indicators

The Midlife Development Inventory (MIDI) was structured to tap three broad dimensions of well-being—psychological health, physical health, and social health—hypothesized to be important for a comprehensive understanding of well-being. To map out both core American and regional ways of being well, we chose twenty-six indicators from the MIDI to reflect these important well-being constructs. These measures and their mean scores can be found in table 1.

THE AMERICAN WELL-BEING CONSENSUS HYPOTHESES

Americans live through an elaborate system of ideas and practices that give form to the most commonly held and endorsed understandings of well-being. Key American cultural ideas can be found, for example, in the Declaration of Independence and the Bill of Rights, the most significant of which are independence from constraint by others and protection of the "natural rights" of each individual (Guisinger and Blatt 1994; Hogan 1975; Markus and Kitayama 1994; Shweder, Mahapatra, and Miller 1987). Indeed, empirical research suggests that Americans are strongly oriented toward self-direction and self-reliance and generally assume an individualist stance on the world (Hofstede 1980; Triandis 1995), manifesting what Bellah et al. (1985) called expressive individualism. The sources of this American form of individualism are a matter of ongoing debate, but most observers agree that this cultural ethos involves a synthesis of three powerful and highly prevalent ideas: (1) the idea of the frontier and the importance of personal independence and self-reliance; (2) the Protestant ethic, which involves a belief in the moral superiority of industriousness and hard work; and (3) the idea that the greatest good is to be as individually successful as possible (Bellah et al. 1985; Kitayama and Markus 1999; Potter 1963; Turner 1920; Weber 1958; Zelinsky 1992). The mindset that claims it is possible to get to the top and achieve almost anything if one works hard enough and with direction and perseverance is often called "the American dream" (Hochschild 1995; Spindler and Spindler 1990), and it has played an unparalleled role in the shaping of the American psyche. Even though the veracity of these ideas may be challenged, they are still powerful in the sense that they are inscribed in and promoted by many American systems and institutions. A variety of empirical evidence suggests that can-do ideology is widely held and that Americans indeed believe strongly in their personal control and their efficacy in the world (Taylor and Brown 1988).

Given the repertoire of ideas and practices that are common to American mainstream experience, as well as some recent empirical findings (Fiske et al. 1998; Herzog et al. 1998; Iyengar and Lepper 1999; Quinn and Crocker 1999), predictions can be made about which understandings of well-being are likely to be commonly represented and endorsed. We expect that constructs related to independence, such as autonomy and

TABLE 1 Well-Being Indicators Used in Analyses

Dimension/Measure	Description	Example	Mean[a]
PSYCHOLOGICAL HEALTH			
Psychological well-being	18-item scale (1 = strongly agree to 7 = strongly disagree)	See the 6 subscales below	5.51
Autonomy	3-item scale (1 = strongly agree to 7 = strongly disagree)	I judge myself by what I think is important, not by the values of what others think is important.	5.50
Environmental mastery	3-item scale (1 = strongly agree to 7 = strongly disagree)	In general, I feel I am in charge of the situation in which I live.	5.33
Self-acceptance	3-item scale (1 = strongly agree to 7 = strongly disagree)	When I look at the story of my life, I am pleased with how things have turned out so far.	5.49
Purpose in life	3-item scale (1 = strongly agree to 7 = strongly disagree)	Some people wander aimlessly through life, but I am not one of them.	5.45
Personal growth	3-item scale (1 = strongly agree to 7 = strongly disagree)	For me, life has been a continuous process of learning, changing, and growth.	5.95
Positive relations	3-item scale (1 = strongly agree to 7 = strongly disagree)	Maintaining close relationships has been difficult and frustrating for me.	5.34
Control			
Mastery	4-item scale (1 = strongly agree to 7 = strongly disagree)	I can do just about anything I really set my mind to.	5.84
Constraint	8-item scale (1 = strongly agree to 7 = strongly disagree)	I have little control over the things that happen to me.	2.74
Satisfaction			
Overall life now	1-item rating (0 = worst to 10 = best)	How would you rate your life overall these days?	7.65
Satisfaction with life	1-item rating (1 = a lot to 4 = not at all)	At present, how satisfied are you with you life?	2.49
Self-satisfaction	1-item rating (1 = a lot to 4 = not at all)	Overall, how satisfied are you with yourself?	2.51
Affect			
Positive affect	6-item scale of ratings of positive feelings (1 = all the time to 5 = none of the time)	During the past 30 days, how much of the time did you feel . . . in good spirits?	3.36
Negative affect	6-item scale of ratings of negative feelings (1 = all the time to 5 = none of the time)	During the past 30 days, how much of the time did you feel . . . so sad nothing could cheer you up?	1.57
Mental and emotional health	1-item rating (1 = poor to 5 = excellent)	What about your mental or emotional health—would you say it is . . .	3.69

TABLE 1 *continued*

Dimension/ Measure	Description	Example	Mean[a]
	PSYCHOLOGICAL HEALTH		
Health Problems Chronic conditions	Yes/no to experience or treatment of 29 chronic conditions	In the past 12 months, have you experienced or been treated for any of the following . . . alcohol or drug problems?	2.56
Subjective health			
Overall health	1-item rating (0 = worst possible to 10 = best possible)	How would you rate your health these days?	7.35
Physical health	1-item rating (1 = poor to 5 = excellent)	In general, would you say your physical health is. . .	3.45
	SOCIAL HEALTH		
Social responsibility			
Contribution to welfare and well-being of other people	1-item rating (0 = worst to 10 = best)	How would you rate your contribution to the welfare and well-being of other people these days?	6.59
Family obligation	8-item scale of ratings of degree of obligation felt toward children, parents, spouse, friends (0 = none to 10 = very great)	How much obligation would you feel . . . to drop your plans when your children seem very troubled?	60.11 (sum)
Work obligation	3-item scale of ratings of degree of obligation felt toward job (0 = none to 10 = very great)	To cancel plans to visit friends if you were asked, but not required, to work overtime?	22.81 (sum)
Civic obligation	4-item scale of ratings of degree of obligation felt toward civic participation (0 = none to 10 = very great)	To vote in local and national elections?	30.75 (sum)
Social support			
Family support	4-item scales of ratings of supportive network interactions (1 = a lot to 4 = not at all)	How much can you rely on them for help if you have a serious problem?	3.42
Friend support			3.22
Partner support			3.55
Social well-being	15-item scale of ratings of social well-being (1 = strongly agree to 7 = strongly disagree)	I feel close to other people in my community.	4.53

[a] Items have been re-coded where necessary so that higher scores indicate higher values of a measure.

mastery, and to the Protestant ethic and the American dream, such as work obligation and purpose in life, compose a set of well-being constructs that most Americans endorse.

A related set of core well-being constructs should also emerge. These are constructs associated with the notion of satisfaction, as measured in this study by ratings of one's overall life and one's satisfaction with life. Individual satisfaction is an important component of the success ethic described above (Zelinsky 1992), and in the last thirty years, feeling good or satisfied with one's self has been a key American idea (Bellah et al. 1985). A large literature on positive illusions and unrealistic optimism provides support for the hypothesis that Americans in general report being satisfied with their lives. In American samples, most people report being happy and satisfied most of the time (Freedman 1978; Herzog et al. 1998; Taylor and Brown 1988; see Markus et al., chap. 10, this volume). Moreover, most mainstream Americans believe that they are even happier and more satisfied than their friends and peers—a pattern that is not common in much of the rest of the world (Heine et al. 1999; Suh 2000).

Because there is marked regional variation in socioeconomic status in our study—for example, the regions in our study range from 16 percent to 35 percent in the number of respondents holding at least a bachelor's degree—and because socioeconomic status has been shown to be powerfully related to health, we do not anticipate that high levels of physical health will be part of the American well-being core (i.e., that Americans regardless of region will show high levels of physical health). Finally, given the conflicted discourse over whether or not Americans are currently responsible and socially engaged (Putnam 1995; Rossi 2001; Wuthnow 1998), we hesitate to make any predictions about consensual trends in Americans' social health.

Regional Variation

Researchers have documented a variety of forces that serve to create and maintain regional cultures, including local religious communities and attitudes and concentration of ethnic groups (Hulbert 1989; Raitz 1979), distinct political cultures (Gastil 1975; Glenn and Simmons 1967; Hulbert 1989), local economic forces (Edgerton 1971; Nisbett 1993), shared histories and environmental conditions (Anderson 1987), and the regional lifestyles and values that have been reinforced through marketing efforts and migration (Borchert 1972; Kahle 1996; Raitz 1979). Although there is likely to be considerable consensus in American

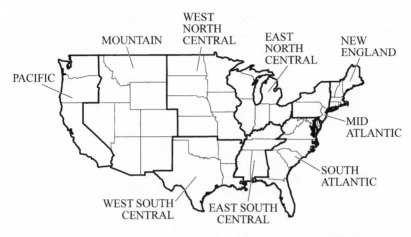

FIGURE 1. U.S. Census Bureau divisions in the continental United States.

well-being (a consensus that can be systematically tied to nationally prevalent ideas and practices), the important role of more local experience in shaping psychological life cannot be ignored. Thus, we expect that regional culture can also have pervasive effects on the well-being of its inhabitants.

For our regional analysis we employ the regional classification scheme used by the U.S. Census Bureau, which has also been the basis for regional comparisons in a variety of other studies (Kahle 1986; Rubenstein 1982).[1] In this chapter we paint a portrait of well-being at midlife, in five—New England, Mountain, West North Central, West South Central, and East South Central—of the nine Census regions of the United States (see fig. 1) for which we have developed some hypotheses about the nature of well-being in that region. Because our goal is to show that differences in well-being can be predicted on the basis of what we know of prevalent ideas and practices, we have chosen to do this thoroughly for five regions. The same could be done for the four remaining regions, but space constraints of a single chapter do not allow us to present a complete description and discussion of all nine regions (see Plaut, Markus, and Lachman 2002 for data for the other four regions).[2]

American Consensus: Results

A well-being variable described in table 1 was classified as a core construct of well-being if it satisfied the criteria that (1) it was highly endorsed and (2) there was no regional variation. We classified a variable

TABLE 2 Variables for Which More Than 50% of Sample Responded in the Top 25% of the Scale[a]

Well-Being Dimension and Scale	Measure	% Endorsing Highest Option(s)	No Across Region Variation
Psychological health			
Psychological	Autonomy	51.0	
well-being	Self-acceptance	50.3	
	Purpose in life	51.7	✓
	Personal growth	69.6	
Control	Mastery	65.8	✓
Satisfaction	Overall life now	63.7	✓
	Satisfaction with life	59.3	✓
	Satisfied with yourself	58.2	
	(Lack of) negative affect	78.5	
Physical health			
	Overall health now	54.3	✓
Social health			
Responsibility	Family obligation	53.8	✓
	Work obligation	58.4	✓
	Civic obligation	59.3	
Social support	Partner support	74.7	✓
	Family support	63.9	✓

[a]This would be the equivalent of circling 4 on a four = point scale.

as highly endorsed if over 50 percent of the sample responded in the top 25 percent of the scale, which is equivalent to circling 4 on a four-point scale. There was no regional variation if a one-way analysis of variance (ANOVA) of region for that variable did not yield a significant F statistic at the $p = .05$ level. In table 2, core well-being constructs are highlighted in boldface.

Most elements that we hypothesized would be important in American well-being are indeed endorsed at the highest levels by more than 50 percent of Americans, although not all of these elements meet the second criterion, which involved no regional variation. Consistent with our predictions, having a purpose is important to many mainstream midlife Americans. Fifty-two percent of Americans responded within the top 25 percent of the purpose-in-life scale. There are no regional differences on this scale. Overall, Americans are also highly concerned with mastery. Sixty-six percent of Americans averaged a response to the four mastery items that falls into the top 25 percent of the scale. We found no regional differences on mastery. In other words, Americans do not vary significantly by region on the extent to which they feel that they can do what they want and have set their mind to.

Despite the fact that health, education, and economic resources are not evenly distributed across regions, the portrait of the United States looks fairly homogeneous with respect to life satisfaction. No significant differences emerged between regions on responses to two separate life satisfaction ratings. Americans are, for the most part, satisfied with their lives. Sixty-four percent circled one of the three highest options on an eleven-point scale in response to "How would you rate your life overall these days?" In response to the question "At present, how satisfied are you with your life?" 59 percent gave the highest possible response (i.e., "a lot") on a four-point scale.

As expected, physical health is not a core aspect of well-being. However, the more global rating of overall health was highly endorsed by 54 percent of respondents and met the criterion for regional invariance.

As predicted, Americans are also very oriented toward work. Fifty-eight percent of Americans responded within the top 25 percent of the work obligation scale. Rossi (2001), who has recently chronicled political and social commentary about American trends in civil responsibility and activism, notes that it is difficult to find any literature suggesting that recent cohorts of Americans are socially responsible. Thus, we were surprised to find a few social responsibility and social support constructs in our core category. For example, 54 percent of respondents perceived themselves as high on family obligation, and there is no regional variation for this variable. In retrospect, however, it makes sense that family obligation would be a core aspect of well-being. Americans may not be broadly concerned with community or society, but they are very obligated to their nuclear families, and this may comprise a special case of social responsibility (Rossi 2001). Philosopher David Potter (1963) claims that in American life, private values have always eclipsed public values, and in his description of this American "privatism," he cites the Old Yankee prayer: "God save me and my wife. / My son John and his wife, / Us four and no more." The presence of family obligation in the core is paralleled by our finding that Americans across regions believe that they receive a lot of social support from their family (64 percent responded in the top 25 percent of the scale) and partner (75 percent). The high endorsement of partner support fits Adams's (2002) observation that, in contrast to cultural settings in many parts of the world, in American contexts the adult man–woman couple is regarded as the most significant social relationship and the one that is essential for well-being. Finally, reflecting Bellah et al.'s (1985) claim that Americans seem more isolated than they actually are, another type of responsibility, civic obligation, was also highly endorsed. More than 50 percent of respondents endorsed the civic obligation items at the highest levels, but this variable did not meet the criterion for regional invariance.

REGIONAL WELL-BEING PATTERNS
Demographic Data and Prevalent Ideas

In this section, we develop hypotheses about the profiles of well-being for each of the five regions being analyzed. These predictions come from an integration of qualitative and quantitative accounts. The qualitative accounts provide a summary of regional values and practices that are prevalent in each region and that we expect will be sources of regional variation in well-being. Our goal here is to draw together suggestions from historical, sociological, and cultural accounts and commentaries about regional differences to formulate a set of hypotheses about which ideas of well-being are likely to be prevalent (i.e., pervasively available and distributed) in a given region. We expect that the ideas that are prevalent in public discourse and representation in a given region (e.g., in daily interpersonal conversations and in the media) will be directly or indirectly active in thinking and feeling about well-being, establishing a local frame of reference for what is good and right. In fact, it is difficult to think or to talk to others about one's well-being without the framework of meaning provided by these ideas. Moreover, these ideas are intrinsically linked with particular practices and institutions (Bourdieu 1977; Giddens 1990; Harris 1979), which also promote some ways of being well rather than others. For example, although not every person who lives in New Hampshire is likely to happily and self-consciously endorse the state motto of "Live Free or Die," this motto is inscribed on the New Hampshire license plate and is a feature of almost everyone's daily environment— part of the collective meaning space. The motto is a widely dispersed idea about what is important for a good life and well-being. To the extent that this idea is fostered and reinforced by a variety of other messages and practices in New England, the well-being profile of this region, in comparison with that of other regions in which this sentiment is not as pervasive or institutionalized, is likely to reflect a concern with a certain type of autonomy.

The quantitative accounts consist of demographic data that provide an outline of the sociostructural features of these regions. These are presented in tables 3 and 4 and include statistics from the U.S. Bureau of the Census (1996) and demographic data from the MIDUS survey.

TABLE 3 Demographic Indicators of Each Region

	New England	West North Central	East South Central	West South Central	Mountain
Population					
Resident population	13,351	18,468	16,193	29,290	16,118
Metro/non-metro population	5.3	1.4	1.4	3.3	2.6
Economy					
Unemployment (%)	4.8	3.7	5.5	5.5	5.3
Personal income per capita ($)	28,633	23,448	20,095	21,144	21,735
Health					
Health care expenditure ($1000/person)	1.43	1.20	1.23	1.15	0.94
Social					
Colleges (/1,000)	1.92	2.15	1.64	1.02	1.32
Divorce rate (/1,000)	3.0	4.1	5.9	4.7	4.7
Crime rate (/100,000)	4091	4562	4601	5738	6357

Source: U.S. Bureau of the Census 1996.

TABLE 4 Demographics of Regional Samples

	New England	West North Central	East South Central	West South Central	Mountain
Sample size (n)	148	323	241	366	218
Gender (%)					
Male	54.7	51.4	46.9	48.6	51.4
Female	45.3	48.6	53.1	51.4	48.6
Education (%)					
<High school	6.8	8.7	17.8	13.9	6.9
High school	26.4	35.1	32.0	28.1	25.2
Some college	32.4	28.6	34.4	28.7	36.7
Bachelor's or higher	34.5	27.6	15.8	29.2	31.2
Household income ($)	66,207	50,080	46,012	48,658	48,988
Race (%)					
White	92.9	94.6	90.1	80.4	91.0
Black	3.2	2.2	7.9	10.0	1.1
Asian	0	1.1	0	0.6	1.6
Native American	0	0.4	1.0	1.9	2.7
Mixed	1.6	0.4	0.5	1.0	0.5
Other	2.4	1.4	0.5	6.1	3.2
Religion (%)					
Protestant[a]	25.0	46.3	64.0	58.8	29.4
Catholic	46.0	31.6	9.5	22.1	23.0
Jewish	4.8	0.4	1.0	0.3	1.1
Agnostic/atheist	14.5	6.3	5.5	8.8	13.9
Other	9.7	15.4	20.0	10.4	32.6

[a]Includes interdenominational, no denomination, Baptist, Episcopalian, Lutheran, Methodist, Presbyterian.

TABLE 5 Well-Being Groupings

Types of Well-Being	Measures
1. Health-focused well-being	• Chronic conditions • Physical health
2. Autonomy-focused well-being	• Autonomy • Environmental mastery • Lack of constraint
3. Self-focused well-being	• Self-acceptance • Self-satisfaction • Personal growth
4. Emotion-focused well-being	• Positive affect • Negative affect • Mental or emotional health
5. Other-focused well-being	• Positive relations with others • Social well-being
6. Social responsibility	• Contribution to others' welfare • Civic obligation

Well-Being Groupings

The well-being variables in table 1, which included some from each of the three well-being dimensions, were regrouped into six separate types of well-being to reflect our expectations about the ways well-being was likely to vary by region (see table 5).[3] We did not include here variables that were regionally invariant because we were interested in highlighting regional variation. Friend support, a variable that showed regional invariance but was not highly endorsed, was also left out of these analyses. The first grouping, *health-focused well-being,* examines whether a person thinks he/she is healthy. The second grouping, *autonomy-focused well-being,* represents those psychological well-being variables that have to do with taking charge and not letting others tell one what to do. The third grouping, *self-focused well-being,* involves being happy with oneself and challenging oneself to change and develop. Our fourth category, *emotion-focused well-being,* gauges people's day-to-day feelings. The fifth grouping, *other-focused well-being,* captures a person's feelings of well-being in relation to other people and society in general. A sixth grouping, *social responsibility,* which we consider to be highly related to other-focused well-being, looks at conceptions of one's societal contribution.

Reporting Regional Variation

In the following sections we compare each region to other regions on aspects of well-being. Regional comparisons are made only for variables

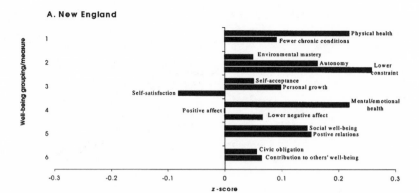

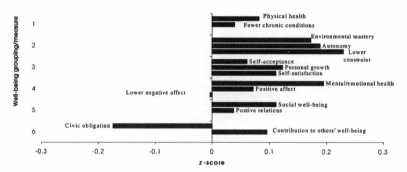

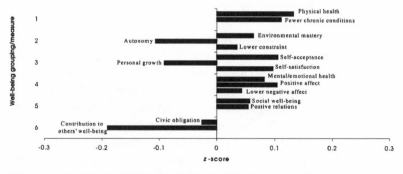

FIGURE 2. Regional profiles compared with the national average. (*Continued on overleaf.*)

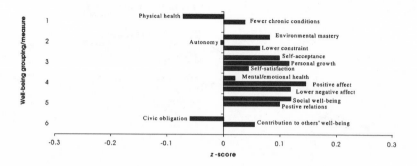

D. West South Central

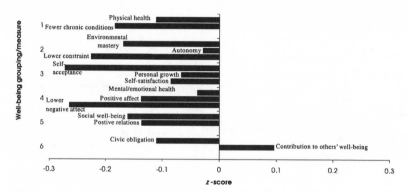

E. East South Central

FIGURE 2. (*Continued*)

that are significantly different by region according to an omnibus *F*-test. All analyses are post hoc, using one-way ANOVAs with least significant difference–adjusted group comparisons. Figure 2 shows a profile for each region in terms of how much it diverges from the national average (i.e., average of all nine regions) on each well-being measure for which we found regional variation. The bars are organized according to the well-being groupings in table 5. The metric used in these charts is a *z*-score, or a standardized score, which allows us to compare variables that have different scales and indicates the amount of standard deviation that a particular regional score varies from the national mean. In reporting our results for each region, we use categories such as "high" or "low" to indicate a region's mean response relative to eight other U.S. Census regions, on the basis of the post-hoc analyses.

NEW ENGLAND

Hypotheses

Demographics and Census data. New England (Maine, New Hampshire, Vermont, Massachusetts, Rhode Island, and Connecticut) has the highest per capita income in the country, high per capita health care expenditure, and a large ratio of colleges per resident (U.S. Bureau of the Census 1996; see table 3). Nearly 67 percent of the New England respondents in our study have completed some amount of higher education, and over one-third hold a bachelor's and/or another advanced degree. On the basis of previous studies showing the strong relationship between social class and health, we can predict that New England's well-being profile will reflect high health-focused well-being. A growing literature on the relationship between social class and health reveals that groups with higher socioeconomic status have lower morbidity and mortality rates (Adler et al. 1994; Marmot et al. 1991). New England is also characterized by low to moderate unemployment, a low crime rate, an average urban/rural (metro/non-metro area) ratio, and an average to low divorce rate. The sample is predominantly white, and a large proportion are Catholic.

Prevalent ideas. The region of New England is known as the home of the Puritan settlers and the birthplace of the American Revolution. Because the nation now known as the United States began in New England, it is reasonable to expect that some of the most significant and foundational American ideas and practices, including freedom and independence, might be pervasively distributed and especially strongly endorsed and reflected in practice in this region. The notion of being free from the imposition of other people's ideas and styles of life so that it is possible to be "one's own person" may be particularly salient in the region of the country that has the largest number of independent voters and is routinely cast as the home of the "cranky Yankee" or as Puritan heaven (Rubenstein 1982). We predict, therefore, that New England respondents may be particularly high on some aspects of autonomy-focused well-being, expressing relatively high feelings of autonomy and low feelings of constraint.

The desire to be unconstrained does not necessarily conflict with maintaining some kinds of social ties, however. New England is the region that developed and fostered the institution of the town meeting and the notion of giving the ideas of others a fair hearing is widely available here. Rubenstein (1982) found that people in New England knew their neighbors, made friends, and rated them positively. We expect to find this affiliative tendency in our analyses of well-being, in particular, on measures of other-focused well-being. Rubenstein (1982) also characterized New Englanders as stoical because of their low ratings on both negative affect and positive affect. We expect to find a similar pattern of emotion-focused well-being in our data.

Well-Being Profile

Health-focused well-being. Various indicators in the survey suggest that New England is doing very well with respect to physical health (see fig. 2A for a well-being profile). Our analyses reveal that as predicted, respondents from New England have the highest subjective ratings of physical health in the country. In addition, New England respondents reported a low number of chronic conditions—the second lowest in the country.

Autonomy-focused well-being. Consistent with our hypotheses, New England respondents reported the lowest levels of constraint, significantly lower than those of respondents from the six other regions. The region scored second highest in autonomy but only average on environmental mastery. These findings suggest that to the extent that autonomy-focused well-being is reported by this region's respondents, it revolves more around the feeling of being one's own person and not being constrained by others rather than a feeling of being in charge of one's situation.

Self-focused well-being. New England is not characterized by self-focused well-being. It ranked third among regions in self-satisfaction and personal growth and fourth in self-acceptance but was not significantly higher than any region on these indexes.

Emotion-focused well-being. As we expected, respondents from New England reported only average positive affect in comparison with respondents from other regions. They reported lower negative affect than all regions except West South Central. In addition, New England respondents rated themselves highest in mental and emotional health.

Other-focused well-being. New England also ranked highest in social well-being. A regional comparison on the social well-being subscales reveals that New England is highest in meaningfulness of society (making sense of the world) and second highest in social actualization (belief in the improvement of society) and social contribution (value of one's contribution to society). New England respondents also scored highest in the country on positive relations with others. However, they scored only just above average on various measures of social responsibility, including civic obligation and their contribution to others' welfare and well-being.

MOUNTAIN

Hypotheses

Demographics and Census data. The Mountain region includes Montana, Wyoming, Idaho, Colorado, Utah, Nevada, New Mexico, and Arizona. This region has the highest crime rate and the lowest health care expenditure. It has a low urban/rural ratio and an average to high divorce rate. Although, according to Census data, this region has low personal income, the respondents in our sample have relatively high levels of education, with two-thirds of the respondents having had some college education. The relatively high education level of this region might suggest that well-being will be characterized by high health-focused well-being; however, the low income and low health care expenditure may well mitigate this relationship. A relatively large number of Mountain region respondents report being atheist or agnostic, and there are almost equal proportions of Protestants and Catholics. The sample is predominantly white, and it has the highest regional percentage of Native American respondents.

Prevalent ideas. The Mountain region has always played a significant role in the American cultural imagination and in the world's imagination about America. This is the land of "Don't fence me in," Gary Cooper in *High Noon,* and the Marlboro man. Bellah et al. (1985, 145) suggested that the cultural significance of the lone cowboy lies in his "unique, individual virtue and special skill." Novelists, journalists, social scientists, and casual observers alike routinely draw a connection between the barren terrain and harsh climate of this region and the psyches of the people who live there. As Farney (1999) claims, "There is something about this sweeping, limitless landscape that tempts inhabitants to believe that here, history is a blank slate—that here, anything is possible." Cultural geographer Zelinsky (1992) describes the man of the frontier region "as the resourceful, isolated fighter against the wilderness, triumphantly carving out his own autonomous barony, the virile libertarian, jack-of-all-trades, and rough-and-ready paragon of all democratic virtues." Kaplan (1998, 168), in his recent book about social and cultural trends in the West, *Empire Wilderness,* describes Tuscon, for example, as a place that "[although it] is becoming increasingly connected to the outside world thanks to immigration and the Internet, its people are increasingly isolated from one another: the houses further and further apart, the public spaces empty. To me, the city's terrain seemed to say 'Leave me alone.'"

The idea that the Mountain region is concerned with autonomy and self and reflects a type of frontier mentality is supported by some previous empirical work. Most recently, Vandello and Cohen (1999), who used a slightly different region classification system, found the Great Plains and Mountain West to be more individualist than all other regions. We expect therefore that respondents of the Mountain region may have high scores on all aspects of autonomy-focused well-being. Further, Kahle's (1986) finding that people living in the Mountain region value self-respect more than do those living in any other region leads us to expect that Mountain respondents will score high on some aspects of self-focused well-being. Specifically, to the extent that the ecology of this region indeed fosters a sense of limitless possibility, respondents may score higher on ratings of personal growth.

Well-Being Profile

Health-focused well-being. The Mountain region did not score as high as New England on health-focused well-being, but its subjective health ratings were fairly high in comparison with the rest of the country (see fig. 2B for a well-being profile). Mountain respondents ranked third on the rating of physical health. The Mountain region ranked sixth in chronic conditions, reporting average to low levels of chronic conditions in comparison with other regions.

Autonomy-focused well-being. As predicted, autonomy-focused well-being characterizes the Mountain region. Respondents from this region reported the highest levels of autonomy and environmental mastery in the country—significantly higher than respondents in six and four other regions, respectively. The Mountain region also reported low feelings of constraint (significantly lower than six other regions); only New England is lower.

Self-focused well-being. The Mountain region is also characterized by self-focused well-being. Levels of personal growth are the highest in the country in this region. Respondents from this region are also the most satisfied with themselves. In addition, they are relatively high on self-acceptance, although not as high as respondents from the West South Central and West North Central regions.

Emotion-focused well-being. Respondents from the Mountain region reported significantly higher mental and emotional health than did respondents from six other regions, lower only than New England. The

Mountain region falls within the top three in terms of positive affect and the lowest three on negative affect.

Other-focused well-being. The picture with respect to other-focused well-being is mixed. The Mountain region scores among the top three regions on social well-being and is significantly higher than two regions on this measure. The Mountain well-being profile reveals a belief in the value of one's contribution to society, a subscale of social well-being. Similarly, with respect to social responsibility, Mountain respondents scored second highest on contribution to others' welfare. However, respondents from the Mountain region did not report high positive relations with others. Moreover, they were lowest of all regions on civic obligation. This relative lack of social responsibility is consistent with Mountain region respondents' emphasis on autonomy and on the importance of being "left alone."

WEST SOUTH CENTRAL

Hypotheses

Demographics and Census data. The West South Central (WSC) region includes Texas, Oklahoma, Arkansas, and Louisiana. It is characterized by a moderate crime rate, divorce rate, and unemployment and a low to moderate urban/rural ratio. This region is relatively poor with respect to personal income and has the lowest number of colleges per 100,000 residents. Census statistics also reveal that this region is moderate in health care expenditure, and according to sample demographics, respondents are only moderately educated in comparison with those of other regions (58 percent have had some higher education). Therefore, we might expect WSC respondents to score relatively low on measures of health-focused well-being in comparison with those from New England, a region that has high income, education, and health care expenditure. The most common religious affiliation of WSC respondents is Protestant. WSC has the lowest percentage of white respondents (80.4 percent), the second highest percentage of Native American respondents, and a large percentage who indicated "other," which probably reflects the large Latino population, a category that was not a response option in the survey.

Prevalent ideas. The majority of what has been written about this region concerns Texas. These accounts routinely note that many Texans like to believe that Texas is really an independent country, claiming that they are fundamentally different from the rest of America and intend to stay that way (Kaplan 1998). This sentiment is well represented by bumper

633

stickers and posters that proclaim "Don't mess with Texas." Conscious self-aggrandizing and self-promotion are common in public representation and symbolism in this area (Garreau 1981).

Garreau (1981) labels this region the "Anglo Plains," but it has also been characterized historically by a strong Hispanic and Mexican presence. The site of constant change and economic upheaval, the West South Central region has been labeled the "Gulf Growth Sphere" (Garreau 1981) or the "Go-getting Gulf" (Rubenstein 1982). Some suspect that in the American Southwest, Mexican values and ways of being may soon be more prevalent than Anglo-Saxon Protestant ones (Kaplan 1998; Zelinsky 1992).

Given that the WSC region is so much in flux, relative to the four other regions we characterize here, it is difficult to predict what forms well-being will assume. Given the hypothesized strong impact of geography as well as the powerful myth of an independent, tough, and invincible Texas, it is likely that some aspects of autonomy and self-focused well-being will be emphasized. Yet, given the presence of Hispanic culture in parts of this region, we might also expect to find conceptions of well-being that reflect some values and perspectives that are common in Mexican cultural contexts. For instance, in keeping with the finding that Hispanic and Latino cultures are more collectivist than European-American cultures (Hofstede 1980; Triandis et al. 1984), we expect that WSC respondents will report high levels of other-focused well-being. In other words, this region's conceptions of well-being and self may reflect a creolization of individualist and collectivist ideas and values. This combination may also result from the interaction of people with the environment. As with the Mountain region, virtually all observers of this region make some link between terrain and psyche. As Kaplan claims, "Texas constitutes just another friendly desert culture . . . where great distances and an unforgiving, water-scarce environment weld people closely to one another at oases, while demanding a certain swaggering individualism out in the open—as well as religious conservatism" (1998, 231).

Finally, given the influence of Hispanic or Mexican culture in this area (Zelinsky 1992), there might also be some greater emphasis on emotionality in reports of well-being. Triandis et al. (1984), for example, report that Mexicans are socialized to emphasize the expression of positive affect and deny the expression of negative affect. This is one element of the more general cultural script of *simpatia*—a pattern of social interaction involving respect toward others and a value of smooth, harmonious social relations.

Well-Being Profile

Health-focused well-being. In contrast with New England, WSC did not score high on health-focused well-being (see fig. 2C for a well-being profile). Respondents from this region reported the third lowest subjective ratings of physical health, significantly lower than those from New England and West North Central. The region only ranked fourth on chronic conditions.

Autonomy-focused well-being. In contrast with the Mountain region, West South Central did not score high on all aspects of autonomy-focused well-being. In fact, the WSC region mean on autonomy is significantly lower than that of the Mountain region mean. However, WSC does rank second on environmental mastery and third lowest on constraint. In comparison with the Mountain region, the autonomy-focused well-being that is salient in this region may be based more on being in charge of one's situation or not feeling out of control than on independent thinking.

Self-focused well-being. The West South Central region ranked high on self-focused well-being. The well-being profile shows the second highest levels of personal growth (significantly higher than four other regions) and self-acceptance (significantly higher than two other regions).

Emotion-focused well-being. The West South Central region is characterized by a focus on emotions. Respondents in this region reported the highest levels of positive affect and the lowest levels of negative affect. In particular, they reported the lowest levels of feeling nervous and restless and the highest levels of feeling cheerful and happy in the past thirty days. However, the WSC ranked fourth in subjective mental and emotional health behind New England, Mountain, and West North Central, and was significantly lower than the first two on this item.

Other-focused well-being. The West South Central region can also be described as having high other-focused well-being. The well-being profile of this region reveals the second highest mean on social well-being, significantly higher than that of four other regions. The WSC was highest on two social well-being subscales: social actualization and social integration (feeling close to one's community). In addition, an important part of this region's other-focused well-being is positive relations with others. The WSC scored second highest (significantly higher than three other regions) on this measure. This region ranked third in the country on a rating of contribution to others' welfare and well-being and on feelings of civic obligation.

WEST NORTH CENTRAL
Hypotheses

Demographics and Census data. Minnesota, North Dakota, South Dakota, Nebraska, Iowa, Kansas, and Missouri compose the West North Central (WNC) region. This region has the highest number of colleges per inhabitant in the country, but our sample has moderate levels of education in comparison with those of other regions. Its health care expenditure and personal income are also average compared with other regions. From these average levels of income and education, we can reasonably predict average levels of physical health relative to other regions. The divorce rate in WNC is also moderate, and it has the lowest urban/rural ratio (along with East South Central). WNC also has the lowest unemployment rate and a low to moderate crime rate. The West North Central region is predominantly Protestant, but it is also home to many Catholics. WNC respondents are predominantly white.

Prevalent ideas. The West North Central region includes much of the area of the country identified as the all-American heartland or the stable core of America. Settled primarily by Scandinavians and Germans, and with one of the lowest rates of recent immigration, this is the area that still most clearly reflects and fosters the white Anglo-Saxon Protestant ideas and practices that were foundational for American culture (Gastil 1975; Spindler and Spindler 1990). This is the region widely believed to be the one that most obviously expresses and demonstrates the American values of hard work, responsibility, helpfulness, and egalitarianism (Bellah et al. 1985; Kahle 1986). Encompassing the central plains, the West North Central region is often referred to as the breadbasket (Garreau 1981) of the nation and is typically symbolized as the solid, stable, productive center of the country. Rubenstein (1982, 26), in summarizing survey data on the West North Central region, dubbed this area the "complacent plains," a place where many people seem "to prefer life on a simple, even keel."

A prevalent idea in journalistic, social, and political commentary on this part of the Midwest is the idea of "averageness" and the representation and cultivation of the importance of being average. This region includes the geographical as well as the statistical center of the country. Kaplan (1998, 31), for example, says of St. Louis that it is the most average American city—"whether it's industry, unemployment, per capita growth rates, whatever, this is the mean level American metropolis." Averageness can connote boredom or a lack of excitement, but for insiders and more expert observers, averageness means being moderate, not too extreme, and resisting self-preoccupation. Ideas of not wanting too much, of being satisfied with what one has, and of adjusting to the life one leads are more frequently expressed and publicly represented in this region than in others. The importance of these ideas to well-being in this region is implied by novelist Jane Smiley:

> Basically, I'm always satisfied to be invited, you know? We try to wipe our mouths after we eat, and keep our hands below the table, and speak when spoken to. But it's a good pattern too, in some ways, because of your own mental health you don't go around saying, "I should have had this, I should have had that," all signs of excellent mental health in New York City. In the Midwest, we say to ourselves, "Gee, I got this; I got that" and "Wow, they didn't have to give me anything." (As quoted in Pearlman 1993, 101)

Similarly, in characterizing the fictional town of Lake Wobegon, Minnesota, the radio humorist Garrison Keillor repeatedly explains and celebrates the value of being solid, average, knowing what one has to do, and being content with one's position in life.

We expect, therefore, that the well-being profile of this region will be characterized by some elements of self-focused well-being, especially self-acceptance and self-satisfaction, and not particularly by attention to possibility or growth. Unlike that of New England or the Mountain region, the well-being profile of this region is unlikely to reflect much concern with autonomy-focused well-being. Further, given the seeming prominence of ideas about the importance of being content and cheerful and not complaining, we anticipate that the well-being profile should also reflect some elements of emotion-focused well-being, revealing a profile that is relatively high in positive affect and relatively low in negative affect.

Well-Being Profile

Health-focused well-being. The inclination toward accepting one's life and its conditions manifests itself in the region's scores on health-focused well-being measures (see fig. 2D for a well-being profile). The West North Central region reported the lowest number of chronic conditions in the country, despite the fact that its health care expenditures and education are only average. In addition, it ranked second on a subjective rating of physical health—lower only than New England and significantly higher than five other regions.

Autonomy-focused well-being. As hypothesized, the West North Central region contrasts with New England and the Mountain region on most aspects of autonomy-focused well-being. The well-being profile of the WNC region shows the lowest ratings of autonomy and reports of feelings of constraint that lie just below the national average, significantly lower on autonomy and significantly higher on constraint than New England and the Mountain region. However, WNC ranked third on environmental mastery, indicating that to the extent that respondents of this region experience autonomy-focused well-being, they do so not as much in terms of independent thinking but rather in terms of being in charge of their situation.

Self-focused well-being. Also consistent with our hypotheses, WNC respondents score particularly high on two of our three self-focused well-being measures. The region ranked highest on self-acceptance, which involves liking oneself and being pleased with one's life. Respondents from this region also ranked high on self-satisfaction, second only to those from the Mountain region. But for WNC respondents, self-focused well-being may be more about being pleased with one's current self than about seeking change and improvement. This region ranked the lowest on personal growth, in sharp and significant contrast with the West South Central and Mountain regions.

Emotion-focused well-being. WNC respondents' tendency toward self-contentedness is further reflected in their scores on emotion-focused well-being. This region ranked third in mental or emotional health and second in positive affect, and just below the national mean on negative affect. In particular, the West North Central region reported the highest levels of feeling calm and peaceful (significantly higher than those of four other regions) and feeling satisfied (significantly higher than those of three other regions) in the past thirty days. Further, it ranked second lowest on feeling nervous and feeling restless in the past thirty days.

Other-focused well-being. Concern with others characterizes the West North Central region but not quite as much as it does New England and West South Central. WNC ranked third after these two regions on positive relations with others and differs significantly from two regions on this measure. WNC respondents ranked fourth on social well-being behind the New England, West South Central, and Mountain regions. In particular, they ranked first in acceptance of others (belief in others' goodness) and second in social integration. However, they ranked eighth in meaningfulness of society. With respect to social responsibility, the WNC well-being profile does not show low scores on the obligation variables; however, unlike some other regions, in WNC respondents do not boast about their contribution—they were the lowest of the regions on contribution to the welfare and well-being of others.

East South Central
Hypotheses

Demographics and Census data. The East South Central (ESC) region consists of Kentucky, Tennessee, Mississippi, and Alabama. According to Census data, ESC has the country's lowest personal income. ESC respondents in the MIDUS study are less educated than those from other parts of the country, with the lowest percentage of college-educated respondents (15.8 percent) and the highest percentage of respondents that did not complete high school (17.8 percent). Thus, although the region is average with respect to the number of colleges per 100,000 in population and health care expenditure, we can expect its respondents to display low levels of physical health relative to respondents from regions with higher per capita incomes and higher levels of education. ESC has the highest divorce rate, an average crime rate and unemployment rate, and the lowest urban/rural ratio (along with WNC) in comparison to the rest of the country. This region's respondents are predominantly Protestant and predominantly white, with 7.9 percent black respondents.

Prevalent ideas. Like the West, the South holds a prominent place in the collective American imagination. As Nisbett and Cohen (1996, 1) note: "The U.S. South has long been viewed as place of romance, leisure, and gentility. Southerners have been credited with warmth, expressiveness, spontaneity, close family ties, a love of music and sport, and an appreciation for the things that make life worth living—from cuisine to love." According to Garreau (1981, 129), "being a Southerner is the most fervent and time-honored regional distinction in North America," and ideas about what it means to be a good or proper Southerner are plentiful and well elaborated. This is Dixie, the land of charm and grace and Southern hospitality, but it is also, according to many theorists of this region, a place where remembering and honoring the past is a well-honed practice. William Faulkner claimed that "the past is alive in the South, in fact, it's not even past." And remembering the Civil War and coming to terms with the South's defeat are especially significant features of public discourse. Many of these ideas about the meaning of the Civil War and what it means to be a Southerner today are prominent features of everyday life and its interpretation in the South.

Previous regional analyses have found high levels of collectivism in the Deep South. Most recently, using somewhat different regional definitions than the Census categories, Vandello and Cohen (1999) found significantly higher collectivism here than in the Mountain West and Great Plains, the Great Lakes and Midwest, or the Northeast. They found, for example, greater endorsement of items such as "It is better to be a cooperative person who works well with others." Vandello and Cohen posited that historical factors and institutional practices such as defeat in the Civil War, slavery, poverty, and the prominence of church life have helped shape the Deep South into a relatively collectivist region. The South is also a place of relative poverty and strict racial segregation, both of which are direct legacies of the Civil War. Other regional analyses have documented that the region's general quality of life is the lowest in the country, and in comparison to other regions, accounts of this part of the South often describe a certain wariness and uncertainty or insecurity about the future (Rubenstein 1982).

Our hypotheses about the East South Central well-being profile are particularly tentative, however, because the average level of education in this region is so different from that of the other four regions we have analyzed. There is nothing in our survey of prevalent Southern ideas about well-being to suggest that autonomy-focused or self-focused well-being, as measured in this study, would be particularly distinctive in the well-being profile of this region. There is certainly a tradition of ideas and values emphasizing the importance of charm, warmth, and positive affect in East South Central. At the same time, ideas that focus on past historical injustices and current uncertainties are also widespread, so negative affect may also be relatively salient in the well-being profile. We anticipate, however, that the well-being profile will reflect some elements of other-focused well-being, particularly positive relations with others, and also some elements of social responsibility, particularly contribution to the welfare and well-being of others.

Well-Being Profile

Health-focused well-being. As we expected, the East South Central region fared worse than all other regions on measures of health (see fig. 2E for a well-being profile). Respondents' ratings of physical health were the lowest in the country, significantly lower than those from three other regions. Moreover, ESC respondents reported the most chronic health conditions, significantly more than respondents from seven other regions.

Autonomy-focused well-being. As we predicted, ESC respondents displayed low levels of autonomy-focused well-being. They gave the highest ratings of feelings of constraint (significantly higher than those of respondents from six other regions) and the lowest ratings of environmental mastery.

Self-focused well-being. Similarly, this region's respondents scored lowest in self-acceptance (significantly lower than respondents from all other regions) and second lowest in self-satisfaction (significantly lower than respondents from three regions).

Emotion-focused well-being. ESC respondents also ranked lowest in positive affect (significantly lower than those from three regions) and highest in negative affect (significantly higher than those from three regions).

Other-focused well-being. Counter to our prediction, the ESC region did not rank high in other-focused well-being. In fact, respondents from this region scored lowest on social well-being and positive relations with others (significantly lower than those from three and four regions, respectively). We were surprised by these findings and hypothesize that perhaps these particular measures of other-focused well-being do not tap into the collectivism and focus on relationships that have been found in previous studies. With respect to social responsibility, in keeping with our prediction, ESC respondents did give the highest ratings of contribution to the welfare and well-being of others.

Conclusion

Overall, our analyses of region profiles of well-being lead us to conclude (a) that there is a strong consensus among Americans at midlife, wherever they live, about what is important for well-being, and (b) that there is considerable diversity by region in how people come to represent and experience well-being at midlife. We have proposed that both the common and the regionally variable well-being responses can be understood by examining some features of the various sociocultural contexts that people engage as they live their lives. Most Americans have some contact with nation-wide media and with the ideas and practices of a common legal, political, and consumer culture. Further, they participate in educational systems that, although often diverse, convey an overlapping set of historically constituted ideas and narratives about being American and the moral desirability of these ideas and ways of being. As a consequence of this pervasive network of ideas and practices, there is what can be called an American well-being profile. As indicated in table 2, a majority (ranging from 51 percent to 78 percent, depending on the question) of a national sample of Americans, regardless of where they live in this country, believe with full certainty (4 on a four-point scale) that they are healthy overall, in control of their lives such that they can do what they set their minds to, purposeful, very satisfied with their lives, and obligated to work and family, and that their partners and families support them. A majority of Americans also believe with full certainty (although there is regional variation in these tendencies) that they are autonomous, self-accepting, and satisfied with themselves, that they have the potential for growth and change, that they feel civic obligation, and that they do not experience negative feelings.

The regional variation in well-being profiles derives from the fact that although Americans share some ideas and practices about well-being, well-being is also substantially patterned by a person's local worlds—worlds that are shaped by regionally distinct ideas of what is the right way to be. In summary, we find the following:

1. The New England well-being profile reveals high levels of physical well-being and is distinctive for its emphasis on the aspect of autonomy-focused well-being that concerns not being constrained. The profile of New England shows the highest levels of social well-being and positive relations with others.

2. The Mountain region profile differs somewhat from that of New England. For example, physical health is not a salient feature of its well-being profile. It is distinctive for its emphasis on self-satisfaction and on all aspects of autonomy-focused well-being, including independent thinking, being in charge of one's situation, and not feeling constrained by others.

3. The West South Central profile is distinguished by self-focused well-being, particularly the possibility of personal growth, a finding consistent with the exaggeration and hyperbole that are often features of the public representations of this part of the West. The WSC profile is also distinguished by high levels of emotion-focused well-being, revealing the lowest levels of feeling nervous and restless and the highest levels of feeling cheerful and happy. This region's profile is also high on other-focused well-being.

4. The West North Central region is not particularly distinguished by any aspect of autonomy. Instead it is distinctive for its levels of self-focused well-being, particularly self-satisfaction and self-acceptance. It ranks lowest of all regions on personal growth, consistent with ideas of being content or satisfied with one's place that are prevalent in this area.

Moreover, like the West South Central, this region is notable for emotion-focused well-being, but instead of being high on feeling cheerful and happy, it ranks the highest on feeling calm, peaceful, and satisfied.

5. The East South Central region's well-being profile is the most distinctive of all. Except for social responsibility, in which the region is highest on contribution to the welfare and well-being of others, this region's profile is distinguished by relatively low scores on all other aspects of well-being.

These regional comparisons allow us to see how various aspects of core well-being are represented and enacted differently in different regions. For example, being in control and being autonomous are key features of American well-being. The Mountain region is perhaps the prototype for autonomy-focused well-being. In New England, however, autonomy-focused well-being seems to take shape as a concern with not being constrained as opposed to being in charge of one's situation.

Similarly, feeling purposeful in the sense of having direction and feeling self-satisfied and self-accepting are core aspects of American well-being, but this self-focused well-being is manifest differently in different regions. The Mountain region is almost a prototype for self-focused well-being; it is distinctive on all aspects including personal growth and self-satisfaction. Self-focused well-being takes almost the same form in the West South Central. In the West North Central, however, self-focused well-being does not revolve around personal growth but centers on self-acceptance and self-satisfaction.

Downplaying negative feelings is another important aspect of the American well-being profile, but emotion-focused well-being also takes distinctive regional forms. The West South Central stands out both in terms of positive affect and lack of negative affect. Positive affect also characterizes the West North Central, yet here the prevalent emotion is feeling calm and satisfied, whereas in the West South Central the salient emotion is feeling cheerful and happy. Notably the two regions—New England and Mountain—that report the highest levels of mental or emotional heath are not the regions that report particularly high affect, a finding that may indicate different regional understandings of mental and emotional health.

Regions also differ with respect to which part of other-focused well-being is most salient. Among the regions, New England stands out, and it is particularly distinctive on positive relations with others and the social well-being subscale, meaningfulness of society (making sense of the world). In the West South Central, other-focused well-being takes the form of social actualization (belief in the improvement of society) and social integration (feeling close to one's community), whereas in the West North Central, it is acceptance of others (belief in the goodness of others) that is distinctive.

Social responsibility in the sense of feeling obligated to family, work, and civic issues and feeling support from partner and family is also a key aspect of core American well-being, but this type of social responsibility also takes different regional forms. For instance, while the Mountain region reports the highest contribution to the well-being and welfare of others, it simultaneously reports the lowest levels of civic obligation. In contrast, the West North Central does not report low levels of obligation to others, but it does report the lowest level by far of contribution to the well-being of others. This suggests a very different interpretation of contributing to others and is consistent with the tendency to be modest or to downplay one's actions or importance that is widely represented in this region.

Overall, we have confirmed our belief that well-being is constituted in part by the cultural contexts, in this case the regional contexts, with which people are engaged. The five regions of the United States that we have examined here vary not only in their geography but also in the topography of ideas and practices about well-being. Knowledge of the prevalent ideas and practices in these regions allowed us to make a variety of accurate predictions about the salient features of the well-being profile in these regions. So, for example, on average the well-being profile of the upper Midwest (West North Central) reflects a sense of contentment, consistent with novelist Jane Smiley's view that one should be "satisfied to be invited." This satisfaction is not particularly evident in the well-being profile of New England, where there is instead a heightened concern with not being constrained, reflective perhaps of a popular notion that one should "live free or die." The differences we have described here are for the most part small in magnitude, but they are highly consistent and revealed on questions that were not specifically designed to reveal such differences.

Regional contexts are constituted by a combination of sociocultural and sociostructural factors, some of which we have highlighted in this chapter. For example, factors such as education, economic position, and ethnic and racial background of a region's inhabitants as well as whether they live predominantly in rural or urban communities contribute to the prevalence of certain ideas and practices of well-being in that region. Because we focus on region as a variable that incorporates all of these influences on people's understandings of how to be and how to be well, we have not controlled for each individual factor. Yet we recognize that it may be useful to examine the role of these factors.

For example, given recent evidence of educational variation in well-being (see Markus et al., chap. 10, this volume), after testing for regional differences in well-being, we asked whether some of these differences might be explained by the different proportions of college-educated respondents in the various regional samples. On the basis of the demographic data (see table 4), we can see that with the exception of the East South Central, which has less than 16 percent college-educated respondents, the other four regions discussed here are quite similar in their distribution of educational level, yet their well-being profiles are quite distinct. To more directly evaluate the contribution of education to the well-being profiles in the various regions, we performed regional comparisons within each of two levels of education—high school graduation or less, and one to two years of college or more. For those with some college or more, three-quarters of the well-being indicators used in our analyses (see table 1) varied significantly by region. In other words, if we look at the effects of education within region, we see that people who are more educated in one region have well-being profiles that look distinct from their highly educated counterparts in another region. Post-hoc analyses reveal that people with some college education in the East South Central region, for example, score significantly lower than do college-educated people from the other regions on various measures across dimensions of well-being. It is notable that among those with a high school education or fewer years of schooling, only one-tenth of the well-being indicators varied significantly by region. This could mean that people with less formal schooling are not influenced by regional meanings and practices. Or these results may lead us to echo the conclusion from Markus et al. (chap. 10, this volume) that the MIDUS instrument does a better job of assessing the well-being of relatively educated respondents than the well-being of the less formally educated.[4]

The systematic patterns of regional variation that we have found may suggest the value of studies specifically designed to assess regional sources of well-being and may underscore the value of a sociocultural analysis of well-being. Given that quantitative instruments such as the one used in this study may not fully capture regional distinctiveness in well-being, it may be necessary to draw on more qualitative sources (e.g., those available in MIDUS), organized by region, that might help define new dimensions of assessment. With a better understanding of some of the cultural sources and mediators of well-being, researchers should be able to develop more refined conceptualizations and measures of well-being.

Future studies could systematically assess the prevalent meanings and practices in these regions and link engagement with them to various well-being ideas and attitudes. Other research could also easily include items constructed to directly assess regional variation in the meanings and practices of well-being. For example, Nisbett and Cohen (1996) find that maintaining one's honor is a key factor at least for men in the South, and thus protecting one's reputation for strength and toughness could well be a key feature of well-being in the South. Items keyed to such important regional differences would provide a more nuanced picture of well-being, an important goal in its own right. Future studies on regional variation could also examine the dynamics of regionalism, or track how the ethos of particular regions evolve and change over time. The intersection between social change and regionalism could prove to be another important extension of this research. Are certain areas of the country particularly slow or quick to endorse social changes (e.g., attitudes about women's rights, acceptance of technology) that may be consequential for some aspects of well-being? Pursuing this line of research may eventually serve to illuminate the ways in which well-being involves a dynamic, finely tailored attunement with the ideas and practices of one's various sociocultural contexts. In sum, an essential element of well-being is its sociocultural particularity such that well-being necessarily assumes a diversity of forms.

Notes

1. For the most part, the existence and maintenance of boundaries of regions within the United States have been documented without a consistent classification scheme. Region researchers have drawn regional boundaries based on a wide set of characteristics, including topography, economics, political values, ethnic background, or religious affiliation of inhabitants (e.g., Garreau 1981; Gastil 1975; Nisbett 1993; Zelinsky 1992). Kahle (1986) has found values to be related to the nine Census Bureau regions, but not to other regional classifications such as Garreau's Nine Nations. For Kahle, the usefulness of the Census scheme lies in the fact that political boundaries tend to develop significance apart from other influences. In particular, shared history and shared loyalties contribute to regional consciousness, and people and the media tend to identify with their states, and therefore perhaps with the collection of surrounding states.

2. We considered collapsing regions into fewer units, but using empirically derived, finer-grained divisions such as the Census divisions has proved more productive in other careful analyses on region (e.g., Kahle 1986; Rubenstein 1982; Vandello and Cohen 1999).

3. The Ryff scale of psychological well-being includes six subscales, each assessing a different dimension of well-being. For our regional comparison, we found it useful to use each subscale as a separate measure. Therefore, we do not include the omnibus psychological well-being scale in our regional analyses. The regions do differ on this overall measure, however, with the Mountain region scoring highest (significantly higher than four regions), followed by New England, and West South Central. West North Central respondents report average levels of psychological well-being, ranking fifth among regions on this measure. East South Central has the lowest psychological well-being mean, significantly lower than that of the six other regions. Note that we did not separate Ryff's social well-being measure into its five subscales—meaningfulness of society, social integration, acceptance of others, social contribution, and social actualization—but we do report some of the regional variation we found for the subscales.

4. To further evaluate the effects of socioeconomic characteristics, we used education and income as covariates in a series of analyses of covariance (ANCOVAs). It is important to note that we found that the classification of well-being variables as consensual well-being constructs did not change with the introduction of these two covariates. We also found that the regional effects reported were not diminished for any of the fifteen well-being variables that showed regional variation (with the exception of personal growth) when education and income were used as covariates in ANCOVAs.

References

Adams, G. 2002. The cultural grounding of personal relationship: Spouseship, kinship, friendship, enemyship. Manuscript. University of Kansas

Adler, N. E., T. Boyce, M. A. Chesney, S. Cohen, S. Folkman, R. Kahn, and L. Symer. 1994. Socioeconomic status and health: The challenge of the gradient. *American Psychologist* 49:15–24.

Anderson, C. A. 1987. Temperature and aggression: Effects on a quarterly, yearly, and city rates of violent and nonviolent crime. *Journal of Personality and Social Psychology* 52:1161–73.

Andersen, P. A., M. W. Lustig, and J. F. Andersen. 1987. Regional patterns of communication in the United States: A theoretical perspective. *Communication Monographs* 54:128–44.

Bellah, R. N., R. Madsen, W. M. Sullivan, A. Swidler, and S. M. Tipton. 1985. *Habits of the heart: Individualism and commitment in American life.* New York: Harper and Row.

Berry, J. W., Y. H. Poortinga, and J. Pandey. 1997. *Handbook of cross-cultural psychology,* vol. 1. *Theory and method.* 2d ed. Boston: Allyn and Bacon.

Borchert, J. R. 1972. America's changing metropolitan regions. *Annals of the Association of American Geographers* 62:352–73.

Bourdieu, P. 1977. *Outline of a theory of practice.* Trans. R. Nice. Cambridge: Cambridge University Press.

Cole, M. 1996. *Cultural psychology: A once and future discipline.* Cambridge: Belknap Press of Harvard University Press.

Diener, E., and E. M. Suh, eds. 2000. *Subjective well-being across cultures.* Cambridge: MIT Press.

Edgerton, R. 1971. *The individual in cultural adaptation.* Berkeley: University of California Press.

Farney, D. 1999. Beyond John Wayne: The West writes itself a new script. *Wall Street Journal,* June 16, A1, A18.

Fiske, A. P., S. Kitayama, H. R. Markus, and R. E. Nisbett. 1998. The cultural matrix of social psychology. In *Handbook of social psychology,* ed. D. T. Gilbert, S. T. Fiske, and G. Lindzey, 915–81. New York: McGraw-Hill.

Freedman, J. 1978. *Happy people: What happiness is, who has it, and why.* New York: Harcourt Brace Jovanovich.

Garreau, J. 1981. *The nine nations of North America.* Boston: Houghton Mifflin.

Gastil, R. D. 1975. *Cultural regions of the United States.* Seattle: University of Washington Press.

Giddens, A. 1990. *The consequences of modernity.* Stanford, Calif.: Stanford University Press.

Glenn, N. D., and J. L. Simmons. 1967. Are regional cultural differences diminishing? *Public Opinion Quarterly* 312:176–93.

Guisinger, S., and S. J. Blatt. 1994. Individuality and relatedness: Evolution of a fundamental dialectic. *American Psychologist* 49:104–11.

Harris, M. 1979. *Cultural materialism: The struggle of for a science of culture.* New York: Random House.

Heine, S. H., D. R. Lehman, H. R. Markus, and S. Kitayama. 1999. Is there a universal need for positive self-regard? *Psychological Review* 1064:766–94.

Herzog, A. R., H. R. Markus, M. M. Franks, and D. Holmberg. 1998. Activities and well-being in older age: Effects of self-concept and educational attainment. *Psychology and Aging* 13:179–85.

Hochschild, J. L. 1995. *Facing up to the American dream: Race, class, and the soul of the nation.* Princeton, N.J.: Princeton University Press.

Hofstede, G. 1980. *Culture's consequences.* Beverly Hills, Calif.: Sage.

Hogan, R. 1975. Theoretical egocentrism and the problem of compliance. *American Psychologist* 30:533–40.

Hulbert, J. S. 1989. The southern region: A test of the hypothesis of cultural distinctiveness. *Sociological Quarterly* 30:245–66.

Iyengar, S. S., and M. Lepper. 1999. Rethinking the value of choice: A cultural perspective on intrinsic motivation. *Journal of Personality and Social Psychology* 76:349–66.

Kahle, L. R. 1986. The Nine Nations of North America and the value basis of geographic segmentation. *Journal of Marketing* 502:37–47.

Kaplan, R. D. 1998. *An empire wilderness: Reflections into America's future.* New York: Random House.

King, L. A., and C. K. Napa. 1998. What makes a good life? *Journal of Personality and Social Personality* 75:156–65.

Kitayama, S., and H. R. Markus. 1999. Yin and yang of the Japanese self: The cultural psychology of personality coherence. In *The coherence of personality:*

Social-cognitive bases of consistency, variability, and organization, ed. D. Cervone and U. Shoda, 242–302. New York: Guilford Press.

———. 2000. The pursuit of happiness and the realization of sympathy: Cultural patterns of self, social relations, and well-being. In *Subjective well-being across cultures*, ed. E. Diener and E. M. Suh. Cambridge: MIT Press.

Lachman, M. E., and S. L. Weaver. 1998. The sense of control as a moderator of social class differences in health and well-being. *Journal of Personality and Social Psychology* 74:763–73.

Markus, H. R., and S. Kitayama. 1991. Culture and the self: Implications for cognition, emotion, and motivation. *Psychological Review* 98:224–53.

———. 1994. A collective fear of the collective: Implications for selves and theories of selves. Special issue: The self and the collective. *Personality and Social Psychology Bulletin* 205:568–79.

Marmot, M. G., G. D. Smith, S. Stansfeld, C. Patel, F. North, J. Head, I. White, E. Brunner, and A. Feeney. 1991. Health inequalities among British civil servants: The Whitehall II study. *Lancet* 337:1387–93.

Nisbett, R. 1993. Violence and U.S. regional culture. *American Psychologist* 48:441–49.

Nisbett, R. E., and D. Cohen. 1996. *Culture of honor: The psychology of violence in the South.* Boulder, Colo.: Westview Press.

Pearlman, M. 1993. *Listen to their voices: Twenty interviews with women who write.* New York: Houghton Mifflin.

Plaut, V. C., H. R. Markus, and M. E. Lachman. 2002. Place matters: Consensual features and regional variation in American well-being and self. *Journal of Personality and Social Psychology* 83:160–84.

Potter, D. M. 1963. American individualism in the twentieth century. *Texas Quarterly* 62:140–51.

Putnam, R. 1995. Bowling alone: America's declining social capital. *Journal of Democracy* 6:65–78.

Quinn, D. M., and J. Crocker. 1999. When ideology hurts: Effects of belief in the Protestant ethic and feeling overweight on the psychological well-being of women. *Journal of Personality and Social Psychology* 77: 402–14.

Raitz, K. B. 1979. Themes in the cultural geography of European ethnic groups in the United States. *Geographical Review* 69:79–94.

Rossi, A. S. 2001. Contemporary dialogue on civil society and social responsibility. In *Caring and doing for others: Social responsibility in the domains of family, work, and community*, ed. A. S. Rossi. Chicago: University of Chicago Press.

Ryff, C. D., and B. Singer. 1998. The contours of positive human health. *Psychological Inquiry* 9:1–28.

Rubenstein, K. 1982. Regional states of mind: Patterns of emotional life in nine parts of America. *Psychology Today* 16:22–30.

Shweder, R. A. 1990. Cultural psychology: What is it? In *Cultural psychology: Essays on comparative human development*, ed. J. W. Stigler, R. A. Shweder, and G. Herdt, 1–46. Cambridge: Cambridge University Press.

Shweder, R. A., M. Mahapatra, and J. Miller. 1987. Culture and moral development. In *The emergence of morality in young children*, ed. J. Kagan and S. Lamb, 1–83. Chicago: University of Chicago Press.

Hazel Rose Markus, Victoria C. Plaut, and Margie E. Lachman

Spindler, G. D., and L. S. Spindler. 1990. *The American cultural dialogue and its transmission.* New York: Falmer Press.

Suh, E. M. 2000. Self, the hyphen between culture and subjective well-being. In *Subjective well-being across cultures,* ed. E. Diener and E. M. Suh. Cambridge: MIT Press.

Taylor, S. E., and J. D. Brown. 1988. Illusion and well-being: A social psychological perspective on mental health. *Psychological Bulletin* 103:193–210.

Triandis, H. C. 1995. *Individualism and collectivism.* Boulder, Colo.: Westview Press.

Triandis, H. C., G. Marin, J. Lisansky, and H. Betancourt. 1984. Simpatia as a cultural script of Hispanics. *Journal of Personality and Social Psychology* 47:1363–75.

Turner, F. J. 1920. *The frontier in American history.* New York: Holt.

U.S. Bureau of the Census. 1996. *Statistical abstract of the United States.* 116th ed. Washington, D.C.: Government Printing Office.

Vandello, J. A., and D. Cohen. 1999. Patterns of individualism and collectivism across the United States. *Journal of Personality and Social Psychology* 77:279–92.

Weber, M. 1958. The Protestant ethic and the spirit of capitalism Trans. T. Parsons. New York: Scribner's. First published in 1904.

Wuthnow, R. 1998. *Loose connections: Joining together in America's fragmented communities.* Cambridge: Harvard University Press.

Zelinsky, W. 1992. *The cultural geography of the United States* Rev. ed. Englewood Cliffs, N.J.: Prentice Hall. First published in 1973.

David M. Almeida is associate professor in the Department of Human Development and Family Studies at the University of Pennsylvania. Topics of recent publications include sources of gender differences in psychological distress and emotional transmission in the daily lives of families. His current research interest focuses on environmental and genetic components of daily stress processes during adulthood.

John Z. Ayanian is associate professor of medicine and health care policy at the Harvard Medical School and director of the General Internal Medicine Fellowship at the Brigham and Women's Hospital. He is also deputy editor of the journal *Medical Care,* a member of the Institute of Medicine Committee on the Consequences of Uninsurance, and a fellow of the American College of Physicians. He has published studies of access to care and quality of care in the fields of cardiovascular disease, breast and colorectal cancer, diabetes, and renal disease. His current research focuses on the relation of patients' sociodemographic characteristics—including gender, race, ethnicity, and socioeconomic status—to the process and outcomes of health care, and the effect of physician and organizational characteristics—such as specialization, teaching status, and volume—on the quality of health care.

Orville Gilbert Brim is past director of the John D. and Catherine T. MacArthur Foundation Research Network on Successful Midlife Development. He is the author and editor of a dozen books on human development. He is the former president of both the Russell Sage Foundation and the Foundation for Child Development. His research focuses on life-span development, particularly on constancy and change in personality from childhood through old age. His most recent book was on the maintenance of ambition after success and failure. Currently he is writing about the origins of the desire for fame and its transformations during middle age.

Larry L. Bumpass was elected to the National Academy of Sciences in 2001. He is currently the N. B. Ryder Professor Emeritus at the University of Wisconsin and co-director of the National Survey of Families and Households, a major national resource for understanding family life in the United States that is longitudinal, interdisciplinary, and structured from a life-course perspective. He has published extensively on the social demography of the family, including cohabitation, marriage, divorce, and fertility, and the consequences of these processes for children's living arrangements and development. His current work involves two major foci. The first is the attempt to understand the implications of unmarried cohabitation and childbearing for the boundaries and definition of families, and how entry into marriage may affect family relationships. The second seeks to place U.S. family patterns in international context with comparisons to European countries, on the one hand, and East Asian countries on the other.

Deborah Carr is assistant professor in the Department of Sociology and the Institute for Health, Health Care Policy, and Aging Research at Rutgers University. Her recent publications have focused on psychological adjustment to late-life widowhood, the effects of work and family roles on midlife psychological well-being, and the work–family strategies of American men and women. Her current research focuses on end-of-life planning and its implications for the well-being of the dying patient and family members.

Paul D. Cleary is professor of health care policy at the Harvard Medical School and the Harvard School of Public Health. He is a member of the Institute of Medicine of the National Academy of Sciences. His research interests include developing better methods for using patient reports about their care and health status to evaluate the quality of medical care and studying the relationships between clinician and organizational characteristics and the quality of medical care. His current research includes a national evaluation of a continuous quality improvement initiative in clinics providing care to HIV-infected individuals and a statewide effort to improve cancer care in Massachusetts. He also is principal investigator of a Consumer Assessment of Health Plans Study (CAHPS II) funded by the Agency for Health Care Policy and Research to develop survey protocols for collecting information from consumers about their health plans and services.

Katherine B. Curhan is a doctoral student in the human development and psychology program at the Harvard University Graduate School of Education. Her research interests include the influence of various sociocultural contexts on strategies for achieving and maintaining well-being, the study of meaning making through narrative analysis, social class and health issues, successful aging and life-span development, and the possible synergistic combinations of qualitative and quantitative research methods.

Alison Earle is project director for the Work, Family and Democracy Initiative and instructor at the Harvard School of Public Health. Her current research focuses on how public policies affect the needs of working families in the United States and worldwide. Her past research has included an examination of the effect of parental working conditions in the United States on children's health and development. Her publications have appeared in *American Educational Research Journal, Journal of the American Public Health Association, Community Work and Family,* and *Journal of the American Medical Women's Association.*

Kimberly M. Prenda Firth is an assistant professor in the Department of Health Care Sciences at George Washington University in Washington, D.C. She is also an adjunct staff member to the Children's National Medical Center Community Research Department, where she serves as an analytic consultant with the Starting Early Starting Smart national intervention project aimed at improving family and school support for minority families through the Head Start Program. She has also served as a social science analyst for the Behavioral and Social Research branch of the National Institute on Aging in Bethesda, Maryland. Her current research interests include the relationship between temporal orientation, perceived control, and life goal facilitation across the adult life span.

William Fleeson is Ollen R. Nalley Associate Professor in the Department of Psychology at Wake Forest University. His research interests include personality, self-regulation, adult development, and psychological well-being. His current research focuses on distinguishing between those human efforts that add to successful, satisfying lives and those that lead to dead ends, frustrated hopes, and wasted resources.

Rebecca Fuhrer is professor of epidemiology and chair of the Department of Epidemiology, Biostatistics, and Occupational Health at McGill University in Montreal. Her previous appointment was as a senior lecturer at University College London Department of Epidemiology and Public Health and a research scientist at INSERM (Institut de la Santé et de la Recherche Médicale) in France. She has co-authored numerous journal articles and book chapters in the field of psychiatric and psychosocial epidemiology. Her present research focuses on the epidemiological study of psychosocial risk factors and mechanisms involved in the occurrence of mental ill health and its relationship to physical ill health and mortality, cognitive decline, and dementia; the role and pathways of the impact of social relations (social support and social networks) on health, illness and mortality, and cognitive ageing; and the role of social inequalities as an effect modifier on the above relationships, and their impact on public health.

Stephen E. Gilman is a research fellow in the Department of Society, Human Development and Health at Harvard School of Public Health and at the Centers for Behavioral and Preventive Medicine at Brown Medical School. His research interests focus on the connection between socioeconomic conditions over the life course and the risk of mood, anxiety, and substance-use disorders.

Lana Hamilton is a graduate student at Kent State University.

S. Jody Heymann is an associate professor at the Harvard School of Public Health and Harvard Medical School. Her recent books include *The Widening Gap: Why America's Working Families Are in Jeopardy and What Can Be Done about It* and *Can Working Families Ever Win?* Heymann is chair of the Work, Family, and Democracy Initiative and the founding director of the Project on Global Working Families. She leads studies in North America, Europe, Latin America, Africa, and Asia on the impact of work and social conditions on the health and development of children, the care of the elderly and disabled, the ability of employed adults to obtain and retain work, and the ability of nations to decrease the number of families living in poverty.

Melanie C. Horn is a research associate and lecturer at the University of California at Irvine and Long Beach State University in California. She is completing her dissertation on the roles of early parental loss and attachment quality on daily well-being and stressor reactivity in adulthood.

Randall Horton is a doctoral candidate in the Committee on Human Development and the Department of Psychology at the University of Chicago. He has completed several years of research and clinical training looking at the mental health and adjustment of immigrants in Chicago. His dissertation, based on long-term fieldwork in South Asia, explores the cultural psychological underpinnings and complexities of the Tibetan political commitment to nonviolence.

Diane L. Hughes is associate professor of psychology at New York University. Her research has focused on the influences of occupational stress on families, racial socialization processes within ethnic minority families, cross-race friendships, and culturally anchored research methods. In her most recent work, she examines parental and other contextual influences on academic engagement and performance among a multi-ethnic sample of adolescents and their parents. She has served on the editorial boards of several journals and on study sections at the National Institute of Mental Health. She is also co-author of *Community Psychology: A Quarter-Century of Theory, Research, and Action.*

Heyjung Jun is a lecturer in the Department of Social Welfare for the Elderly at Hoseo University in Korea. Topics of her recent publications include the effects of productive role activity on the mental and physical health of older adults and parent–child relationships across the life course. Her current research interest focuses on religiousness and spirituality among older adults, and social and psychological factors of successful aging.

Kenneth S. Kendler is the Rachel Brown Banks Distinguished Professor of Psychiatry and professor of human genetics at Virginia Commonwealth University. He also directs the Virginia Institute for Psychiatric and Behavioral Genetics. He has received an honorary doctor of science from the University of Birmingham, England, and is a member of the Institute of Medicine of the National Academy of Sciences. He has received a number of prestigious awards, most recently including the Edward Strecker Award (2000) for outstanding contributions to psychiatric care and treatment, the Edward J. Sachar Award (2001) for outstanding contributions to psychiatric research, and the Rema Lapouse Award (2002) for contributions to understanding of epidemiology and control of mental disorders. Recent research projects include molecular genetic studies focusing on nicotine and alcohol dependence and major depression.

Ronald C. Kessler is professor of health care policy at the Harvard Medical School and director of the World Health Organization's World Mental Health Survey

Initiative. His research deals broadly with the psychosocial determinants of mental health and with the comparative societal costs of illness. He is the author of more than three hundred publications and the recipient of numerous awards for his research. He is a member of the Institute of Medicine.

Corey L. M. Keyes holds joint appointments in the Departments of Sociology and of Behavioral Sciences and Health Education in the Rollins School of Public Health at Emory University. He is a member of the steering committee of the Society for the Study of Human Development. His recent books include *Flourishing: Positive Psychology and the Life Well-Lived* (American Psychological Association, 2003) and *Well-Being: Positive Development throughout the Life Course* (Erlbaum, 2003). His research focuses broadly on the domains of successful human development and aging, and the diagnosis and etiology of mental health and illness.

Margie E. Lachman is professor of psychology and director of the Life-Span Developmental Psychology Laboratory at Brandeis University. She is editor of the *Journal of Gerontology: Psychological Sciences* (2000–2004) and the recent *Handbook of Midlife Development.* Her research focuses on personality and cognitive changes in middle and later adulthood, with a specific emphasis on the sense of control over the aging process. With funding from the National Institute on Aging, she is currently exploring how the sense of control is related to memory and physical activity.

Nadine F. Marks is professor and chair of Human Development and Family Studies at the University of Wisconsin, Madison. Her research and publications focus on how psychosocial factors—including gender, socioeconomic status, race-ethnicity, marital status, caregiving, parenting, and the work–family interface—influence mental and physical health across adulthood. Her current research is exploring linkages between social inequalities, psychological factors, health behaviors, and adult physical health.

Hazel Rose Markus is professor of psychology and co-director of the Research Institute for Comparative Studies in Race and Ethnicity at Stanford University. Her research has focused on the role of the self in regulating behavior. The topics of her published work are self-schemas, possible selves, the influence of the self on the perception of others, and the constructive role of the self in adult development. Her most recent research is in the area of cultural psychology and explores the mutual constitution between psychological structures and processes and sociocultural practices and institutions.

Michael G. Marmot is professor of epidemiology and public health and director of the International Centre for Health and Society at University College London. He has been at the forefront of research into health inequalities for the past twenty years, as principal investigator of the Whitehall studies of British civil servants, investigating explanations for the striking inverse social gradient in morbidity and mortality. He is a foreign associate member of the Institute of Medicine. He was awarded a knighthood in 2000 by Her Majesty the Queen for services to epidemiology and understanding of health inequalities.

Kristin D. Mickelson is assistant professor of psychology at Kent State University. Her recent publications have focused on three areas: the relation of stress to social support and mental health in various populations (e.g., parents of children with special needs, the elderly, the poor, and homeless women); the correlates and patterns of adult attachment in a nationally representative sample; and coping as a communal process. Her current research examines differential vulnerability to life events by socioeconomic status and whether social support may serve as an explanatory mechanism.

Daniel K. Mroczek is an associate professor of psychology at Fordham University in New York City. His publications focus primarily on well-being and personality development across the life span. Specific research interests include stability and change in personality traits and psychological well-being across the life span, as well as personality predictors of physical health. His research on estimating trajectories of personality change has been funded by the National Institute on Aging. He has several statistical and methodological interests as well, including the use of mixed models, issues in longitudinal design and data analysis, and psychometrics.

Karen A. Palmersheim is an assistant researcher at the Institute on Aging at the University of Wisconsin. Her research interests are understanding socioeconomic influences on health-related behaviors, and the prevention of disease and disability in relation to health behaviors in the aging population.

Joy E. Pixley is assistant professor in the Department of Sociology at the University of California, Irvine. Her research examines the intersection of work and family trajectories over the life course, with a focus on how spouses in dual-earner couples prioritize their two careers when making major decisions. She also works on problems of representation and comparison for life history data.

Victoria C. Plaut is assistant professor of psychology at the College of the Holy Cross in Worcester, Massachusetts. Her research interests include the sociocultural shaping of well-being and self, sociocultural models of racial and ethnic diversity, and the influence of social representations of computer science on women's participation.

Alice S. Rossi is professor emerita of sociology at the University of Massachusetts, Amherst, and has been the recipient of six honorary degrees. She edited two earlier volumes in the Midlife Series of the University of Chicago Press: *Caring and Doing for Others: Social Responsibility in the Domains of Family, Work, and Community* (2001), and *Sexuality across the Life Course* (1994). Her research interests are in family and kinship, sex and gender, and human development, with special interest in the reproductive phase of women's lives from menarche through menopause.

Carol D. Ryff is director of the Institute on Aging and professor of psychology at the University of Wisconsin, Madison. She is a fellow of the American Psychological

Association (division 20) and the Gerontological Society of America, and was a former fellow at the Center for Advanced Study in the Behavioral Sciences. Her research centers on the study of psychological well-being, for which she developed assessment instruments that have been translated to more than twenty different languages and are used in numerous scientific fields. Her empirical studies, involving longitudinal and national samples, have probed how well-being varies by age, gender, socioeconomic status, ethnicity, and culture, as well as how diverse life experiences (critical events and transitions) impact well-being. How psychosocial resources and strengths are linked with physical health, including diverse biomarkers, is also a current focus. An integrative theme across these studies is resilience—the capacity to maintain or regain health and well-being in the face of cumulative life adversity. Such work seeks to identify the protective factors (biological, psychological, social) that underlie such resilience.

Adam Shapiro is an associate professor of sociology at the University of North Florida in Jacksonville, Florida. His recent publications have focused on the social epidemiology and etiology of adult well-being within the contexts of marital status transitions, intergenerational family relationships, and community-based care programs. His current research involves understanding the ways in which family and community networks help explain social disparities in health.

Richard A. Shweder is the William Claude Reavis Distinguished Service Professor of Human Development at the University of Chicago. His recent research examines the scope and limits of pluralism and the moral challenge of multiculturalism in Western liberal democracies. He examines the norm conflicts that arise when people migrate from Africa, Asia, and Latin America to countries in the "North." His publications include *Thinking Through Cultures: Expeditions in Cultural Psychology, and Why Do Men Barbecue? Recipes for Cultural Psychology.* He is editor of *Welcome to Middle Age! (And Other Cultural Fictions)* and co-editor (with Martha Minow and Hazel Markus) of the book *Engaging Cultural Differences: The Multicultural Challenge in Liberal Democracies.*

Burton H. Singer is the Charles and Marie Robertson Professor of Public and International Affairs at Princeton University. He was formerly a professor at Yale University (public health, economics, and statistics) and Columbia University (statistics), and an adjunct professor at Rockefeller University (Laboratory of Populations). His research has had three interrelated foci: (1) development of mathematical and statistical methods for analysis of longitudinal surveys in sociology, economics, and epidemiology; (2) identification of social, biological, and environmental risks associated with vector-borne diseases in the tropics and chronic diseases of the elderly; and (3) integration of psychosocial and biological evidence to characterize pathways to alternate states of health. He recently co-authored (with Heping Zhang) "Recursive Partitioning in the Health Sciences" and co-edited (with Carol Ryff) "Emotion, Social Relationships, and Health."

Laura M. Thornton is senior program coordinator for eating disorders research at the University of Pittsburgh Medical Center. Her current research concerns phenotypic aspects and genetic associations of anorexia and bulimia nervosa.

Ellen E. Walters is senior biostatistician in the Department of Health Care Policy at the Harvard Medical School. Her main projects include analysis of data from the National Comorbidity Survey suite of studies and the World Health Organization's World Mental Health Survey Initiative, a series of coordinated psychiatric epidemiological surveys currently in progress in twenty-five countries throughout the world. These studies investigate cross-national psychosocial risk factors for and consequences of psychiatric morbidity and comorbidity.

Elaine Wethington is associate professor of human development and of sociology at Cornell University and a faculty affiliate of the Bronfenbrenner Life Course Center. Her research has focused on stress processes and mental health among adults. She is currently director of two projects on social support, life change, well-being, and mental health among aging adults. Her current research focuses on the measurement of chronic and accumulated stressor exposure across the life course.

Lawrence B. Zaborski is a statistical programmer and analyst in the Department of Health Care Policy at the Harvard Medical School. His current research focuses on the assessment of quality of care in Medicare managed care health care plans.

Shanyang Zhao is associate professor in the Department of Sociology at Temple University. His research interests include mental health, life satisfaction, and the impact of the Internet on human relationships.

DATE DUE

JUN 9 '04			
	SUBJECT TO		
	RECALL		